AAOS
AMERICAN ACADEMY OF ORTHOPAEDIC SURGEONS

AF813841

Eighth Edition

Emergency Medical Responder

Your First Response in Emergency Care

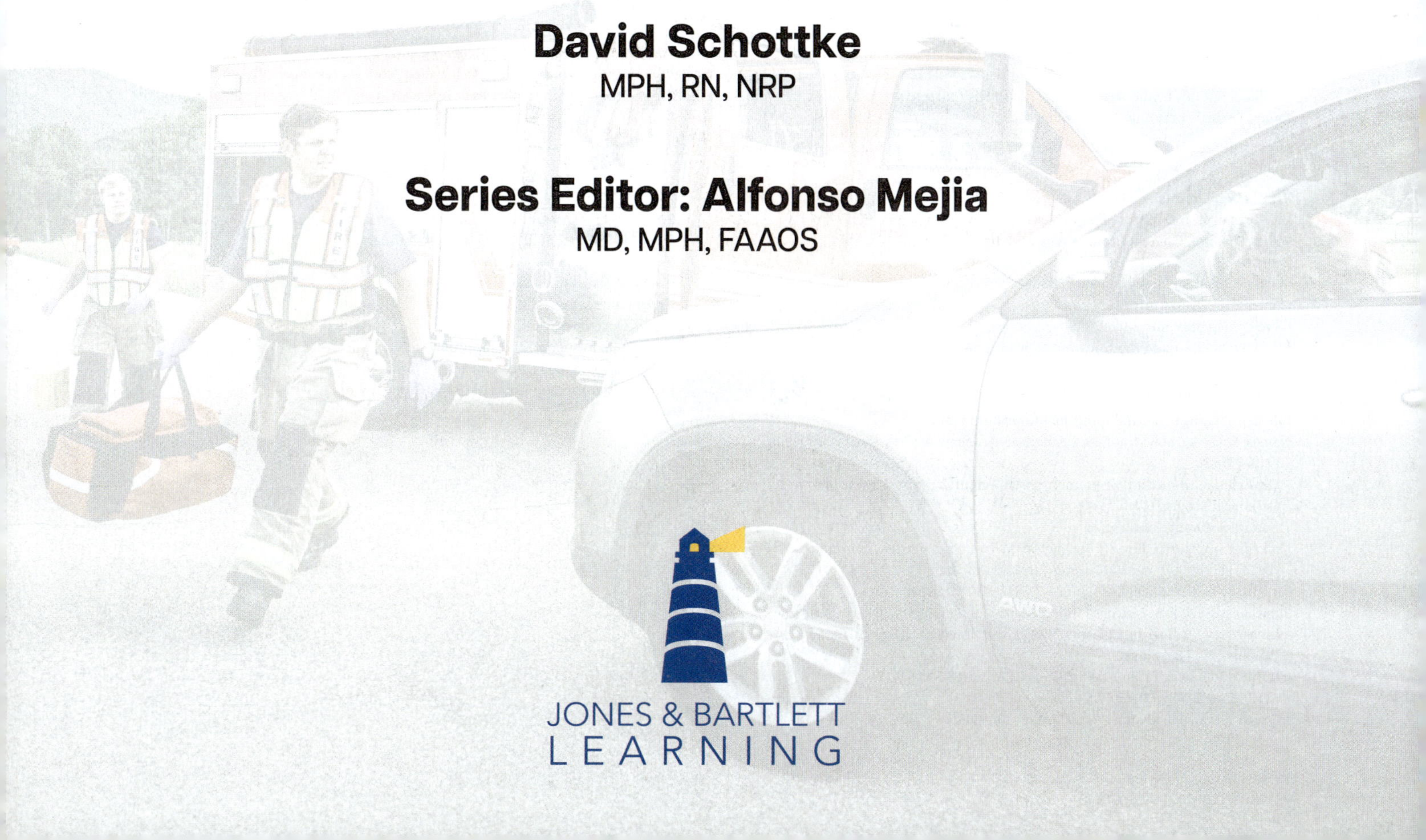

David Schottke
MPH, RN, NRP

Series Editor: Alfonso Mejia
MD, MPH, FAAOS

JONES & BARTLETT
LEARNING

World Headquarters
Jones & Bartlett Learning
25 Mall Road
Burlington, MA 01803
978-443-5000
info@jblearning.com
www.jblearning.com
www.psglearning.com

AMERICAN ACADEMY OF ORTHOPAEDIC SURGEONS

AAOS Board of Directors 2025–2026
President: Annunziato Amendola, MD, FAAOS
First Vice President: Wilford K. Gibson, MD, FAAOS
Second Vice President: Michael L. Parks, MD, FAAOS
Treasurer: Mininder S. Kocher, MD, MPH, FAAOS
Past President: Paul Tornetta III, MD, PhD, FAAOS
BOC Chair: Michael J. Leddy III, MD, FAAOS
BOC Chair-Elect: James W. Barber, MD, FAAOS
BOC Secretary: Jeffrey R. McLaughlin, MD, FAAOS
BOS Chair: Adolph J. Yates, Jr, MD, FAAOS
BOS Chair-Elect: Julie B. Samora, MD, PhD, MPH, FAAOS
BOS Secretary: Reid B. Nichols, MD, FAAOS
Members-at-Large:
Evalina L. Burger, MD, FAAOS
John T. Gill, MD, FAAOS
Monica M. Payares, MD, FAAOS
Sean Tabaie, MD, MBA, FAAOS, FAOA
Public Board Members
Timothy J. Constantine
Lily Marks
Chief Executive Officer (ex-officio): Thomas E. Arend, Jr, Esq, CAE

Editorial Credits
Chief Commercial Officer: Anna Salt Troise, MBA
Director, Publishing: Hans J. Koelsch, PhD
Senior Manager, Editorial: Lisa Claxton Moore
Senior Editor: Steven Kellert

Jones & Bartlett Learning books and products are available through most bookstores and online booksellers. To contact the Jones & Bartlett Learning Public Safety Group directly, call 800-832-0034, fax 978-443-8000, or visit our website, www.psglearning.com.

Substantial discounts on bulk quantities of Jones & Bartlett Learning publications are available to corporations, professional associations, and other qualified organizations. For details and specific discount information, contact the special sales department at Jones & Bartlett Learning via the above contact information or send an email to specialsales@jblearning.com.

Copyright © 2027 by Jones & Bartlett Learning, LLC, an Ascend Learning Company

All rights reserved. Unauthorized use is prohibited. Materials protected by this copyright may not be reproduced, adapted, transmitted, stored in a retrieval system, or utilized in whole or part, in any form or any means, electronic, mechanical, photocopied, recorded, or otherwise, without prior written permission from the copyright owner, except as permitted by U.S.A. copyright law.

The content, statements, views, and opinions herein are the sole expression of the respective authors and not that of Jones & Bartlett Learning, LLC. Reference herein to any specific commercial product, process, or service by trade name, trademark, manufacturer, or otherwise does not constitute or imply its endorsement or recommendation by Jones & Bartlett Learning, LLC and such reference shall not be used for advertising or product endorsement purposes. All trademarks displayed are the trademarks of the parties noted herein. *Emergency Medical Responder: Your First Response in Emergency Care, Eighth Edition* is an independent publication and has not been authorized, sponsored, or otherwise approved by the owners of the trademarks or service marks referenced in this product.

There may be images in this book that feature models; these models do not necessarily endorse, represent, or participate in the activities represented in the images. Any screenshots in this product are for educational and instructive purposes only. Any individuals and scenarios featured in the case studies throughout this product may be real or fictitious but are used for instructional purposes only.

The procedures and protocols in this book are based on the most current recommendations of responsible medical sources. The AAOS and the publisher, however, make no guarantee as to, and assume no responsibility for, the correctness, sufficiency, or completeness of such information or recommendations. Other or additional safety measures may be required under particular circumstances.

This textbook is intended solely as a guide to the appropriate procedures to be employed when rendering emergency care to the sick and injured. It is not intended as a statement of the standards of care required in any particular situation, because circumstances and the patient's physical condition can vary widely from one emergency to another. Nor is it intended that this textbook shall in any way advise emergency personnel concerning legal authority to perform the activities or procedures discussed. Such local determination should be made only with the aid of legal counsel.

The manufacturer's authorised representative in the EU for product safety is Mare Nostrum Group B.V., Mauritskade 21D, 1091 GC Amsterdam, The Netherlands.
Email: gpsr@mare-nostrum.co.uk

Production Credits
Vice President, Innovative Learning and Assessment Solutions: Ada Woo
Senior Director, Content Production and Delivery: Christine Emerton
Director, Product: Cathy Esperti
Manager, Content Development: Tiffany Sliter
Content Manager: Carly Mahoney
Developmental Editor: Mike Boblitt
Manager, Intellectual Properties and Content Production: Kristen Rogers
Content Production Manager: Erin Bosco
Intellectual Property Specialist: Angela Dooley
Senior Product Marketing Manager: Elaine Riordan
Director, Product Fulfillment: Aaron McKinzie
Purchasing Manager: Wendy Kilborn
Composition: S4Carlisle Publishing Services
Cover and Text Design: MPS Limited
Media Developer: Faith Brosnan
Intellectual Property Specialist: Robin Silverman
Cover Image (Title Page): Courtesy of Bryan Ware
Printing and Binding: Lakeside Book Company

Library of Congress Cataloging-in-Publication Data
Names: Schottke, David, author. | American Academy of Orthopaedic Surgeons, issuing body.
Title: Emergency medical responder / David Schottke ; American Academy of Orthopaedic Surgeons.
Other titles: Orange book series
Description: Eighth edition. | Burlington, MA : Jones & Bartlett Learning, [2027] | Series: Orange book series | Includes index.
Identifiers: LCCN 2025003699 | ISBN 9781284301212 (paperback)
Subjects: MESH: Emergencies | Emergency Medical Technicians--education | Emergency Medical Technicians--standards | Emergency Treatment | Examination Questions
Classification: LCC RC86.7 .S35 2025 | NLM WB 18.2 | DDC 616.025--dc23/eng/20250715
LC record available at https://lccn.loc.gov/2025003699

6048

Printed in the United States of America
29 28 27 26 25 10 9 8 7 6 5 4 3 2 1

Brief Contents

SECTION 1 Preparatory 1

1 **EMS Systems** 3

2 **Workforce Safety and Wellness** 19

3 **Lifting and Moving Patients** 39

4 **Medical, Legal, and Ethical Issues** 67

5 **Communications and Documentation** 79

6 **The Human Body** 97

SECTION 2 Airway 113

7 **Airway Management** 115

8 **Professional Rescuer CPR** 151

SECTION 3 Patient Assessment 175

9 **Patient Assessment** 177

SECTION 4 Medical 211

10 **Medical Emergencies** 213

11 **Poisoning and Substance Use** 241

12 **Behavioral Emergencies** 259

13 **Environmental Emergencies** 279

SECTION 5 Trauma 293

14 **Bleeding, Shock, and Soft-Tissue Injuries** 295

15 **Injuries to Muscles and Bones** 331

SECTION 6 Special Patient Populations 367

16 **Childbirth** 369

SECTION 7 EMS Operations 387

17 **Transport Operations** 389

18 **Vehicle Extrication and Special Rescue** 399

19 **Incident Management** 421

Appendix 441

Glossary 446

Index 457

Contents

SECTION 1 Preparatory 1

1 EMS Systems 3
Introduction 4
Overview of the EMS System 4
Public Health and EMS 6
The History of EMS 7
A Word About Patient Transport 8
EMR Training 9
Goals of EMR Training 10
Additional Skills 11
Roles and Responsibilities of the EMR 12
Medical Oversight 14
Quality Management 14
Your Certification 14

2 Workforce Safety and Wellness 19
Introduction 20
General Wellness Principles 20
Crew Resource Management 25
Workforce Safety 25

3 Lifting and Moving Patients 39
Introduction 40
General Principles 40
Recovery Position 40
Body Mechanics 41
Emergency Movement of Patients 42
Equipment 48
Treatment of Patients With Suspected Head or Spine Injuries 53

4 Medical, Legal, and Ethical Issues 67
Introduction 68
Duty to Act 68
Standard of Care 68
Scope of Practice 68
Ethical Responsibilities and Competence 68
Consent for Treatment 69
Patient Refusal of Care 70
Advance Directives 70
Legal Concepts 70
Good Samaritan Laws 73
Reportable Events 73
Crime Scene Operations 73
Documentation 74

5 Communications and Documentation 79
Introduction 80
Data and Communications Systems 80
Verbal Communication 84
Medical Terminology 90
Documentation 92

6 The Human Body 97
Introduction 98
Topographic Anatomy 98
Body Systems 98
Stages of Life: Growth and Development 105

SECTION 2 Airway 113

7 Airway Management 115
Introduction 116
Anatomy and Function of the Respiratory System 117
A Is for Airway 120
B Is for Breathing 126
Airway and Breathing Review 133
Foreign Body Airway Obstruction 136
Oxygen Administration 141
Pulse Oximetry 144
Special Considerations 145

8 Professional Rescuer CPR 151
Introduction 152
Anatomy and Function of the Circulatory System 152
Cardiac Arrest 154
Components of CPR 154
The Cardiac Chain of Survival 155
When to Start CPR 155
When to Stop CPR 156
Cardiac Compression 156
Adult CPR 158
Infant CPR 162
Child CPR 163
Signs of Effective CPR 164
Complications of CPR 164
Creating Sufficient Space for CPR 166
Early Defibrillation by EMRs 166
CPR Training 170
Legal Implications of CPR 170

SECTION 3 Patient Assessment 175

9 Patient Assessment **177**
Introduction 178
Patient Assessment Sequence 178
Scene Assessment 180
Primary Assessment 184
History Taking 188
Secondary Assessment 191
Reassessment 203
The Handoff Report 204
A Word About Medical and Trauma Patients 204

SECTION 4 Medical 211

10 Medical Emergencies **213**
Introduction 214
Patient Assessment in Medical Emergencies 214
Medications 215
General Medical Complaints 215
Specific Medical Conditions 218
Infectious Diseases and Epidemics 230
Pharmacology 231
Patients With Advanced Medical Needs 233
Advanced Medical Devices 233

11 Poisoning and Substance Use **241**
Introduction 242
Patient Assessment for Poisoning 242
Ingested Poisons 243
Inhaled Poisons 245
Injected Poisons 246
Absorbed Poisons 248
Nerve Agents 249
Substance Misuse 250
Intentional Self-Poisoning 254

12 Behavioral Emergencies **259**
Introduction 260
Patient Assessment in Behavioral Emergencies 260
Behavioral Emergencies 260
Phases of a Situational Crisis 261
Crisis Management 262
Mental Health Considerations in Geriatric Patients 272
Medical and Legal Considerations 272
Coping With Work-Related Stress 273

13 Environmental Emergencies **279**
Introduction 280
Patient Assessment for Environmental Emergencies 280
Exposure to Heat 281
Exposure to Cold 282
Drowning and Submersion 285
Other Environmental Emergencies 287

SECTION 5 Trauma 293

14 Bleeding, Shock, and Soft-Tissue Injuries **295**
Introduction 296
Patient Assessment for Bleeding, Shock, and Soft-Tissue Injuries 297
Standard Precautions and Soft-Tissue Injuries 297
Parts and Function of the Circulatory System 298
Shock 299
Bleeding 304
Wounds 310
Burns 320
Multisystem Trauma 324

15 Injuries to Muscles and Bones **331**
Introduction 332
Patient Assessment of Injuries to Muscles and Bones 332
The Anatomy and Function of the Musculoskeletal System 333
Mechanism of Injury 335
Types of Injuries 336
Standard Precautions and Musculoskeletal Injuries 337
Examination of Musculoskeletal Injuries 337
Treatment of Musculoskeletal Injuries 340
Injuries of the Head (Skull and Brain) 353
Injuries of the Face 356
Injuries to the Spine 356
Injuries of the Chest 360

SECTION 6 Special Patient Populations 367

16 Childbirth **369**
Introduction 370
The Anatomy and Function of the Female Reproductive System 370
Assessing the Birth Situation 370
Standard Precautions and Childbirth 372
Equipment 372
Assisting With Delivery 372
Aftercare of the Mother and Newborn 376
Resuscitating the Newborn 376
Complications of Pregnancy and Childbirth 378
Trauma and Pregnant Patients 381

SECTION 7 EMS Operations 387

17 Transport Operations **389**
Introduction 390
Preparing for a Call 390

Phases of an EMR Call 390
Helicopter Operations 391

18 Vehicle Extrication and Special Rescue 399
Introduction 400
Extrication 400
Water and Ice Rescue 408
Confined Space Rescue 412
Farm Rescue 412
Bus Rescue 415

19 Incident Management 421
Introduction 422
Hazmat Incidents 422
Mass-Casualty Incidents 424
Terrorism Awareness 431

Appendix 441

Glossary 446

Index 457

Skill Drills

Skill Drill 2-1	Removing Medical Gloves	30
Skill Drill 3-1	Performing a Direct Ground Lift	46
Skill Drill 3-2	Using a Scoop Stretcher	52
Skill Drill 3-3	Applying a Short Backboard Device	55
Skill Drill 3-4	Performing a Four-Person Log Roll	56
Skill Drill 3-5	Preparing a Blanket Roll	59
Skill Drill 3-6	Applying the Blanket Roll to Stabilize the Patient's Head and Neck	60
Skill Drill 7-1	Clearing the Airway Using Finger Sweeps	122
Skill Drill 7-2	Inserting an Oral Airway	125
Skill Drill 7-3	Inserting an Oral Airway in a Child	126
Skill Drill 7-4	Inserting a Nasal Airway	127
Skill Drill 7-5	Performing Mouth-to-Mask Rescue Breathing	130
Skill Drill 7-6	Performing Mouth-to-Barrier Rescue Breathing	132
Skill Drill 7-7	Using a Bag-Mask Device With One Rescuer	134
Skill Drill 7-8	Performing Infant Rescue Breathing	135
Skill Drill 7-9	Managing Airway Obstruction in an Alert Patient	138
Skill Drill 8-1	Performing Adult Chest Compressions	157
Skill Drill 8-2	Performing One-Rescuer Adult CPR	159
Skill Drill 8-3	Performing Two-Rescuer Adult CPR	160
Skill Drill 8-4	Performing Automated External Defibrillation	169
Skill Drill 9-1	Performing a Secondary Assessment	193
Skill Drill 14-1	Controlling Bleeding With a Tourniquet	306
Skill Drill 15-1	Checking Circulation, Sensation, and Movement in an Injured Extremity	338
Skill Drill 15-2	Applying a Vacuum Splint	342
Skill Drill 15-3	Stabilizing the Forearm	345
Skill Drill 15-4	Applying a Zippered Air Splint	345
Skill Drill 15-5	Applying an Unzippered Air Splint	346
Skill Drill 15-6	Applying a Traction Splint	349
Skill Drill 15-7	Applying an Air Splint to the Leg	350
Skill Drill 15-8	Applying a Pillow Splint for Ankle or Foot Injury	351
Skill Drill 15-9	Stabilizing the Cervical Spine and Maintaining an Open Airway	358
Skill Drill 15-10	Removing the Mask on a Sports Helmet	359
Skill Drill 15-11	Removing a Helmet	359
Skill Drill 16-1	Putting on Sterile Gloves	373
Skill Drill 16-2	Resuscitating a Newborn	377
Skill Drill 18-1	Airway Management in a Vehicle	407
Skill Drill 18-2	Turning a Patient in the Water	410

Let Navigate Take Your Course to New Heights

Navigate comprises a suite of mobile-ready course materials that will change the way you teach and the way your students learn and access course content. Whether you teach an online, hybrid, or traditional classroom-based course, you can use **Navigate** to improve results and deliver unbeatable value to your students, including:

- Market-leading interactive resources
- Proven preparatory and educational tools that improve success
- Personalized support and training to get you up and running

Try It Today

Contact your Public Safety Group Account Manager today at 1-978-443-5000 or visit **www.jblearning.com/navigate**

Acknowledgments

AAOS
AMERICAN ACADEMY OF ORTHOPAEDIC SURGEONS

The American Academy of Orthopaedic Surgeons and the Public Safety Group would like to acknowledge the contributors and reviewers of *Emergency Medical Responder: Your First Response in Emergency Care, Eighth Edition.*

Series Editor

Alfonso Mejia, MD, MPH, FAAOS
Program Director, Orthopedic Surgery Residency Program
Vice Head, Department of Orthopedic Surgery
University of Illinois at Chicago College of Medicine
Medical Director
Tactical Emergency Medical Support Physician
South Suburban Emergency Response Team
Chicago, Illinois

Author

David Schottke, MPH, RN, NRP
Fairfax Volunteer Fire Department
Fairfax, Virginia

Contributor

Rhonda J. Hunt, MEd, NRP
Albany State University
Darton College of Health Professions
Albany, Georgia

Reviewers

Aref Abdellatif, MSc TRM, Firefighter/Paramedic, LI
Oakton College
Skokie, Illinois
Chicago Fire Department
Chicago, Illinois

Daniel Benard, MBA, Paramedic IC
Kalamazoo Valley Community College
Kalamazoo, Michigan

Derrick Bunge, EMT-P/IC
Brighton Area Fire Authority
Brighton, Michigan

Brian W. Buzzella, AS, Firefighter/Paramedic
Broward College
Davie, Florida

Helen T. Compton, NRP
Southside Rescue Squad
South Hill, Virginia

Glenn Faught, MS, NREMT-P
Arkansas State University Mid-South
West Memphis, Arkansas

Anthony S. Harbour, MEd, BSN, RN, NRP
Virginia Commonwealth University, School of Medicine, Center for Trauma and Critical Care Education
Richmond, Virginia

Mark A. Huckaby, NRP, LP, CADS
OhioHealth EMS
Columbus, Ohio

Matt Hunt, BSEd, EMT-P
Albany State University
Albany, Georgia

Joseph Hurlburt, BS, NREMT-P
Northwest Wexford Emergency Authority
Mesick/Buckley, Michigan

Michael Kaduce, MPS, NRP
The Falck Health Institute
Orange County, California

Chris Kroboth, MS, FP-C
LifeLine EMS Training and Consulting
Boston, Virginia

Josh Lopez, MA, BS, NRP
University of New Mexico, School of Medicine, Department of Emergency Medicine–EMS Academy
Albuquerque, New Mexico

Kristen McKenna, MA, NRP
University of South Alabama
Mobile, Alabama

Richard M. Saalsaa, EMT
Philomath Fire and Rescue
Philomath, Oregon

John C. Schwab, EMT-B
Castleton Community Volunteer Fire Company
Castleton, Virginia

Jameel Sylvia, MPA, NRP
David Geffen School of Medicine at UCLA
Los Angeles, California

Michael Tarantino, MAS, BA
Bergen County EMS Training Center
Paramus, New Jersey

Brian Turner, RN, CCEMT-P
Princeton, Iowa

Matthew G. Watson, BS
Haymarket Police Department
Haymarket, Virginia

Niki Whitehead, NREMT
Oklahoma State University
Oklahoma City, Oklahoma

Thomas Worthington, MEd, EMTP, EMSIC
Schoolcraft College, Department of Emergency Medical Technology
Livonia, Michigan

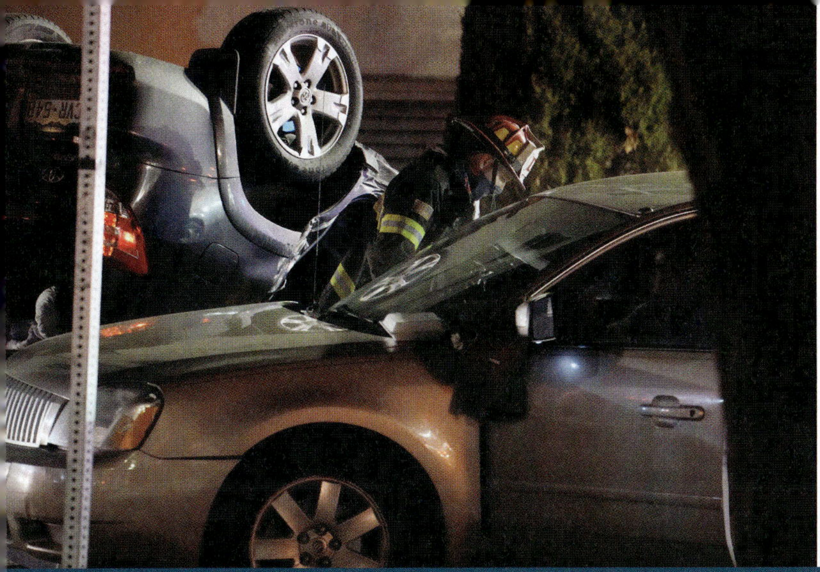

SECTION 1

Preparatory

1 EMS Systems

2 Workforce Safety and Wellness

3 Lifting and Moving Patients

4 Medical, Legal, and Ethical Issues

5 Communications and Documentation

6 The Human Body

© David Zalubowski/AP Photo

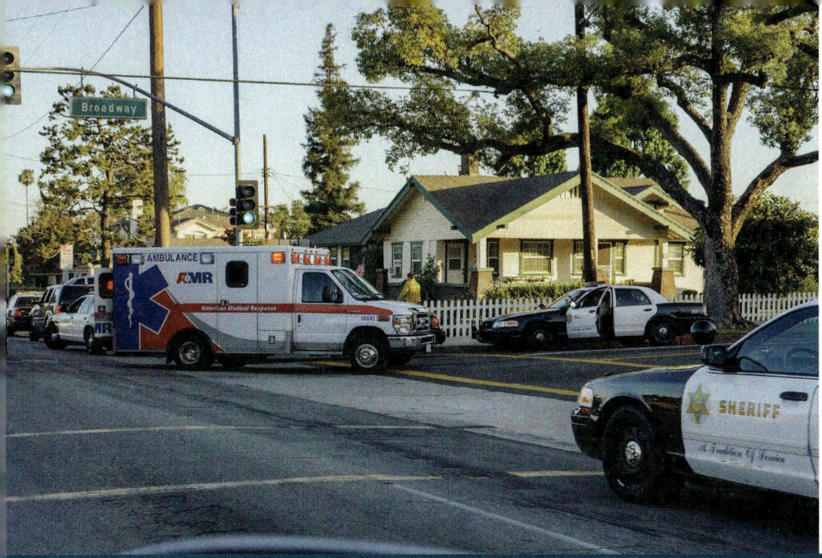

CHAPTER 1

EMS Systems

National EMS Education Standard Competencies

Preparatory

Uses simple knowledge of the emergency medical services (EMS) system, safety/well-being of the emergency medical responder (EMR), medical/legal issues, and ethical issues at the scene of an emergency while awaiting a higher level of care.

EMS Systems

- EMS systems (pp 4–15)
- Roles/responsibilities/professionalism of EMS personnel (pp 4–6)
- Quality improvement vs. quality assurance (p 14)
- Role of medical oversight (p 14)
- Culture of safety/patient safety (Chapter 2, *Workforce Safety and Wellness*)
- Continuum of care (p 4)

Research

- Impact of research on EMR care (p 14)
- Data collection (pp 4, 14)

Public Health

Has an awareness of local public health resources and their role in public health.

Public Health Overview

- EMS roles in public health (pp 6–7)
- Infection prevention and control (Chapter 2, *Workforce Safety and Wellness*)
- Human trafficking (p 7)

Knowledge Objectives

1. Describe the different elements of an emergency medical services (EMS) system. (pp 4–16)
2. Discuss the four levels of EMS training and licensure. (pp 5–6)
3. Describe the role of public health resources and how this role applies to EMS clinicians. (pp 6–7)
4. Discuss the history of the EMS system. (pp 7–8)
5. List the 11 standard components of an EMS system. (p 8)
6. Describe how the seriousness of the patient's condition is used to determine the urgency of transport to an appropriate medical facility. (pp 8–9)
7. Describe the general goals of emergency medical responder (EMR) training. (p 9)
8. Define the roles and responsibilities of EMRs. (p 12)
9. Describe the attributes that EMRs are expected to possess. (p 12)
10. Define medical oversight. (p 14)
11. Discuss the EMR's role in relation to medical oversight. (p 14)
12. Explain the quality management process and how it helps to improve patient care. (p 14)
13. Describe the impact of research on evidence-based patient care. (p 14)

Skills Objectives

There are no skills objectives for this chapter.

© Chon Kit Leong/Alamy Stock Photo

Introduction

An **emergency medical responder (EMR)** is often the first medically trained person to arrive on the scene of an emergency. As an EMR, the care you give could mean the difference between life and death. Your care is usually followed by care given by an **emergency medical technician (EMT)**, **paramedic**, nurse, physician, or other type of allied health professional.

Overview of the EMS System

The EMS system was developed to improve patient outcomes. Evidence showed that patients who received appropriate emergency medical care before they reached the hospital had a better chance of surviving a major injury or sudden illness than patients who did not receive such care. Over time, EMS has continued to improve its ability to quickly reach patients and provide prompt care and transport toward definitive care. EMS has become a vital component of the overall medical system.

It is important that you understand the operation and complexity of your EMS system. EMS systems can be organized in many different ways. Different agencies may provide different parts of the system. For example, first responders in one community may be law enforcement officers. In another community, the first responders may be firefighters. Another community may contract with a private EMS company to provide emergency services for that community. All three function similarly from a medical care perspective.

Problems during an EMS operation often result from a lack of coordination between resources and personnel. Agencies and personnel need to share an understanding of their roles for an EMS system to operate smoothly. This understanding develops through close cooperation, careful planning, communication, and continual effort.

The following sections explain how an EMS system typically works, from the time an emergency is reported to the time an injured or ill patient receives definitive care (**FIGURE 1-1**). Throughout this process, members of the entire health care team must work together with a unified goal. This concept is referred to as the **continuum of care**. Maintaining the continuum of care results in improved individual and team performance, better patient and responder safety, and improved patient outcomes.

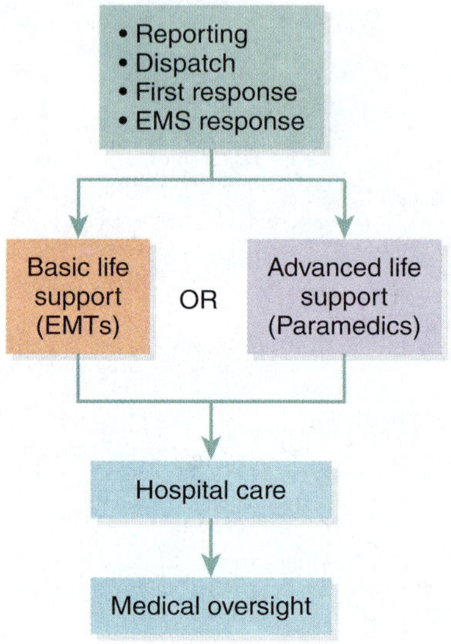

FIGURE 1-1 The EMS system.

© Jones & Bartlett Learning

Reporting

The first step in reporting an emergency is recognizing that an emergency exists. Often, the patient, a relative, or a bystander sees a serious illness or injury and decides to call for help. Other times, you may be the first to observe and report the emergency in the course of your primary job duties. Most 9-1-1 calls today are made using cell phones. Some other calls are still made using landline telephones, two-way radios, or personal emergency call systems. An **emergency response communications center** or **public safety answering point (PSAP)** usually receives the telephone call reporting an incident (**FIGURE 1-2**). The communications center may be a fire, police, or EMS agency; a 9-1-1 center; or a seven-digit emergency telephone number used by one or all of the emergency agencies. Enhanced 9-1-1 centers use computers to determine the location of landline telephones as soon as the telephone in the 9-1-1 center is answered. Under FCC guidelines, cellular carriers are required to also provide PSAPs with some information about the location of a cellular caller. The ability of different PSAPs to receive this information and incorporate it into dispatch information remains variable.

YOU are the EMR **CASE 1**

A few weeks after completing your EMR course, you are traveling along a freeway in your town. Suddenly the traffic slows down. At the right side of the road you see a car that has just crashed into the wall of a concrete overpass. As you pull over to stop, you see two people dragging a woman by her arms and legs away from the wrecked car.

1. Why is your role as an EMR so important during the first minutes after a crash?
2. Why is it important to know how the components of your EMS system work?
3. How does good interaction between different levels of the EMS team improve the quality of care?

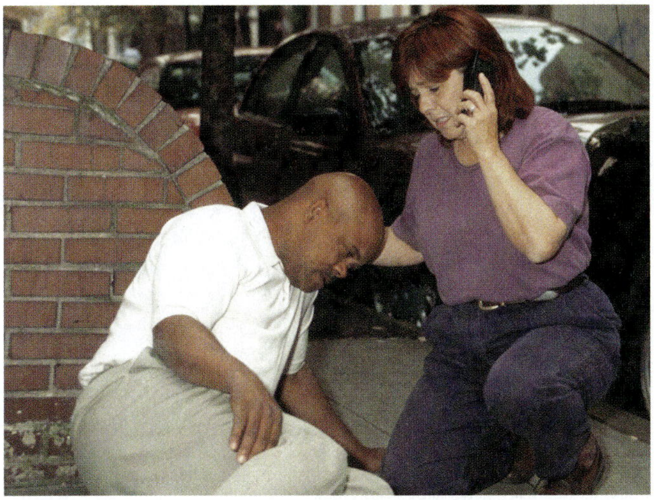

FIGURE 1-2 Reporting an emergency is the first step in EMS response.
© Jones & Bartlett Learning. Courtesy of MIEMSS.

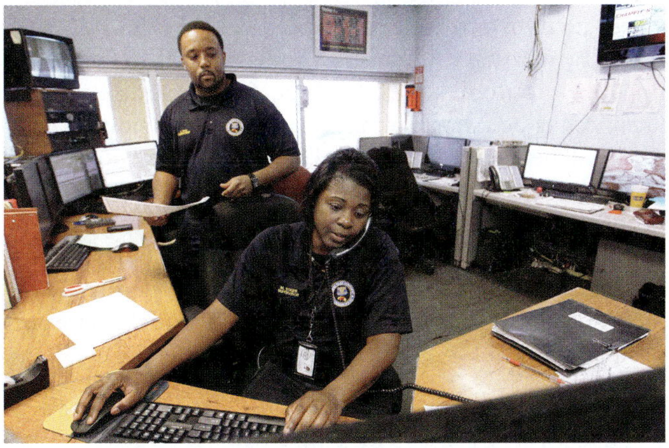

FIGURE 1-3 An emergency response communications center receives the call.
© Nikki Boertman/The Commercial Appeal/AP Photo

Some communities are beginning to implement Next Generation 9-1-1 (NG9-1-1) systems. These systems use broadband technology to transmit voice, text, data, and multimedia information. NG9-1-1 systems have the capacity to transmit valuable data such as medical information and building plans to first responders. Upgraded systems will be able to better pinpoint the location of cell phone callers.

Dispatch

Once the emergency response communications center is notified of an incident, appropriate equipment and personnel are dispatched to the scene (**FIGURE 1-3**). Dispatch may occur by landline telephone, cell phone, pager, public safety radio system, computer, or other means. Agencies, personnel, and equipment that are involved in the emergency medical first response vary by community.

First Response

Firefighters (paid or volunteer) or law enforcement personnel, because of their location or speed in responding, are in many cases the first EMRs on scene (**FIGURE 1-4**). Most communities have many EMRs but fewer EMTs, and even fewer paramedics. EMRs may be employed as lifeguards, security officers, teachers, or workers in an industrial setting. A community with four or five fire stations may have only two or three ambulances. The patient's first and perhaps most crucial contact with the EMS system occurs when the trained EMR arrives. For example, a key survival factor for people in cardiac arrest is the length of time between when the heartbeat stops and when manual cardiopulmonary resuscitation (CPR) starts.

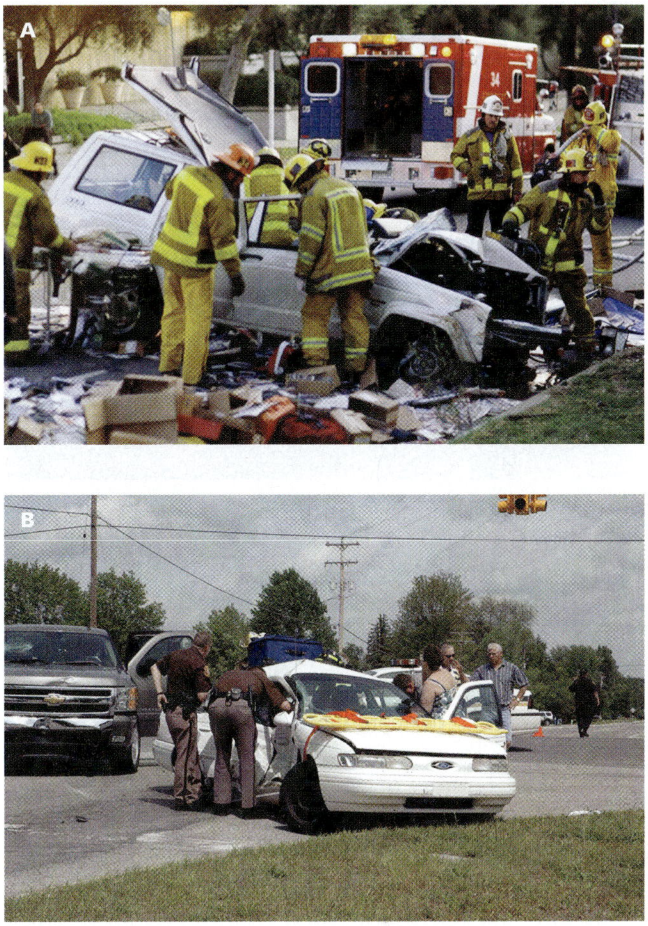

FIGURE 1-4 Firefighters (**A**) and law enforcement personnel (**B**) are EMRs in many emergencies.
A: © Corbis/Getty Images; **B:** Courtesy of Captain David Jackson, Saginaw Township Fire Department.

EMS Response

The arrival of an emergency medical vehicle (usually an ambulance) staffed by EMTs or paramedics is the patient's second contact with the EMS system (**FIGURE 1-5**). A properly equipped vehicle and the EMT staff make up a **basic life support (BLS)** unit. Each EMT has completed at least 150 hours of training. Many complete even longer training programs.

EMTs continue the care begun by EMRs. EMTs stabilize the patient's condition further and prepare the patient for transport to the hospital's emergency department (ED). Well-trained emergency personnel who can carefully move the

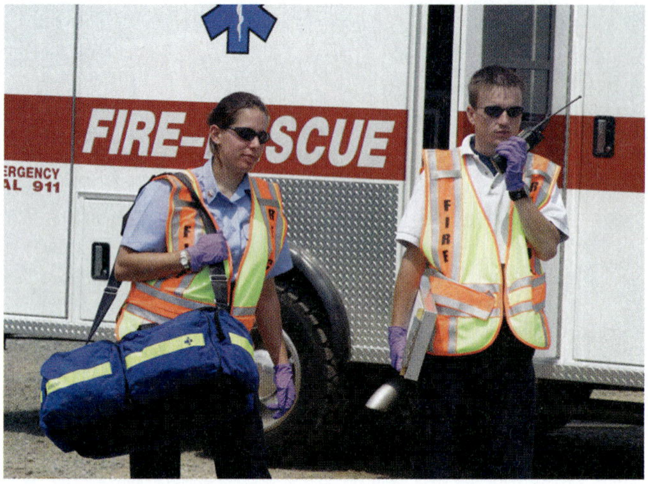

FIGURE 1-5 EMS responds.
© Jones & Bartlett Learning. Courtesy of MIEMSS.

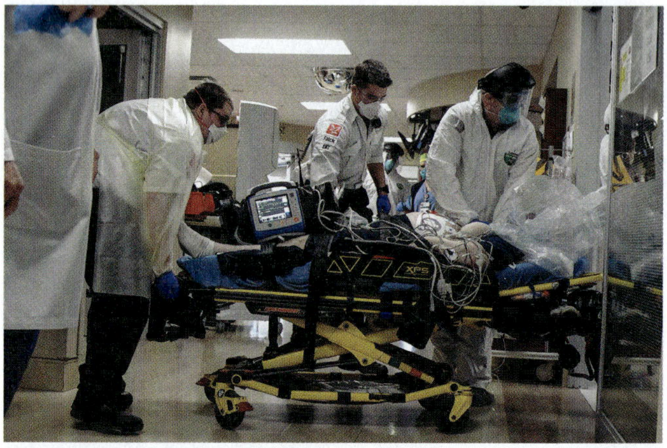

FIGURE 1-6 Hospital emergency care.
© AAron Ontiveroz/MediaNews Group/*The Denver Post*/Getty Images

patient and provide proper treatment increase the chance that the patient will arrive at the ED in the best possible condition.

An **advanced emergency medical technician (AEMT)** is able to perform limited **advanced life support (ALS)** skills. These clinicians have completed at least 200 hours of training beyond the EMT level. AEMTs may work alone or with a paramedic on an ALS unit.

Paramedics provide ALS services. They have usually received more than 1,000 hours of additional training. They can administer intravenous fluids and certain medications. They can also monitor and treat heart conditions with medications and electrocardiographic monitoring. **Defibrillation** is the administration of an electric shock to the heart of a patient who is experiencing a highly irregular heartbeat, known as ventricular fibrillation. Defibrillation can be accomplished using an automated external defibrillator (AED) by trained bystanders, EMRs, or EMTs. AEDs are present in many public settings and are carried by many emergency responders. Paramedics and in-hospital personnel use more sophisticated devices that can perform both defibrillation and cardiac monitoring. Paramedics are also trained in other advanced skills such as inserting special airway tubes (endotracheal tubes) to keep the patient's airway open.

Each level of skill builds on the one that precedes it: the paramedic's skills originate from those of the EMT, and the techniques used by the EMT depend on those of the EMR. All skill levels are based on what is learned in the EMR course: airway maintenance, bleeding control, and prevention, recognition, and treatment of shock.

The EMS system involves more than emergency medical care. For example, law enforcement personnel may provide protection and control at the scene of an incident. Fire units provide fire protection, specialized rescue, and patient extrication.

Hospital Care

The patient's third contact with the EMS system occurs in the hospital, primarily in the ED. After being treated at the scene, the patient is transported to an appropriate hospital, where definitive treatment can be provided (**FIGURE 1-6**). It may be necessary to transport some patients to the closest **appropriate medical facility** first. An appropriate medical facility may be a hospital, trauma center, or medical clinic. They will be stabilized there and then transported to a hospital that provides specialized treatment. Specialized treatment facilities include trauma centers, spinal cord injury centers, hand centers, cardiac centers, stroke centers, burn centers, pediatric centers, poison control centers, and perinatal centers. You must learn and follow your local patient transport protocols.

Public Health and EMS

The EMS system holds a unique place in our society. In most communities, it is considered part of the public safety function of government. EMS can also be considered a part of public health because these services are available to all people in a community. It is important for you to understand the basic functions of public health agencies because EMS personnel need to interact with public health practitioners.

Public health departments monitor restaurant cleanliness, conduct immunization programs, and determine the incidence of contagious diseases such as influenza, tuberculosis, and hepatitis. Public health departments also work to prevent the incidence or progression of diseases. They monitor the spread of contagious diseases and inform other members of the medical community about the scope of a disease. When people's actions can affect the spread of a disease, public health personnel work hard to educate the community about how to limit the spread of that disease.

EMS Roles in Public Health

Because prevention is better than treatment, public health and public safety departments provide education and screening programs to help prevent injuries and illness. They conduct car seat installation programs, programs to encourage seat belt use, alcohol awareness programs, programs to encourage bicycle and motorcycle helmet use, blood pressure screenings, and diabetes screenings. Public health departments provide support to EMS in certain situations. For example, EMS personnel may receive vaccinations at a public health clinic.

In some cases, EMS may be called on to support certain functions of a public health department. In the event of an epidemic such as influenza, EMS systems may need to work with public health departments to determine the number of people who are sick. The US Centers for Disease Control and Prevention (CDC) is one public health agency that monitors the incidence of diseases. Public health departments provide the standard precaution guidelines used to limit the spread of contagious diseases.

Words of Wisdom

An example of how EMS can help with public health efforts was seen during the coronavirus disease 2019 (COVID-19) pandemic. By evaluating patients in their homes and nursing facilities, EMS clinicians helped keep patients out of hospitals. Some EMS clinicians were trained and permitted to administer vaccines and treatments for COVID-19. Moreover, EMS clinicians staffed emergency operations centers, hospitals, and other medical facilities.

Human Trafficking

As a first responder, you will be in a position to detect and report criminal activity. **Human trafficking**, the illegal exploitation of a person through force, fraud, or coercion, is a growing problem in our society, requiring public health efforts to increase awareness and provide support to victims. It may be defined as sex trafficking or forced labor. This crime can happen anywhere and can involve people of either sex (although more than three-fourths are women) and any age or nationality. Traffickers can be strangers or acquaintances, such as family members, gang members, intimate partners, or employers.

You may encounter people being exploited at truck stops, rest areas, or workplaces or in private homes. Signs of human trafficking are subtle and may include the following:

- A person who has recently been disconnected from their family or social network
- A child who stops attending school
- A child younger than 18 years who is involved in commercial sex acts
- Signs of mental or physical abuse
- A child who seems fearful, timid, or submissive
- Signs of physical or medical neglect
- Brands or tattoos

Do not confront a suspected trafficker if you are not qualified to do so, but notify law enforcement as soon as possible. Questions to consider when evaluating a person you suspect is involved in human trafficking might include the following:

- Does the person appear to be controlled by another person?
- Does the person seem to be coached about what to say?
- Are the living conditions inappropriate?
- Does the person appear to lack personal possessions?
- Does the person not appear to be free to move about or leave (ie, existence of surveillance equipment or unusual locks or security measures)?

Remember that your primary role is to care for the patient's medical needs, not investigate a potential crime.

The Department of Homeland Security has developed awareness and educational materials through its Blue Campaign. It also provides support hotlines. To report suspected human trafficking, the number is 1-866-347-2423. To ask for help, the number is 1-888-373-7888, or the person may text HELP or INFO to BeFree (233733).

The History of EMS

As an EMS clinician, you should have some understanding of the history of EMS. Many advances in civilian EMS have followed progress initially established in the military medical system. Horse-drawn ambulances were first used to remove wounded patients from the battlefield during the Civil War. Traction splints were first used in World War I, which greatly reduced the death rate from fractured femurs (thigh bones). During World War II, well-trained medical corpsmen and field hospitals helped reduce battlefield mortality (deaths). In the 1950s, during the Korean Conflict, timely helicopter evacuations to Mobile Army Surgical Hospital (MASH) units further reduced battlefield mortality. Additional medical advances were made in the 1960s and 1970s during the Vietnam War. Improved protocols for use of tourniquets, chemical blood-clotting agents, and fluid resuscitation protocols helped improve survival during the conflicts in Iraq and Afghanistan.

In the United States during the 1950s and 1960s, funeral homes, hospitals, and volunteer rescue squads provided most ambulance services. The only training available for ambulance attendants was basic first aid.

Even interns who staffed hospital-based ambulances had no special training for their prehospital duties. Hearses were commonly used to transport ill and injured patients. The mortality rate from trauma to civilians was much higher than the mortality experienced by military personnel.

Some physicians recognized that civilian prehospital medical care lagged behind military emergency medical care. They urged the National Academy of Sciences to investigate this situation. In 1966, the National Academy of Sciences/National Research Council published a landmark paper, *Accidental Death and Disability: The Neglected Disease of Modern Society*. This paper described the deficiencies in emergency medical care. It recommended the development

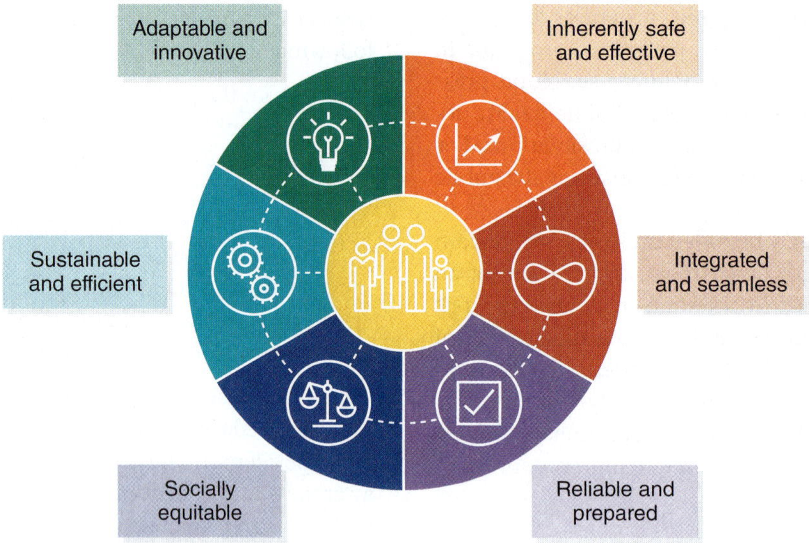

FIGURE 1-7 The six guiding principles from the National Highway Traffic Safety Administration's *EMS Agenda 2050*.
Courtesy of EMS.Gov/U.S. Department of Transportation.

of a national course of instruction for prehospital emergency care personnel. It also called for nationally accepted textbooks, ambulance vehicle design guidelines, ambulance equipment guidelines, state regulations for ambulance services, and improvements in hospital EDs. As a result, in the early 1970s, the US Department of Transportation developed a national standard curriculum for training EMS clinicians. This curriculum was the precursor of the education guidelines currently in use, the *National EMS Education Standards*.

During the 1970s and 1980s, the use of ALS within EMS became common. Currenty, paramedics are able to perform many procedures that were limited to physicians in the early days of EMS. Cities, counties, fire departments, third-party EMS departments, rescue squads, and hospitals currently provide most EMS. EMS clinicians are now trained through standardized courses conducted at accredited training centers. Certified personnel use standardized vehicles to transport patients to hospital EDs, where patients receive a high level of care.

As EMS systems have become increasingly sophisticated, the EMS community has recognized the need for oversight to ensure optimal performance and alignment with standards and guidelines. The National Highway Traffic Safety Administration evaluates EMS systems based on the following 11 criteria:

1. Regulation and policy
2. Resource management
3. Human resources and training
4. Transportation equipment and systems
5. Medical and support facilities
6. Communications system
7. Public information and education
8. Medical direction
9. Trauma system and development
10. Evaluation
11. Preparedness

States can request assessment of their EMS systems as well as other programs, such as their 9-1-1 systems.

In January 2019, the National Highway Traffic Safety Administration (NHTSA) of the US Department of Transportation released a report titled *EMS Agenda 2050: A People-Centered Vision for the Future of Emergency Medical Services*. This report focuses on bold, ambitious ideas for the future of EMS and provides ideas for today while looking toward the future. To achieve this vision, EMS systems of the future must be people centered and designed around six guiding principles: they must be (1) inherently safe and effective, (2) integrated and seamless, (3) reliable and prepared, (4) socially equitable, (5) sustainable and efficient, and (6) adaptable and innovative (**FIGURE 1-7**).

Words of Wisdom

To prevent confusion, in this text the term *clinician* is used to refer to a person certified at any EMS level: EMR, EMT, AEMT, or paramedic. The term *public safety provider* includes firefighters, law enforcement personnel, and EMS clinicians. The term *rescuer* refers to public safety providers engaged in the rescue and care of patients at an incident.

A Word About Patient Transport

As an EMR, your primary goal is to provide immediate care for a sick or injured patient. As more highly trained EMTs or paramedics arrive on scene, you will assist them in treating the patient and preparing the patient for transport. Although other EMS personnel usually transport patients, you need to understand when a patient must be transported quickly to a hospital or other medical facility (**FIGURE 1-8**).

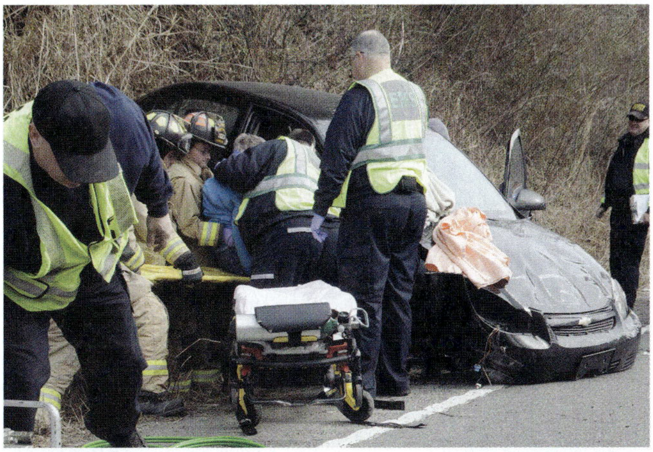

FIGURE 1-8 Ambulance transport to a hospital or medical facility.
© Curt Habraken/The Mountain Press/AP Photo

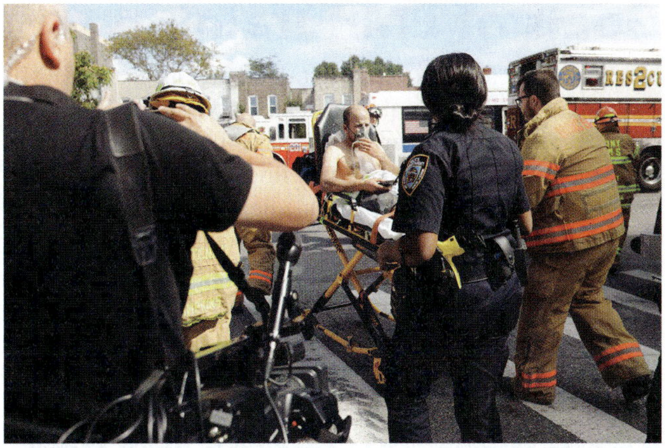

FIGURE 1-9 A typical emergency scene with injured patients.
© Spencer Platt/Getty Images News/Getty Images

This text uses three terms to describe the proper method of transporting a patient to an appropriate medical facility:

- **Transport.** This term means the patient's condition requires care by medical professionals, but speed in getting the patient to a medical facility is not the most important factor. For example, *transport* might describe the method of transporting a patient who has sustained an isolated injury to an extremity but whose condition is otherwise stable.
- **Prompt transport.** This phrase is used when a patient's condition is serious enough that the patient needs to be taken to an appropriate medical facility in a short time. If the patient is not transported quickly, the condition may get worse and the patient may die.
- **Rapid transport.** This phrase is used when EMS personnel are unable to give the patient adequate lifesaving care in the field. The patient may die unless transported immediately to an appropriate medical facility. *Rapid transport* is rarely used in this text.

Each of these three terms refers to transport to an appropriate medical facility. An appropriate medical facility may be a hospital, trauma center, or medical clinic. It is essential that you be familiar with the services provided by the medical facilities in your community and that you follow the protocols for your department.

EMS personnel must work closely with their medical director to establish transport protocols that ensure patients are transported to the closest medical facility capable of providing adequate care. To provide the best possible patient care, all members of the EMS team must remember that they are key components in the total system. Smooth operation of the team ensures the best care for the patient.

EMR Training

This text is written for an EMR training course. Although the text alone can teach you many things, it is best to use it as part of an approved EMR course. In this EMR course, you will learn how to examine patients and how to use basic emergency medical skills. These skills are divided into two main groups: (1) those needed to treat injured trauma patients and (2) those needed to care for patients experiencing illness or serious medical problems. The skills and knowledge you will gain from this course provide the foundation for the entire EMS system (**FIGURE 1-9**). Your actions can prevent a minor situation from becoming serious and will sometimes determine whether a patient lives or dies.

You will learn the following skills to stabilize conditions and treat persons who have been injured:

- Controlling airway, breathing, and circulation (Chapter 7, *Airway Management*, and Chapter 8, *Professional Rescuer CPR*)
- Controlling external bleeding (hemorrhage), treating shock, and managing wounds (Chapter 14, *Bleeding, Shock, and Soft-Tissue Injuries*)
- Splinting injuries to stabilize extremities (Chapter 15, *Injuries to Muscles and Bones*)

In addition to these trauma skills, you will learn to recognize, stabilize, and provide initial treatment for the following medical conditions:

- Heart attacks (Chapter 10, *Medical Emergencies*)
- Seizures and altered mental status (Chapter 10, *Medical Emergencies*)
- Poisonings, including alcohol/drug use and bites/stings (Chapter 11, *Poisoning and Substance Use*)
- Behavioral or psychological crises (Chapter 12, *Behavioral Emergencies*)
- Problems associated with excessive heat or cold (Chapter 13, *Environmental Emergencies*)
- Emergency childbirth (Chapter 16, *Childbirth*)

In addition, this text covers the fundamental knowledge required of any EMS clinician at any level, including workplace safety, patient lifting, effective communication, and basic human anatomy. The final chapters will apply these principles to specific, commonly encountered EMS situations.

Goals of EMR Training

It is important for you to understand the basic goals of EMR training. This training aims to teach you how to evaluate, stabilize, and treat patients using a minimum of specialized equipment. As an EMR, you will find yourself in situations in which little or no emergency medical equipment is readily available. You must know how to improvise using materials and objects already present at an emergency scene to serve in place of otherwise unavailable medical equipment. Finally, EMR training teaches you what you can do to help EMTs and paramedics when they arrive on the scene.

Know What You Should Not Do

The first lesson you must learn as an EMR is what not to do. For example, it may be better for you to leave a patient in the position found rather than attempt to move the person without the proper equipment or an adequate number of trained personnel. Sometimes the first priority at an emergency scene is to stabilize the scene or call for more help before beginning patient care. It is also critical that you not judge patients based on their cultural background, religion, skin color, gender, sexual orientation, age, or socioeconomic status. Doing so may undermine the quality of care you provide. Treat all your patients as you would treat a member of your own family.

Know How to Use Your EMR Life Support Kit

The second goal of EMR training is to teach you to treat patients using limited emergency medical supplies. An EMR life support kit, also known as a jump bag, should be small enough to fit in the trunk of an automobile or on almost any police, fire, or rescue vehicle. Although the contents of the kit are limited, such supplies are all you need to provide immediate care for most patients you will encounter. The suggested contents of an EMR life support kit are shown in **FIGURE 1-10** and described in **TABLE 1-1**.

Know How to Improvise

The third goal of EMR training is to teach you how to improvise. As a trained EMR, you will often be in situations with little or no emergency medical equipment. Therefore, it is important that you know how to improvise. This text gives examples of improvisation that can be applied to real-life situations. You will learn, for example, how to use articles of clothing and handkerchiefs to stop bleeding and how to use wooden boards, magazines, or newspapers to immobilize injured extremities.

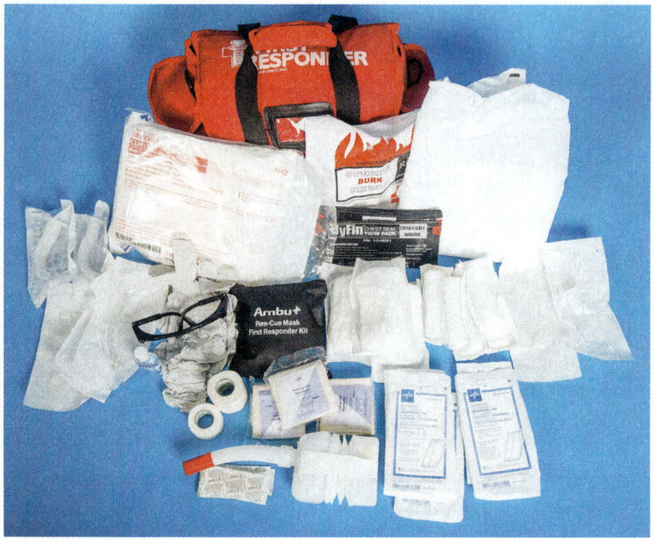

FIGURE 1-10 An EMR life support kit, also called a jump bag.
© Jones & Bartlett Learning

> **Words of Wisdom**
>
> An EMR life support kit, or jump bag, should include personal protective equipment as well as those things immediately needed to control bleeding, manage the airway, and assist with breathing.

Know How to Assist Other EMS Clinicians

Finally, EMR training teaches you how to assist EMTs and paramedics once they arrive on the scene. Many procedures that EMTs and paramedics use require at least three people to be performed correctly. Thus, you may have to assist with these procedures and you must know what to do.

YOU are the EMR — CASE 2

You are dispatched to 11 North Fourth Street for a report of an injured woman. Your dispatcher reports that the woman was excited and that he was not able to get additional information from her. He indicates that the patient will meet you in front of her house. You arrive at the address and find a 38-year-old woman sitting on the front porch steps crying. After you introduce yourself, you ask her why she called EMS. She tells you that she had a skillet of grease, and as she tried to move it, it caught on fire. She has some blisters and reddening on both hands and redness on her face. You ask her if the fire is out. She says she does not know. She says there is no one else in the house.

1. Why is it so important to get correct information from the emergency dispatcher?
2. What are the first actions you need to take at this emergency scene?

TABLE 1-1 Suggested Contents of an EMR Life Support Kit

Patient examination equipment	1 flashlight
Personal safety equipment	5 pairs of gloves 5 face masks 1 bottle of hand sanitizer Eye protection 1 disposable gown
Resuscitation equipment	1 mouth-to-mask resuscitation device 1 portable hand-powered suction device 1 set oral airways 1 set nasal airways
Bandaging and dressing equipment	10 gauze adhesive strips (1-inch [3-cm]) 10 gauze pads (4 × 4–inch [10 × 10–cm]) 5 gauze pads (5 × 9–inch [13 × 23–cm]) 2 universal trauma dressings (10 × 30–inch [25 × 76–cm]) 1 occlusive dressing for sealing chest wounds 4 conforming gauze rolls (3 inches × 15 feet [8 cm × 5 m]) 4 conforming gauze rolls (4.5 inches × 15 feet [11 cm × 5 m]) 6 triangular bandages 1 adhesive tape (2-inch [5-cm]) 1 burn sheet 1 tourniquet
Patient immobilization equipment	2 (each) cervical collars: small, medium, large, *or* 2 adjustable cervical collars 3 rigid conforming splints (SAM splints), *or* 1 set air splints for arm and leg, *or* 2 (each) cardboard splints (18-inch [46-cm] and 24-inch [61-cm])
Extrication equipment	1 spring-loaded center punch 1 pair of heavy leather gloves
Miscellaneous equipment	2 blankets (disposable) 2 cold packs 1 pair of bandage scissors 1 obstetric kit
Other equipment	1 set of personal protective clothing (helmet, EMS jacket) 1 American National Standards Institute (ANSI)–approved reflective vest 1 fire extinguisher (5-pound [2-kg] ABC dry chemical) 1 *Emergency Response Guidebook* (might be carried as book, or might be accessed via electronic app or dispatcher) 6 flares 1 pair of binoculars
Optional equipment (based on the protocols of your service)	Oral glucose Naloxone intranasal spray (for opioid overdoses) Saline

© Jones & Bartlett Learning

Additional Skills

EMRs operate in a variety of settings. Many problems encountered in urban areas differ sharply from those found in rural settings. Regional variations in climate not only affect the situations you encounter, but also require you to use different skills and equipment in treating patients. Certain skills and equipment mentioned in this text are beyond the essential minimum knowledge you need to successfully complete an EMR course. However, these supplemental skills and equipment may be required in your local EMS system.

Roles and Responsibilities of the EMR

As an EMR, you have several roles and responsibilities. Depending on the emergency situation, you may need to:

- Maintain your body in a healthy physical and mental condition.
- Maintain equipment in a ready state.
- Respond promptly and safely to the scene of an accident or sudden illness.
- Ensure that the scene is safe from hazards.
- Protect yourself.
- Protect the incident scene and patients from further harm.
- Summon appropriate assistance (EMTs, fire department, rescue squad).
- Gain access to the patient.
- Perform patient assessment.
- Administer emergency medical care.
- Provide reassurance to patients and family members.
- Move patients (only when necessary).
- Seek and then direct help from bystanders, if necessary.
- Control activities of bystanders.
- Assist EMTs and paramedics, as necessary.
- Maintain continuity of patient care.
- Document your care.
- Keep your knowledge and skills up to date.

Concern for the patient is primary; you should perform all activities with the patient's well-being in mind. Prompt response to the scene is essential if you are to provide quality care to the patient. It is important that you know your response area well so you can quickly determine the most efficient route to the emergency scene.

Attitude and Conduct

As an EMR, you will be judged on your attitude and conduct, as well as on the medical care you provide. It is important to understand that professional behavior has a positive impact on your patients. To be a good EMR, you need to reflect certain characteristics. You need to be honest and conduct yourself with integrity. You need to be aware of the patient's feelings and have empathy for your patients. You need to be motivated to get the job done and to understand the limits of your training and skills. You must advocate for patients. Unresponsive patients depend totally on your skills, knowledge, and the concern you bring to the emergency scene.

Because you will often be the first medically trained person to arrive on the scene of an emergency, it is important to be calm and caring. You will gain the confidence of patients and bystanders more easily by using a courteous and caring tone of voice. Introduce yourself by name and title or position. Show an interest in your patients. Avoid embarrassing your patients and help protect their privacy. Talk with your patients and let them know what you are doing. A good rule to follow is to treat all of your patients the way you would treat a close family member. This attitude will go a long way in helping patients through the emergency and will make your job easier, too.

Remember, medical information about patients is confidential and should not be discussed with your family or friends. This information should be shared only with other medical personnel who are involved in the care of that patient.

Your appearance should be neat and professional at all times. You should be well groomed and clean. A uniform helps identify you as an EMR. If you are a volunteer who responds from home, always identify yourself as an EMR. Your professional attitude and neat appearance help provide much-needed reassurance to patients (**FIGURE 1-11**). Good EMS personnel learn to keep a cool head and maintain a warm heart while caring for a patient.

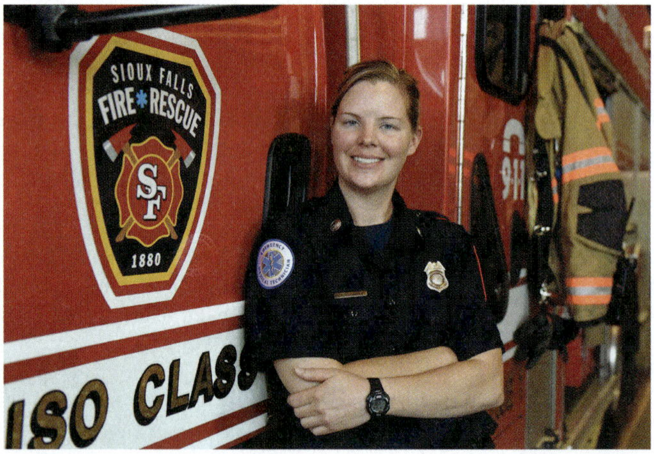

FIGURE 1-11 A professional attitude and neat appearance reassure patients.
© Emily Spartz Weerheim/Argus Leader/AP Photo

YOU are the EMR **CASE 3**

It is shortly after 1000 hours on a sunny Sunday morning when dispatch interrupts your breakfast with a report of a 37-year-old man who has slipped on a dock and fallen at the local marina. You arrive on scene to find the man lying on the dock clutching his foot, breathing normally. You notice the ankle is deformed.

1. How might you be asked to assist advanced EMS personnel?
2. Why is it important that EMRs know how to improvise?

Voices of Experience

One day, while running errands, I stopped by the local coffee shop for my usual double latte with extra cream and sugar. While standing in line waiting to place my order, I saw my neighbor, Mrs. Jones. We were talking about her family (who did not live nearby) when she started to experience some type of medical emergency. I was very concerned by this and asked Mrs. Jones if she was okay. She responded, "My, what a gorgeous day it is outside," and began to fall down. I quickly caught her, lowered her to a chair, and told someone to call 9-1-1. After the EMS crew arrived and I told them what I saw, I left.

As I was walking back home, I thought, "I have lived here for 25 years and think it's time I gave something back to the community." That afternoon I called the EMS system that transported Mrs. Jones. They helped me sign up for an EMR course at the local community center. On completion of the course, I volunteered for a couple shifts a month for the EMS system. During the course, I learned how to protect myself while responding to a medical emergency or a traumatic event. I also learned how the EMS system works, how they are notified, how to prepare myself to respond to a call safely and effectively, which skills and procedures I can and cannot do, and what happens when the patient is transported to the hospital. These are all parts of an effective EMS system, starting with personnel training and moving to vehicle staffing and transport of patients. It is important to remember that the system is like a circle that is complete only when the patient is discharged from the facility.

"Because of you, I am here today."

That day at the coffee shop, the EMS crew showed up about 2 or 3 minutes after they were called. They assessed the situation, called for a higher level of care, loaded the patient on the stretcher, and, due to the long transport time, met ALS clinicians on the way. What I didn't see was what happened when Mrs. Jones arrived at the hospital. A couple of days later, I saw Mrs. Jones back at the coffee shop. She came over to me, gave me a big hug, and said, "Thank you for saving my life. I had an ischemic stroke, but because of you, I am here today."

Greg LaMay, BS, NREMT-P
Education Coordinator
East Texas Medical Center–EMS
Tyler, Texas

Adapted from the personal Medical Identification Symbol of the American Medical Association.

Medical Oversight

The overall leader of the medical care team is the physician or medical director. To ensure that the patient receives appropriate medical treatment, it is important that EMRs receive direction from a physician. Each EMS agency should have a physician who directs training courses, helps set medical policies and procedures, and ensures quality management of the EMS system. This type of medical direction is known as indirect (or off-line) medical control.

A second type of medical control is known as direct (or online) medical control. A physician who is in contact with prehospital EMS clinicians, usually paramedics or EMTs, by two-way radio or wireless telephone provides online medical control. In cases where large numbers of people are injured or in cases of prolonged entrapment, physicians may respond to the scene of the incident to provide on-scene medical control.

Quality Management

Quality management is an umbrella term that encompasses the distinct processes of quality assurance and quality improvement. The purpose of **quality assurance** is to monitor compliance against a standard. Thus, it is a reactive process that identifies problems after they have already occurred. The goal of **quality improvement** is to make changes in medical care systems to improve the effectiveness and safety of current treatments and procedures.

Quality management is used in all parts of the health care system, including EMS. The Institute of Medicine has identified six aims in ensuring quality care:

1. **Safety.** The actions of EMRs must not cause harm to patients, bystanders, or EMS clinicians.
2. **Effectiveness.** EMS care should be based on scientific knowledge and provide the desired benefit to the patient. Refrain from any treatment that does not benefit the patient.
3. **Patient centeredness.** Emergency medical care must be responsive to the patient's needs. Be responsive to the patient's physical needs as well as to values, religion, and heritage.
4. **Timeliness.** Provide care in a timely manner. Timely patient care is an especially important component of EMS.
5. **Efficiency.** Always strive to deliver care without wasting supplies, equipment, or time.
6. **Equitability.** Strive to deliver your best care to all people. This means patient care should not vary between people of different genders, different sexual orientations, different ethnic backgrounds, different geographic locations, or different socioeconomic levels.

EMS systems should have quality assurance programs to evaluate the care they provide. Evaluations should include the six preceding components. They should consider whether errors have occurred because of a gap in skills or knowledge. Your organization uses protocols, continuing medical education, and call debriefing to help improve the quality of care being given to your patients. As part of the quality assurance process, you may be asked to participate in a research study or in data collection in your service. EMS research is an important part of ensuring good patient care.

Words of Wisdom

Virtually all aspects of health care currently rely on evidence-based medicine (EBM). EBM ensures that interventions advocated within EMS have clear, unbiased proof of improving patient outcomes. An example of how EBM can benefit EMS agencies can be seen in the decision to adopt a new device. Before a product becomes part of the standard of care, the process for new product adoption should include rigorous impartial scientific evaluation of manufacturer claims.

As an EMR, you will likely contribute to EMS research. Your documentation may include details that are incorporated into research studies to help support EBM efforts. As you advance in your EMS career, you should stay abreast of current EMS research so that you can help contribute to evidence-based decisions and patient care.

Your Certification

Most states require certification, registration, or licensure of EMS clinicians. **Certification** is the process by which a person, institution, or program is evaluated and recognized as meeting certain standards to ensure safe and ethical patient care. Your state has a lead agency that administers regulations relating to EMS operations. Once certified as an EMR, you must follow the national or state standards for your level

YOU are the EMR — CASE 4

You are dispatched to a local big box store for a report of a sick man. You are close to this location and arrive on the scene within 2 minutes. A store employee meets you at the front door and directs you to a 73-year-old man who is sitting on a chair close to the checkout area. As you approach, you notice that the patient is pale and sweaty and seems to be short of breath. His wife tells you that he started to have severe chest pains just before she called 9-1-1. She says that the pain he described to her before your arrival is just like the pain he had 3 years ago when he had a heart attack.

1. What should you say as you approach this patient?
2. What level of emergency medical care do you think is best for this patient?
3. With whom can you share information about this patient's history, symptoms, and treatment?

of practice. Your employer may set additional requirements for your conduct and practice. You must keep your certification current by meeting continuing education requirements and keeping your skills up to date. Failure to keep your certification current can result in penalties.

In 2020, the National Registry of Emergency Medical Technicians launched the National EMS ID number system. An EMS ID is a 12-digit identification number issued at no charge to all EMS professionals, from EMR to paramedic, and to students entering the profession. The number is automatically generated by the National Registry when a person creates an account. For EMS clinicians with an existing account, an EMS ID is retroactively created. Unlike the number issued by the National Registry (Registry Number) when an individual becomes certified, EMS IDs do not change as the person's certification level changes. Thus, the various certification numbers that individuals may obtain in their career are all tied back to the single EMS ID.

YOU are the EMR — SUMMARY

You are the EMR: CASE 1

1. Why is your role as an EMR so important during the first minutes after a crash?

In the first few minutes after a crash or other emergency, you may be the only person on the scene who has been trained to deal with a medical emergency. Your initial actions can keep the scene safe until other responders arrive and make a difference in the patient's outcome. Also, you can determine whether additional resources need to be dispatched.

2. Why is it important to know how the components of your EMS system work?

It is important to understand the components of the EMS system because you are a part of the system. You provide a vital function in the system and are supported by and interact with people who fulfill other functions within the system.

3. How does good interaction between different levels of the EMS team improve the quality of care?

Good interactions between different levels of the EMS team improve patient care by relaying vital patient information and improving the efficiency of patient care.

You are the EMR: CASE 2

1. Why is it so important to get correct information from the emergency dispatcher?

You need the correct address to get to the emergency scene. Responding to an incorrect address will result in a delay in stabilizing the scene and providing care for the patient.

2. What are the first actions you need to take at this emergency scene?

Ensure that the scene is safe. Do not enter the building to see if the fire is out unless you are properly trained and equipped. Protect yourself. Do not let the patient reenter the house. Call for additional assistance. In this case, that would include fire suppression personnel. You should also verify that EMS transportation has been dispatched.

You are the EMR: CASE 3

1. How might you be asked to assist advanced EMS personnel?

Given the man's location, responding EMTs may need assistance with lifting and moving the patient onto a stretcher and into an ambulance.

2. Why is it important that EMRs know how to improvise?

EMRs occasionally face situations where they have little or no medical gear available and must find solutions, such as using a pillow to stabilize a broken ankle when a conventional splint is not available.

You are the EMR: CASE 4

1. What should you say as you approach this patient?

Introduce yourself by name and title. Sometimes it is helpful to say, "I'm here to help you." Include the patient's wife in your introduction to put her at ease. Asking the patient his name can also be helpful. Patients respond better to your questions when you use their name.

2. What level of emergency medical care do you think is best for this patient?

Experienced emergency medical care clinicians learn to listen to what the patient and patient's family tell them. When the man's wife tells you that the pain is just like the pain he had with a heart attack, there is a good chance that he might be having a heart attack now. When you combine that information with his pallor, sweating, and shortness of breath, you can conclude that this is a serious condition that would benefit from ALS care, if it is available. It is reasonable for you to relay your findings to the emergency dispatcher and request ALS personnel to stabilize this patient and promptly transport him to an appropriate medical facility.

YOU are the EMR — SUMMARY

3. With whom can you share information about this patient's history, symptoms, and treatment?

You can share information about this patient, such as signs and symptoms of his illness, his medical history, and treatment, with other members of the prehospital EMS system who are involved with his care. It is also necessary to share this information with health care workers who are caring for him at the hospital. In addition, it is important to have someone talk with the patient's wife.

Prep Kit

Ready for Review

- The EMR is often the first medically trained person to arrive on the scene. The initial care provided is essential because it is available sooner than more advanced emergency medical care and could mean the difference between life and death.
- EMRs should understand the EMS system. The typical sequence of events of the EMS system is reporting, dispatch, emergency medical response, EMS vehicle response, and hospital care. Throughout this process, members of the entire health care team must work together with a unified goal, a concept known as the continuum of care.
- As an EMR, you may be asked to help with public health efforts and will be expected to help ensure the safety and wellness of your community.
- The basic goals of EMR training are to know what not to do, how to provide care using your EMR life support kit, how to improvise, and how to assist other EMS clinicians.
- As an EMR, your primary goal is to provide immediate care for a sick or injured patient. As more highly trained personnel (EMTs or paramedics) arrive on the scene, you will assist them in treating and preparing the patient for transport.
- Remember that medical information about a patient is confidential and should be shared only with other medical personnel who are involved in the care of that particular patient.
- The overall leader of the medical care team is the physician or medical director. To ensure that the patient receives appropriate medical treatment, it is important that EMRs receive direction from a physician.
- Quality management helps to ensure that a high level of care is rendered by an EMS system. EMS systems should have a method of assessing the quality of care provided (quality assurance) and making necessary changes (quality improvement) to address problems.

Vital Vocabulary

advanced emergency medical technician (AEMT) A person who is qualified to perform basic life support skills and limited advanced life support skills.

advanced life support (ALS) The use of specialized equipment (such as cardiac monitors and defibrillators) and specialized techniques (such as intravenous fluid administration, drug infusion, and endotracheal intubation) to stabilize a patient's condition.

appropriate medical facility A hospital or medical clinic with adequate medical resources to provide continuing care to sick or injured patients who have been transported after field treatment by emergency medical responders.

basic life support (BLS) Emergency lifesaving procedures performed without advanced emergency procedures to stabilize the condition of patients who have experienced sudden illness or injury.

certification The process by which a person, institution, or program is evaluated and recognized as meeting certain standards to ensure safe and ethical patient care.

continuum of care The concept of consistent patient care across the entire health care team from first patient contact to patient discharge.

defibrillation The process of delivering an electric shock through a person's chest wall and heart to establish normal heart contraction rhythms.

Prep Kit

emergency medical responder (EMR) A person who is qualified to provide basic lifesaving interventions until a more highly trained clinician arrives on the scene.

emergency medical technician (EMT) A person who is qualified to provide basic life support and certain other noninvasive prehospital medical procedures.

emergency response communications center A fire, police, or emergency medical services agency; a 9-1-1 center; or a seven-digit telephone number used by one or all of the emergency agencies to receive and dispatch requests for emergency care; also called a public safety answering point.

human trafficking The illegal exploitation of a person through force, fraud, or coercion.

paramedic A person trained and certified to provide advanced life support.

public safety answering point (PSAP) A fire, police, or emergency medical services agency; a 9-1-1 center; or a seven-digit telephone number used by one or all of the emergency agencies to receive and dispatch requests for emergency care; also called an emergency response communications center.

quality assurance A reactive process that involves monitoring compliance against a standard to identify problems that have already occurred.

quality improvement A proactive process that involves making changes to a system to improve performance.

References

Donnelly EA, Oehme K, Barris D, Melvin R. What do EMS professionals know about human trafficking? An exploratory study. *J Hum Trafficking*. 2019;5(4):325–335.

Emergency medical services: more than a ride to the hospital. Centers for Disease Control and Prevention website. https://blogs.cdc.gov/publichealthmatters/2022/05/ems-week/. Published May 18, 2022. Accessed November 19, 2024.

Indicators of human trafficking. US Department of Homeland Security website. https://www.dhs.gov/blue-campaign/indicators-human-trafficking. Updated March 21, 2022. Accessed November 19, 2024.

National Academy of Sciences (US) and National Research Council (US) Committee on Trauma; National Academy of Sciences (US) and National Research Council (US) Committee on Shock. *Accidental Death and Disability: The Neglected Disease of Modern Society.* Washington (DC): National Academies Press (US); 1966. https://www.ncbi.nlm.nih.gov/books/NBK222962/doi: 10.17226/9978

National Association of State EMS Officials. *National EMS Scope of Practice Model 2019.* Washington, DC: National Highway Traffic Safety Administration; February 2019. Report No. DOT HS 812-666. https://www.ems.gov/assets/National_EMS_Scope_of_Practice_Model_2019.pdf. Accessed November 19, 2024.

National Association of State EMS Officials. *National Model EMS Clinical Guidelines: Version 3.0.* https://nasemso.org/wp-content/uploads/National-Model-EMS-Clinical-Guidelines_2022.pdf. Published March 2022. Accessed November 19, 2024.

National Highway Traffic Safety Administration. *National Emergency Medical Services Education Standards*. EMS.gov website. https://www.ems.gov/assets/EMS_Education-Standards_2021_FNL.pdf. Published 2021. Accessed November 19, 2024.

National Highway Traffic Safety Administration (NHTSA), US Department of Transportation. *EMS Agenda 2050: A People-Centered Vision for the Future of Emergency Medical Services.* EMS.gov website. https://www.ems.gov/issues/planning-for-the-future-ems-agenda-2050/. Updated October 18, 2023. Accessed November 19, 2024.

Next generation 911 (NG911) roadmap progress report. The National 911 Program website. https://www.911.gov/assets/NPD-220126-004National911Program_RoadmapStatus_2022_01FEB2022_FINAL.pdf. Published February 2022. Accessed November 19, 2024.

State EMS systems. EMS.gov website. https://www.ems.gov/issues/state-ems-systems/. Updated October 18, 2023. Accessed November 19, 2024.

Wakefield MK. The quality chasm series: implications for nursing. In: Hughes RG, ed. *Patient Safety and Quality: An Evidence-Based Handbook for Nurses*. Rockville, MD: Agency for Healthcare Research and Quality; 2008.

Assessment IN ACTION

A call comes in on a Friday evening at 1943 hours. You and your partner are dispatched to a local high school for a report of an injured soccer player. As you arrive on the scene you are directed to a 17-year-old female soccer player who is trying not to cry. She states she is in a lot of pain. On questioning her, you learn that she was hit from the right side as she was running and now her knee is very painful. She states that she tried to walk, but she cannot put any weight on her right knee. Her right knee shows some deformity and swelling. She tells you nothing else seems to be hurt.

1. What is your initial responsibility when arriving on scene?
   - **A.** Document your patient care.
   - **B.** Summon appropriate assistance.
   - **C.** Protect the incident scene and the patient from further harm.
   - **D.** Move the patient inside a building.
2. If a patient's first contact with the EMS system is interaction with an EMR, and the second occurs when EMTs arrive, the third would be when the patient:
   - **A.** arrives in the emergency department at the hospital.
   - **B.** sees a personal physician.
   - **C.** is discharged.
   - **D.** is moved to the ambulance.
3. How can you assist EMS clinicians with more advanced training?
   - **A.** Maintain command of the incident scene.
   - **B.** Interpret cardiac rhythms.
   - **C.** Help prepare the patient for transport.
   - **D.** Give epinephrine.
4. All of the following are standard components of an EMS system EXCEPT:
   - **A.** medical and support facilities.
   - **B.** communications system.
   - **C.** testing.
   - **D.** transportation systems.
5. In the EMS system, a medical director does all of the following EXCEPT:
   - **A.** help set medical policies and procedures.
   - **B.** ensure that the EMRs are properly trained.
   - **C.** direct the staffing for the ambulance fleet.
   - **D.** ensure the quality management of the EMS system.
6. The roles and responsibilities of the EMR include all of the following EXCEPT:
   - **A.** ensuring that the scene is safe from hazards.
   - **B.** sharing the patient's medical condition with the public media.
   - **C.** gaining access to the patient.
   - **D.** protecting the incident scene and patients from further harm.
7. Why is it important for you to know how to improvise certain medical equipment?
8. With whom can you share information about the patient's injuries, illness, and treatment?
9. What should you tell EMTs arriving on the scene about the condition of this soccer player?
10. Why is it important to tell responding EMS personnel about your assessment and treatment of this patient?

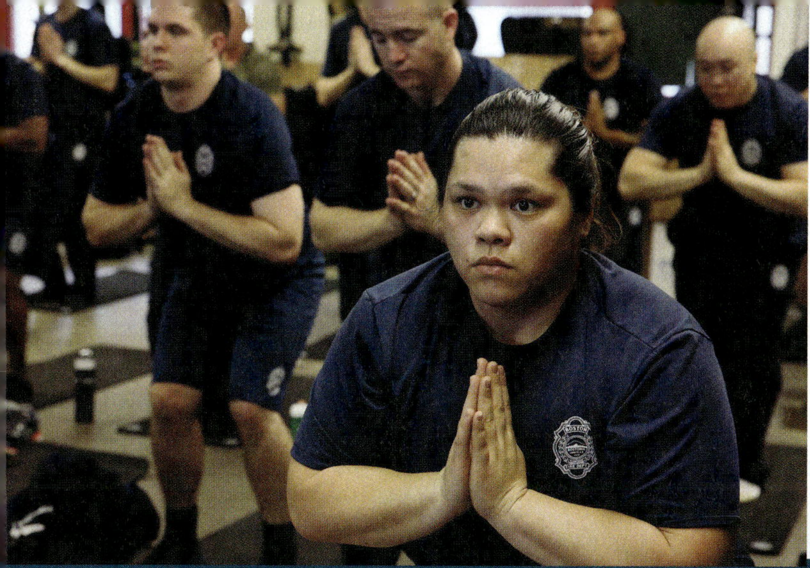

CHAPTER 2

Workforce Safety and Wellness

National EMS Education Standard Competencies

Preparatory

Uses knowledge of the emergency medical services (EMS) system, safety/well-being of the emergency medical responder (EMR), medical/legal issues, and ethical issues at the scene of an emergency while awaiting a higher level of care.

Workforce Safety and Wellness

- Standard safety precautions (pp 25–34)
- Personal protective equipment (p 30)
- Lifting and moving patients (Chapter 3, *Lifting and Moving Patients*)
- Crew resource management (p 25)
- Stress management (pp 23–25)
- Prevention of work-related injuries and illnesses (pp 31–32)
- Responder mental health, resilience, and suicide prevention (pp 23–24)
- Wellness principles (pp 20–24)
- Disease transmission (pp 25–28)

Medicine

Recognizes and manages life threats based on assessment findings of a patient with a medical emergency while awaiting additional emergency response.

Infectious Diseases

- Awareness of a patient who may have an infectious disease (pp 25–28)
- How to disinfect and decontaminate equipment after treating a patient (pp 28–31)

Knowledge Objectives

1. Describe the general wellness principles that enable emergency medical responders (EMRs) to stay physically and emotionally healthy. (pp 20–25)
2. Discuss the importance of physical fitness for the EMR. (p 20)
3. Discuss the importance of nutrition and sleep for the EMR. (p 21)
4. Describe emotional aspects of emergency care encountered by patients, patients' families, and EMRs. (p 22)
5. Describe five stages a person may experience when dealing with grief or death. (p 23)
6. Explain how to confront death and dying with integrity, empathy, respect, and careful delivery of service. (p 23)
7. Describe reactions to stress and grief that EMRs must face concerning care of the dying patient, death, and the grieving process of family members. (pp 23–24)
8. List signs and symptoms of stress. (pp 23–34)
9. Explain actions EMRs can take to reduce or alleviate stress. (pp 23–24)
10. List hazards commonly encountered by EMRs. (p 25)
11. Describe common routes of disease transmission. (pp 25–27)
12. Discuss the importance of standard precautions for preventing infectious diseases from airborne and bloodborne pathogens. (pp 25–27)
13. Explain proper handwashing techniques. (p 29)
14. Explain how to remove gloves properly. (p 30)
15. Describe the order in which you should don and doff personal protective equipment. (pp 30–32)
16. List the steps to take if clothing comes in contact with body fluid from a patient. (p 31)
17. Describe the safety equipment that EMRs should have available for their protection. (pp 31–32)
18. Describe safety considerations when responding to the scene. (pp 31–32)
19. Describe types of hazards to look for when assessing the scene for unsafe conditions. (pp 32–34)

Skills Objectives

1. Demonstrate integrity, empathy, respect, and careful delivery of service when confronted with the death of a patient. (pp 30–32)

© Craig F. Walker/The Boston Globe/Getty Images

2. Demonstrate proper handwashing techniques. (p 29)
3. Demonstrate the safe removal of medical gloves. (p 30; Skill Drill 2-1)
4. Demonstrate the proper order and procedure for donning and doffing personal protective equipment. (pp 30–32)
5. Demonstrate proper treatment of clothing that has come into contact with a patient's body fluid. (p 25)
6. Demonstrate the proper use of safety equipment needed for EMRs. (pp 25–34)
7. Demonstrate scene assessment of a real or simulated rescue event for safety hazards. (pp 25–34)

Introduction

This chapter provides information that will help you understand the factors that may affect your physical or emotional well-being as an emergency medical responder (EMR).

You, your patients, and their families can experience varied degrees of stress and grief during and following a medical emergency. This chapter addresses methods for recognizing, preventing, and reducing stress resulting from emergency incidents. It also discusses hazards you may encounter from infectious diseases and outlines procedures you should follow to reduce your risk of infection. Finally, this chapter covers scene safety and how to prevent injury to yourself and further injury to your patients.

General Wellness Principles

Before discussing specific safety concerns you may encounter as an EMR, such as scenes involving infectious disease or hazardous materials, this chapter will review some basic principles of physical and emotional well-being. Only by taking care of yourself will you be able to enjoy a long career of caring for others.

Physical Fitness

To fulfill your duties as an EMR, you must be in good physical condition. As a new EMR, you should have a complete physical examination to ensure that you are healthy enough to do your job. Most public safety departments require this examination as part of their hiring process. If your department does not have this requirement, you should still have periodic physical examinations to ensure continuing good health.

Emergency medical services (EMS) can be a physically demanding profession. As an EMR, your primary job may be firefighting, which may involve wearing heavy firefighter turnout gear, carrying equipment, and working in extremely hot environments. Or it may be law enforcement, which may involve pursuing or restraining individuals who are resisting arrest. Regardless of your primary job function, all EMS clinicians share one physically demanding task: lifting and moving patients. The importance of strength and conditioning for all of these functions cannot be overstated. This topic is discussed further in Chapter 3, *Lifting and Moving Patients*.

Regular exercise will increase your strength and endurance and decrease your risk of sustaining injury. Your exercise routine should involve aspects of cardiovascular endurance, muscular strength building, mobility, and flexibility. Endurance will ensure your cardiovascular system is able to provide your muscles and brain with needed oxygen. Strength training, also known as resistance training, helps build muscles and protect joints. Mobility training and stretching improve your body's range of motion, flexibility, and functional movement, which can reduce joint deterioration and help you stay active and healthy.

To maintain good health, the American Heart Association recommends the following:

- Each week, engage in at least 150 minutes of moderate-intensity aerobic activity, 75 minutes of vigorous aerobic activity, or a combination of both, preferably spread across multiple days.
- At least 2 days per week, incorporate moderate- to high-intensity muscle-strengthening exercises.
- Limit the time you spend being sedentary. Even light-intensity exercise may improve your fitness level.
- Try to improve these minimum recommendations over time.

While achieving exercise goals may seem daunting, there are strategies you can use to set yourself up for success. Plan activities ahead of time and use strategies that make your exercise sessions convenient. Allow yourself to start small. Exercise should not be a punishment, so try to find activities you enjoy. For some, the key to maintaining a routine is working out with others. Doing so can increase your sense of accountability, increase your enjoyment of exercising, and build social relationships, which can also improve your emotional resilience.

Nutrition

Maintaining a healthy, well-balanced diet and adequate hydration will help ensure you have the energy needed to do your job. Moreover, it will give your body the strength to fight off illness and avoid injury.

Diet

According to the American Heart Association, you should eat a variety of fruits and vegetables, whole-grain products, and healthy proteins (such as legumes, nuts, fish, and lean meat/poultry) and avoid processed foods, heavily salted foods, foods with added sugar, and alcohol. An illustration of a healthy diet compiled by the US Department of Agriculture (USDA) is shown in **FIGURE 2-1**.

The amount of food you need is related to several factors, including your body type, your weight, and your level of physical activity. Many people need to cut down on the amount of sweets in their diet. Eating large quantities of sweets puts your energy level on a roller coaster. Your blood glucose level quickly rises, but in a few hours, the level drops and you crave more sweets. To maintain more consistent glucose levels, it is much better to eat an adequate amount of whole-grain breads, cereals, rice, and pasta. These foods provide a steady energy source over a longer period. Reducing your intake of sugars also may lower your risk of type 2 diabetes later in life.

EMS clinicians often find it hard to maintain regular meal schedules. By planning your food intake and having healthy foods available, you can improve your eating habits. Healthy eating not only helps to cut down on your stress level, it also helps reduce your risk of heart and blood vessel diseases, which are the most common causes of death in public safety workers. Keeping your weight at recommended levels helps your body cope with stress.

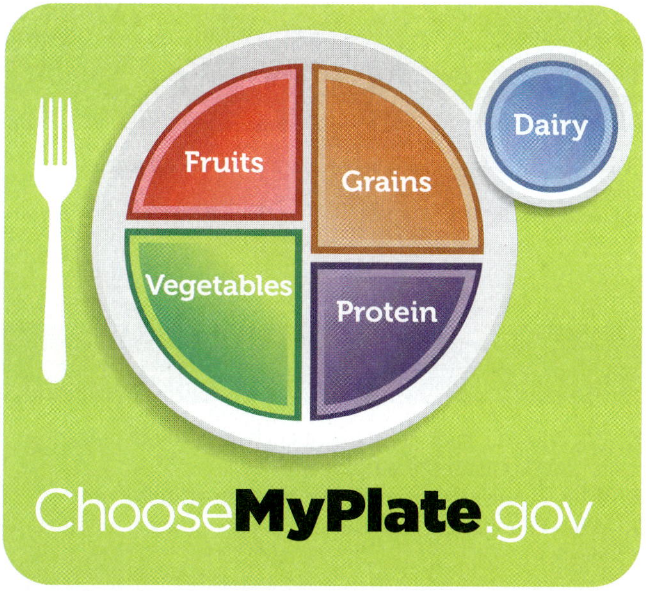

FIGURE 2-1 A healthy diet is illustrated by the USDA MyPlate food guidance system.
Courtesy of USDA.

Hydration

Active EMS clinicians need to drink adequate amounts of fluids every day, including while they are on duty (**FIGURE 2-2**). Law enforcement officers, firefighters, and EMS clinicians who work in hot environments or wear hot bunker gear or ballistic vests are at special risk for dehydration. The typical adult loses about eight glasses of water per day through sweat, exhaling, and elimination. Consuming an adequate quantity of water is essential for maintaining proper body function. Natural fruit juices and sports drinks are also good sources of fluids.

Dehydration can cause headaches, muscle cramps, light-headedness, dizziness, and even loss of consciousness or cardiac emergencies. These symptoms are dangerous not just for you but also for your patient if they affect your ability to provide care. You do not want the onset of dehydration to serve as a reminder to drink water. Be proactive and prevent dehydration by drinking adequate amounts of water throughout the day.

Avoid consuming excessive amounts of caffeine and alcohol. Caffeine is a stimulant that causes adrenaline to be released in your body. Adrenaline raises your blood pressure and increases your stress level. Thus, limiting your intake of caffeine-containing beverages such as coffee, tea, soft drinks,

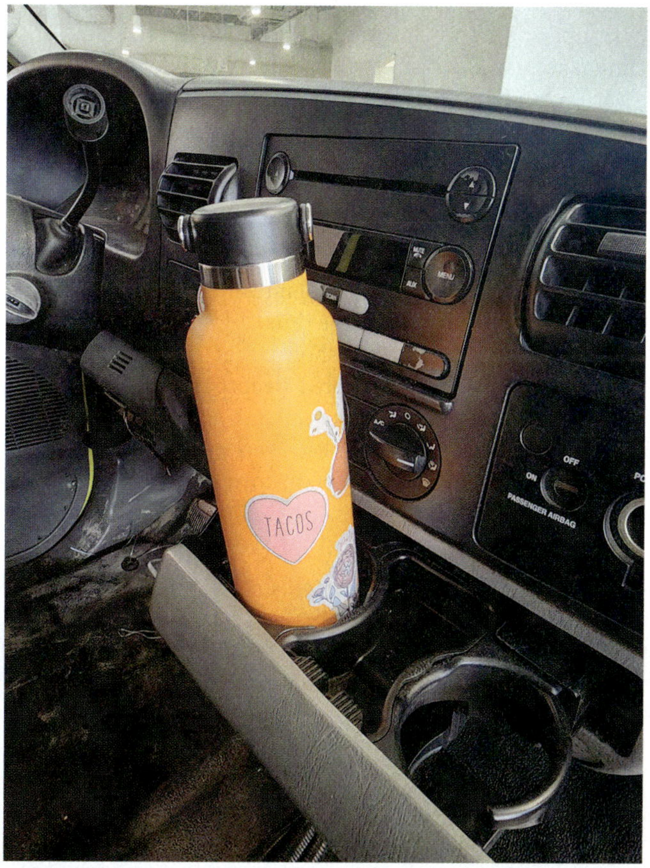

FIGURE 2-2 Drinking adequate quantities of water is important. Carrying a reusable water bottle to refill during your shift can help you stay hydrated.
Courtesy of Remle Crowe.

and energy drinks can help reduce stress. Caffeine and alcohol also cause dehydration.

Words of Wisdom

Tobacco products and alcoholic beverages are often used as a means to relieve stress. However, nicotine and alcohol are both harmful drugs that can lead to serious health problems. Although alcoholic drinks may initially create a feeling of relaxation, the aftereffects of alcohol use may include depression and anxiety, including a reduced ability to deal with stress. Some people who drink alcohol become addicted to it. Bottom line: drinking too much alcohol can end your career.

Words of Wisdom

Some of the most important concepts relating to personal wellness are embodied in the expression "eat, drink, and be merry." A balanced, nutritious diet and proper hydration will help keep you healthy and strong, both physically and mentally. Finding pleasure in life, both at work and in your personal life, will help give you the emotional resilience to keep performing at your highest level.

Sleep

When you are off duty, remember to get an adequate amount of sleep. Because public safety services must be provided 24 hours per day, many law enforcement, fire, EMS, and security personnel work rotating shifts. Firefighters and EMS clinicians may work shifts that are 24 hours or longer with a variety of days off. They may be required to alternate between day and night shifts. These work schedules disrupt normal sleep patterns. In addition, many people in public safety work overtime shifts, have a second job, or commute long distances to work. This combination of factors often means that many public safety personnel do not get enough sleep. If you are working in a volunteer agency, it is best that personnel not be on call all the time.

Scientific studies have shown that most people need about 8 hours of uninterrupted sleep per night. If you are not meeting this need, your mental and physical health may suffer. In addition, the care you give to patients may be compromised. It is important to make sleep a priority in your life.

Emotional Aspects of Emergency Medical Care

Providing emergency medical care as an EMR is stressful. This stress may persist even after the incident has been resolved. In addition, your patients, their families and friends, and bystanders will often show signs and symptoms of stress.

Although all emergency medical calls produce a certain level of stress, some types of calls are more stressful than others. Some calls will affect you on an emotional level. For example, maybe the patient reminds you of a friend or family member, or is a young child who has been badly injured; or maybe the call evokes memories of a particularly stressful past experience (**FIGURE 2-3**). Some calls will affect you because of the high level of pressure and uncertainty involved. Examples may include a mass shooting involving several critical patients or casualties, or a call in which you find yourself in physical danger.

Because stress cannot be completely eliminated, you must learn how to avoid unnecessary stress, how to prevent your stress level from getting too high, and what services and resources are available to help you. Some of the stress-reduction techniques discussed in this chapter will also be helpful when interacting with your patients and their families and friends.

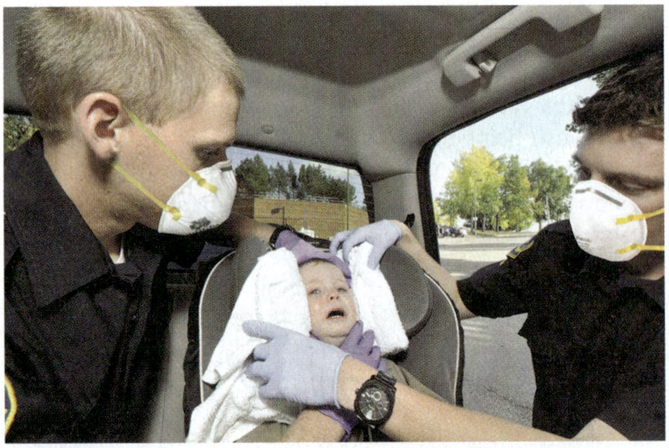

FIGURE 2-3 Certain types of patients may produce a high level of stress.

© Kevin Link/Science Source

YOU are the EMR **CASE 1**

The past week has been especially busy for you and the other members of your shift. You have been dispatched to an unusually large number of serious medical emergencies. You and your crew have cared for a seriously burned infant, an older woman who was found dead by her caregiver, and a motorcyclist about your age who had severe head injuries. As your crew reviews these calls, you realize that crew members were affected differently by these calls.

1. Why do you think crew members had different reactions to the events of the past week?
2. Which types of calls would be most stressful for you?
3. What changes should you consider to reduce your stress level?

> **Safety**
>
> Do not underestimate the effect that stress can have on you. As a firefighter, EMS clinician, or law enforcement officer, you may see more suffering in a year than many people will see in their entire lifetime.

Normal Reactions to Stress

You need to understand how stress can affect you and the people for whom you provide emergency medical care. It is important to realize that a wide variety of stressful events may trigger a grief reaction. These events include the death of a loved one, a major injury or traumatic experience, a serious illness, substance or alcohol use disorder, incarceration, the end of a relationship or divorce, the loss of a job or income, or a major personal rejection. As an EMR, you need to understand how stress is affecting the people for whom you are caring. Moreover, you and your coworkers will experience some of these grief triggers, such as the death of a patient. You need to know how to stay emotionally healthy in this often stressful profession.

One well-recognized model for understanding people's reactions to grief and stress was proposed by Dr. Elisabeth Kübler-Ross. This model defines five stages of grief: denial, anger, bargaining, depression, and acceptance. In studying this model, it is important to understand that people will experience grief in a variety of ways. Some people will exhibit no outward signs of grief. Other people will experience only some of these stages. People do not experience these stages of grief in any predetermined order. They can occur at any time during the grieving process.

- **Denial ("Not me!").** The first stage in the grieving process is denial. A person experiencing denial cannot believe what is happening. This stage may serve as a protection for the person experiencing the situation, and it may also serve as a protection for you as the caregiver. Realize that this reaction is normal.
- **Anger ("Why me?").** The second stage of the grieving process is anger. Understanding that anger is a normal reaction to stress can help you deal with anger that is directed toward you by a patient or the patient's family. Do not become defensive; this anger is likely a result of the situation and not a result of your patient care. This realization can enable you to tolerate the situation without letting the patient's anger distract you from performing your duties of providing care.
- **Bargaining ("Okay, but . . .").** The third stage of the grieving process is bargaining. Bargaining is the act of trying to make a deal to postpone death and dying. If you encounter a patient or family member who is in this stage, try to respond with a truthful and helpful comment such as, "We are doing everything we can and the paramedics will be here in just a few minutes." Remember that bargaining may be a normal part of the grieving process.
- **Depression ("Heavy-hearted").** The fourth stage of the grieving process is depression. Depression is often characterized by sadness or despair. A person who is unusually silent or who seems to retreat into their own world may have reached this stage. This may also be the point at which a person begins to accept the situation. It is not surprising that patients and their families get depressed about a situation that involves death and dying, nor is it surprising that you as a rescuer also get depressed. Our society tends to consider death a failure of medical care rather than a natural event that happens to everyone. A certain amount of depression is a natural reaction to a major threat or loss. The depression can be mild or severe, and it can be of short duration or long-lasting. If you have depression that continues, it is important for you to contact qualified professionals who can help you.
- **Acceptance.** The final stage of the grieving process is acceptance. Acceptance does not mean that you are satisfied with the situation. It means that you understand that an undesired outcome, such as death or disease, cannot be changed. It may require a lot of time to work through the grieving process and arrive at this stage. As an EMS clinician, you may see acceptance in family members who have had time to realize that their loved one's illness is terminal. However, not all people who experience grief are able to work through it and accept the loss.

By understanding these five stages, you can better understand the grief reaction experienced by patients, their families, and their friends. You can also better understand your own reaction to stressful situations.

The techniques used when caring for a grieving individual may be similar to those used when caring for a person experiencing a behavioral or situational crisis. These techniques are presented in Chapter 12, *Behavioral Emergencies*.

> **Street Smarts**
>
> As you go through the anger phase of the grieving process, you may want to direct your anger at the patient, the patient's family, your coworkers, or your own family. Anger is a normal reaction to unpleasant events. Sometimes it helps to talk out your anger with coworkers, family members, or a counselor. By talking through your anger, you avoid keeping it bottled up inside where it can cause unhealthy physical symptoms or emotional reactions. Directing the energy from your anger in positive ways may help you move forward. For example, at the scene of a motor vehicle crash, you may be angry because a child was not properly restrained in a car seat and sustained injuries. Focusing your energy on providing the best medical care for the injured child may help you deal with your feelings.

Stress Management

Stress management has three components: recognizing stress, preventing stress, and reducing stress.

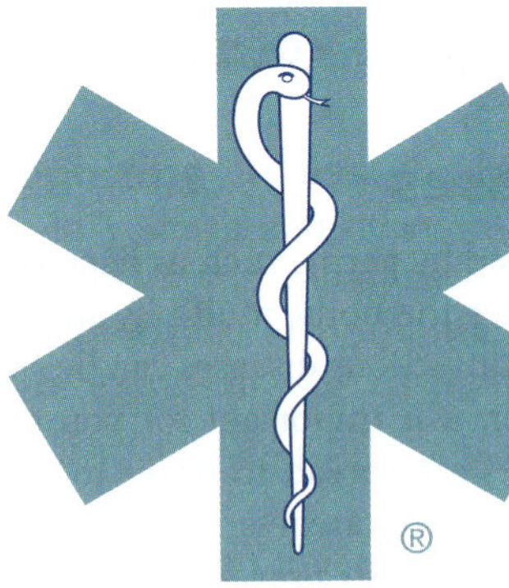

Voices OF Experience

It was the middle of the night, and we were dispatched to a domestic violence event. The scene was not secure, so we staged 1 mile from the scene and waited until police arrived and declared the scene secure. The wife was complaining of head and neck injuries and had been beaten pretty badly. She stated her husband had come home from a bar and started beating her. The husband was not around and could not be found, although his vehicle was still in the driveway. The wife stated that her husband ran out the door when he heard sirens coming. The neighbors had called 9-1-1 as a result of all of the yelling and noise coming from this home.

> **"It was a very scary moment—the husband had a shotgun."**

We treated the wife for her injuries. As we proceeded outside to load her into the ambulance, the husband jumped out from the backseat of his car and came toward us. It was a very scary moment. The husband had a shotgun and was waiting to shoot his wife and anyone treating her. Luckily the police were walking with us, and they were able to subdue the husband and secure his firearm.

We then proceeded to load the wife into the ambulance and leave the scene heading toward the hospital. We drove down the road, stopped, and finished treating our patient with an IV and pain medication. The call could have been so much worse, but fortunately we had police on scene, and they quickly took care of the shooter and kept us safe.

Any domestic violence scene, even one that is considered secure, can change quickly and without warning. Situations occurring in the middle of the night may also contribute to questionable security. Always watch your back in any situation, as the scene could change for the worse quickly and at any time.

Julia Chamberlain, BSN, RN, Paramedic, I/C
Onondaga Fire Department
Onondaga, Michigan

Adapted from the personal Medical Identification Symbol of the American Medical Association.

person touches a surface that has been contaminated with the virus.

When you encounter a patient with an airborne disease, you may need to protect yourself by donning a high-efficiency particulate air (HEPA) respirator. HEPA respirators are commonly called N95 masks because they filter out at least 95% of infectious particles (**FIGURE 2-5**). To be effective, they must be fit-tested to ensure that there is an effective seal between the mask and the health care clinician's face.

The steps for donning an N95 mask are shown in **FIGURE 2-6**. When removing an N95 mask, first remove your gloves according to the steps listed in Skill Drill 2-1, then carefully follow the steps in **FIGURE 2-7** to remove the N95 mask by touching only the straps.

To prevent an infected or potentially infected patient from infecting caregivers, you should place a surgical-type mask on the patient. This type of mask prevents droplets from being released into the air and infecting other people. It protects the people around the person wearing the mask. A surgical mask fastens around the patient's ears or around the back of the patient's head (**FIGURE 2-8**). If a surgical mask is not available, placing an oxygen mask on the patient may provide some protection to caregivers.

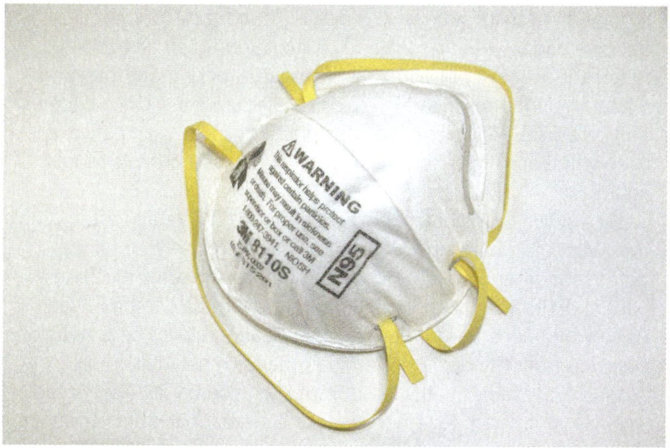

FIGURE 2-5 An N95 HEPA respirator.
© Honeycruller/Shutterstock

Bloodborne Pathogens. Bloodborne **pathogens** are infectious microorganisms in blood that can cause disease. The viruses that cause AIDS and hepatitis B and C are bloodborne pathogens.

Human immunodeficiency virus (HIV) is transmitted by contact with infected blood, semen, vaginal secretions, or breast milk. There is no scientific documentation that the virus is transmitted by contact with sweat, saliva, tears, sputum, urine, feces, vomitus, or nasal secretions, unless these fluids contain visible signs of blood. Exposure can take place in the following ways:

- The patient's blood is splashed or sprayed into your eyes, nose, or mouth or into an open sore or cut.
- You have blood from the infected patient on your hands and then touch your own eyes, nose, mouth, or an open sore or cut.
- A needle that was used to inject the patient breaks your skin.
- Broken glass at a motor vehicle crash or other incident that is covered with blood from an infected patient penetrates your glove and skin.

Remember that some patients who are infected with HIV do not know they are infected. Others who are infected do not show any symptoms. Therefore, the US Centers for Disease Control and Prevention (CDC) recommends that health care workers wear latex or nitrile gloves any time they are likely to come into contact with secretions or blood from any patient. Whenever you are on the job, you should also cover any open wounds you have.

Hepatitis B is also spread by direct contact with infected blood, and it is far more contagious than HIV. EMRs should take standard precautions as described in the following section to reduce their chance of contracting hepatitis B. Check with your medical director about receiving injections of hepatitis vaccine to protect you against this infection. This vaccine should be made available to you. Meningitis and syphilis are two other diseases that can be spread by contact with contaminated blood.

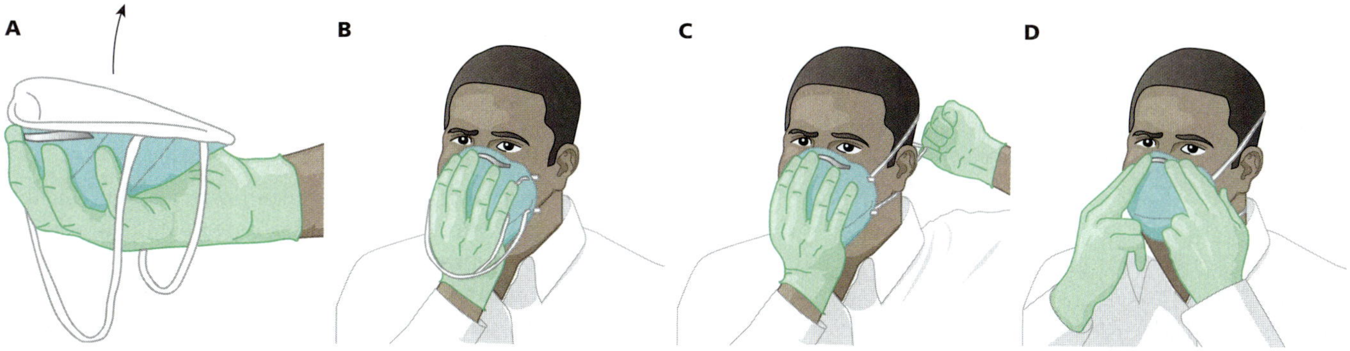

FIGURE 2-6 Steps used to don a disposable respirator. **A.** Position the respirator in your hands with the nose piece at your fingertips. **B.** Cup the respirator in your hand and hold it under your chin, allowing the bands to hang below your hand. **C.** Pull the straps over your head. The top strap rests at the top back of your head. The bottom strap is positioned around the neck, below the ears. **D.** Use your fingertips to mold the metal strip to the shape of your nose.
© Jones & Bartlett Learning

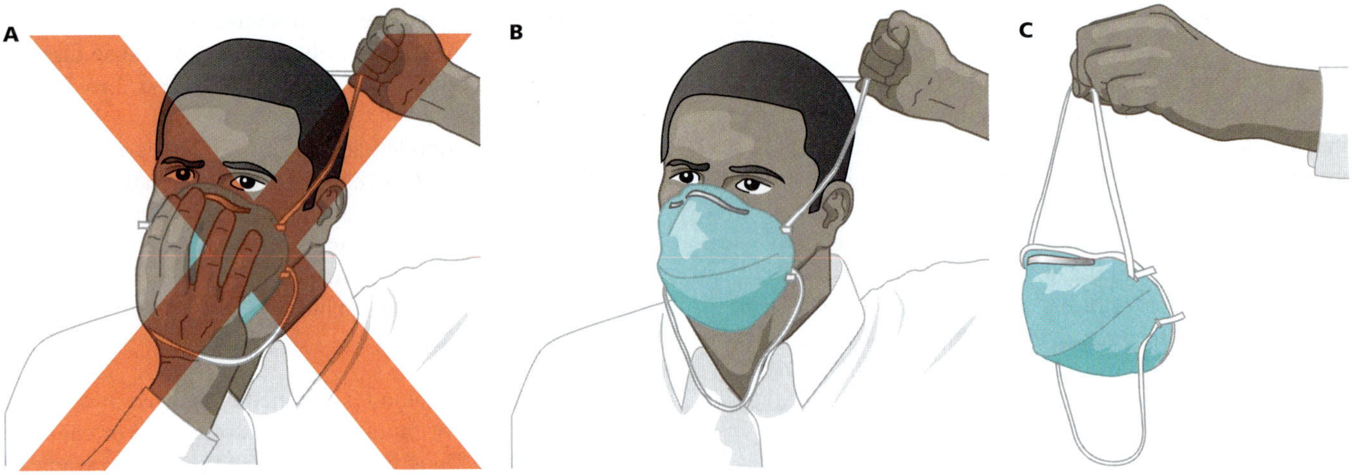

FIGURE 2-7 Steps used to doff a disposable respirator. **A.** Do not touch the front of the respirator. **B.** Remove by pulling the bottom strap over the back of your head, followed by the top strap, without touching the respirator. **C.** Discard the respirator in a waste container or in an appropriate receptacle for reprocessing, depending on local procedure, and wash your hands.

© Jones & Bartlett Learning

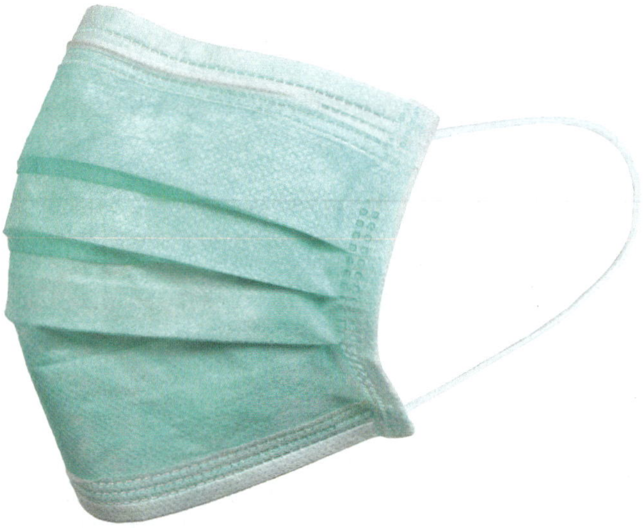

FIGURE 2-8 A surgical mask.

© Sanit Fuangnakhon/Shutterstock

Safety

The most important step you can take to remain healthy and reduce the transmission of any disease is to wash your hands. Bacteria and viruses are picked up when you touch any contaminated surface. Examples include keyboards, doorknobs, steering wheels, telephones, headsets, and EMS equipment. Once bacteria and/or viruses are on your hands, touching your eyes, mouth, or nose with your fingers can introduce these microorganisms into your body.

Wash your hands before and after eating, before and after using the toilet, after blowing your nose or sneezing into your hands, before and after preparing food, and before and after touching a patient. After you touch something that might be contaminated, wash your hands as soon as possible. Wearing gloves does not excuse you from the need to wash your hands regularly.

Wash your hands with clean, warm, running water. Apply soap and rub your hands together to make a substantial lather. The soap does not have to be antibacterial; regular soap is sufficient. Be sure to scrub all the surfaces, working the soap between the fingers and thumbs and clearing debris from under the nails. Keep rubbing your hands together for at least 20 seconds, about the time it takes to sing "Happy Birthday!" Thoroughly rinse your hands and dry them with a paper towel. When it is not possible to wash your hands, use an alcohol-based hand sanitizer to clean your hands until you can wash them.

Words of Wisdom

COVID-19 is a respiratory illness that can spread easily from person to person. The virus that causes COVID-19 spreads through respiratory droplets, the same way influenza and other respiratory diseases spread.

Symptoms of COVID-19 appear 2 to 14 days after exposure and include fever, cough, and shortness of breath. In severe cases of COVID-19, pneumonia has developed in both lungs. Gastrointestinal (GI) symptoms, including nausea, vomiting, and diarrhea, may also be present. COVID-19 can be fatal, especially in those with a depressed immune system. To decrease the risk of contracting COVID-19, or to limit the severity of its effects, it is recommended that EMS clinicians receive the COVID-19 vaccine and boosters.

Standard Precautions

Federal regulations require all health care workers, including EMRs, to assume that all patients are potentially infected with pathogens that can be spread by direct contact, airborne transmission, or blood. These regulations require that all health care workers use gloves and other protective equipment to prevent possible exposure to infectious agents.

Standard Precautions for Bloodborne Pathogens. You will not always be able to tell whether a patient's body fluids contain blood. Therefore, the CDC recommends that all health care workers take the following standard precautions:

1. Always wear approved latex or nitrile gloves when handling patients, and change gloves after contact with each patient. Wash your hands with soap and water immediately after removing gloves. If soap and water are not available, a hand sanitizer can be used as a temporary cleansing agent until soap and warm water are available. Note that leather gloves are not considered safe: leather is porous and traps fluids.
2. Always wear a protective mask, eyewear, and/or a face shield when you anticipate that blood or other body fluids may splatter (**FIGURE 2-9**). Wear a gown/apron, head covering, and shoe covers if you anticipate splashes of blood or other body fluids such as those that occur with childbirth and major trauma.
3. Wash your hands and other skin surfaces immediately and thoroughly with soap and water if they become contaminated with blood and other body fluids (**FIGURE 2-10**). Change contaminated clothes and wash exposed skin thoroughly.
4. Do not recap, cut, or bend used needles. Place them directly into a puncture-resistant container designed for sharps.

Precautions for Airborne Pathogens. When caring for patients who may have respiratory diseases, you need to take additional precautions to prevent the spread of infectious droplets. The exact steps recommended by CDC and the Occupational Safety and Health Administration (OSHA) vary with specific disease outbreaks. You need to stay current with these recommendations and follow your local protocols.

Precautions to prevent the spread of airborne diseases such as influenza or COVID-19 should include the previously discussed steps and the following steps, which are designed to provide protection against the inhalation of larger infectious droplets during direct patient care activities.

1. Be aware of any community-based outbreaks of influenza, COVID-19, or other epidemic disease that requires droplet precautions.
2. Assess the patient on arrival from a distance. A distance of at least 6 feet (1.8 m) is often recommended.
3. Inquire specifically about influenza, COVID-19, or other specific exposures.
4. Perform hand hygiene before and after patient care activities.
5. A disposable surgical mask should be placed on the patient if the person shows signs of respiratory illness such as coughing, sneezing, or a fever.
6. Health care clinicians may need to don an N95 mask to protect themselves from exposure to infected droplets.

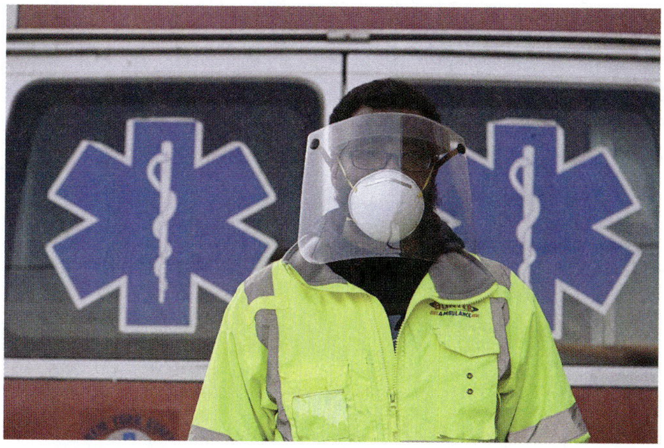

FIGURE 2-9 EMRs must wear a protective mask, eyewear, and/or a face shield when there is a risk of blood or other body fluids splattering.

© Anthony Behar/Sipa USA/AP Photo

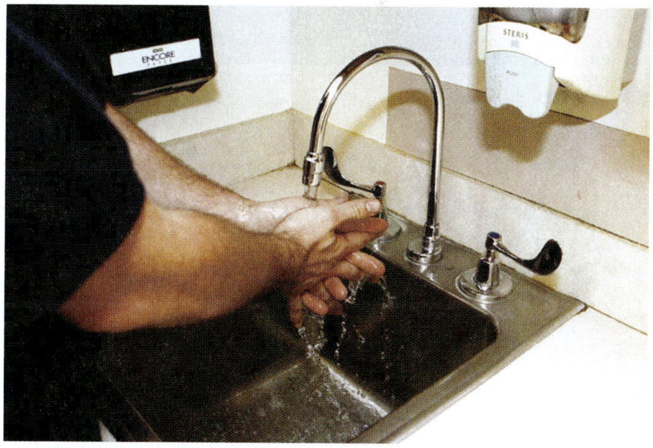

FIGURE 2-10 Wash your hands thoroughly with soap and water if you are contaminated with blood or other body fluids.

© Jones & Bartlett Learning. Courtesy of MIEMSS.

YOU are the EMR — CASE 2

Three days after being dispatched to the home of a teenage mother whose 4-month-old child had died, you notice your partner is not as upbeat as normal. You have also noticed that in the past 2 days your partner has stopped eating during the usual station house meals and has become irritable.

1. What may be causing the changes in your partner's behavior?
2. What can your partner do to alleviate the signs and symptoms?
3. During the initial incident, the mother repeatedly asked rescuers, "Why me?" Which stage of grief was she experiencing?

7. For eye protection, use cleanable goggles or disposable face shields to protect the eyes, nose, and mouth during procedures that are likely to generate splashes or sprays of blood or body secretions.

Personal Protective Equipment (PPE)

The standard precautions listed previously can be effective in preventing the spread of diseases only if you follow proper procedures in donning and doffing needed protective equipment. The steps for removing gloves are listed in **SKILL DRILL 2-1**.

To don infectious disease PPE, follow these steps (**FIGURE 2-11**):

1. Select gloves, mask, and eye protection and ensure they are proper for the situation and the correct size.
2. Wash the hands.
3. Put on a gown, if one is indicated.
4. Put on a mask.
5. Put on eye protection.
6. Put on gloves.

SKILL DRILL 2-1

Removing Medical Gloves

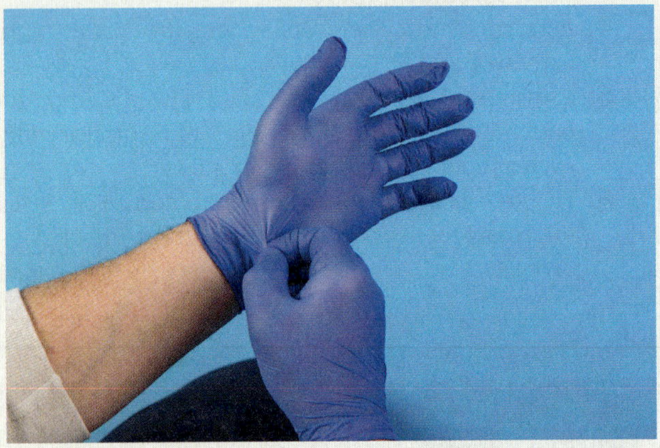

STEP 1 Begin by removing one glove. Pinch one glove on the outside near the wrist.

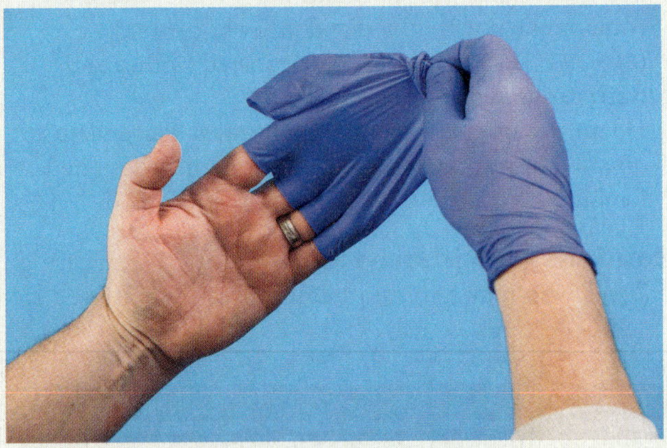

STEP 2 Gently pull the glove off, turning it inside out as you pull with the hand that is still gloved. Hold the removed glove in your gloved hand.

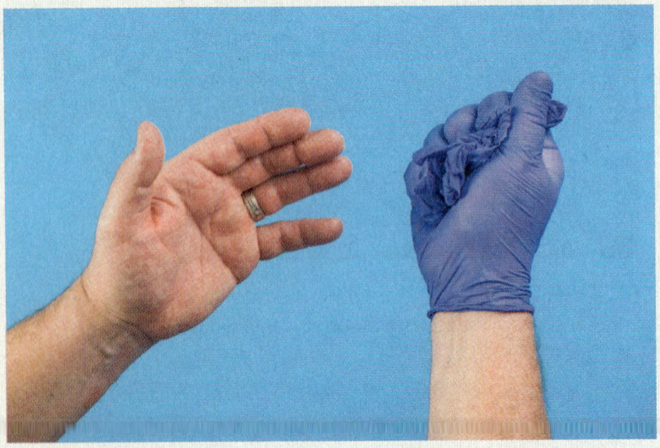

STEP 3 To remove the second glove, slide two fingers of your bare hand inside the remaining glove at the wrist.

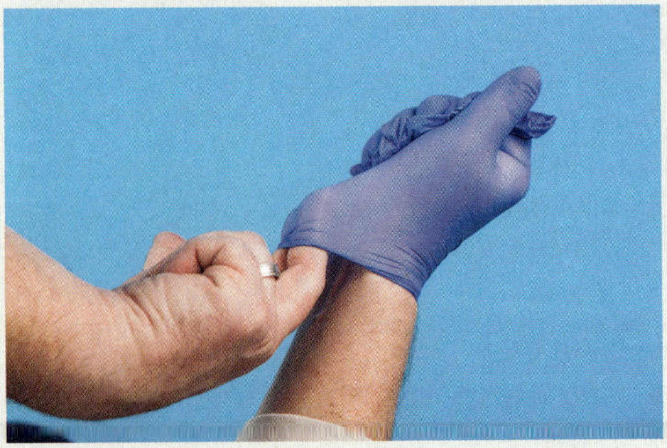

STEP 4 Gently stretch the glove away from the hand and pull the glove off, keeping it inside out. The first glove remains inside the second glove.

If possible, dispose of the gloves in a biohazard container or a sealed plastic bag. If one is not available, use a trash can. Wash your hands with soap and running water. If they are not available, use an alcohol-based hand sanitizer.

© Jones & Bartlett Learning

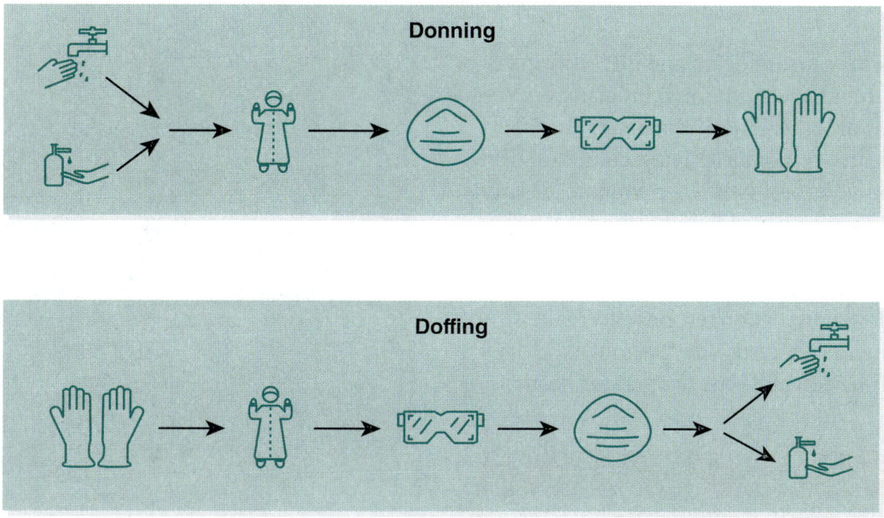

FIGURE 2-11 Sequence for donning and doffing personal protective equipment.
© Jones & Bartlett Learning

To doff infectious disease PPE, follow these steps:

1. Remove and discard gloves using the steps listed in Skill Drill 2-1. Take care not to contaminate your hands. Dispose of the gloves in a biohazard bag.
2. Remove the gown, if one was worn.
3. Remove eye protection. Remove by the strap and avoid touching the front surface of the eye protection. Discard in a biohazard bag or prepare for reprocessing.
4. Remove the mask by tilting the head slightly forward, grasping the elastic straps, and sliding them off your ears and head. Remove the mask without touching the front fabric. Discard the mask in a biohazard bag or in a receptacle for reprocessing.
5. Perform hand hygiene by washing with soap and warm water or by using alcohol-based hand sanitizer.

Federal agencies, such as CDC and OSHA, and state agencies, such as state public health departments, have regulations regarding standard precautions. Because these regulations are constantly changing, it is important for your department to stay updated and provide continuing education to keep you current with the latest changes related to infectious disease precautions.

Safety

If your clothing comes in contact with body fluid from a patient, remove the clothing as soon as possible. If body fluids have contacted you through your clothing, take a shower, washing thoroughly with hot, soapy water. Your clothing should be placed in a marked plastic bag or handled so that the body fluids are contained. Clothing should be washed as soon as possible in hot, soapy water. Always follow the protocols of your department and the CDC's most recent recommendations for these situations.

Immunizations

Certain immunizations are recommended for EMS clinicians. These include COVID, seasonal flu, tetanus prophylaxis, and hepatitis B vaccines. You also should check the status of your varicella (chickenpox) vaccine and your measles, mumps, and rubella (German measles) vaccines. Tuberculin testing may also be recommended. Your medical director can determine which immunizations and tests are needed for members of your department. Being properly immunized protects you from contracting these diseases from patients. In certain cases, such as influenza, it also helps to protect patients from contracting influenza from you.

Safety

Flu shots are required by many health care organizations and public safety agencies. Flu shots reduce your chance of contracting influenza. In addition, by getting a flu shot, you minimize the chance that you will pass the influenza virus to your patients or family. Getting a flu shot is of benefit to you and to others.

Responding to the Scene

Scene safety is a key consideration to you as an EMR. You must consider your safety and the safety of all the other people at the scene of an emergency. An injured or dead EMR cannot help those in need. This person instead becomes someone who needs help, increasing the difficulty of a rescue. Drive safely and always fasten your seat belt when you are in your vehicle. Paying close attention to safety factors can help prevent unnecessary illness, injuries, and death.

Dispatch

Safety begins when you are dispatched to an emergency. Be sure you have correct dispatch information, including the address, before you begin your response. Use your dispatch information to anticipate hazards that may be present and to determine the best way to approach the scene of the emergency.

Response

Vehicle crashes are a major cause of death and disability in law enforcement officers, firefighters, and EMS clinicians. As you respond to the scene of an emergency, remember the safety information that you learned in your driving courses. Drive safely and always fasten your seat belt when you are in your vehicle. Your seat belt can save your life only when it is properly fastened. Plan the best route and drive quickly but safely to the scene. Be especially careful during periods of rain, snow, or high wind. Slow down your response to make sure you arrive safely. All emergency responders who will be driving should complete an emergency vehicle operator's course.

Safety

Simple, portable safety equipment can help prevent injuries and illnesses:

- Medical gloves, masks, and eye protection prevent the spread of infectious diseases.
- Brightly colored clothing or reflective vests make you more visible to drivers in the daytime; reflective striping or vests make you more visible in the dark.
- Heavy gloves can help prevent cuts at a motor vehicle crash scene.
- A hard hat or helmet is needed when you are at an industrial or motor vehicle crash scene.

Some situations require additional safety equipment. Do not hesitate to call for additional equipment as needed.

Parking Your Vehicle

When you arrive at the emergency scene, park your vehicle so that it protects the area from traffic hazards but does not block the ambulance or firetruck from reaching the scene. Check to be sure that the emergency warning lights are operating correctly. Be careful when getting out of your vehicle, especially if you must step into a traffic area.

Federal safety standards require approved safety vests any time you are working on an active highway. These vests enhance your visibility in the daytime, and the reflective material on your safety vest helps make you more visible in the dark (**FIGURE 2-12**). If your vehicle is not needed to protect the incident scene, park it out of the way of traffic. Leave room for other arriving vehicles such as ambulances to be positioned near the patient. Above all else, make sure you have protected the emergency scene from further incidents.

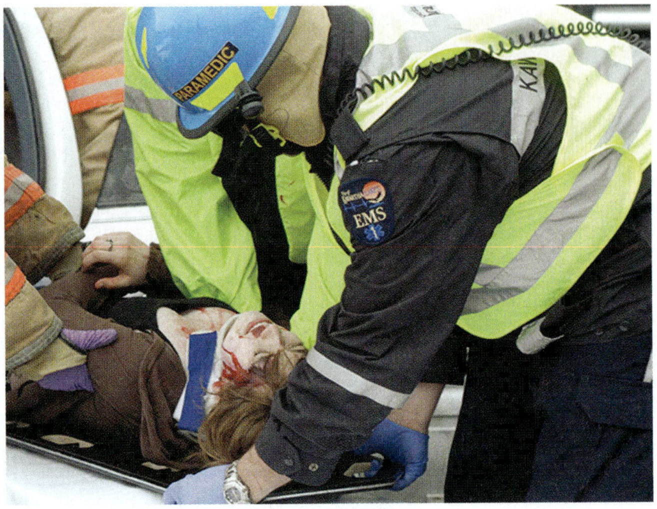

FIGURE 2-12 Reflective clothing helps make you more visible.

© Murray Wilson/Fotolia.com

Safety

Unless your headlights are needed to light up the scene, turn them off when parked at the scene. Your headlights can blind approaching vehicles, making it difficult for the drivers to see rescue personnel walking around the scene.

Assessing the Scene

As you approach the emergency scene, scan the entire area carefully to determine what hazards are present. Consider the following hazards based on the type of emergency; address them in the most appropriate order. For example, assess the scene of a motor vehicle crash for downed electrical wires before you check for broken glass.

Traffic

Consider whether traffic is a problem. Sometimes the most important first step you need to take at a motor vehicle crash scene is to control traffic to prevent further collisions. If you need more help to handle traffic, call for assistance before you get out of your vehicle.

YOU are the EMR — CASE 3

You are sent to the home of a 76-year-old man with an unknown medical illness. You walk in and identify yourself as an EMR. You notice that the man is sweating, even though the room temperature is cool. You start your assessment. Each time he starts to answer a question, you notice that he is stopped by a productive cough. He tells you that he has had a temperature of 104°F (40°C) for a few days.

1. Which route of disease transmission are you most concerned about with this patient?
2. What precautions should you take to protect yourself when caring for this patient?
3. What steps do you need to take to protect yourself and others after caring for this patient?

Crime or Violence

If your dispatch information leads you to believe that the incident involves violence or a crime, follow your department's protocols for approaching the scene. If you are trained in law enforcement procedures, follow your local protocols. If you are not a law enforcement official, proceed very carefully. If you have any doubts about the safety of the scene, it is better to wait at a safe distance and request help from law enforcement officers. If the scene involves a crime, remember to take a mental picture of the scene so that you can provide an accurate description later in your documentation. Avoid disturbing anything at the scene unless it is absolutely necessary to move objects to provide patient care.

Crowds

Crowds may range in size from a few neighbors or bystanders to a huge mass gathering at a large parade or sporting event. The mood of a crowd may range from friendly and helpful to hostile. Friendly neighborhood crowds may interfere very little with your duties. Unfriendly, unruly, or hostile crowds may require a police presence before you are able to begin assessing and treating patients. Assess the crowd's mood before you get in a position from which there is no exit. Request help from law enforcement officers before the crowd is out of control. Safety considerations may require you to wait for the arrival of police before you approach the patient.

Electrical Hazards

Electrical hazards can be present at many types of emergency scenes. Patients located inside buildings may be in contact with a wide variety of electrical hazards. These can range from a faulty extension cord in a house to high-voltage machinery in an industrial setting. Patients located outside may be in contact with high-voltage electrical power lines that have fallen because of a motor vehicle crash or a storm. Assess the emergency scene for any indications of electrical problems. Inside a building, look for cords, electrical wires, or electrical appliances near or in contact with the patient. When you are outside, look for damaged electrical poles and downed electrical wires. Do not approach an emergency scene if there are indications of electrical problems. Keep all other people away from the source of the hazard. Because electricity cannot be seen, make sure the electrical current has been turned off by a qualified person before you get close to the source of the current. Always wear a helmet with a chin strap and face shield in situations that may involve electrical hazards. Remember, contact with a power source can result in severe injury or death.

Fire

Fire is a hazard to both you and the patient. Any time there appears to be a fire, immediately call for fire department assistance. If you are a trained firefighter, follow rescue and firefighting procedures for your department. If you are not a trained firefighter, do not exceed the limits of your training, because any attempt to rescue a person from a burning building is a high-risk undertaking. Do not enter a burning building without proper PPE, including self-contained breathing apparatus (SCBA). Recent fire research has shown that, during a fire, keeping doors and windows closed until hose streams are in place will slow the growth and spread of fire. Do not open doors and windows before the firefighters arrive.

Vehicles that have been involved in collisions also may present a fire hazard from fuel or other spilled fluids. Keep all ignition sources such as cigarettes and road flares away. Carefully assess the fire hazard before you determine your course of action.

Hazardous Materials

Hazardous materials may be found almost anywhere. Motor vehicle crashes with large trucks may involve hazardous materials. Hazardous materials may also be found in homes, businesses, and industries. Chapter 19, *Incident Management*, discusses the signs that a hazardous material may be present at a scene, sources of information relating to these substances, and resources and safety precautions that will help keep you safe at these scenes.

Unstable Objects

Unstable objects may include vehicles, trees, poles, buildings, cliffs, and piles of materials. Motor vehicle collisions, wind storms, ice storms, explosions, fires, building collapses, and earthquakes may result in unstable objects. After a crash, a motor vehicle may be located in an unstable position. You may need to stabilize the vehicle before you assess the patient or begin patient extrication. Do not attempt to enter or get under an unstable vehicle. Motor vehicle collisions may result in other unstable objects, including trees or poles that were hit in the collision. Fires and explosions can result in unstable buildings. Assess a building for stability before attempting to

YOU are the EMR — CASE 4

You and your partner are returning to headquarters after lunch when dispatch sends you to the scene of a rented box truck that has rolled over. Injuries are reported, but dispatch is unable to tell you the extent of the injuries or the number of people involved. As you pull up to the scene, you spot a hazardous materials placard.

1. Where should you park your vehicle?
2. What other issues should you consider before leaving your vehicle?
3. Why is your safety a concern?

enter it. If you are in doubt about the safety of the building, follow your local protocols and call for trained personnel rather than attempting to enter an unsafe building alone.

Safety

Other hazards after a motor vehicle crash include undeployed airbags and the high-voltage batteries found in hybrid or electric vehicles. Rescuers need to be careful around these hazards as they stabilize a vehicle. These topics are covered more fully in Chapter 18, *Vehicle Extrication and Special Rescue*.

Sharp Objects

Sharp objects are frequently present at an emergency scene. These objects range from broken glass at the scene of a motor vehicle crash to hypodermic needles in the pocket of an intravenous drug user. Being aware of sharp objects can reduce the chance of injury to you and to your patients. Latex and nitrile medical gloves can help prevent the spread of disease from blood contamination, but they provide no protection against sharp objects. When glass or other sharp objects are present, wear heavy leather or firefighting gloves over your medical gloves to prevent injuries.

Safety

After working at a scene that involves potential infectious exposure, you should clean and disinfect your equipment. Cleaning refers to the removal of dirt, dust, blood, or other visible contaminants. Disinfection requires special chemicals that kill pathogenic agents when applied directly to a surface. Disposable equipment and supplies should be disposed of in a manner that prevents contamination of other objects. Follow your local protocols and the latest recommendations of the CDC and OSHA. It is also important to complete the appropriate documentation of the exposure.

Animals

Animals, whether they are house pets, farm stock, or wild, are found indoors and outdoors. Pets can become very upset in the confusion of a medical emergency. When you need to enter a house to take care of a patient, be sure excited pets have been secured in another part of the house away from the patient. People often travel with their pets, so pets can be part of the scene of a motor vehicle crash. Service dogs may be protective of their owners. Farm animals, too, can be a safety hazard; be careful when entering a field that may contain livestock. Animals may present hazards such as bites, kicking, or even trampling. Careful assessment of the incident scene can prevent unnecessary injuries.

Environmental Conditions

Weather cannot be changed or controlled; therefore, you should consider the effect weather will have on rescue operations. Dress appropriately for the expected weather and be prepared for precipitation and temperature extremes for you and your patients. Be alert for possible damage from high winds. Keep your patients dry and comfortable. Darkness makes it hard to see all the hazards that may be present, so use any emergency lighting that is available. A bright flashlight is a valuable tool in many rescue situations.

Special Rescue Situations

Special safety considerations are required in situations involving water rescue, ice rescue, confined space or below-grade rescue, terrorism, and mass-casualty incidents. Do not enter an emergency situation that is unsafe unless you have the proper training and equipment. These situations are covered in Chapter 18, *Vehicle Extrication and Special Rescue.*

YOU are the EMR — SUMMARY

You are the EMR: CASE 1

1. Why do you think crew members had different reactions to the events of the past week?

The specific dynamics of a call may resonate differently with the individuals involved. Calls involving young children can produce a sense of outrage or injustice because these patients are not able to take care of themselves or fully understand what is happening. Moreover, they have not yet had the opportunity to live a full, healthy life. Calls involving older patients may remind us of parents, neighbors, or grandparents. These calls may cause us to identify with the individuals involved and thereby experience the situation on a more emotional level. Likewise, calls involving someone our own age may heighten our emotional response by reminding us of our own vulnerability. Certain calls will be more difficult for some team members than for others because each of us has different life experiences.

2. Which types of calls would be most stressful for you?

It is sometimes helpful to consider which types of calls may be most stressful for you. By engaging in this type of self-reflection, you may be able to reduce your stress on these calls. Talking about your concern with a close friend or supervisor may also be helpful.

YOU are the EMR **SUMMARY**

3. What changes should you consider to reduce your stress level?

Consider your current lifestyle and the stressors in your life. Evaluate your diet, your type and amount of fluid intake, the amount and type of exercise you get, the quality and quantity of sleep you get, and how you deal with the stressors at work and away from work. Then consider how to make changes to reduce your stress level and improve your health.

You are the EMR: CASE 2

1. What may be causing the changes in your partner's behavior?

Your partner may be showing signs of job-related stress in connection with the emergency call that involved the death of an infant. Calls involving children are among the most stressful for many people. Signs of postevent stress-related problems include irritability directed at coworkers, family, and friends; a change in the person's normal disposition; and possibly a loss of appetite.

2. What can your partner do to alleviate the signs and symptoms?

There are many methods of handling stress, but it is important to first recognize the signs of job-related stress. EMS personnel experiencing stress also need to maintain proper nutrition when the body's resources are strained. Finally, EMS clinicians experiencing postevent stress should consider contacting their supervisor or their employee assistance program representative for help.

3. During the initial incident, the mother repeatedly asked rescuers, "Why me?" Which stage of grief was she experiencing?

The mother may have been in the second of the five stages of grief, which is anger. The other stages are denial, bargaining, depression, and acceptance.

You are the EMR: CASE 3

1. Which route of disease transmission are you most concerned about with this patient?

The primary means by which this patient could infect others is through airborne droplets of infected secretions. If this patient is coughing up secretions, you need to avoid contact with the secretions.

2. What precautions should you take to protect yourself when caring for this patient?

By placing a mask on this patient, you may prevent the spread of infectious airborne droplets. However, if the patient is coughing up secretions, this may not be a good option. A second option is for you and the other caregivers to put on masks. You should don gloves and consider donning gowns and eye protection, if available. It also might be helpful to supply the patient with tissues to cover his mouth when coughing.

3. What steps do you need to take to protect yourself and others after caring for this patient?

After caring for this patient, it is important to dispose of your mask, gloves, gown, and any other objects that may have come in contact with the patient's airborne droplets or secretions. You need to learn your agency's policy for disposing of potentially infected materials. Do not forget to thoroughly wash your hands. Consider changing your uniform if it has come in contact with any infected secretions.

You are the EMR: CASE 4

1. Where should you park your vehicle?

The vehicle should be parked to protect the area from traffic hazards. However, because the truck is displaying a hazardous materials placard, you need to consider additional risks. The placard indicates the types of materials that may be carried on the truck. Before approaching the vehicle, check your *Emergency Response Guidebook* to determine the type of hazardous materials that may be involved. You should try to park your vehicle uphill and upwind from the crash site. Follow your local protocols.

2. What other issues should you consider before leaving your vehicle?

Motor vehicle crashes present many potential hazards for EMRs. Broken glass presents an injury risk to rescuers. Likewise, leaking fluids and fumes from hazardous materials can also be considered potential hazards.

3. Why is your safety a concern?

An injured or dead EMR will not be able to help people in need. Furthermore, an injured EMR adds to the number of victims, increasing the difficulty of the situation for the other EMRs.

Prep Kit

Ready for Review

- Providing care as an EMR is physically and emotionally demanding. EMRs must keep themselves physically prepared by exercising, eating right, staying hydrated, and getting enough sleep. Doing so provides the strength and energy that EMRs need to do their job and helps them to avoid injury. It also improves their emotional resilience to stressful situations.
- EMRs should understand the role that stress plays in the lives of emergency care clinicians and patients who have experienced a sudden illness or injury. Stress is a normal part of an EMR's life.
- The five stages of the grieving process following different kinds of loss, including death and dying, are denial, anger, bargaining, depression, and acceptance. Patients and rescue personnel may experience some or all of these stages. People experience these stages in different orders and at different rates.
- Stress management consists of recognizing, preventing, and reducing critical incident stress.
- According to the concept of crew resource management, each member is responsible for maintaining awareness of the current patient situation and sharing any critical information with the team leader.
- Scene safety is an important part of your job. You should understand how airborne and bloodborne diseases are spread and how standard precautions prevent the spread of infection. You should also know the steps you can take to protect yourself from infectious diseases.
- As you arrive on the scene of a motor vehicle crash or illness, you must assess the scene for a wide variety of hazards. Potential hazards include traffic, crime, crowds, unstable objects, sharp objects, electrical problems, fire, hazardous materials, animals, environmental conditions, special rescue situations, and infectious disease exposure. You should understand the safety equipment and precautions needed for the various types of rescue situations.

Vital Vocabulary

crew resource management (CRM) A set of procedures for use in environments where human error can have disastrous consequences. It empowers people within a team to communicate effectively with one another with a goal of improving team situational awareness, patient and crew safety, and overall communication.

critical incident stress debriefing (CISD) A system of psychological support designed to reduce stress on emergency personnel after a major stress-producing incident.

critical incident stress management (CISM) A process that confronts the responses to critical incidents and defuses them, directing the emergency services personnel toward physical and emotional equilibrium.

on-scene peer support Stress counselors at the scene of stressful incidents who help emergency personnel deal with stress.

pathogens Microorganisms that are capable of causing disease.

preincident stress education Training about stress and stress reactions conducted for public safety personnel before they are exposed to stressful situations.

standard precautions An infection control concept that treats all body fluids as potentially infectious.

References

Clinical overview of methicillin-resistant *Staphylococcus aureus* (MRSA) in healthcare settings. Centers for Disease Prevention and Control website. https://www.cdc.gov/mrsa/hcp/clinical-overview/index.html. Published April 12, 2024. Accessed December 13, 2024.

EMS infectious disease playbook. Version 2.0. Administration for Strategic Preparedness and Response website. https://files.asprtracie.hhs.gov/documents/aspr-tracie-transport-playbook-508.pdf. Revised 2023. Accessed December 13, 2024.

Gregory ME, Powell JR, MacEwan SR, et al. COVID-19 vaccinations in EMS professionals: prevalence and predictors. *Prehosp Emerg Care*. 2022;26(5):632–640.

The American Heart Association diet and lifestyle recommendations. American Heart Association website. https://www.heart.org/en/healthy-living/healthy-eating/eat-smart/nutrition-basics/aha-diet-and-lifestyle-recommendations. Reviewed July 30, 2024. Accessed December 13, 2024.

Vaccine efficacy, effectiveness, and protection. World Health Organization website. https://www.who.int/news-room/feature-stories/detail/vaccine-efficacy-effectiveness-and-protection. Published July 14, 2021. Accessed February 21, 2025.

Assessment IN ACTION

You and your partner are dispatched to a motor vehicle crash on a secondary rural road. When you arrive at the scene, you see a car sitting in the roadway with the driver's door open. A man is kneeling beside a 17-year-old boy who is lying in the road. A crumpled bicycle is positioned about 50 feet (15 m) from them. You note that the teenager is wearing a helmet. He is bleeding from a scrape on his forearm, and he complains of pain from his left leg, which is bent at an abnormal angle.

1. Which of the following hazards should you be most concerned about when attempting to help this patient?

A. Vehicle instability
B. Downed electrical lines
C. Broken glass
D. Uncontrolled traffic

2. What is another hazard you will need to consider when arriving at the scene of a motor vehicle crash?

A. Airborne pathogens
B. Environmental conditions
C. Bloodborne pathogens
D. Traffic

3. Because the patient is bleeding, what are the minimum standard precautions you should take?

A. Handwashing and a mask
B. Gloves
C. Shoe covers and a gown
D. Leather gloves

4. All of the following are signs and symptoms of job-related stress EXCEPT:

A. irritability.
B. difficulty sleeping.
C. alcohol or drug misuse or abuse.
D. working too hard.

5. A stress-reducing diet includes all of the following EXCEPT:

A. fruits.
B. vegetables.
C. low-fat milk, yogurt, and cheese.
D. fried fast foods.

6. What PPE would you incorporate into your care of the patient in this scenario?

7. How stressful do you think this call would be for you?

8. What should you do if your clothing comes in contact with body fluid from a patient?

9. What are some of the emotional aspects that could affect an EMR's reaction to this call?

10. If, on arrival, you find the patient is trapped by the car, what additional resources would you need to call?

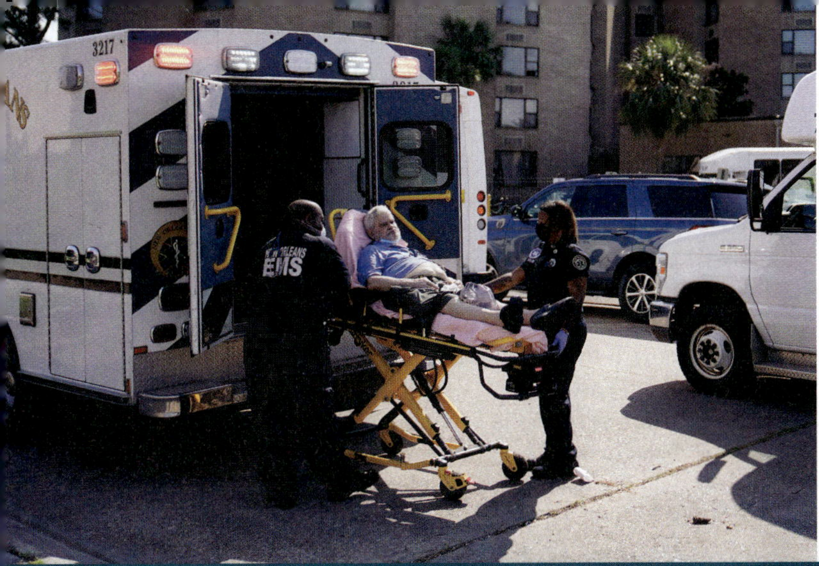

© Matt Slocum/AP Photo

CHAPTER 3

Lifting and Moving Patients

National EMS Education Standard Competencies

Preparatory

Uses knowledge of the EMS system, safety/well-being of the EMR, medical/legal issues, and ethical issues at the scene of an emergency while awaiting a higher level of care.

Workforce Safety and Wellness

- Standard safety precautions (pp 40–61)
- Personal protective equipment (Chapter 2, *Workforce Safety and Wellness*)
- Lifting and moving patients (pp 42–44)
- Crew resource management (Chapter 2, *Workforce Safety and Wellness*)
- Stress management (Chapter 2, *Workforce Safety and Wellness*)
- Prevention of work-related injuries and illnesses (pp 40–61)
- Responder mental health, resilience, and suicide prevention (Chapter 2, *Workforce Safety and Wellness*)
- Wellness principles (Chapter 2, *Workforce Safety and Wellness*)
- Disease transmission (Chapter 2, *Workforce Safety and Wellness*)

Knowledge Objectives

1. Describe the general guidelines for moving patients. (p 40)
2. Explain the purpose and indications for use of the recovery position. (p 40)
3. Discuss the components of good body mechanics. (p 41)
4. Explain how emergency medical responders should decide when emergency movement of a patient is necessary. (p 42)
5. Describe the purpose of each of the following pieces of equipment:
    - Wheeled ambulance stretcher (p 49)
    - Portable stretcher (p 49)
    - Stair chair (p 49)
    - Long backboard (p 50)
    - Short backboard (p 54)
    - Scoop stretcher (p 52)

Skills Objectives

1. Demonstrate the components of good body mechanics. (p 41)
2. Demonstrate the steps needed to perform the following emergency patient drags:
    - Clothes drag (p 42)
    - Blanket drag (p 42)
    - Arm-to-arm drag (p 42)
    - Firefighter drag (p 43)
    - Emergency drag from a vehicle (p 43)
3. Demonstrate the steps needed to perform the following carries for nonambulatory patients:
    - Two-person extremity carry (p 44)
    - Two-person seat carry (p 44)
    - Cradle-in-arms carry (p 44)
    - Two-person chair carry (p 44)
    - Pack-strap carry (p 45)
    - Direct ground lift (pp 46–47; Skill Drill 3-1)
    - Transfer from a bed to a stretcher (p 47)
4. Demonstrate the steps needed to perform the following walking assists for ambulatory patients:
    - One-person walking assist (p 47)
    - Two-person walking assist (p 47)
5. Demonstrate the steps in each of the following procedures for patients with suspected spinal injuries:
    - Moving the patient using a long backboard (p 50)
    - Moving the patient using a scoop stretcher (p 52; Skill Drill 3-2)
    - Applying a cervical collar (p 53)
    - Assisting with a short backboard device (pp 53–54; Skill Drill 3-3)
    - Log rolling (pp 54–55; Skill Drill 3-4)
    - Strapping (p 57)
    - Stabilizing the patient's head (pp 58–60; Skill Drill 3-5 and Skill Drill 3-6)

Introduction

As an emergency medical responder (EMR), you must analyze a situation, quickly evaluate a patient's condition (under stressful circumstances and often by yourself), and perform effective, lifesaving emergency medical procedures. These procedures sometimes include lifting, moving, or positioning patients as well as assisting other emergency medical services (EMS) clinicians in moving patients and preparing them for transport.

Usually, you will not have to move patients. In most situations, you can treat the patient in the position found and later assist other EMS personnel in moving the patient. However, in some cases, the patient's survival may depend on your knowledge of emergency movement techniques. You may have to move patients for their own protection (for example, to remove a patient from a burning building), or you may have to move patients before you can provide needed emergency care (for example, to administer cardiopulmonary resuscitation [CPR] to a patient in cardiac arrest who was found in a bathroom). You can perform some of the techniques presented in this chapter with no equipment, whereas other techniques require simple objects that are often available at emergency scenes. With other techniques, you can assist other EMS clinicians in using the specialized equipment they bring to the emergency scene.

General Principles

Every time you move a patient, keep the following general guidelines in mind:

- Do no further harm to the patient.
- Move the patient only when necessary for treatment or protection.
- Move the patient as few times as possible.
- Move the patient's body as a unit.
- Use proper lifting and moving techniques to ensure your own safety.
- Do not rush the moving process.
- Have one rescuer give commands when moving a patient (usually the rescuer at the patient's head).

Also consider the following recommendations:

- Delay moving the patient, if possible, until additional EMS personnel arrive.
- Treat the patient before moving unless the patient is in an unsafe environment.
- Try not to step over the patient (your shoes may drop sand, dirt, or mud onto the patient or you might fall onto the patient).
- Explain to the patient what you are going to do and how. If the patient's condition permits, they may be able to assist you.
- If you suspect the patient has sustained trauma to the head or spine, apply spinal motion restriction, which will discourage patient movement (discussed later in the chapter).

Safety

Whatever technique you use for moving patients, keep these rules of good body mechanics in mind:

- Know your own physical limitations and capabilities. Do not try to lift too heavy a load.
- Keep yourself balanced when lifting or moving a patient.
- Maintain a firm footing.
- Lift and lower the patient by bending your legs, not your back. Maintain the natural curve of your spine; do not bend at the waist. Use your large leg muscles to do the work.
- Try to keep your arms close to your body for strength and balance.
- Move the patient as few times as possible.

Recovery Position

Place unresponsive patients who have not sustained suspected trauma in the side-lying **recovery position** to help keep the airway open (**FIGURE 3-1**). The recovery position

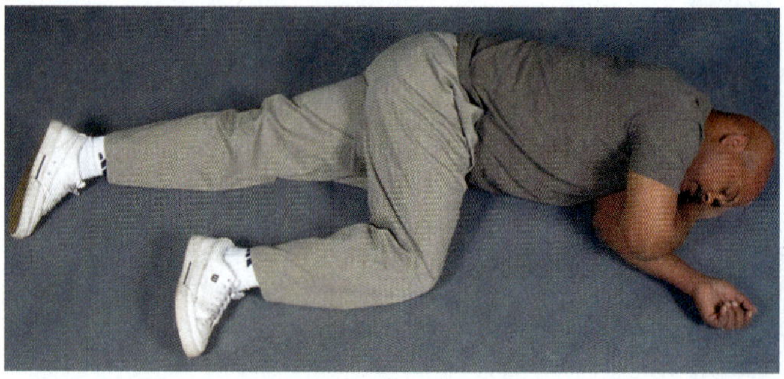

FIGURE 3-1 A patient in the recovery position.

© Jones & Bartlett Learning. Courtesy of MIEMSS.

YOU are the EMR — **CASE 1**

At 1023 hours, you and your partner are dispatched to a large discount supermarket for the report of a 64-year-old woman who has slipped and fallen in one of the aisles. As you assess the patient, she tells you she has some tenderness in her right leg. Her right wrist is noticeably deformed and painful. You also note she has a large abrasion and some swelling on her forehead. The nearest ambulance is 8 to 10 minutes away.

1. Under what circumstances would it be necessary to move this patient before the EMS transport unit arrives?
2. Why is it often better for EMRs to delay moving a patient until the arrival of an EMS transport unit?

also allows secretions to drain from the mouth. The indications for the use of the recovery position are discussed in Chapter 7, *Airway Management*, as well as other chapters.

Body Mechanics

Your top priority is to ensure your own safety. Improperly lifting or moving a patient can result in injury to you or to the patient. By exercising good body mechanics, you reduce the possibility of injuring yourself. **FIGURE 3-2** shows how to lift using good body mechanics.

> **Safety**
>
> Don't forget to breathe out when lifting!

Good body mechanics means using the strength of the large muscles in your legs to lift patients instead of using your back muscles. This practice prevents strains and injuries to weaker muscles, especially in your back. Get as close to the patient as possible so that your back is in a straight and upright position, and maintain the natural curve of your spine as you lift. Do not lift when your back is bent over a patient. Lift, using your legs, without twisting your body. Keep your feet in a secure position and be sure you have a firm footing before you start to lift or move a patient.

To lift safely, keep certain guidelines in mind. Before attempting to move a patient, assess the weight of the patient. Know your physical limitations, and do not attempt to lift or move a patient who is too heavy for you to handle safely. Call for additional personnel if needed for your safety and the safety of the patient. Discuss the route of travel prior to lifting. Because you will sometimes need to assist other EMS clinicians, practice with them so that lifts are handled in a coordinated and helpful manner.

As you lift, make sure you communicate with the other members of the lifting team. Failure to give clear commands or failure to lift at the same time can result in serious injuries to both rescuers and patients. You can never practice too much; perfect your lifts and moves until they become smooth for you and your partner and for the patient.

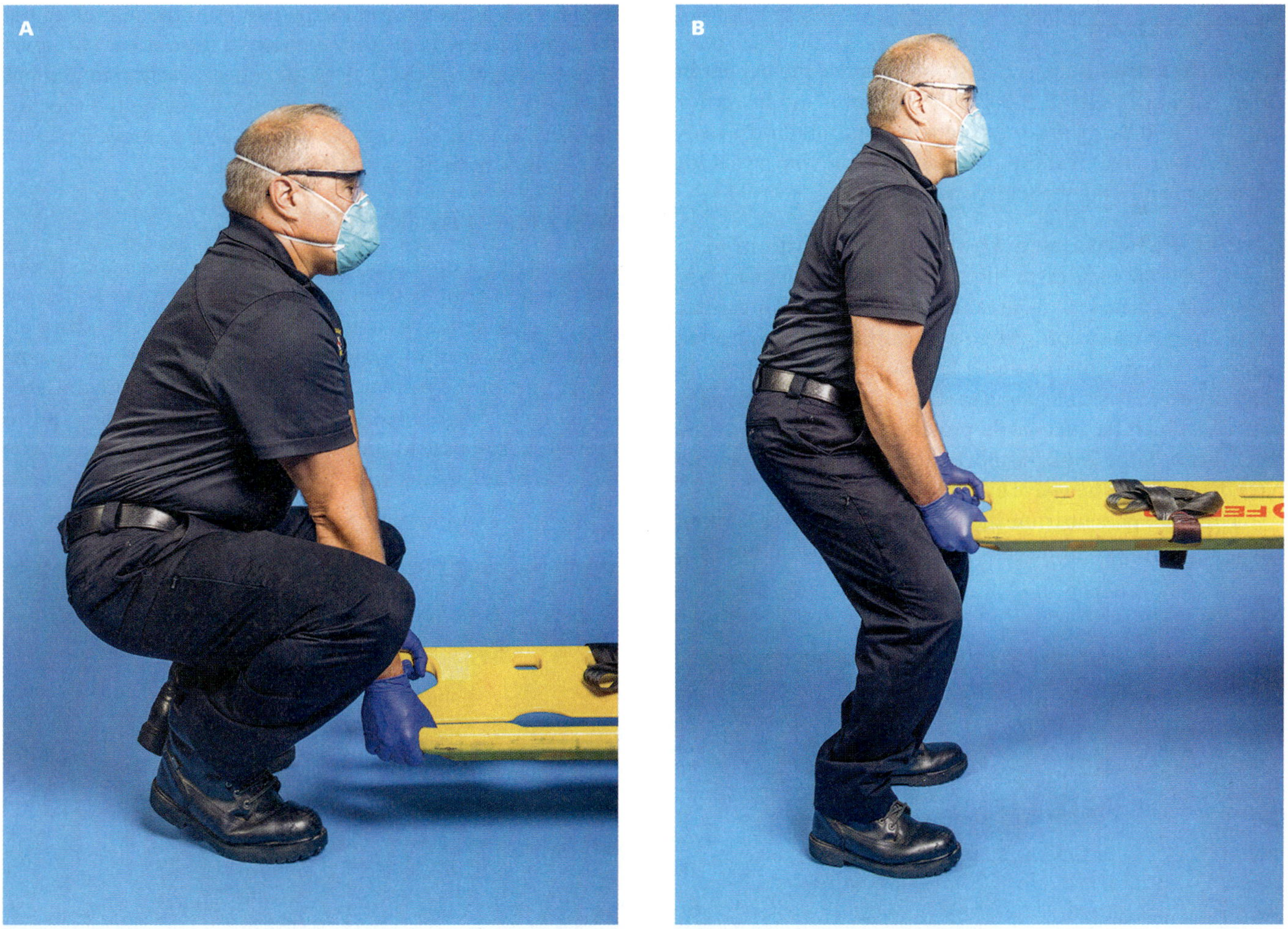

FIGURE 3-2 Use good body mechanics when lifting a patient. **A.** Keep your head and neck in proper alignment with your spine, maintain the natural curve of your spine, and do not bend at the waist. **B.** Keep your feet shoulder width apart to maintain your balance. Keep the patient who is being lifted close to your body. Use the muscles in your legs to lift. Avoid twisting your body when carrying a patient.

© Jones & Bartlett Learning

Emergency Movement of Patients

Although it is preferable to avoid moving the patient until additional EMS personnel arrive, emergency movement of a patient is sometimes necessary. Immediately move a patient in the following situations:

- Danger of fire, explosion, or structural collapse exists.
- Hazardous materials are present.
- The emergency scene cannot be protected.
- It is otherwise impossible to gain access to other patients who need lifesaving care.
- The patient has experienced cardiac arrest and must be moved so you can begin CPR.

Emergency Drags

If the patient is lying on the floor or ground during an emergency situation, you may have to drag the person away from the scene instead of trying to lift and carry the patient. Make every effort to pull the patient in the direction of the long axis of the body to protect the spine as much as possible.

Clothes Drag

The **clothes drag** is the simplest way to move the patient in an emergency (**FIGURE 3-3**). If the patient is too heavy for you to lift and carry, grasp the patient's clothing in the neck and shoulder area, rest the patient's head on your arms for protection, and drag the patient out of danger.

Cardiac Patients and the Clothes Drag. In most situations, you can easily determine whether emergency movement is necessary. Cases involving patients in cardiac arrest are the exception. Patients in cardiac arrest are often found in a bathroom or small bedroom. You will have to judge whether basic life support (BLS) or advanced life support (ALS) can be adequately provided in that space. If the room is not large enough, move the patient as soon as you have determined they have experienced cardiac arrest.

Drag the patient from the tight space to a larger room (such as a living or dining room) that has space to perform CPR and ALS procedures (**FIGURE 3-4**). Quickly make adequate room before you begin CPR. Move furniture out of the way so you and other EMS personnel have room to work. By doing so, you will be able to provide care with increased efficiency, which will more than make up for the time it took to move the patient or any objects.

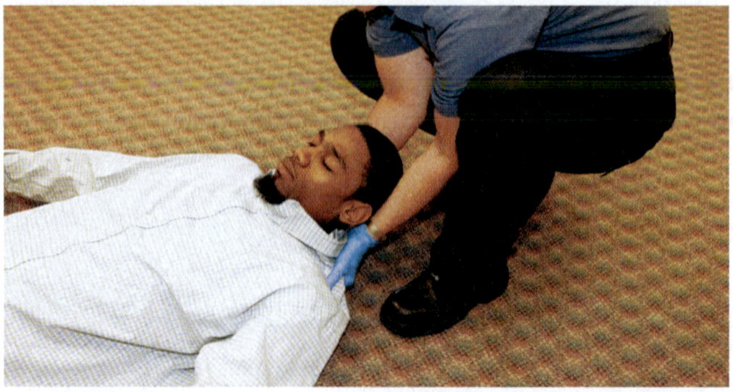

FIGURE 3-3 Clothes drag.

© Jones & Bartlett Learning. Courtesy of MIEMSS.

> **Words of Wisdom**
>
> To eliminate distractions at the scene, take a second to turn off any televisions or audio devices. Emergency scenes are calmer and less stressful when you are not competing to be heard over a loud television program or music.

Blanket Drag

If the patient is not dressed or is dressed in clothing that could tear easily during the clothes drag (for example, a nightgown), move the patient by using a large sheet, blanket, or rug (**blanket drag**). Place the sheet, blanket, rug, or similar item on the floor next to the patient and roll the patient onto their side. Tuck the item close to the patient's side on the ground, and then roll the patient onto the item. Pull the remainder of the item from the side of the patient (you may need to briefly roll the patient the other direction to pull out the item). Pull the patient to safety by dragging the sheet or blanket. You can also use the blanket drag to move a patient who weighs more than you do (**FIGURE 3-5**).

Arm-to-Arm Drag

If the patient is on the floor, you can place your hands under the patient's armpits from the back of the patient and grasp the patient's wrists or forearms. The **arm-to-arm drag** allows you to move the patient by carrying the weight of the upper part of the patient's body as the lower trunk and legs drag on the floor (**FIGURE 3-6**). This drag enables you to move a heavy patient and it offers some protection for the patient's head and neck.

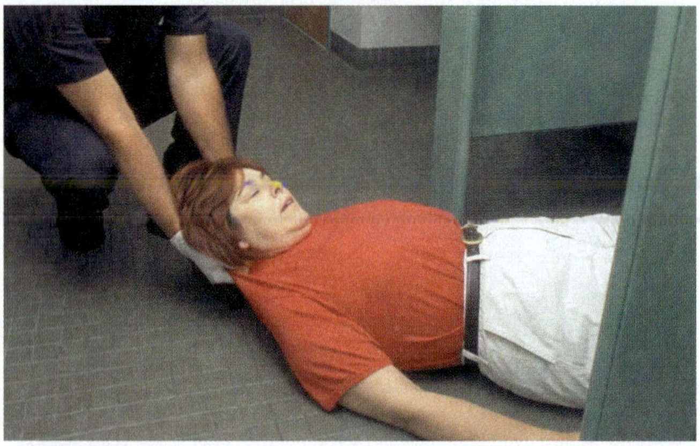

FIGURE 3-4 Remove the patient from a tight space to administer CPR.

© American Academy of Orthopaedic Surgeons

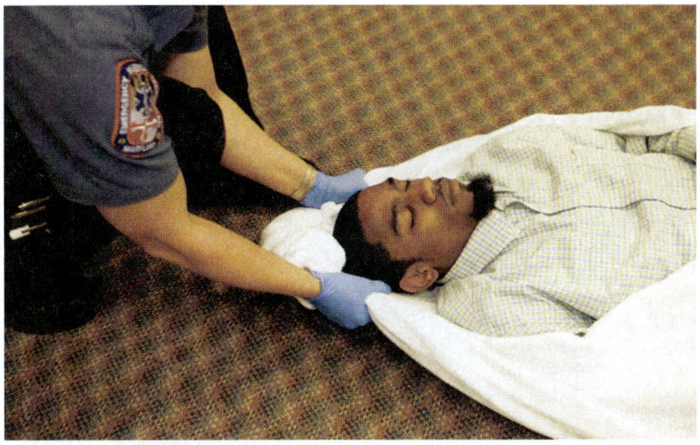

FIGURE 3-5 Blanket drag.
© Jones & Bartlett Learning. Courtesy of MIEMSS.

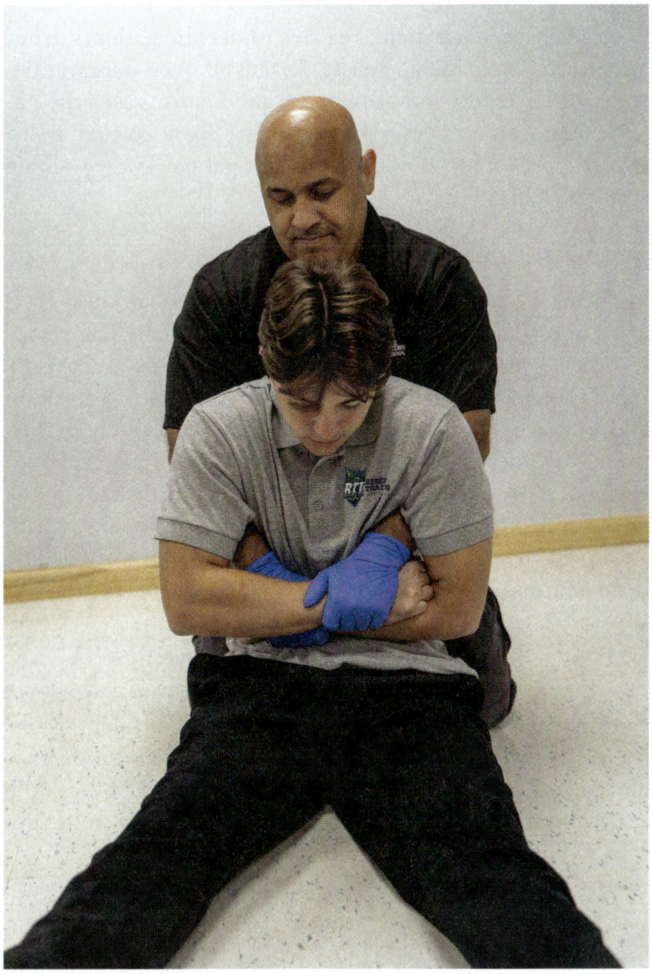

FIGURE 3-6 Arm-to-arm drag.
© Jones & Bartlett Learning

Firefighter Drag

The **firefighter drag** enables you to move a patient who is heavier than you are because you do not have to lift or carry the patient. Tie the patient's wrists together with any material that is handy, such as a cravat (a folded triangular bandage), strip of gauze, belt, or necktie, being careful not to impair circulation. Then get down on your hands and knees and straddle the patient. Pass the patient's tied hands around your neck, straighten your arms, and drag the patient across the floor by crawling on your hands and knees (**FIGURE 3-7**).

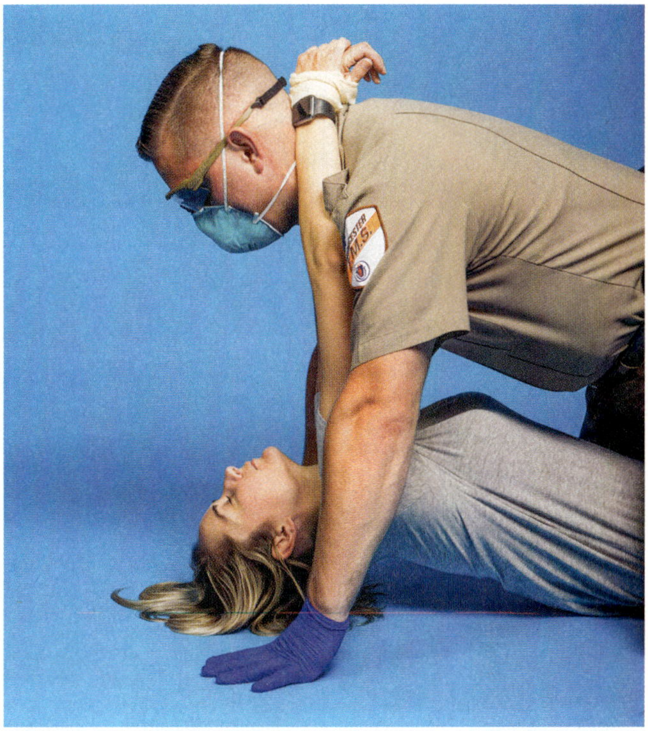

FIGURE 3-7 Firefighter drag. Tie the patient's wrists together, then drag the patient across the floor by crawling on your hands and knees with the patient's arms around your neck.
© Jones & Bartlett Learning

Emergency Drag From a Vehicle

Sometimes you have to use emergency movement techniques in life-threatening situations when no equipment is immediately available (for example, to remove a patient from a motor vehicle that is on fire or to administer CPR). All the basic movement principles apply, but the techniques need to be slightly modified because the patient is sitting instead of lying down. Emergency drags from a vehicle can be performed with one or more rescuers.

One Rescuer. Grasp the patient under the arms and cradle the patient's head between your arms (**FIGURE 3-8**). Pull the patient down into a horizontal position as you ease the person from the vehicle. Although there is no effective way to remove a patient from a vehicle by yourself without causing some movement, it is important to prevent excessive movement of the patient's neck.

Two or More Rescuers. If you must immediately remove a patient from a vehicle and two or more rescuers are present, have one rescuer support the patient's head and neck, while the second rescuer moves the patient by lifting under the arms. The patient can then be removed in line with the long axis of the body, with the head and neck manually

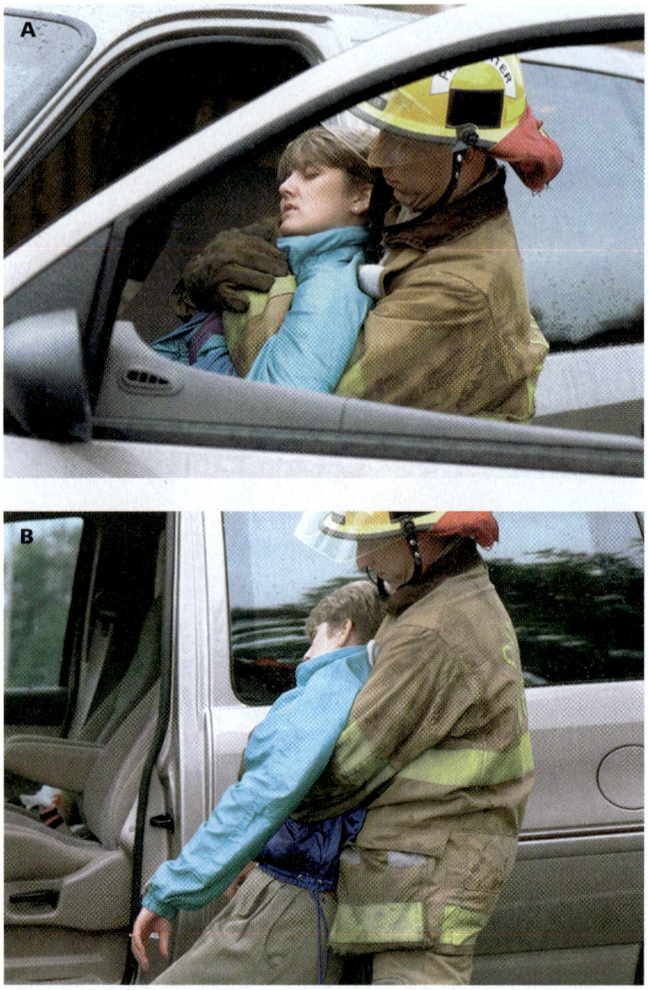

FIGURE 3-8 Emergency removal from a vehicle. **A.** Grasp the patient under the arms. **B.** Pull the patient down into a horizontal position.
© Jones & Bartlett Learning. Courtesy of MIEMSS.

stabilized in a neutral position. If time permits and if you have one available, use a long backboard for patient removal. Procedures for using a long backboard are covered later in this chapter.

Carries for Nonambulatory Patients

Many patients are unable or should not be allowed to move without your assistance. Patients who are unable to move because of injury or illness must be carried to safety. This section describes several useful carrying techniques for nonambulatory patients. Whatever technique you use, remember to follow the rules of good body mechanics.

Two-Person Extremity Carry

The **two-person extremity carry** enables two rescuers with no equipment to move a patient in tight or narrow spaces, such as mobile home corridors, small hallways, and narrow spaces between buildings (**FIGURE 3-9**). The focus of this carry is to use the patient's **extremities** to move the patient. First, the rescuers help the patient sit up. Rescuer 1 kneels behind the patient, reaches under the patient's arms, and grasps the patient's wrists. Rescuer 2 then backs in between the patient's legs, reaches around, and grasps the patient behind the knees. At a command from rescuer 1, the two rescuers stand up and carry the patient away, walking straight ahead.

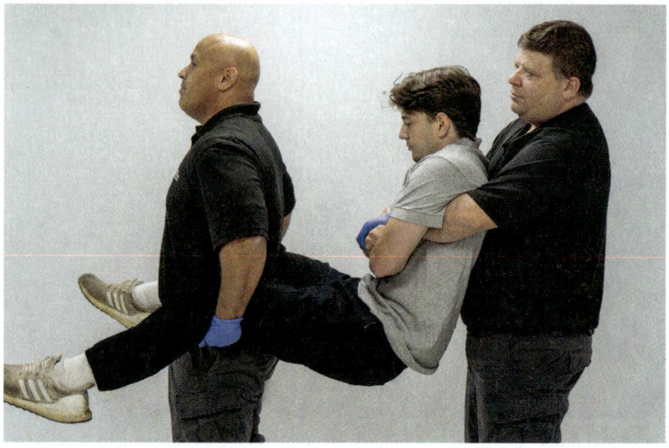

FIGURE 3-9 Two-person extremity carry.
© Jones & Bartlett Learning

Two-Person Seat Carry

With the **two-person seat carry**, two rescuers use their arms and bodies to form a seat for the patient. The rescuers kneel on opposite sides of the patient near the patient's hips. The rescuers then raise the patient to a sitting position and link arms behind the patient's back. The rescuers then place the other arm under the patient's knees and link with each other. If possible, the patient puts their arms around the necks and shoulders of the rescuers for additional support. Although the two-person seat carry requires two rescuers, it does not require any equipment (**FIGURE 3-10**).

Cradle-in-Arms Carry

The **cradle-in-arms carry** can be used by one rescuer to carry a small patient, typically a young child or infant. Kneel beside the patient and place one arm around the child's back and the other arm under the thighs. Lift slightly and roll the child into the hollow formed by your arms and chest. Be sure to use your leg muscles to stand (**FIGURE 3-11**).

> **Safety**
>
> Maintain the natural curve of your spine and use the large muscles in your legs to do the lifting.

Two-Person Chair Carry

In the **two-person chair carry**, two rescuers use a chair to support the weight of the patient. Do not use a folding chair. Test the strength of the chair using a healthy person before moving an ill or injured patient using the chair. The chair carry is especially useful for taking patients up

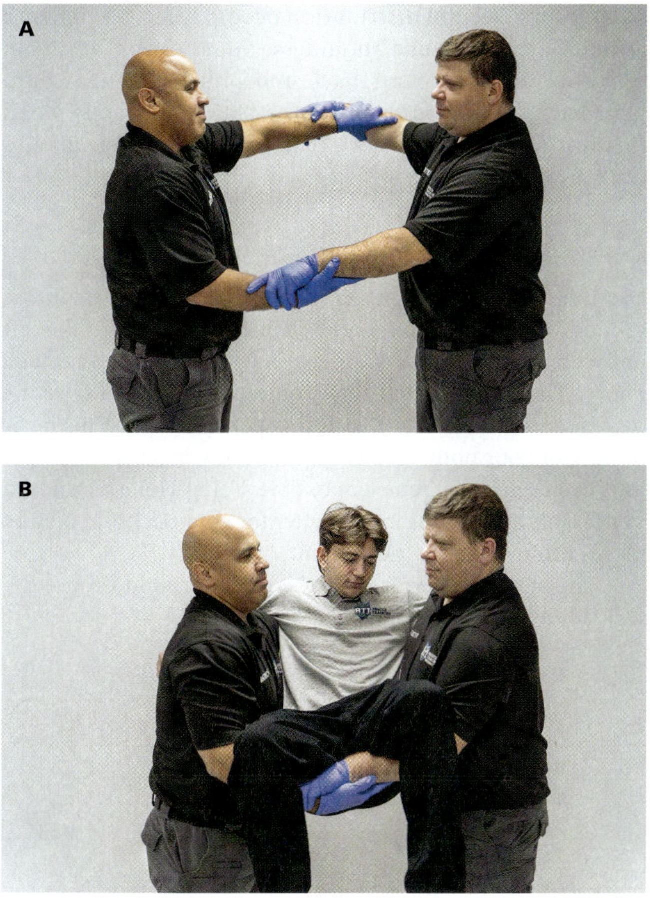

FIGURE 3-10 Two-person seat carry. **A.** Link arms. **B.** Raise the patient to a sitting position.
© Jones & Bartlett Learning

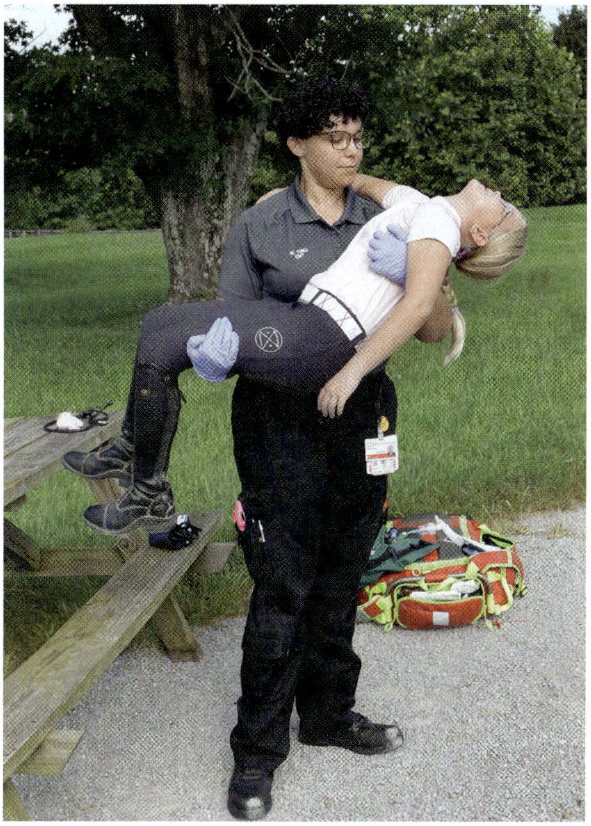

FIGURE 3-11 Cradle-in-arms carry.
© Jones & Bartlett Learning

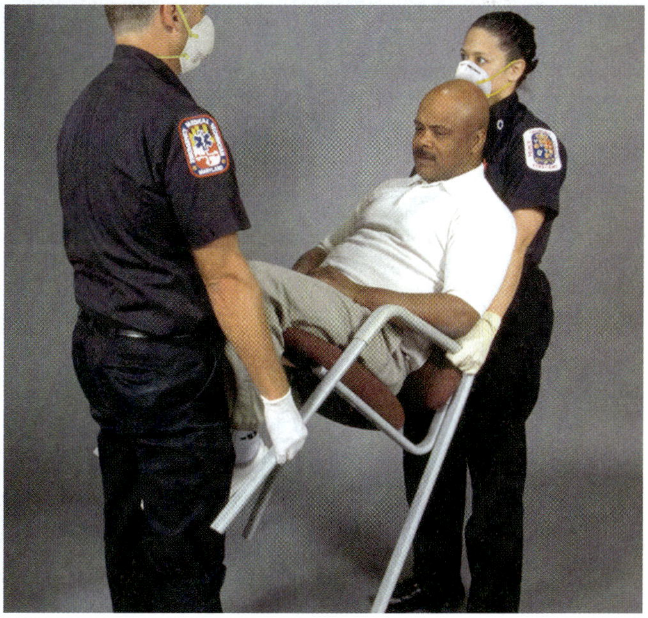

FIGURE 3-12 Two-person chair carry.
© Jones & Bartlett Learning. Courtesy of MIEMSS.

or down stairways or through a narrow hallway. An additional benefit is that because the patient is able to hold on to the chair (and should be encouraged to do so), the individual feels much more secure than with the two-person seat carry.

Rescuer 1 stands behind the seated patient, reaches down, and grasps the back of the chair close to the seat. Rescuer 1 then tilts the chair slightly backward on its rear legs so rescuer 2 can face the chair and grasp the chair's front legs. The patient's legs should be between the legs of the chair. When both rescuers are correctly positioned, rescuer 1 gives the command to lift and walk away (**FIGURE 3-12**).

Safety

Because the two-person chair carry may force the patient's head forward, have rescuer 2 watch the patient for airway problems.

Pack-Strap Carry

The **pack-strap carry** is a one-person carry that allows you to carry a patient while keeping one hand free. Have the patient stand (or have other rescue personnel support the patient) and back into the patient so your shoulders fit into the patient's armpits. Grasp the patient's wrists and cross the arms over your chest (**FIGURE 3-13**). Now you can hold both wrists in one hand and your other hand remains free.

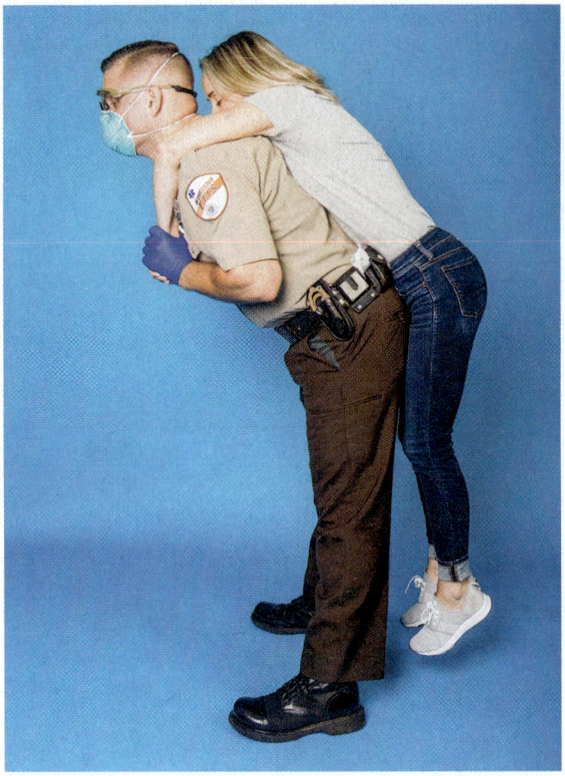

FIGURE 3-13 Pack-strap carry. After the patient's arms are crossed in front of your chest, you can hold the patient's wrists in one hand, leaving the other hand free, if needed.

© Jones & Bartlett Learning

Optimal weight distribution occurs when the patient's armpits are over your shoulders. Squat deeply to avoid potential injury to your back and pull the patient onto your back. After you position the patient correctly, bend forward to lift the patient off the ground, stand up, and walk away.

Direct Ground Lift

Use the direct ground lift to move a patient who is on the ground or the floor to an ambulance stretcher. Use this lift only for those patients who have not sustained a traumatic injury. The direct ground lift requires you to bend over the patient and lift with your back in a bent position. This positioning of your body results in poor body mechanics; therefore, avoid this lift whenever possible. Using a long backboard or portable stretcher is much better for your back and may be more comfortable for the patient.

The steps for performing the direct ground lift are described in **SKILL DRILL 3-1**.

Safety

The direct ground lift requires you to use poor body mechanics, so avoid using it whenever possible. Never use the direct ground lift with a patient who may have sustained any injury to the head, spine, or legs.

SKILL DRILL 3-1

Performing a Direct Ground Lift

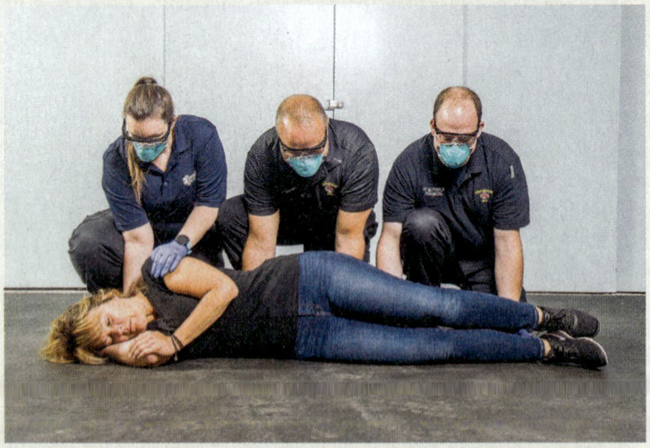

STEP 1 Line up on one side of the patient, with one provider at the head, one at the waist, and one at the patient's knees. Place a soft stretcher underneath the patient. All providers should be kneeling. Place the patient's arms on their chest, if possible.

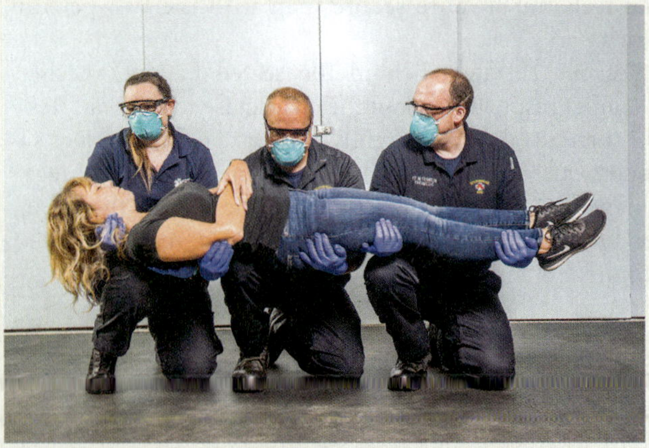

STEP 2 The first provider places one arm under the patient's neck and shoulders and cradles the patient's head. This provider places the other arm under the patient's low back. The second provider places one hand under the patient's waist and the other under the knees. The third provider places one arm under the patient's knees and the other under the ankles. On command, the team lifts the patient up to knee level as each provider rests an arm on their knee.

SKILL DRILL 3-1 (continued)

Performing a Direct Ground Lift

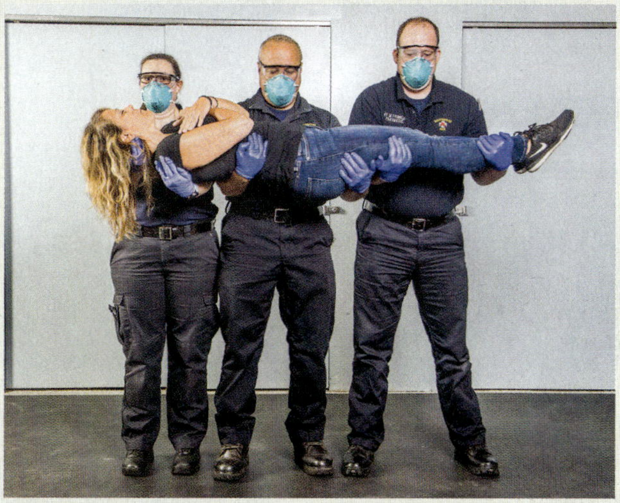

STEP 3 As a team and on command, each provider rolls the patient in toward their chest. Again on command, the team stands and carries the patient to the stretcher.

© Jones & Bartlett Learning

> **Words of Wisdom**
>
> Using a scoop stretcher (discussed later in this chapter) is an excellent alternative to using the direct ground lift.

Transferring a Patient From Bed to Stretcher

Patients who are ill are often found in their beds. If EMS personnel need to transport these patients to the hospital, they may request your assistance with transferring a patient from the bed to the ambulance stretcher using the draw sheet method (**FIGURE 3-14**).

Place the stretcher next to the bed, making sure it is at the same height as the bed and that the rails are lowered and straps unbuckled. Hold the stretcher to keep it from moving. Loosen the bottom sheet underneath the patient or log roll the patient onto a blanket. Reach across the stretcher and grasp the sheet and blanket firmly at the patient's head, chest, hips, and knees. Gently slide the patient onto the stretcher. Use this method with caution because it requires you to reach across the stretcher to get to the patient. This action results in poor body mechanics.

An alternative method for moving a patient is to loosen the bottom sheet of the patient's bed, place the ambulance stretcher parallel with the bed, and reach across the stretcher to pull the sheet and the patient onto the stretcher. Again, use this method with caution because reaching across the stretcher to get to the patient results in poor body mechanics.

Walking Assists for Ambulatory Patients

Frequently, patients simply need assistance to walk to safety. Either one or two rescuers can perform this task. Choose a technique after you have assessed the patient's condition and the scene of the incident. The technique you might use to help a patient walk to a chair is probably not appropriate to help a patient walk up a highway embankment.

One-Person Walking Assist

Use the **one-person walking assist** if the patient can bear their own weight. Help the patient stand. Have the patient place one arm around your neck so their wrist hangs over your shoulder. Hold the patient's wrist with one hand and put your free arm around the patient's waist, then help the patient to walk (**FIGURE 3-15**).

Two-Person Walking Assist

The **two-person walking assist** is the same as the one-person walking assist, except that a rescuer supports the

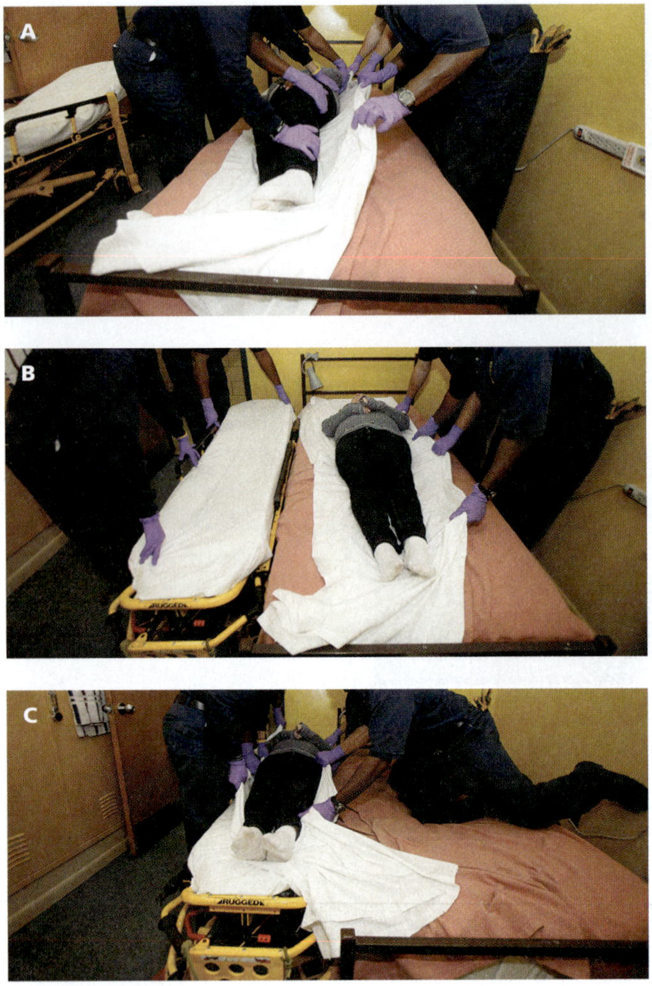

FIGURE 3-14 The draw sheet method. **A.** Log roll the patient onto a sheet or blanket. **B.** Bring the stretcher in parallel with the bed. Gently slide the patient to the edge of the bed. **C.** Transfer the patient to the stretcher.

© Jones & Bartlett Learning. Courtesy of MIEMSS.

patient from both sides. This technique is useful if the patient cannot bear weight. The two rescuers completely support the patient (**FIGURE 3-16**).

> **Safety**
>
> Do not use any of the lifts or carries explained in this chapter if you suspect the patient has a spinal injury, unless it is absolutely necessary to remove the patient from an immediately life-threatening situation.

Equipment

Most of the lifts and moves described in the previous section are performed without the use of any specialized equipment. However, EMS departments commonly use various types of patient-moving equipment. To be able to assist other EMS clinicians, familiarize yourself with the following equipment.

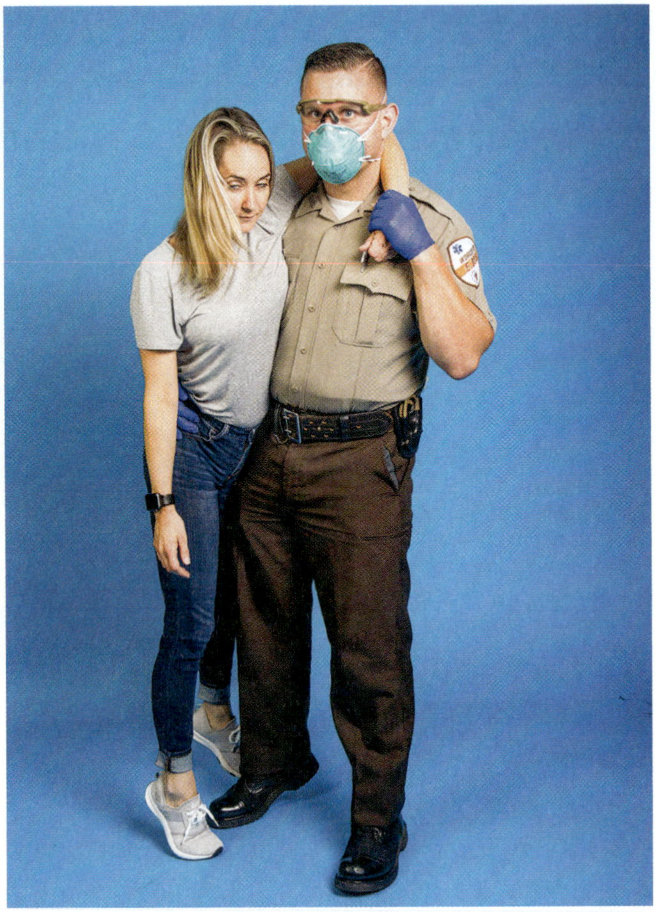

FIGURE 3-15 One-person walking assist.

© Jones & Bartlett Learning

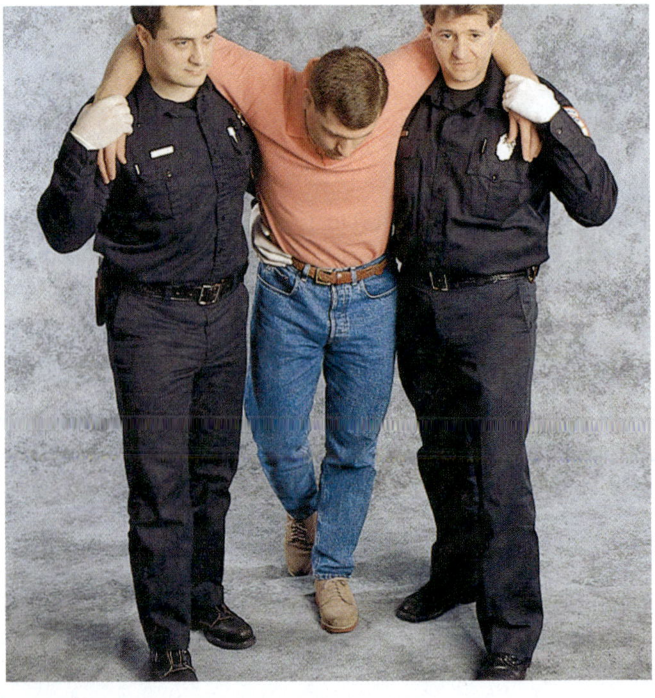

FIGURE 3-16 Two-person walking assist.

© Jones & Bartlett Learning. Courtesy of MIEMSS.

Wheeled Ambulance Stretchers

Wheeled ambulance stretchers are carried by ambulances and are one of the most commonly used EMS devices (**FIGURE 3-17**). These stretchers are also called cots. Each type of stretcher has its own set of levers and controls for raising and lowering the stretcher to different heights. The head end of the stretcher can be raised to elevate the patient's upper body. These stretchers have belts to secure the patient. Some EMS departments use electronic stretchers, which can be raised and lowered using a battery-powered system. These stretchers reduce the strain on EMS clinicians and operate smoothly for patient comfort. If you regularly work with the same EMS unit, it will be helpful for you to learn how their particular type of stretcher operates.

Stretchers can be rolled, or they can be carried by two or four people. If the surface is smooth, a wheeled stretcher can be rolled, typically with one clinician pushing the head of the stretcher while another clinician guides the foot end. If the loaded stretcher must be carried, it is best to use four people, one person at each corner. The use of four people offers more stability, and less strength is required to carry the stretcher. If the stretcher must be carried through a narrow area, only two people will be able to carry it. The two rescuers should face each other from opposite ends of the stretcher. Carrying the stretcher with two people requires that each person be strong enough to maintain the balance of the stretcher. As an EMR, you may also be asked to assist with loading a patient into the ambulance. Learn the method of loading ambulance stretchers that your EMS unit uses, and practice this procedure with the EMS unit. It is important to lift as a team to avoid injury to yourself or to the other rescuers.

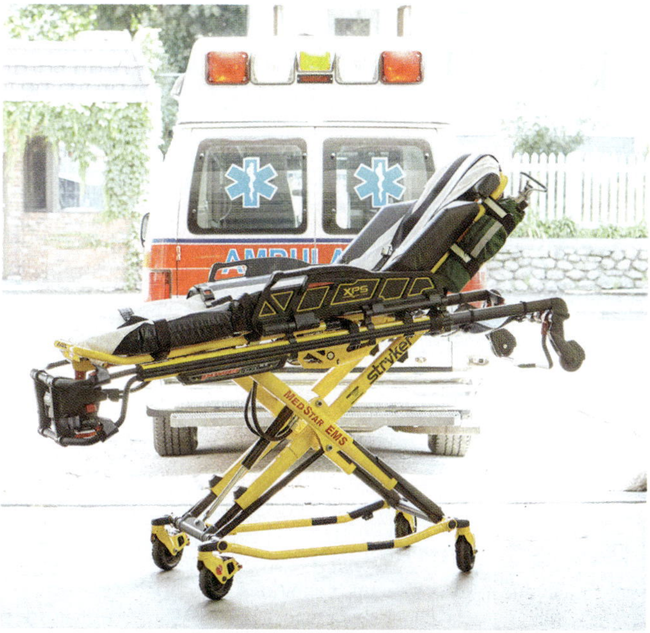

FIGURE 3-17 A wheeled ambulance stretcher.

© Jones & Bartlett Learning

> **Special Populations**
>
> **Bariatric Stretchers**
>
> Some EMS systems have specialized stretchers for moving patients with obesity. These are called **bariatric** stretchers. They are designed to safely handle patients who exceed the weight limit of standard equipment. In addition, some EMS systems have specialized bariatric ambulances that are equipped not only with heavy-duty stretchers but also with ramps for loading and unloading bariatric patients. It will be helpful to notify other emergency responders when you are caring for a bariatric patient in case they need to call for specialized equipment or additional personnel to move the patient.

Portable Stretchers

Use a **portable stretcher** when you cannot move the wheeled ambulance stretcher into a small space. They are smaller and lighter to carry than wheeled stretchers. You can carry a portable stretcher in the same ways that you carry a wheeled stretcher. An example of one type of portable stretcher is shown in **FIGURE 3-18**.

Stair Chairs

A **stair chair** is a portable moving device that is used to carry a patient in a sitting position. The stair chair is useful for patients who are short of breath or who are more comfortable in a sitting position. They are small, lightweight, and easy to carry in narrow spaces. This type of stretcher will sometimes fit in a small elevator where there is insufficient room for a regular wheeled stretcher. Do not use the stair chair with patients who have experienced a major trauma. When carrying a stair chair, the rescuers face each other and lift on a set command. If you are going to assist your local EMS unit with this device, learn how to unfold it and how to assist with carrying it. One type of stair chair is shown in **FIGURE 3-19**.

> **YOU are the EMR** — **CASE 2**
>
> As you are driving to work, you are shocked to see a driver ahead of you suddenly swerve to the left, cross over the oncoming lane of traffic, and collide with a tree. You park your vehicle in a safe location and rush toward the wreck. As you approach the crashed vehicle, you find a man slumped against the deflated airbag, and he does not seem to be moving. You see smoke starting to come from the engine compartment and can smell burning plastic and oil.
>
> 1. How can you quickly remove this patient from the burning vehicle?
> 2. How do you determine where to place this patient after removal?

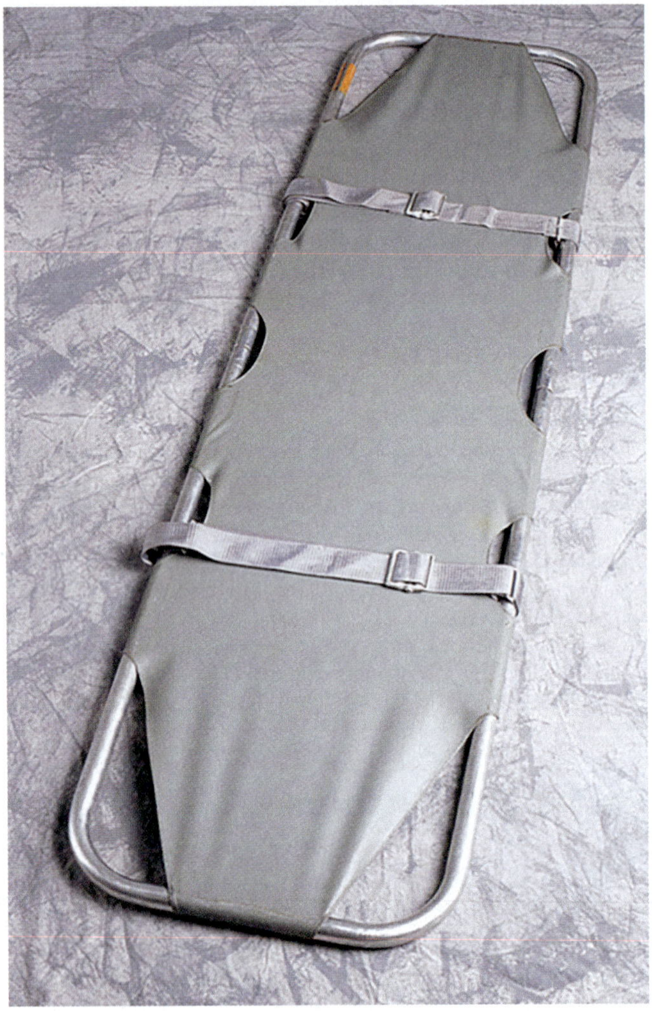

FIGURE 3-18 A portable stretcher.
© American Academy of Orthopaedic Surgeons

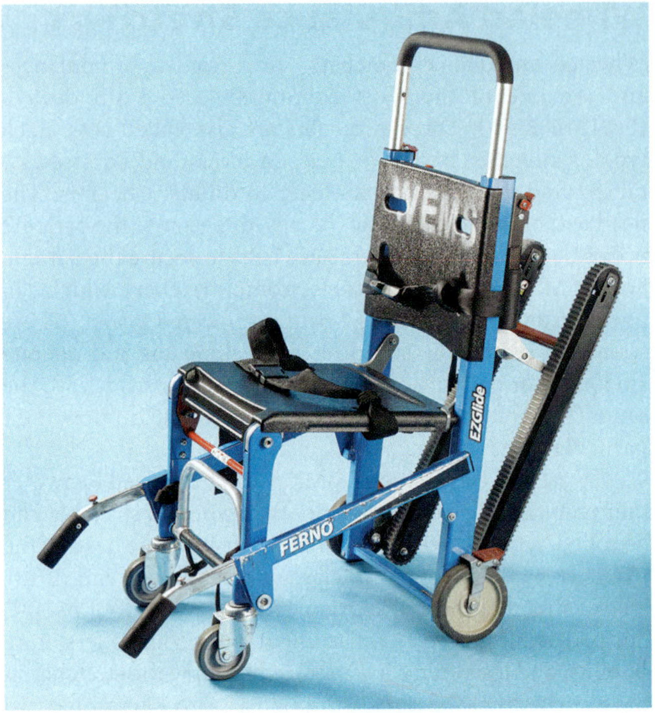

FIGURE 3-19 A stair chair.
© Jones & Bartlett Learning. Courtesy of Darren Stahlman.

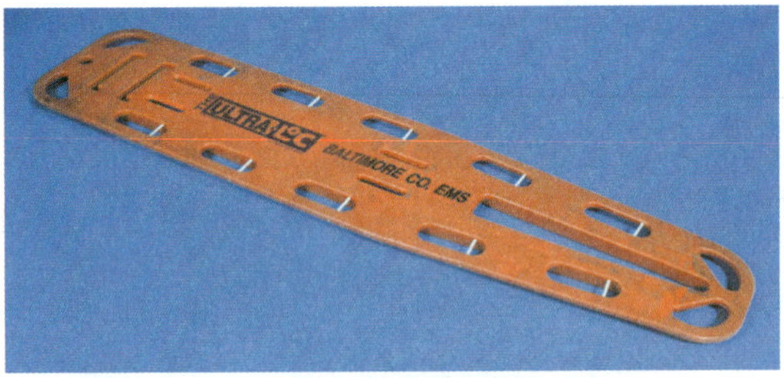

FIGURE 3-20 A long backboard.
© Jones & Bartlett Learning. Courtesy of MIEMSS.

Devices Used for Spinal Motion Restriction

Use backboards to ensure spinal motion restriction in patients who have neck or back injuries. You can also use such devices to assist in lifting patients and as an aid in immobilizing lower extremity injuries. This section discusses the use of long backboards and scoop stretchers.

Long Backboards

Use long backboards to move patients who have experienced trauma, especially if they may have neck or back injuries. You can also use long backboards for lifting and moving patients who are in tight spaces or who need to be moved off the ground or floor. Long backboards make lifting a patient much easier for the rescuers. Most long backboards are made of plastic or fiberglass. Secure the patient with straps after the individual is placed on the long backboard; if the patient has sustained back or neck injuries, stabilize the head. Procedures for assisting EMS clinicians with these devices are covered later in this chapter. One type of long backboard is shown in **FIGURE 3-20**.

Special Populations

Moving Geriatric Patients

When you move older patients, be mindful that they may have fragile bones due to osteoporosis. Move older patients carefully to avoid further injuries.

Words of Wisdom

You may be asked to assist with the removal of deceased patients, especially in mass-casualty incidents. Usually, deceased patients are placed in specifically designed body bags before removal. Body bags are flexible and difficult to carry. Removal of a deceased person is much easier for rescuers if the body is placed on a backboard or portable stretcher after being placed in a body bag. This process greatly reduces the risk of injury to rescuers. It also creates a more respectful image of the deceased person for family members, bystanders, and members of the media.

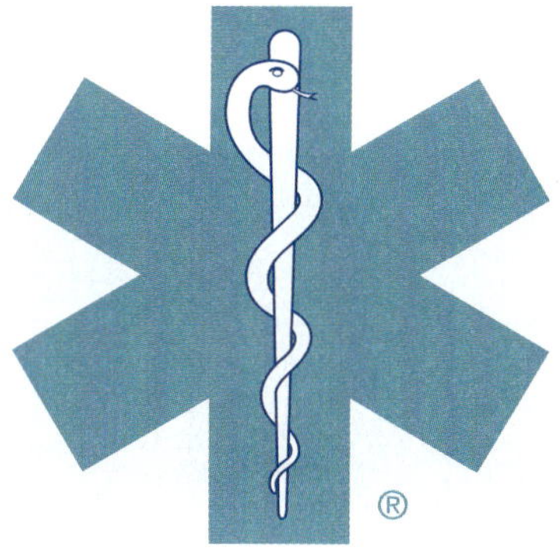

Voices OF Experience

"How are you going to get me to the ambulance? I'm a big guy!" *Good question*, I thought. He was 350 pounds (159 kg) and had experienced a stroke while in the shower in a dark, upstairs motel room. The stroke had rendered him nonambulatory. He had no clothes to grab onto and was positioned on the floor between the bed and the wall in a right lateral recumbent position. He also needed manual stabilization because of a fall. There was a four-person fire crew, my partner, and myself on scene. The small space was limiting in that not all of us would fit around the patient to appropriately care for or move him.

"Throughout the move, we stayed in constant communication with each other and with the patient."

With everyone working together, we used two sheets from the bed: one to cover him and one to position under him. The sheet under the patient would be used for the draw sheet method. The patient was moved with the long axis of his body onto the backboard while manual stabilization was maintained. A firefighter put his tarp/carry-all under the backboard prior to moving the patient, giving us more handles to safely carry him after he was secured to the backboard. The limited space around the patient allowed for only one crew member at the patient's head and one at the feet. The two of them worked together to push and pull, respectively, with the tarp/carry-all to move the patient across the balcony to the landing of the stairs. On the landing, we were able to add two crew members: one on the patient's right side and one on the left. One of the two remaining crew members went to the bottom of the stairs to position and stabilize the gurney while the other stood behind the person who was going backwards down the stairs while moving the patient to ensure the safety of his fellow crew member.

For any successful patient move, the cornerstone is communication. Prior to walking down the stairs, we discussed how the move would be executed and shared our plan with the patient. Throughout the move, we stayed in constant communication with each other and with the patient. This communication reduced the chance of injuring him or ourselves. We successfully made it to the gurney, where we continued to work as a team using a four-person lift to elevate the gurney and load the patient into the ambulance.

Once he was loaded, the patient said, "I didn't think you were going to be able to do it, but that wasn't bad at all!" That was the nicest thing I had heard all night.

Lori Gallian, Paramedic
American Medical Response
Sacramento, California

Adapted from the personal Medical Identification Symbol of the American Medical Association.

Scoop Stretchers

A **scoop stretcher,** or orthopaedic stretcher, is a rigid device that separates into a right half and a left half. Apply these devices by placing one half on each side of the patient and then attaching the two halves together. These devices are helpful when moving patients out of small spaces. Scoop stretchers are another effective tool for maintaining spinal motion restriction in patients at risk for having sustained spinal injury and for lifting patients with suspected hip dislocations or fractures. One type of scoop stretcher is shown in **FIGURE 3-21**.

If your EMS department uses scoop stretchers, practice using them. The steps for applying a scoop stretcher are shown in **SKILL DRILL 3-2**.

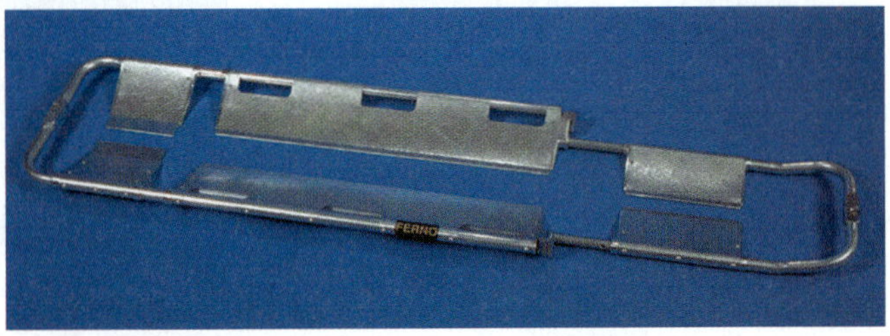

FIGURE 3-21 A scoop stretcher.

© Jones & Bartlett Learning. Courtesy of MIEMSS.

SKILL DRILL 3-2

Using a Scoop Stretcher

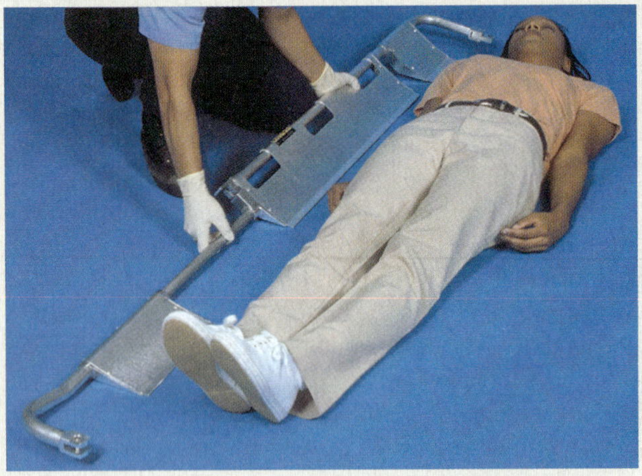

STEP 1 With the scoop stretcher separated, adjust the stretcher's length to match the patient's length.

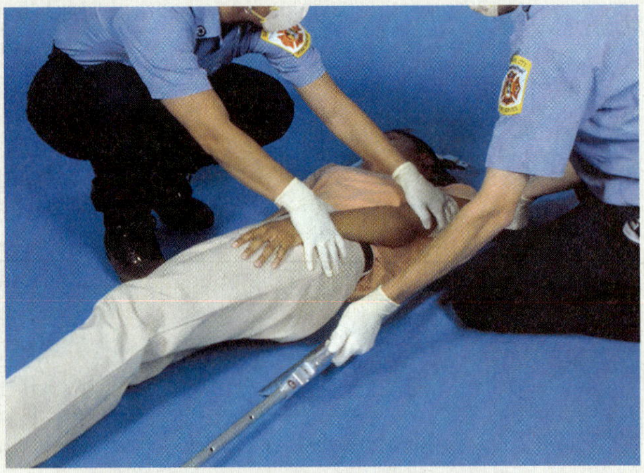

STEP 2 Position the stretcher, one side at a time. Lift the patient's side slightly by pulling on the far hip and upper arm, while your partner slides the stretcher into place.

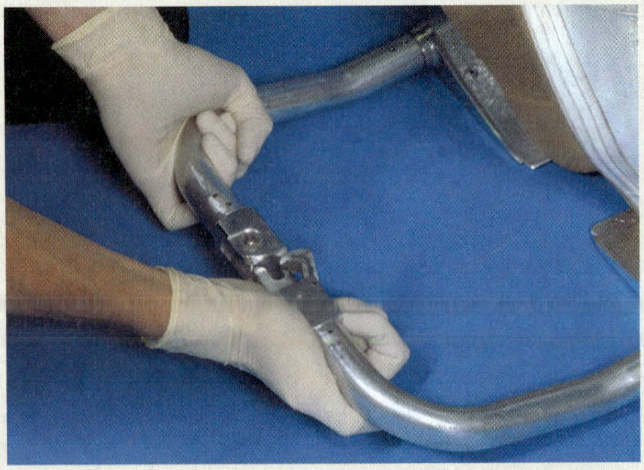

STEP 3 Lock the stretcher ends together by engaging its locking mechanisms one at a time. Continue to lift the patient slightly as needed to avoid pinching the patient and/or your fingers.

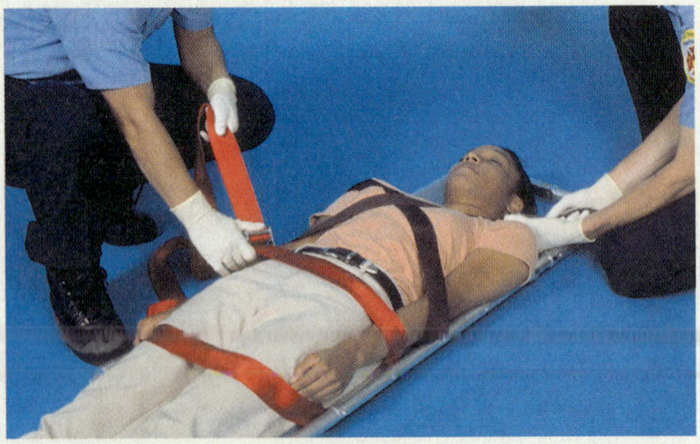

STEP 4 Apply and tighten the straps to secure the patient to the scoop stretcher before transferring it to the wheeled stretcher.

© Jones & Bartlett Learning. Courtesy of MIEMSS.

Words of Wisdom

In an emergency situation, you can use the following objects for improvised backboards:

- Wide, sturdy planks
- Doors
- Ironing boards
- Sturdy folding tables
- Full-length lawn chair recliners
- Surfboards or snowboards

Treatment of Patients With Suspected Head or Spine Injuries

Any time a patient has sustained a traumatic injury, you should consider the possibility that the patient also has an injury to the head, neck, or spine. Improper treatment can lead to permanent damage or paralysis. Provide spinal motion restriction by stabilizing the patient's head and neck in a neutral position using your hands (manual stabilization), a blanket roll, or foam blocks. It is also important that you be able to assist other EMS personnel in caring for patients who may have sustained head or spine injuries. The following sections show you how to stabilize a patient's head and neck and how to assist other EMS clinicians in placing a patient on a backboard or other device. More information on spinal cord injuries is presented in Chapter 15, *Injuries to Muscles and Bones*.

Applying a Cervical Collar

Use a **cervical collar** to minimize (but not completely prevent) movement of the patient's head and neck (**FIGURE 3-22**). These collars do not totally prevent head and neck movement; rather, they minimize the movement. After you apply a cervical collar, it is still necessary for you to manually stabilize the patient's head and neck.

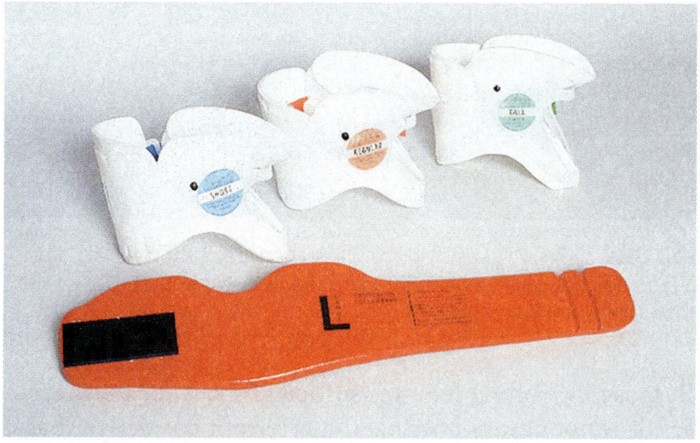

FIGURE 3-22 Types of cervical collars.

© Jones & Bartlett Learning. Courtesy of MIEMSS.

Soft cervical collars do not provide sufficient support for trauma patients. Many different types of rigid cervical collars for trauma patients are available. **FIGURE 3-23** shows how one common style of rigid cervical collar is applied. Apply the cervical collar before the patient is placed on a backboard.

Moving Patients Using Backboards

Placing a patient on a backboard is not your primary responsibility, but you may be required to assist other EMS personnel with this task. Therefore, be familiar with the proper handling of patients who must be moved on backboards. Although the specific technique you will use depends on the circumstances, the general principles described in the remainder of this chapter are relevant in nearly all cases.

The following principles of patient movement are especially important if you suspect the patient has a spinal injury:

1. Move the patient as a unit.
2. Transport the patient faceup (supine), the only position that provides adequate spinal motion restriction. However, because patients involved in acute traumatic events often vomit, be prepared to turn the patient and backboard quickly as a unit to permit the vomitus to drain from the patient's mouth.
3. Keep the patient's head and neck in a neutral position.
4. Be sure all rescuers understand what is to be done before attempting any movement.
5. Be sure one rescuer, typically the one at the head, is responsible for giving commands.

Special Populations

Securing the Geriatric Patient to a Backboard

Many older patients have irregular curves in their spine. When securing these patients to a backboard, you may need to add extra padding to conform to the unusual shape of their spine.

Words of Wisdom

In some EMS departments, EMTs or paramedics may be permitted to remove spinal motion restriction from a patient if, after following a well-defined protocol, they have determined these precautions are not necessary. As an EMR, you may not be authorized to make this decision; you should ensure spinal motion restriction is maintained until the patient has been evaluated by a more highly qualified clinician.

Assisting With Short Backboard Devices

Short backboard devices are used to provide spinal motion restriction for patients who are found in a sitting position, are alert and oriented, and have sustained isolated trauma

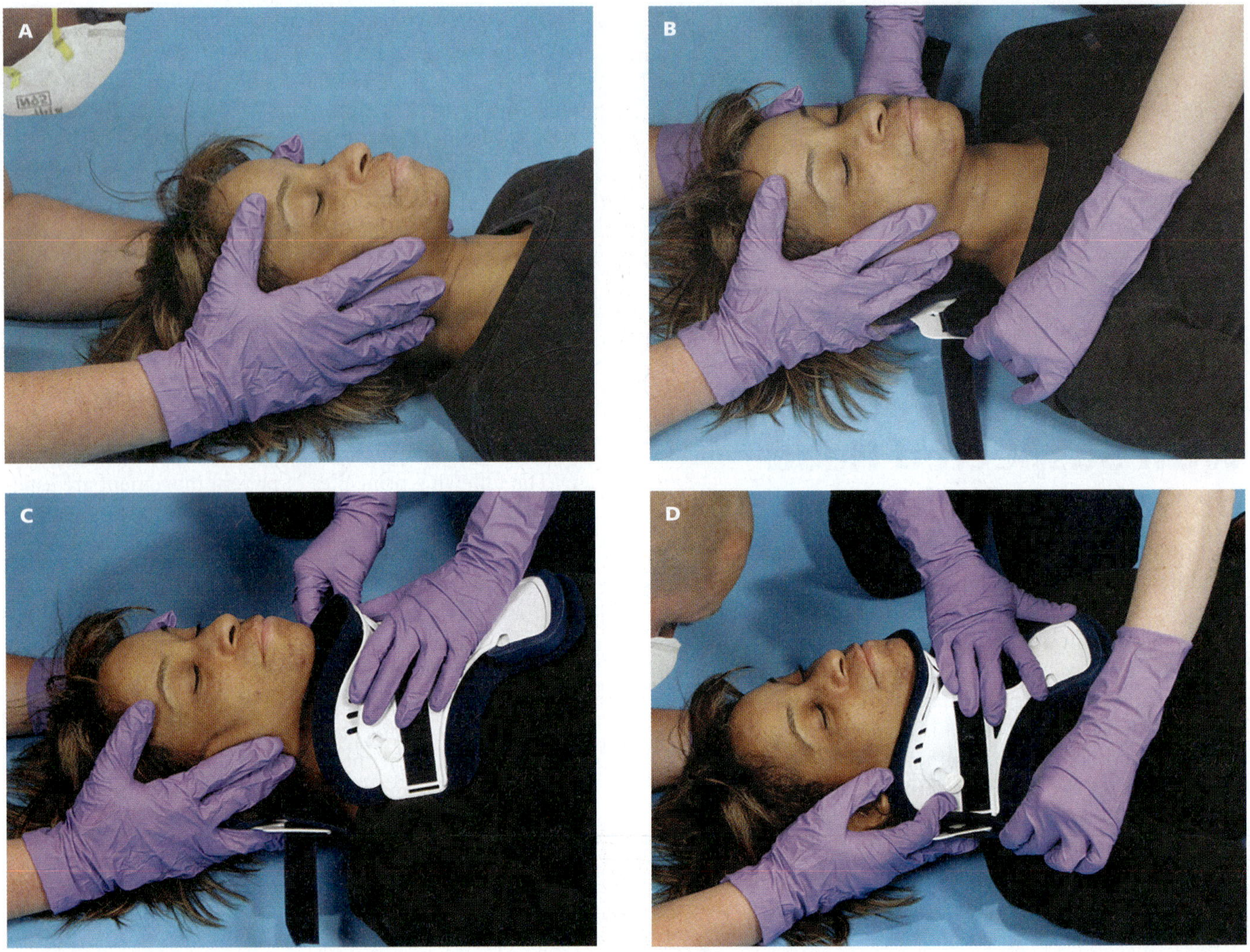

FIGURE 3-23 Applying a cervical collar. **A.** Stabilize head and neck. **B.** Insert back part of collar. **C.** Apply front part of collar. **D.** Secure collar together.

© Jones & Bartlett Learning. Courtesy of MIEMSS.

to the head, neck, or spine. Short backboard devices allow rescuers to stabilize the patient before moving. After the short backboard device is applied, the patient is carefully placed on a long backboard. As an EMR, you will not be applying a short backboard device by yourself but you may need to assist with its application. Some of these devices are in the form of a vestlike garment that wraps around the patient, sometimes called a Kendrick Extrication Device, or KED (**FIGURE 3-24**). Note that in some areas KEDs are not used, as other methods of spinal motion restriction are preferred.

SKILL DRILL 3-3 illustrates how one common type of short backboard device is applied.

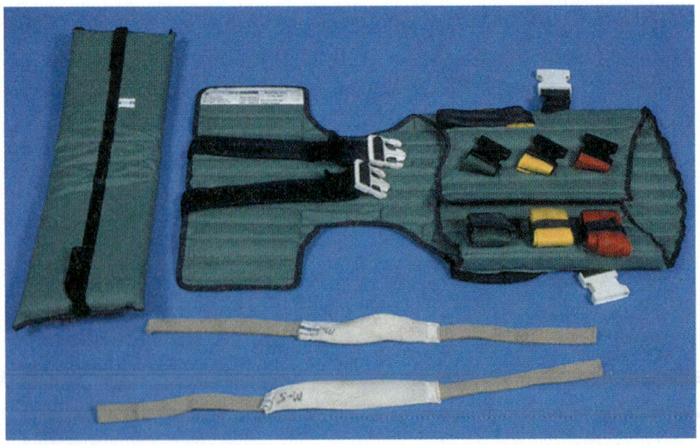

FIGURE 3-24 This vest-type device is one type of short backboard. It is sometimes called a Kendrick Extrication Device, or KED.

© Jones & Bartlett Learning. Courtesy of MIEMSS.

Log Rolling

Log rolling is the primary technique you will use to move a patient onto a long backboard. It is usually easy to accomplish, but it requires a team of four rescuers for safety and effectiveness: three to move the patient and one to maneuver the backboard. Log rolling is the movement technique of choice in all patients with suspected spinal injury. Because log rolling requires sufficient space for four rescuers, it is not always possible to perform it correctly. That is why the principles of movement, rather than specific rules, are stressed here.

SKILL DRILL 3-3

Applying a Short Backboard Device

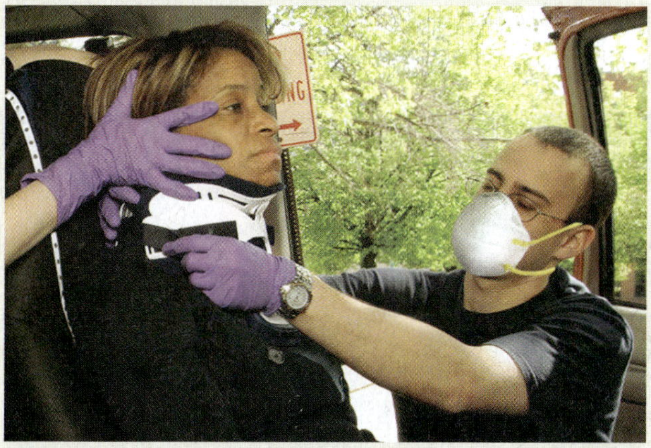

STEP 1 Position rescuer 1 behind the patient to stabilize the head. Rescuer 2 then applies a cervical collar.

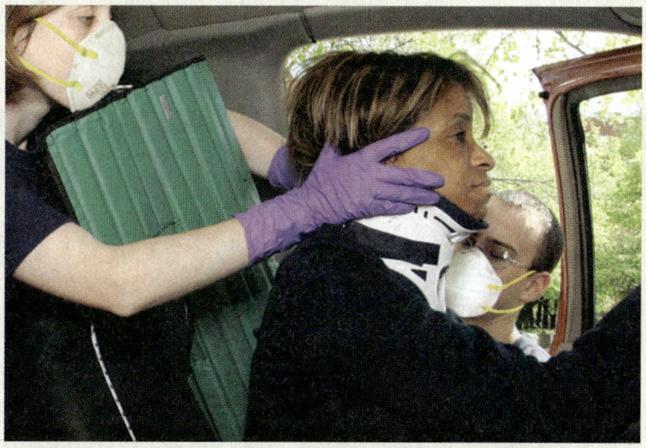

STEP 2 While both rescuers are careful to maintain neutral, in-line manual stabilization, rescuer 2 leans the patient forward and inserts the device behind the patient, starting with the head portion.

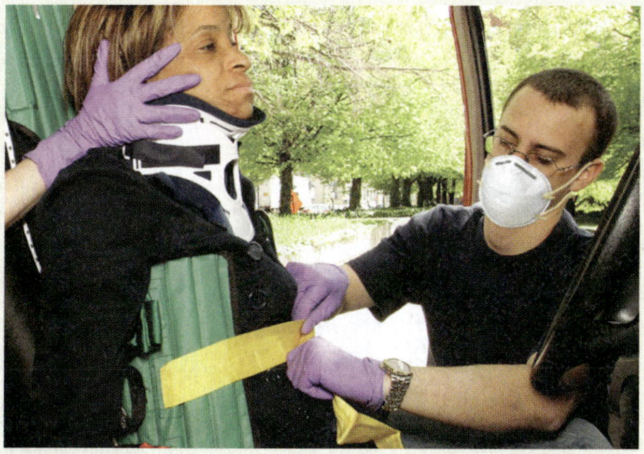

STEP 3 Rescuer 2 carefully eases the patient back against the device. Rescuer 2 fastens the middle strap of the device.

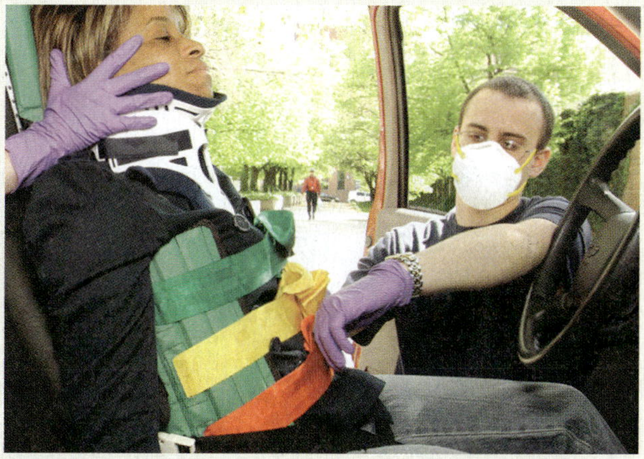

STEP 4 Rescuer 2 fastens the rest of the straps.

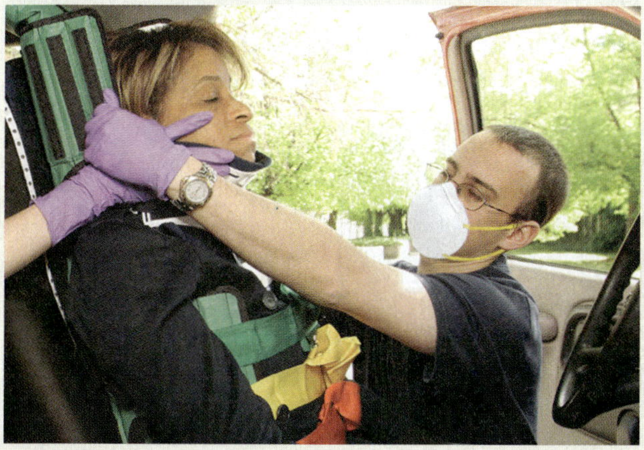

STEP 5 Rescuer 2 places the wings of the device around the patient's head.

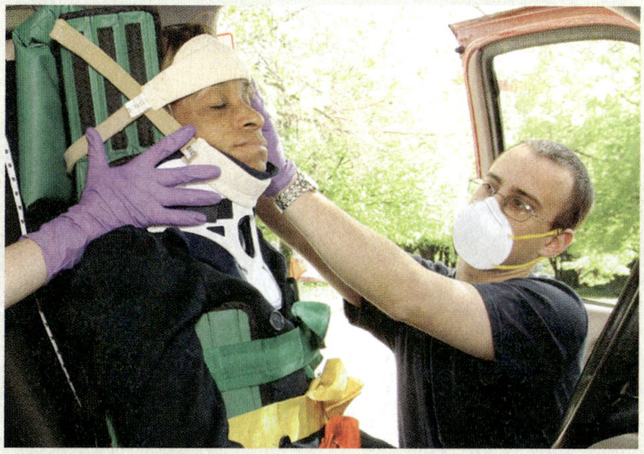

STEP 6 Rescuer 1 maintains in-line manual stabilization until rescuer 2 has secured the head strap of the device.

© Jones & Bartlett Learning. Courtesy of MIEMSS.

The procedure for the four-person log roll is shown in **SKILL DRILL 3-4**.

When using any patient movement technique, everyone must understand who is directing the maneuver, especially if you suspect the patient has a spinal injury. The rescuer holding the patient's head (rescuer 1) should always give the commands so all rescuers can better coordinate their actions. All team members must understand their specific position and function.

Although the specific wording of the command is not important, patient movement commands should have two parts: a question and the order for movement. Rescuer 1 says, "The command will be 'Ready? Roll!'" When everyone is ready to roll the patient, rescuer 1 says, "Ready?" (This

SKILL DRILL 3-4

Performing a Four-Person Log Roll

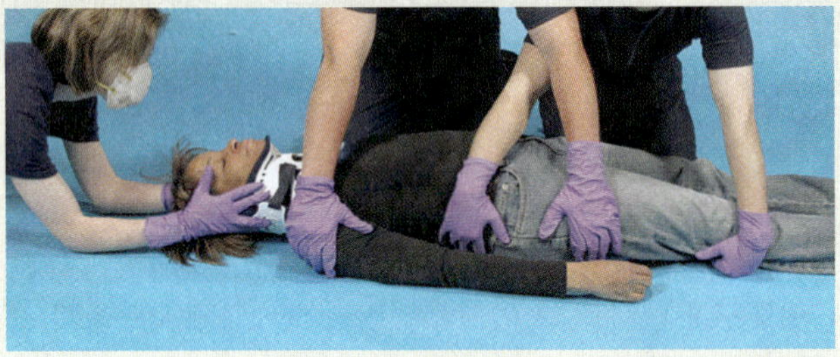

STEP 1 All rescuers get into position to roll the patient.

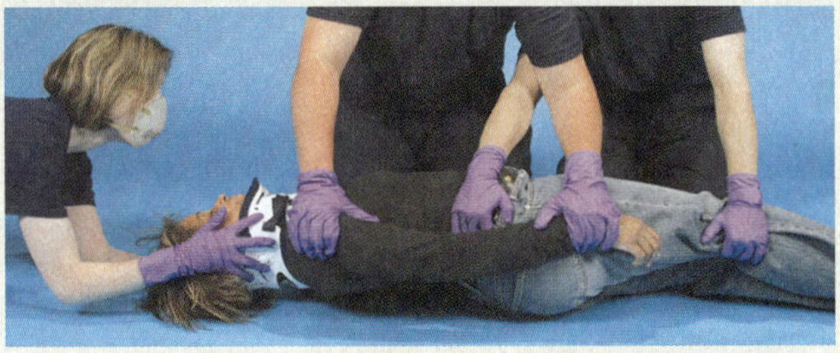

STEP 2 Rescuer 1 stabilizes the head and instructs the team. Once rescuer 1 gives the command, rescuers 2 and 3 roll the patient onto the side. All rescuers are careful to maintain spinal alignment throughout this process.

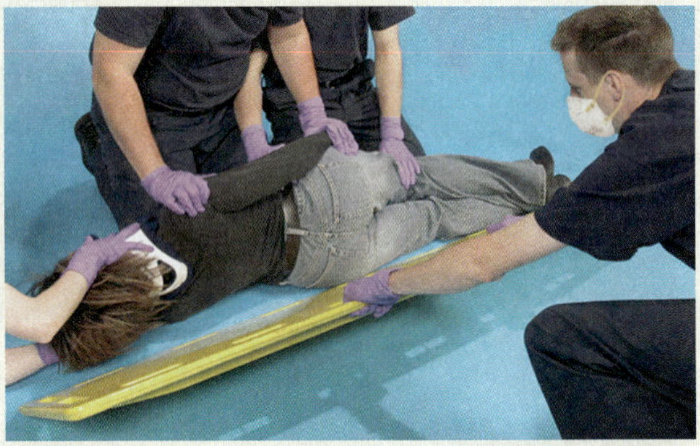

STEP 3 The fourth rescuer slides the backboard toward the patient.

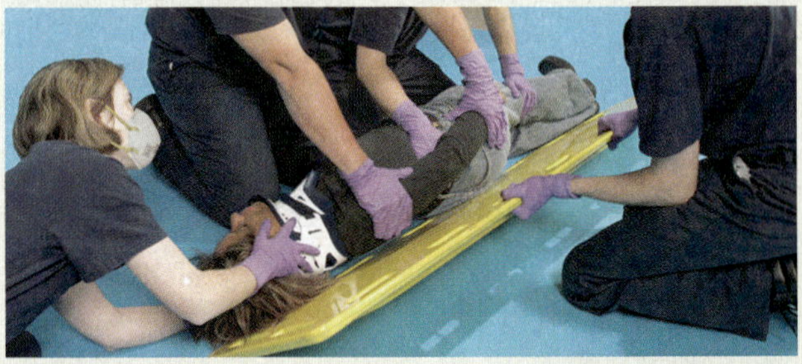

STEP 4 Once rescuer 1 gives the command, rescuers 2 and 3 roll the patient onto the backboard.

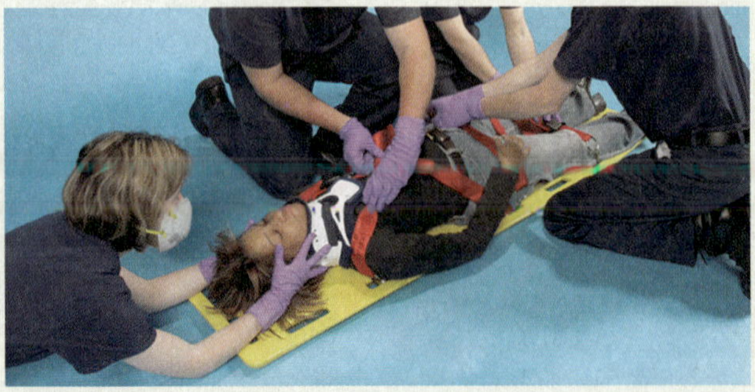

STEP 5 Rescuers center the patient on the backboard, without lateral movement, and secure the patient before moving.

© Jones & Bartlett Learning. Courtesy of MIEMSS.

question is followed by a short pause to allow for response from the team.) Then rescuer 1 says, "Roll!"

In any log-rolling technique, you must move the patient as a unit. Keep the patient's head in a neutral position at all times. Do not allow the head to rotate, move backward (extend), or move forward (flex). Sometimes this is simply stated as, "Keep the nose in line with the belly button at all times."

Car Seats and Children

The effect of mandatory child restraint laws means that EMRs are finding more children still strapped into car seats after motor vehicle crashes. You should become familiar with child restraint seats and understand how to gain access to children restrained in them. If you find a child properly restrained in a car seat, leave the child in the car seat until the ambulance arrives (**FIGURE 3-25**). In many situations, a child can be secured in the seat, the seat removed from the vehicle, and both the seat and the child transported together to the hospital (**FIGURE 3-26**).

Children younger than 9 years who are not in a booster seat but are wearing a seat belt are at risk of sliding out of the lap belt during a crash. Rapid, jackknife bending of the child's body increases the chances of intra-abdominal, spinal cord, and brain injuries.

Straps and Strapping Techniques

Secure every patient who is on a backboard with straps to prevent the patient from sliding or slipping off the backboard. There are many ways to strap a patient to a backboard. The straps should be long enough to go around the backboard and a large patient. Straps that are 6 to 9 feet (2 to 3 m) long with seat belt–type buckles work well (**FIGURE 3-27**).

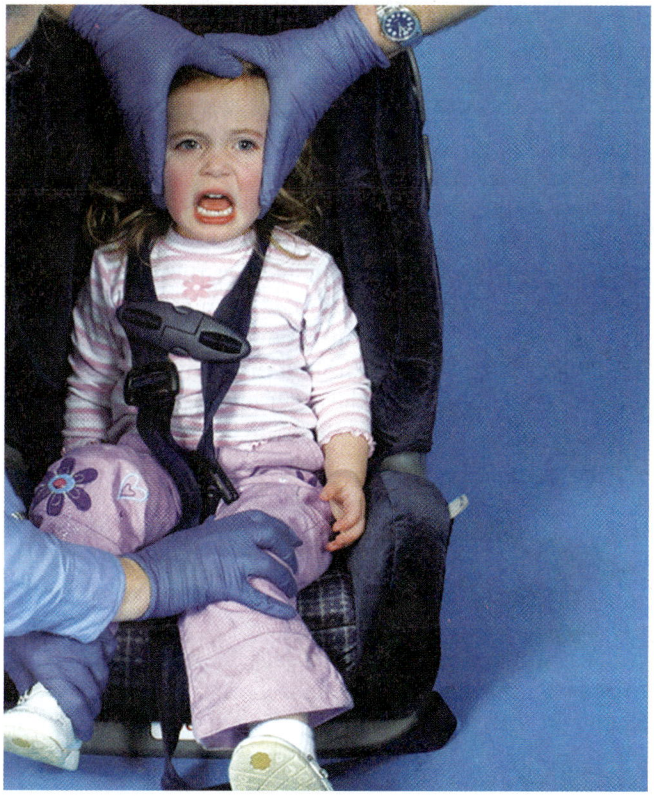

FIGURE 3-25 Leave the child in the car seat if possible.

© Jones & Bartlett Learning. Courtesy of MIEMSS.

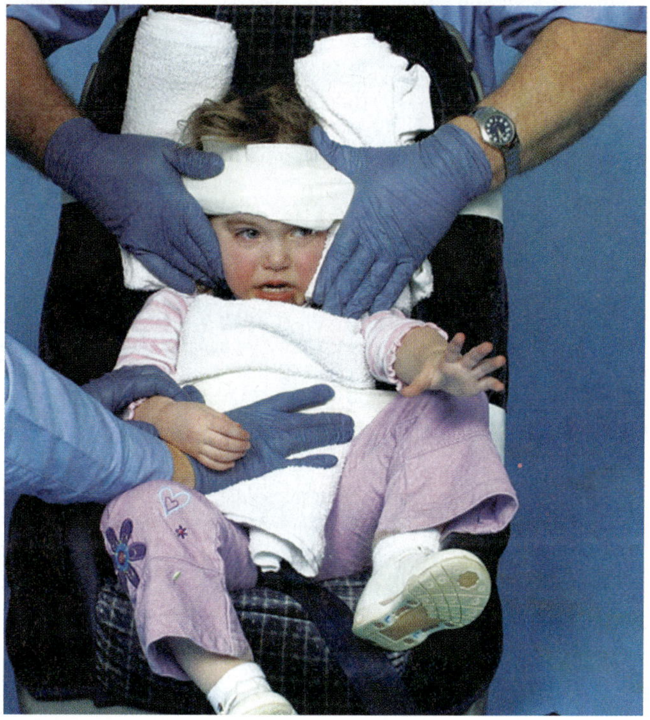

FIGURE 3-26 A child can be immobilized in the car seat.

© Jones & Bartlett Learning. Courtesy of MIEMSS.

YOU are the EMR — CASE 3

You are at the scene of a motor vehicle crash involving a vehicle that has collided with a tree. An EMS clinician is sitting behind the driver and is holding manual cervical spine stabilization. As other team members gather and prepare to put the patient on a backboard, the EMS clinician asks you to put a cervical collar on the patient.

1. What type of cervical collar should be placed on the patient?
2. Explain how you would apply a cervical collar to the patient.

Once the patient is centered on the board, secure the upper torso with straps. Consider padding voids between the patient and the backboard. Next, secure the pelvis and upper legs, using padding as needed. To reduce the risk of head movement, secure the straps around the wrist and hip area and the knees before securing the head to the backboard. Strap placement is shown in **FIGURE 3-28**. Different EMS systems use many different types of straps and strapping techniques. Learn and implement the method used by your EMS department.

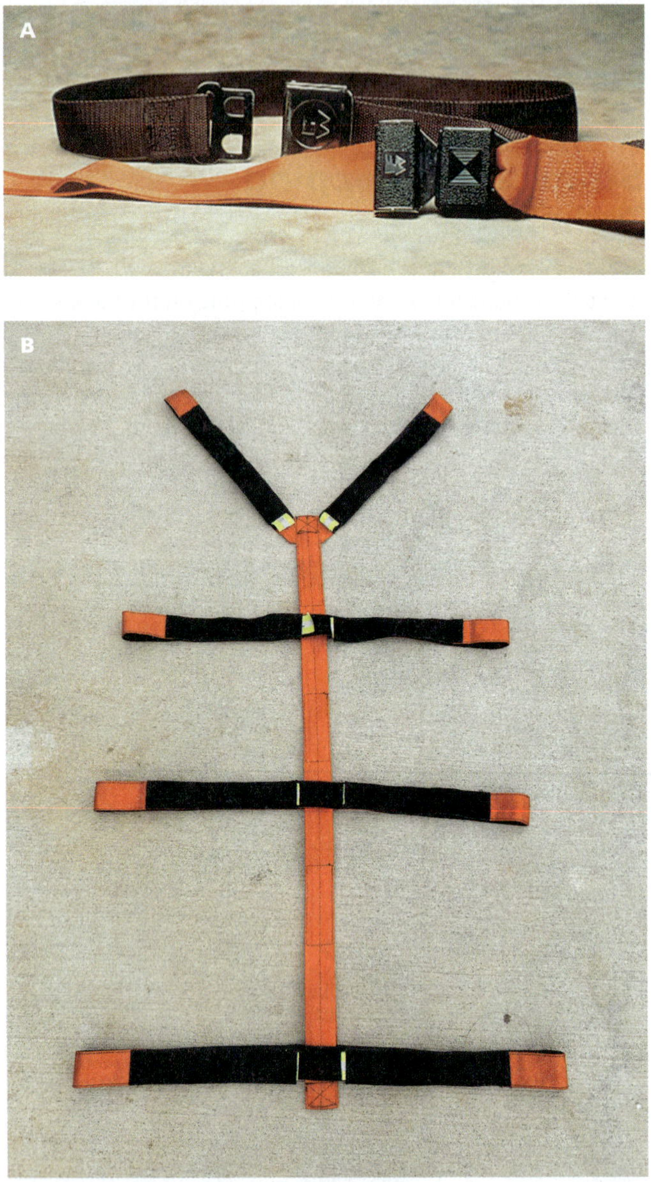

FIGURE 3-27 A. Seat belt–type straps. **B.** Spider straps.
A: © American Academy of Orthopaedic Surgeons; **B:** Courtesy of Rhonda Hunt.

Stabilizing the Patient's Head

After a patient has been secured to the backboard, stabilize the head and neck using commercially available devices (such as foam blocks) or improvised devices (such as a blanket roll). The use of a blanket roll is explained here because it works well and because a blanket is almost always available. Assemble the blanket roll ahead of time. Fold and roll the blanket (with towels as bulk filler) as shown in **SKILL DRILL 3-5**.

To place the blanket roll under a patient's head, one rescuer unrolls it enough to fit around the patient's head as another rescuer maintains manual stabilization. The rescuer holding the patient's head (rescuer 1) carefully slides their hands out from between the blanket and the patient's head, and spinal alignment is maintained by the blanket roll as shown in **SKILL DRILL 3-6**.

Provide motion restriction throughout the entire procedure (first by manually stabilizing the patient's head, then by using the blanket roll). The blanket roll must be fitted securely against the patient's shoulders to widen the base of support for the patient's head. Secure the blanket roll to the head with two cravats tied around the blanket roll: one over the patient's forehead and the other under the chin. Use two more cravats in the same positions to bind the head and the blanket roll to the backboard. The patient's head and neck are now adequately stabilized against the backboard. This head stabilization technique, coupled with proper placement of straps around the backboard, ensures spinal motion restriction of an injured patient and packages the patient for movement as a unit.

As an alternative to blanket rolls, foam blocks are quick to apply and provide good stabilization of the patient's head and neck. The use of one type of foam block is shown in **FIGURE 3-29**.

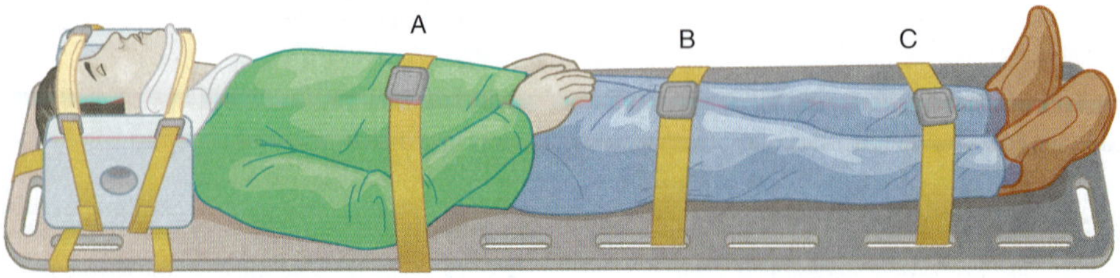

FIGURE 3-28 Strap placement for effective spinal motion restriction on a backboard. **A.** Arms. **B.** Upper legs. **C.** Below the knees.
© Jones & Bartlett Learning

SKILL DRILL 3-5

Preparing a Blanket Roll

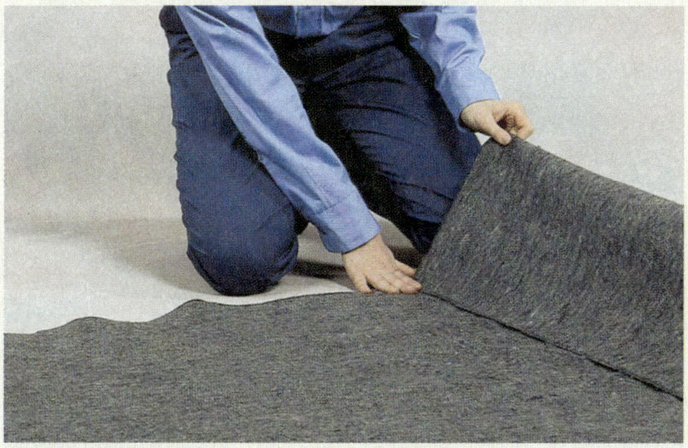

STEP 1 Fold the blanket into a long rectangular shape.

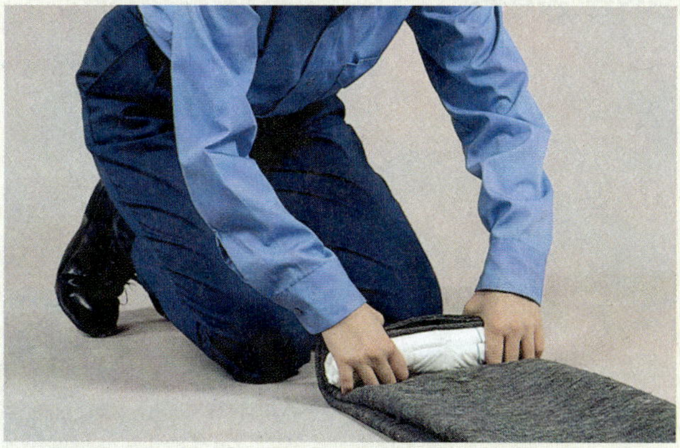

STEP 2 Insert a rolled towel and roll the blanket from each end.

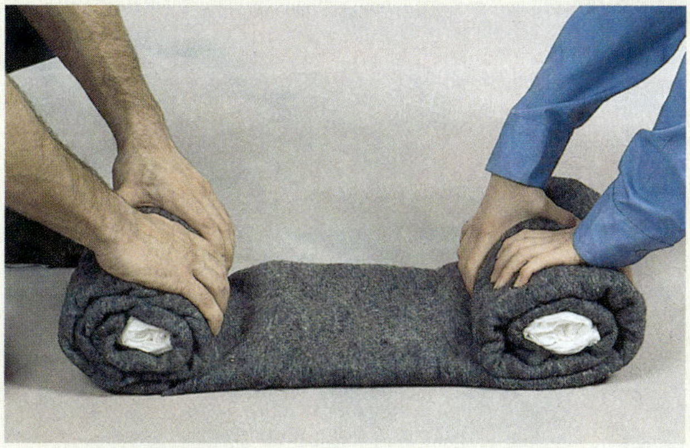

STEP 3 Roll the ends together.

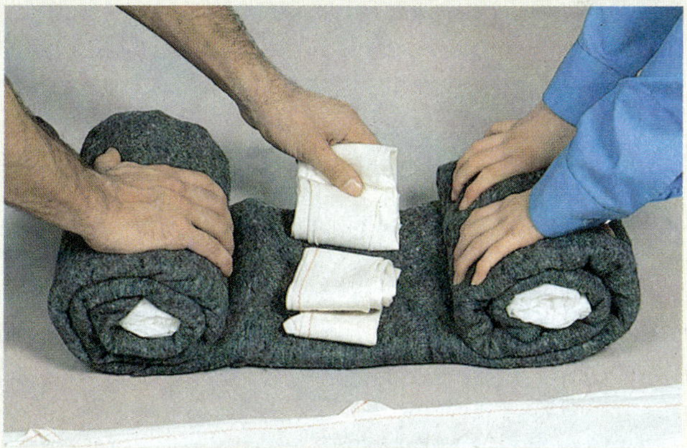

STEP 4 Place extra cravats in between the two rolled ends.

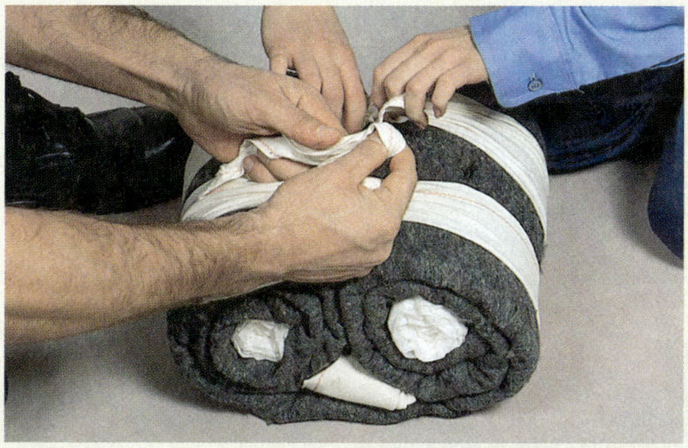

STEP 5 Tie the rolled ends together with two cravats.

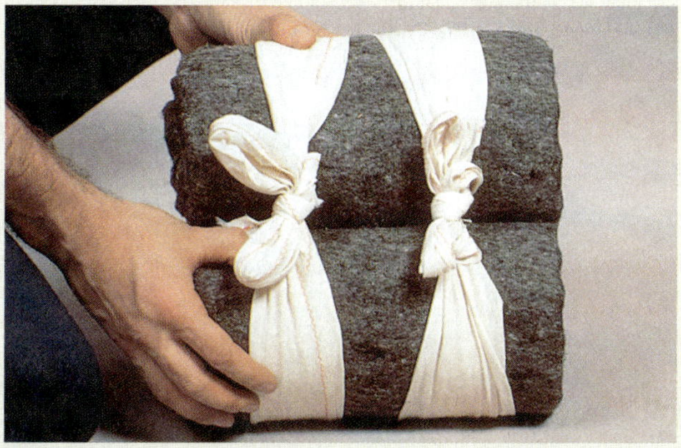

STEP 6 The finished blanket roll.

© Jones & Bartlett Learning. Courtesy of MIEMSS.

SKILL DRILL 3-6

Applying the Blanket Roll to Stabilize the Patient's Head and Neck

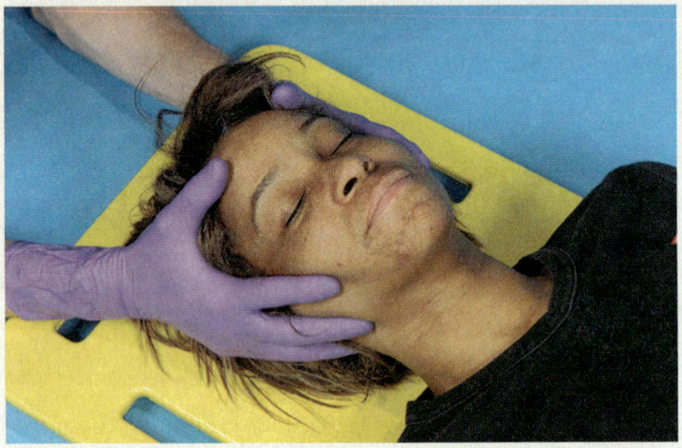

STEP 1 Rescuer 1 stabilizes the patient's head.

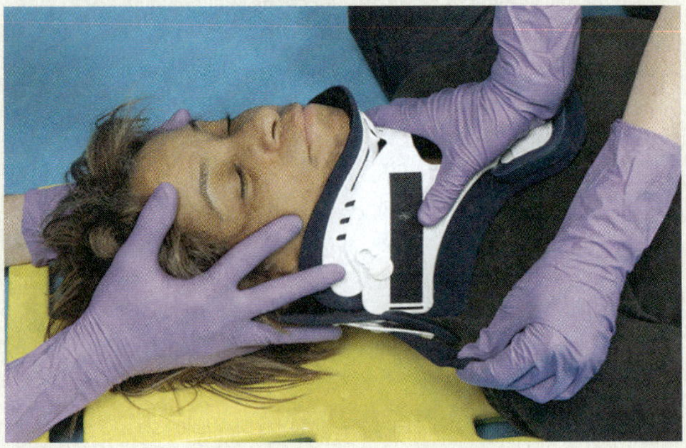

STEP 2 Rescuer 2 applies a cervical collar.

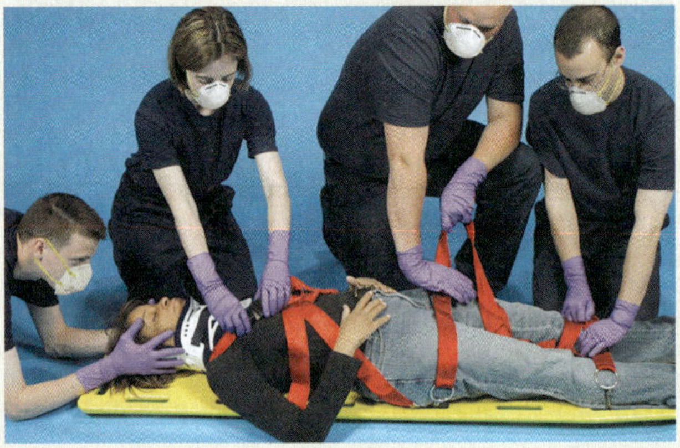

STEP 3 Place straps around the backboard and the patient.

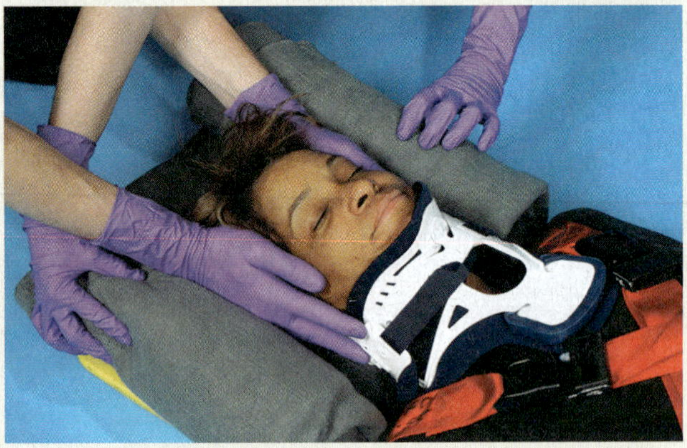

STEP 4 Insert the blanket roll under the patient's head. Roll the blanket snugly against the patient's neck and shoulders.

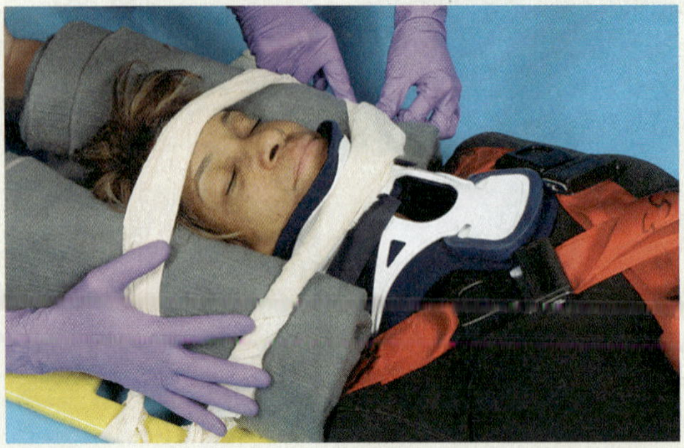

STEP 5 Tie two cravats around the blanket roll. Continue to stabilize the patient's head. Tie two more cravats around the blanket roll and backboard. Assess sensory and motor function after stabilization is completed.

© Jones & Bartlett Learning. Courtesy of MIEMSS.

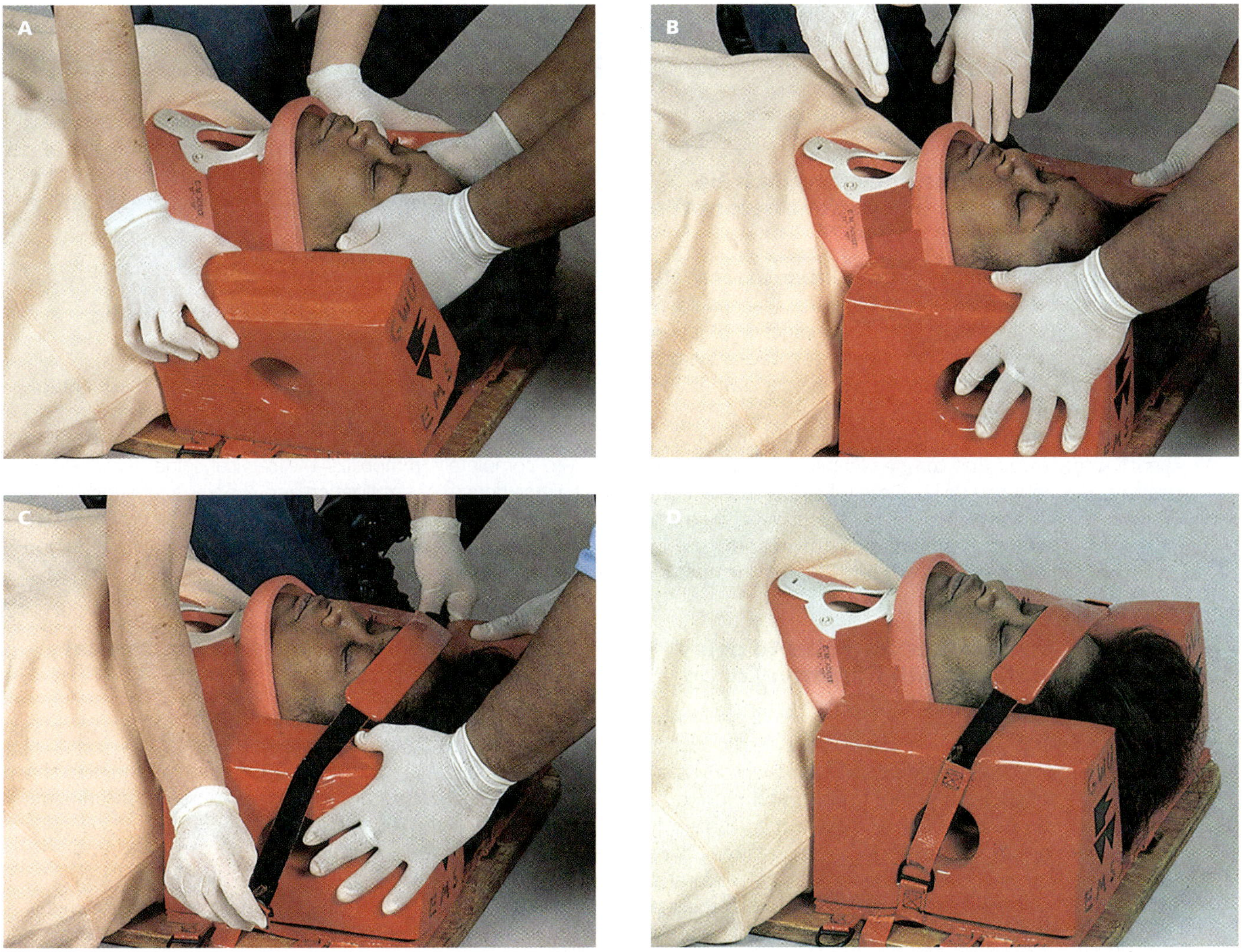

FIGURE 3-29 Application of a commercial device to stabilize a patient's head and neck. **A.** Apply the foam blocks. **B.** Secure the device. **C.** Apply the straps. **D.** The head is stabilized.
© American Academy of Orthopaedic Surgeons

In an extreme emergency where a patient must be moved from a dangerous environment and a commercially available backboard is unavailable, improvise. Make sure the improvised backboard is strong enough to hold the patient without breaking. Use improvised devices only when a patient must be moved to prevent further injury or death and when a commercially available backboard is not available.

Words of Wisdom

Before stabilizing the head, check for obvious injuries as well as blood or fluid draining from the ears. Once a blanket roll or other device is in place, you will not be able to visualize those covered areas.

YOU are the EMR — CASE 4

You are dispatched to a nearby apartment for a report of an unresponsive man. After a short drive, you arrive at the apartment and are directed to a bathroom by the man's wife. She appears to be about 70 years old. As you enter the tiny bathroom, you find a man who appears to have been sitting on the toilet. He is now slumped against the wall. He does not respond to verbal stimuli. He does not appear to be breathing, and you determine he has no carotid pulse.

1. How do you decide whether or not to move this patient before you begin further assessment and treatment?
2. If you decide you need to move this patient, what method would you use?

YOU are the EMR SUMMARY

You are the EMR: CASE 1

1. Under what circumstances would it be necessary to move this patient before the EMS transport unit arrives?

One of the most important decisions facing you as an EMR is whether to move a patient. Generally, you should not move a patient except in extreme emergency situations. These include fires, explosions, structural collapse, the presence of hazardous materials, unsafe vehicle crash scenes, and situations where you need to move a patient to perform CPR. In general, when an imminent threat to the patient's safety exists that can be eliminated by moving the patient, it is better to do so. Otherwise, it is usually better to wait for additional personnel before moving a patient. Place the patient in a comfortable position and cover her with a blanket to preserve body heat. Treat the injuries you are equipped to treat.

2. Why is it often better for EMRs to delay moving a patient until the arrival of an EMS transport unit?

There are several reasons why it is usually better to wait for additional EMS clinicians before moving a patient. EMTs and paramedics have more training in lifting and moving patients. EMS transport units carry a variety of equipment for lifting and moving patients. The expression "Many hands make light work" is certainly true here. Injuries to rescuers are less likely and patient safety is enhanced when there are enough people to move a patient. Because EMRs usually do not transport patients, there is no hurry to move patients before the arrival of an EMS transport unit unless one of the emergency situations discussed in the chapter is present.

You are the EMR: CASE 2

1. How can you quickly remove this patient from the burning vehicle?

First, decide if you can safely rescue the driver from this vehicle without risk of harm to you. If you determine a rescue attempt is feasible, approach the vehicle and try to open a door. Determine if the patient can assist with his own rescue. If the patient is unresponsive, you will need to grasp the patient under his arms. Cradle the patient's head between your arms. Pull the patient down into a horizontal position as you ease him from the vehicle. Although there is no effective way to remove a patient from a vehicle by yourself without causing some movement, it is important to try to prevent excess movement of the patient's neck. Use this technique only if the patient is in danger and must be moved.

2. How do you determine where to place this patient after removal?

Move the patient only as far as you need to get him to a safe place. In this case, you need to get the patient far enough from the burning vehicle that the vehicle fire will not pose a danger to either you or the patient. You also need to consider traffic hazards. Place the patient where distracted drivers will not cause further harm to the patient.

You are the EMR: CASE 3

1. What type of cervical collar should be placed on the patient?

A variety of cervical collars are available in the prehospital environment. Trauma patients should receive a rigid cervical collar. Although these devices are not designed to completely immobilize the cervical spine, they provide some degree of stabilization and serve as a reminder to the patient not to move the head and neck. The proper size of the collar is key. Most commercial cervical collars allow you to adjust the size of the collar; therefore, adjust the collar to create the best fit for the patient.

2. Explain how you would apply a cervical collar to the patient.

Begin by selecting the appropriate cervical collar and size. Make sure someone is maintaining manual in-line cervical spine stabilization during this procedure, and remind this person to continue providing stabilization even after the collar is in place. Then, slide the back portion of the collar along the posterior portion of the patient's neck. Wrap the front portion of the collar around the anterior aspect of the neck, making sure the chin is properly seated in the chin-groove of the collar. Finally, secure the collar in place using the straps.

You are the EMR: CASE 4

1. How do you decide whether or not to move this patient before you begin further assessment and treatment?

It is not unusual to discover a patient in cardiac arrest in a small bathroom. This patient will require a lot of care to give him the best chance for recovery. If the bathroom is too small for all the necessary rescuers to enter and provide adequate treatment, then it is better to quickly move the patient to a larger room. It is easier to move this patient before you begin treatment than to start treatment in a tight space and then try to move the patient.

2. If you decide you need to move this patient, what method would you use?

If the patient is wearing sufficient clothing, then grasp the patient's clothing in the neck and shoulder area, rest the patient's head on your arms, and quickly drag the patient from the tight space to a larger room that has space to perform CPR and ALS skills. You may also need to move furniture out of the way to provide enough space. You can accomplish these actions in a short time.

Prep Kit

Ready for Review

- In most situations, you can treat the patient in the position found and later assist other EMS personnel in moving the patient. In some situations, however, the patient's survival may depend on your knowledge of emergency movement techniques.
- Every time you move a patient, keep the following general guidelines in mind:
  - Do no further harm to the patient.
  - Move the patient only when necessary.
  - Move the patient as few times as possible.
  - Move the patient's body as a unit.
  - Use proper lifting and moving techniques to ensure your own safety.
  - Have one rescuer give commands when moving a patient.
- Always use good body mechanics when you move patients, including:
  - Know your own physical limitations and capabilities.
  - Keep yourself balanced when lifting or moving a patient.
  - Maintain a firm footing.
  - Lift and lower the patient by bending your legs, not your back. Keep your back as straight as possible at all times and use your leg muscles to do the work.
  - Keep your arms close to your body for strength and balance.
- Place unresponsive patients who have not sustained trauma in the recovery position.
- If a patient is lying on the floor or ground during an emergency situation, you may have to drag the person away from the scene instead of trying to lift and carry the person. Make every effort to pull the patient in the direction of the long axis of the body to protect the patient's spine.
- Do not lift or move a patient if you suspect a spinal injury, unless it is necessary to remove the patient from a life-threatening situation.
- EMS departments typically use wheeled ambulance stretchers, portable stretchers, stair chairs, long backboards, short backboards, and scoop stretchers to help stabilize and/or move patients.
- Any time a patient has sustained a traumatic injury, you should consider the possibility of an injury to the head, neck, or spine. Keep the patient's head in a neutral position and restrict motion. Use a cervical collar, along with manual stabilization, to prevent excessive movement of the head and neck.
- Log rolling is the primary technique you will use to move a patient onto a backboard. Secure every patient who is on a backboard with straps to prevent sliding or slipping.
- After you secure a patient to the backboard, provide spinal motion restriction using commercially available devices or improvised devices.

Vital Vocabulary

arm-to-arm drag An emergency move that consists of the rescuer grasping the patient's arms from behind; used to remove a patient from a hazardous environment.

bariatric Relating to or specializing in the prevention and treatment of obesity.

blanket drag An emergency move in which a rescuer encloses a patient in a blanket and drags the patient to safety.

cervical collar A neck brace that partially stabilizes the neck following injury.

clothes drag An emergency move used to remove a patient from a hazardous environment; performed by grasping the patient's clothes and moving the patient headfirst from the unsafe area.

cradle-in-arms carry A one-rescuer patient movement technique used primarily for children; the patient is cradled in the hollow formed by the rescuer's arms and chest.

extremities The arms and legs.

firefighter drag A method of moving a patient without lifting or carrying; used when the patient is heavier than the rescuer. The rescuer places the patient's tied hands around their neck and drags the patient by crawling on the hands and knees.

log rolling A technique used to move a patient onto a long backboard; four rescuers work together to ensure spinal alignment while turning the patient onto a side.

Prep Kit

one-person walking assist A method in which one rescuer supports the patient from a side while walking; used if the patient is able to bear their own weight.

pack-strap carry A one-person carry in which the rescuer backs into the patient and positions the patients such that their armpits are over the rescuer's shoulders and the arms hang over the rescuer's chest; the rescuer holds the patient's wrists with one hand and carries the patient, with one hand free.

portable stretcher A lightweight, nonwheeled device for transporting a patient; used in small spaces where the wheeled ambulance stretcher cannot be used.

recovery position A side-lying position that helps an unresponsive patient maintain an open airway.

scoop stretcher A firm device used to carry a patient; can be split into halves and applied to the patient from both sides.

stair chair A small portable device used for transporting a patient in a sitting position.

two-person chair carry A method of carrying a patient in which two rescuers use a chair to support the weight of the patient.

two-person extremity carry A method of carrying a patient out of tight quarters in which two rescuers use the patient's extremities, one reaching under the patient's arms and holding the wrists and the other backing between the patient's legs and holding the legs, to carry the patient; requires no equipment.

two-person seat carry A method of carrying a patient in which two rescuers link arms behind the patient's back and under the patient's knees; requires no equipment.

two-person walking assist A method in which two rescuers support the patient's full weight from each side while walking; used when a patient cannot bear their own weight.

References

Emergency medical services clinician injury data. Centers for Disease Control and Prevention website. https://www.cdc.gov/niosh/ems/data/?CDC_AAref_Val=https://www.cdc.gov/niosh/topics/ems/data.html. Published February 16, 2024. Accessed November 19, 2024.

EMS safety. NAEMT website. https://www.naemt.org/initiatives/ems-safety. Accessed November 19, 2022.

National Association of State EMS Officials. *National EMS Scope of Practice Model 2019.* Washington, DC: National Highway Traffic Safety Administration; February 2019. Report No. DOT HS 812-666. https://www.ems.gov/assets/National_EMS_Scope_of_Practice_Model_2019.pdf. Accessed November 19, 2024.

National Association of State EMS Officials. *National Model EMS Clinical Guidelines: Version 3.0.* https://nasemso.org/wp-content/uploads/National-Model-EMS-Clinical-Guidelines_2022.pdf. Published March 2022. Accessed November 19, 2024.

National Highway Traffic Safety Administration. *National Emergency Medical Services Education Standards.* EMS.gov website. https://www.ems.gov/assets/EMS_Education-Standards_2021_FNL.pdf. Published 2021. Accessed November 19, 2024.

Reichard AA, Marsh SM, Tonozzi TR, Konda S, Gormley MA. Occupational injuries and exposures among emergency medical services workers. *Prehosp Emerg Care.* 2017;21(4);420–431.

Assessment IN ACTION

You and your partner have been called to an assisted-living facility to help evacuate patients because flood-waters caused by a hurricane are threatening to cut off the access road to the facility. The officer in charge assigns you and your partner to one wing that has four patients. He asks you to bring the patients to the front lobby where they will be assigned to vehicles for evacuation.

1. Which of the following techniques is NOT an example of good body mechanics when moving patients?
   - **A.** Lift and lower by bending your legs, not your back.
   - **B.** Do not try to lift too heavy a load.
   - **C.** Try to keep your arms away from your body for strength and balance.
   - **D.** Move the patient as few times as possible.
2. Which of the following situations is NOT a reason for using an emergency drag to move a patient?
   - **A.** To begin CPR on a patient who has experienced cardiac arrest
   - **B.** To remove the patient from a scene that cannot be protected
   - **C.** To remove the patient from a noisy environment
   - **D.** To remove the patient from the scene of an explosion, fire, or structural collapse
3. The first resident tells you he can walk slowly, but he is weak. Which technique would you use to move this man to the lobby?
   - **A.** Two-person walking assist
   - **B.** One-person walking assist
   - **C.** Two-person extremity carry
   - **D.** Pack-strap carry
4. The second room is occupied by a woman who has a brace on her ankle. She is not supposed to put weight on her broken ankle. Which of the following carries would you consider using for this patient?
   - **A.** Two-person extremity carry
   - **B.** Pack-strap carry
   - **C.** Two-person chair carry
   - **D.** Direct ground lift
5. On the third floor, you find an 82-year-old woman who says she has a heart condition and gets short of breath if she walks very far. The elevator is not working. How would you move this person, assuming the following equipment is available?
   - **A.** Scoop stretcher
   - **B.** Long backboard
   - **C.** Stair chair
   - **D.** Portable stretcher
6. The fourth person is confined to bed because she experienced a stroke 2 years ago. A nurse brings you a stretcher and asks you to use it to move the patient. How would you move this woman to the stretcher?
   - **A.** Draw sheet method
   - **B.** Log roll
   - **C.** Clothes drag
   - **D.** Direct ground lift

Assessment IN ACTION

7. Which of the following is an important consideration when lifting and moving older adults?
   A. Their bones may be more fragile, and thus more susceptible to injury, than those of younger adults.
   B. More rescuers will be required to maintain spinal motion restriction.
   C. They tend to weigh less than younger adults, so maintaining proper lifting mechanics is less important.
   D. Because older adults often take multiple medications, ALS presence is always required before moving an older adult.

8. Why is it important for you and your partner to communicate when lifting and moving patients?

9. You are assigned to assist with getting patients from the front lobby into emergency medical services vehicles for evacuation. What type of devices can be used for patients who are supine?

10. When you are moving a patient on a portable stretcher, what are some important lifting techniques to keep in mind?

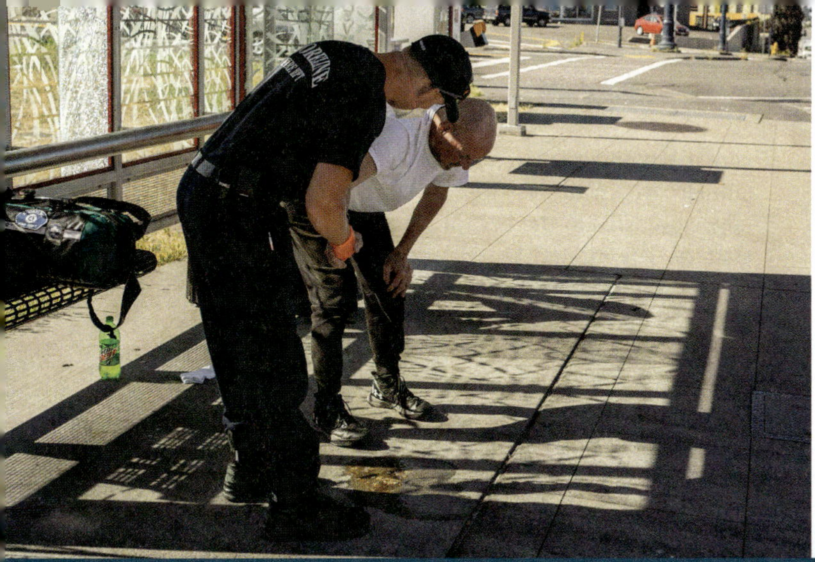

CHAPTER 4

Medical, Legal, and Ethical Issues

National EMS Education Standard Competencies

Preparatory

Uses knowledge of the emergency medical services (EMS) system, safety/well-being of the emergency medical responder (EMR), medical/legal issues, and ethical issues at the scene of an emergency while awaiting a higher level of care.

Medical/Legal and Ethics

- Consent/refusal of care (pp 69–70)
- Confidentiality (p 73)
- Advance directives (p 70)
- Tort and criminal actions (p 68)
- Evidence preservation (p 74)
- Statutory responsibilities (pp 68–72; pp 73–74)
- Mandatory reporting (p 73)
- Ethical principles/moral obligations (pp 68–74)
- End-of-life issues (pp 68–74)

Knowledge Objectives

1. Describe the legal duty to act for an emergency medical responder (EMR). (p 68)
2. Explain how to comply with the standard of care. (p 68)
3. Discuss the ethical responsibilities of an EMR. (p 68)
4. Define *consent*, and include how it relates to decision making. (p 69)
5. Differentiate between expressed consent and implied consent. (pp 69–70)
6. Discuss consent as it relates to minors who require treatment or transport. (p 69)
7. Discuss consent as it relates to patients with a mental illness. (p 69)
8. Discuss the EMR's role and obligations if a patient refuses treatment or transport. (p 70)
9. Discuss the three types of advance directives and how they impact patient care. (p 70)
10. Explain the legal concepts of abandonment, people dead at the scene, negligence, and confidentiality. (pp 70–72; p 73)
11. Recognize that most patient information is confidential and protected by the Health Insurance Portability and Accountability Act (HIPAA). (p 73)
12. Describe the role of Good Samaritan laws. (p 73)
13. Explain the requirements for reportable events, including crimes and certain infectious diseases. (p 73)
14. Explain the reasons for documentation. (p 74)

Skills Objectives

There are no skills objectives for this chapter.

© David Ryder/Getty Images News/Getty Images

Introduction

As an emergency medical responder (EMR), you need to know some basic legal principles that guide how you provide care to patients. Knowing these principles can help you provide the best possible care for your patients and prevent situations that could result in legal difficulties for you, your public service agency, or your department. Because some laws differ from one location to another, you will need to learn the specific laws of your state and your local jurisdiction (ie, the area in which you work). It is easy to become concerned about the legal consequences of providing emergency medical care or immediate care or treatment. Remember the following concepts when providing patient care:

- Above all else, do no harm.
- Provide all your care in good faith, keeping the patient's best interest uppermost in your mind.
- Provide proper, consistent care; be compassionate; and maintain your composure.

These concepts can help prevent many of the legal issues that are discussed in this chapter.

Duty to Act

The first legal principle to consider is the **duty to act**. An uninvolved citizen (bystander) who arrives on the scene of a motor vehicle crash is not required by law to stop and give emergency care to injured people. However, if you are employed by an agency that has designated you as an EMR and you are dispatched to the scene of an injury or illness, then you do have a duty to act. You must proceed quickly to the scene and provide emergency medical care within the limits of your training and available equipment (**FIGURE 4-1**). Any failure to respond or provide necessary emergency medical care leaves both you and your agency vulnerable to legal action.

Standard of Care

What level of care are you expected to give to a patient? As a trained EMR, you cannot provide the same level of care as a physician, but you are responsible for providing the level of care that a person with similar training would provide under similar circumstances. You are expected to use your knowledge and skills to the best of your ability under the circumstances. The circumstances under which you must provide care may affect the standard of care. The **standard of care** is the manner in which you must act or behave. To comply with the standard of care, you must meet two criteria. First, you must treat the patient to the best of your ability. Second, you must provide care that a reasonable, prudent person with similar training would provide under similar circumstances. It is important to know your local standards of care and what statutes affect your community. Failure to provide proper care because of a wrongful act could result in legal action being taken against your public safety agency or against you as an individual health care clinician. A wrongful act is called a tort by the legal community.

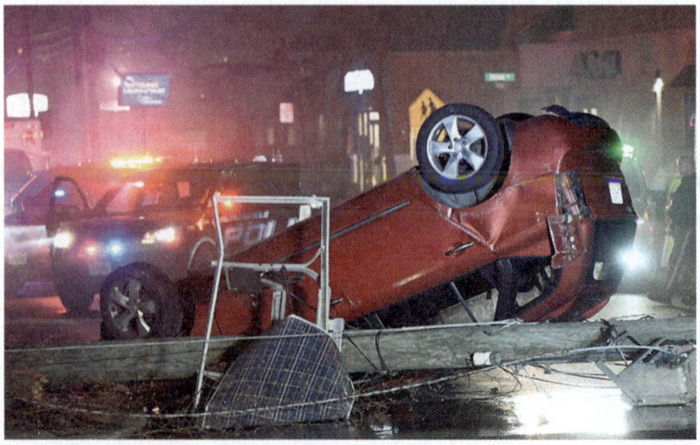

FIGURE 4-1 EMRs have a duty to act when dispatched to an emergency scene.
© Kyle Mazza/NurPhoto/AP Photo

Scope of Practice

The scope of practice that guides an EMR is defined on several levels. The *Emergency Medical Responder Education Standards*, originally developed by the US Department of Transportation, specify the skills taught in this course and the way those skills should be performed. These standards have evolved into the current *National Emergency Medical Services (EMS) Education Standards*. States also have scope-of-practice laws that may modify the specifications in the education standards. In most states, a law outlines the roles and responsibilities of EMRs. You are required to operate under the direction of a medical director. The medical director for your department may use medical protocols, or **standing orders**, to specify your scope of practice. In some cases, online medical direction is provided by radio or telephone. Your state gives you the responsibility to practice within the limits specified within the law. You have a professional responsibility to your patients, to your medical director, and to the public you serve.

Ethical Responsibilities and Competence

Your community and your department have entrusted you, as an EMR, with certain moral and ethical responsibilities. This moral responsibility means that the community expects you to follow the established codes of what is right and wrong. It is your ethical responsibility as an EMR to follow these codes. Treating a patient ethically means doing so in a manner that conforms to accepted professional standards of conduct. These standards include staying up to date on the EMR skills and knowledge you need to provide high-quality patient care. You are also responsible for reviewing your performance and assessing the techniques you use. Evaluate your response times, and try to follow up on patient care outcomes with your medical director or hospital personnel. Always look for ways to improve your performance. Continuing education classes and refresher courses are designed to keep your knowledge and skills current. It is in your best interest to make the most of these opportunities. It is also a good idea to participate in quality improvement activities within your department.

Words of Wisdom

Certification as an EMR is itself a legal process that is subject to a variety of federal, state, local, and agency regulations. To assume the professional responsibilities of an EMR, you must properly attain certification and keep it up to date. Chapter 1, *EMS Systems*, discusses the certification and registration process.

Ethical behavior requires honesty. Your reports should accurately reflect the conditions found at the scene. Always provide complete and correct reports to other EMS clinicians. If you make a mistake on the report or document information incorrectly, do not try to cover it up. Never change a report except to correct an error. See Chapter 5, *Communications and Documentation*, for more information about reporting.

Remember, the actions you take in the first few minutes of an emergency may make the difference between life and death for a patient. Your ethical behavior and competence will be invaluable to both you and your patient.

Consent for Treatment

Consent simply means giving approval or permission. Legally, there are a few key concepts the EMR should understand regarding consent. With **expressed consent**, the patient explicitly, whether verbally or nonverbally, accepts the treatment you are offering. Expressed consent is based on the idea that the patient has the right to determine what will be done to their body. The patient must be of legal age (in most states, 18 years or older) and able to make a rational decision. Expressed consent is sometimes called actual consent.

Ideally, from both a legal and an ethical standpoint, the patient's consent will be not only clearly expressed but also well informed. Thus, you should understand the concept of **informed consent**. As you approach a patient, be sure the patient understands who you are, tell them what you are going to do, and be sure they agree to treatment. For example, if you say, "You have a cut on your arm. I need to bandage it to stop the bleeding," and the response is "OK," then the patient has given you both expressed consent and informed consent.

In situations in which a patient is under the influence of alcohol or other drugs, has a mental impairment, or has a medical condition that affects their mental status, it may be hard to determine whether the patient is capable of making decisions about their health care. In these situations, carefully explain to the patient what needs to be done and try to provide the necessary care.

Any patient who is not in a position to specifically refuse emergency medical care can be treated under the principle of **implied consent**. The principle of implied consent is best understood in the situation of an unresponsive patient. Because an unresponsive patient is unable to communicate, the law assumes the patient would agree to treatment if they were able to do so. Therefore, never hesitate to treat an unresponsive patient.

Consent for Minors

A minor is a person who has not yet reached the legal age designated by a particular state. Under the law, minors (usually people younger than 18 years) are not considered capable of speaking for themselves. Many states have laws that permit a minor to have the rights of an adult if the minor is considered emancipated. Learn the laws of your state related to the issues surrounding emancipated minors. If a minor requires emergency medical care in the field (out of the hospital) and you cannot quickly get the permission of a parent or legal guardian, then do not hesitate to give appropriate emergency medical care. Never delay or withhold emergency medical treatment of a minor just to obtain permission from a parent or legal guardian (**FIGURE 4-2**). Let hospital officials determine what treatment can be postponed until permission is obtained. Remember, good prehospital patient care is your first responsibility. By following the course of action that is best for the patient, you will stand on firm legal ground.

Consent of Patients With a Mental Illness

An adult who is alert, oriented, and mentally in control is said to have **decision-making capacity**. This person may legally refuse to be treated, even if doing so may result in serious injury or death. The legal issues are more complicated if the patient who refuses to be treated appears to be out of touch with reality and is a danger to themself or others. The difficult part, even for highly trained medical personnel, is determining whether such a patient is rational and has decision-making capacity. Generally, if the person appears to be a threat to self or others, then arrangements need to be made to place this person under medical care. The legal means by which these arrangements are made vary from state to state. You and other members of the EMS system should

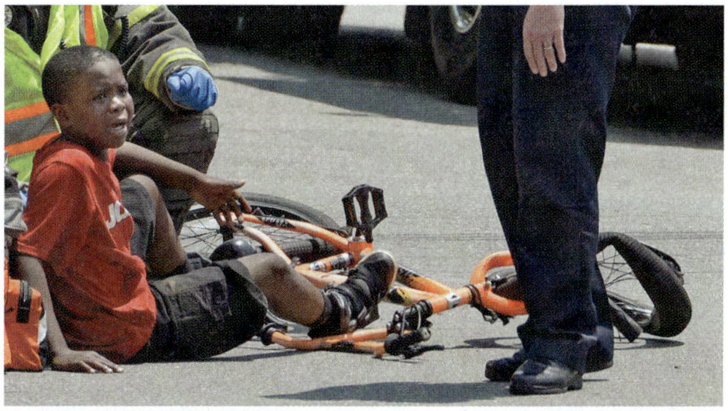

FIGURE 4-2 Do not delay or withhold emergency medical treatment from a patient who is a minor.

© Sam Roberts/The Times-News/AP Photo

know your local policies for patients who refuse to be treated and do not appear to be making rational and reasonable decisions. Do not hesitate to involve law enforcement agencies, because this process may require the issuance of a warrant or an order of protective custody.

Patient Refusal of Care

An adult with decision-making capacity has a legal right to refuse treatment from emergency medical personnel at any time. You can continue to talk with a person who refuses treatment and try to help them understand the consequences of this action. Explain the treatment to the person, why it is needed, the potential risks if treatment is not provided, and any alternative treatments that may help. Sometimes another EMS clinician or a law enforcement officer may have more success in convincing a patient of the need to receive treatment. When patients are firm in their refusal, tell them they should call EMS again if they change their mind. Carefully document patient refusals on your patient care report according to your agency protocols. Many agencies require a second person to witness a refusal. Follow all local EMR protocols related to patient refusal of care.

Advance Directives

An **advance directive** is a document that specifies what a person would like to be done if the person becomes unable to make their own medical decisions. Three kinds of advance directives exist. The first is called a **living will**. A living will is a written document drawn up by a patient, a physician, and a lawyer. A living will states the types of medical care a person wants, or wants withheld, if the person becomes unable to make their own treatment decisions. Living wills are often written when a patient has a terminal (incurable) condition. A living will does not let the person select someone to make decisions for them.

A second type of advance directive is a **durable power of attorney for health care** or medical power of attorney. A durable power of attorney for health care allows a patient to designate another person to make decisions about medical care for the patient if they cannot make decisions for themselves. The person designated to be a patient's health care representative is often a family member. This representative may be referred to as the patient's health care agent or health care proxy.

A **do not resuscitate (DNR) order** is the third type of advance directive. It is a written request giving permission to medical personnel to withhold resuscitation in the event of cardiac arrest. Additional terms for these types of orders that are often used include medical orders for life-sustaining treatment (MOLST) or physician's orders for life-sustaining treatment (POLST). You should be familiar with the types of forms used in your area and with how to identify if they have been properly completed and validated. Advance directives may include DNR orders but are not required to include them. DNR orders are most frequently used for patients who are in hospitals or nursing homes and are most common in cases of terminal disease or medical futility.

If you are unable to determine whether an advance directive is legally valid, then begin appropriate medical care and leave the questions about advance directives to physicians. Some states have systems, such as bracelets, to identify patients with advance directives. Know your local policies and protocols.

Legal Concepts

As an EMR, it is important for you to understand some legal concepts that relate to your work. These concepts include abandonment, death of a patient at the scene, negligence, and confidentiality. Each of them is explained in this section.

Abandonment

Abandonment occurs when a trained person begins emergency medical care and then leaves the patient before another trained person arrives to take over. After you have started treatment, you must continue that treatment as long as the scene is safe and until a person who has skills and/or training at the same or a higher level arrives on the scene and takes over or until you deliver the patient to another medical care clinician at a medical facility. Never leave a patient without

> **Safety**
>
> In the event of a scene that becomes unsafe, try to take the patient with you. If the patient is unable to walk, or you are unable to move the patient, leave the patient at the scene and return when it is safe to do so. Personal safety comes first, even after patient care has been initiated.

YOU are the EMR — CASE 1

You respond to a call for an unresponsive 85-year-old man who is not breathing. Over the phone, dispatch attempted to guide family members through the steps of cardiopulmonary resuscitation (CPR). The family members are not able to follow the dispatcher's instructions. On your arrival, family members say they think the man has a DNR order; however, they are unable to provide you with the document.

1. What should you do in this situation?
2. What level of emergency medical care should you provide?

care after you begin treatment. The most common abandonment scenario occurs when an EMS clinician responds to a call, examines the patient, assesses the patient's condition, fails to transport the patient to a hospital, and finds out later that the patient died. Emergency medical care began, but the patient was abandoned.

Patient Death at the Scene

If you see any signs that a person is alive when you arrive on the scene, then begin providing necessary care. People who are obviously dead should be handled according to the laws of your state and the protocols of your service. Generally, you cannot assume a person is dead unless one or more of the following conditions exist:

- **Decapitation.** Decapitation means that the head is separated from the body. When this occurs, there is obviously no chance of saving the patient.
- **Rigor mortis.** Rigor mortis is the temporary stiffening of muscles that occurs several hours after death. The presence of this stiffening indicates the patient is dead and cannot be resuscitated.
- **Tissue decomposition.** Once body tissue begins to decompose and flesh begins to decay, any attempt at resuscitation is futile.
- **Dependent lividity.** **Dependent lividity** is the red or purple color that occurs in the parts of the patient's body that are closest to the ground. It is caused by blood seeping into the tissues in the dependent, or lower, part of the person's body. Dependent lividity occurs after a person has been dead for several hours.

If one or more of these signs are present, then you can consider the patient to be dead. Know the protocol your department uses in dealing with patients who are dead on the scene (**FIGURE 4-3**). Chapter 8, *Professional Rescuer CPR*, covers these criteria as they relate to starting CPR.

Words of Wisdom

You must understand how these legal concepts guide your patient care and behavior on scene:

- Abandonment
- Patient death at the scene
- Negligence
- Confidentiality

Negligence

Negligence is the failure of a medical clinician at any level to meet the required standard of care. For a legal claim of negligence to be sustained, four conditions must be present:

1. Duty to act
2. Breach of duty
3. Resulting injuries
4. Proximate cause

As an EMR who has been dispatched or otherwise called to the scene of an incident to provide patient care, you will have a duty to act to help the patient. This means that you have a duty to provide care within your scope of training and certification, in a manner in which a reasonable, similarly trained and certified clinician would, under similar circumstances. Failure to provide such care represents breach of duty. If the patient sustains injury that can be directly attributed to your actions (proximate cause), then you may be considered negligent and therefore considered responsible for causing those injuries. For example, if you drag a patient with a neck injury out of a vehicle without providing spinal

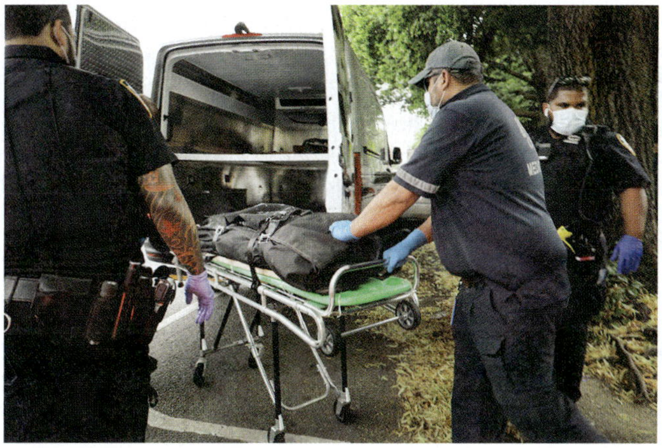

FIGURE 4-3 Learn the protocol for dealing with patients who are obviously dead at the scene.

© Spencer Platt/Getty Images News/Getty Images

YOU are the EMR — CASE 2

You are dispatched to a call for a 9-year-old boy who was bitten by a dog. When you arrive, the child is crying and holding his head. He is bleeding from a gash on the side of his cheek. He tells you his parents are not home. A police officer is nearby, and she reports that she has also been unsuccessful in reaching the parents. The child says he has no other relatives in the area that he can call.

1. You ask the child if you can help and he says yes. What should you do next?
2. You have finished applying a bandage to the wound on the boy's cheek when the police officer tells you she still cannot reach the parents. Because you treated the bite wound, can you now leave the child alone?

Voices OF Experience

I was the attendant-in-charge dispatched to a rollover motor vehicle crash at about 0230 hours one dreary, rainy night. Dispatch information told me a sport utility vehicle (SUV) was involved and our county sheriff's department was already at the scene. We were sent to direct aid with an adjoining fire department engine that arrived on scene first. We arrived on scene a couple of minutes after the engine and discovered there were multiple patients. I made contact with the engine company lieutenant and became the medical group supervisor.

The story was a sad one. The sheriff deputy already had taken the driver of the SUV into custody. He told me there were four occupants in the SUV who were taking methamphetamines and drinking alcohol. They were not wearing any vehicle restraints. When the sheriff had tried to pull the vehicle over, the driver evaded the pursuit and in the ensuing chase, the SUV rolled over and ejected three of the four occupants.

> **"I can recall thinking to myself that this was not what I had come into this profession to do."**

I began triage and found one passenger on the roadside, screaming in pain from an open femur fracture. There were already EMTs preparing her for transport. I immediately called for a second EMS unit. The other two occupants had been thrown from the vehicle in opposite directions. They were approximately 25 feet (8 m) from the vehicle, sustaining fatal injuries. These two patients were teenagers. To this day, I can recall thinking to myself that this was not what I had come into this profession to do. I didn't like the tremendous responsibility of declaring someone dead. I was there to save the lives of people. Look at this tragedy; these two young people had no futures ahead of them. Did their parents know where they were?

I persuaded the sheriff's department to release the driver into my care for evaluation at the emergency department. Due to the mechanism of injury and the deaths of the other occupants as risk factors, it was important to have the driver examined for any hidden injuries. As I transferred the patient to the bed in the emergency department, a vial of methamphetamines fell out of his pocket. He lay there laughing, displaying no remorse for the deaths of his friends.

As an EMS provider, it is difficult to respond to situations like this one. Ethically, it can be a challenge to treat patients who act irresponsibly and put their own lives and the lives of others in unnecessary danger. However, we must put our own personal feelings aside and treat the patient regardless of our feelings. In situations like this one, it is helpful to have the assistance of a law enforcement officer to ensure scene safety while the patients are triaged and treated. Police assistance is especially important in cases where drug and alcohol use may affect the behavior of the patients.

T. J. Bishop, NREMT-P
Clinical Officer
North Country EMS
Yacolt, Washington

Adapted from the personal Medical Identification Symbol of the American Medical Association.

motion restriction and that patient becomes paralyzed as a direct result of your actions, then you could be considered negligent and responsible for causing the spinal cord injury. In contrast, if the patient later falls during physical therapy and breaks a leg, you would not be responsible for the broken leg because your action in dragging the patient from the vehicle was not the direct cause of the broken leg.

Confidentiality

Most patient information is confidential. Confidential information includes the patient history, assessment findings, and treatment provided, as well as your communication with the patient. This information should be shared only with other medical personnel who are directly involved in the patient's care. Do not discuss this private information with your family or friends. Most departments have strict policies prohibiting the release of any patient information over social media.

In certain situations, you may release confidential information to designated people. In most states, records may be released when a legal subpoena is presented or the patient signs a written release. The patient must have decision-making capacity and fully understand the nature of the release.

Some information about a patient's care may be classified as public information. This information often includes the patient's name, address, and age and the hospital to which they were transported. Learn what patient information is considered public information in your state. Public information can be released to the news media through your department's approved process.

HIPAA

HIPAA is the acronym for the Health Insurance Portability and Accountability Act of 1996. Although this act had many aims, including improving the portability and continuity of health insurance coverage and combating waste and fraud in health insurance and in the provision of health care, the section of the act that most affects EMS relates to patient privacy. The aim of this section was to strengthen laws for the protection of the privacy of health care information and to safeguard patient confidentiality. It provides guidance on what type of information is protected, the responsibility of health care clinicians regarding that protection, and the penalties for breaching that protection.

Most personal health information is protected and should not be released without the patient's permission. If you are not sure, then do not give any information to anyone other than those directly involved in the care of the patient. For specific policies, each EMS agency is required to have a manual and a privacy officer who can answer questions. You can expect to receive further training on how HIPAA affects your specific response agency and resource hospital.

Words of Wisdom

In this time of ever-present digital devices and phones with cameras, realize that patient confidentiality extends to photographs and videos. Do not take or send images of a patient without permission of both the patient and your supervisor.

Good Samaritan Laws

Most states have adopted **Good Samaritan laws**, which protect citizens from liability for errors or omissions in giving good faith emergency medical care. These laws vary from state to state, and they may or may not apply to EMRs in your state.

Any properly trained EMR who practices the skills and procedures learned in an EMR course should not be overly concerned about lack of protection under Good Samaritan statutes.

Reportable Events

State and federal agencies have requirements for reporting certain events, including crimes and certain infectious diseases. Reportable crimes vary by state and often include knife wounds, gunshot wounds, motor vehicle crashes, suspected child abuse, intimate partner violence, elder abuse, dog bites, and rape. Learn which crimes are reportable in your area and know your agency's procedures for reporting these crimes. It is important that you learn how this process is handled in your agency and what you are required to do. Failure to notify proper authorities of reportable events may result in penalties against you or your agency.

Crime Scene Operations

Many emergency medical situations are also crime scenes. As an EMR, keep the following considerations in mind:

- Protect yourself. Be sure the scene is safe before you try to enter.

YOU are the EMR **CASE 3**

As a new EMR, you have mastered the knowledge and skills covered in your course. However, you are concerned about the possibility of making a mistake that might result in legal action against you or your department.

1. How does the concept of a standard of care protect you?
2. Why is the concept of confidentiality so important for you to follow?

- If you determine that a crime scene is unsafe, then wait in a safe location until law enforcement personnel tell you the scene is safe for entry.
- Your first priority is patient care. Nothing except your personal safety should interfere with that effort.
- When you assess the scene, document anything you see that seems unusual.
- Move the patient only if necessary, such as for rapid transport to the hospital, for administration of CPR, or for treatment of severe shock. If you must move the patient, then take a mental snapshot of the scene.
- Touch only what you need to touch to gain access to the patient.
- Preserve the crime scene for further investigation (**FIGURE 4-4**). Do not move furniture or objects unless they interfere with your ability to provide care. If you must move anything out of the way, then move it no further than necessary to provide care.
- Be careful not to cut through knife or bullet holes in the patient's clothing.
- Be careful where you put your equipment to avoid changing or destroying evidence.

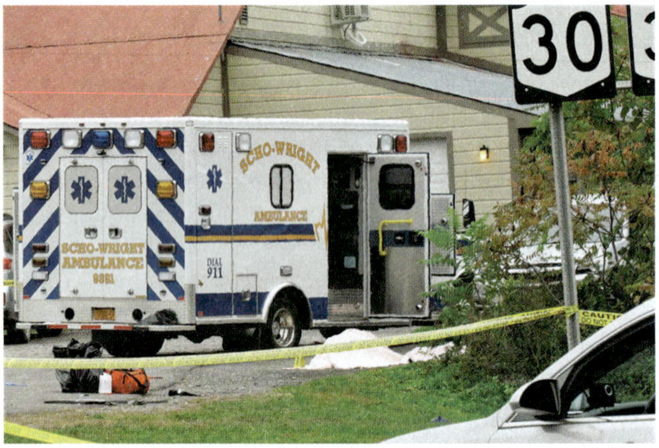

FIGURE 4-4 Try to cause as little disruption to a crime scene as possible without compromising patient care.
© Tom Heffernan Sr./AP Photo

- Keep nonessential people, such as curious bystanders, away from the scene.
- Work with the appropriate law enforcement authorities on the scene to ensure that everyone has the information they need.
- After you have attended to a patient at a crime scene, write a report about the incident as soon as possible and make a sketch of the scene that shows how and where you found the patient. This may be useful information if you are required to recall the incident 2 or 3 years later.

Documentation

After you have finished treating the patient, record your observations about the scene, the patient's condition, and the treatment you provided. Complete your documentation according to the policies of your organization. These policies should follow appropriate local and state laws. Your documentation is important because it is the initial account describing the patient's condition and the care administered. You will not be able to remember the treatment you provide to each patient without documentation. It also serves as a legal record of your treatment, and it will be required in the event of a lawsuit. Documentation also provides a basis for evaluating the quality of care you provided.

Documentation should be clear, concise, accurate, and readable. Documentation may be completed using a paper form or an electronic device. Documentation should include the following information:

- A description of the scene
- The condition of the patient when found
- The patient's description of the injury or illness
- The patient's initial and repeat vital signs
- The treatment you gave the patient
- The agency and personnel who took over treatment of the patient
- Any reportable conditions present
- Any infectious disease exposure
- Anything unusual regarding the situation

More information on documentation is presented in Chapter 5, *Communications and Documentation.*

YOU are the EMR — CASE 4

You and your partner are sent to the home of a 63-year-old woman who is reporting difficulty breathing and minor chest pain. She is in a part of the house that will require you to use a stair chair to get her to the street. While your partner is inside beginning to deliver emergency care to the woman, a neighbor stops you outside of the home. "Is Marie okay?" she asks.

1. How does HIPAA affect the way you respond to the neighbor?
2. Does this patient have the right to refuse treatment? If so, what should you do?

YOU are the EMR SUMMARY

You are the EMR: CASE 1

1. What should you do in this situation?

Without a copy of a legally executed living will or DNR order in hand, you must begin to provide care for the patient. On arrival at the nearest hospital, inform the hospital staff about the patient's condition and the care provided and let them continue appropriate medical care.

2. What level of emergency medical care should you provide?

As with any patient, provide treatment that is in line with the scope of care as outlined by the *National EMS Education Standards* and those set by local medical protocols.

You are the EMR: CASE 2

1. You ask the child if you can help and he says yes. What should you do next?

Although the child has given you expressed consent to treat him, the child is considered a minor and the law requires that a parent or legal guardian give consent for treatment or transport. However, in this situation, the parents cannot be reached, so do not delay treatment because the child is an unaccompanied minor. Provide emergency care in the field and transport the patient to a local hospital.

2. You have finished applying a bandage to the wound on the boy's cheek when the police officer tells you she still cannot reach the parents. Because you treated the bite wound, can you now leave the child alone?

Leaving the child after you have begun treatment would be considered abandonment and would leave you and your organization legally vulnerable. After you have started treatment, you must stay with the patient until he is delivered to a hospital or until someone of an equal or higher level of training arrives and takes over his care.

You are the EMR: CASE 3

1. How does the concept of a standard of care protect you?

The standard of care is the manner in which you act and behave when treating a patient. A standard of care requires that you treat all patients to the best of your ability and training. This concept takes into account your level of training and the conditions under which you provide care to the patient. It does not hold you to the standard of a person who has received more advanced training than you have.

2. Why is the concept of confidentiality so important for you to follow?

The concept of confidentiality is one of the cornerstones on which the health care system is based. Confidential patient information includes the patient history, assessment findings, and the treatment provided. The federal HIPAA law safeguards the right of patients to keep their personal and medical information private. Remember, this information can be shared only with other medical clinicians who are directly participating in the patient's care. Consider how you would want your private medical information to be safeguarded.

You are the EMR: CASE 4

1. How does HIPAA affect the way you respond to the neighbor?

HIPAA, which stands for the Health Insurance Portability and Accountability Act of 1996, prevents you from sharing any details about the patient with the neighbor.

2. Does this patient have the right to refuse treatment? If so, what should you do?

Yes, the patient has the right to refuse treatment even though it appears she needs immediate medical attention. If the patient has decision-making capacity, then she can refuse treatment. As an EMR, it is your responsibility to try to convince the patient to consent to treatment and transport. If you are unsuccessful in convincing the patient, then follow your organization's guidelines for patients who refuse medical treatment and advise the woman to call EMS immediately if she changes her mind and decides she needs help. Carefully document patient refusals in your patient care report according to your agency's protocols. Many agencies require a second person to witness this refusal.

Prep Kit

Ready for Review

- As an EMR, you have a duty to act when you are dispatched on a call as a part of your official duties.
- You are held to a certain standard of care, which is related to your level of training, and you are expected to perform to the level to which a similarly trained person would perform under similar circumstances.
- You should understand the differences among expressed consent, implied consent, consent for minors, consent of mentally ill persons, and the right to refuse care.
- Advance directives consist of living wills, durable powers of attorney, and do not resuscitate orders. They give a patient the right to have care withheld and to appoint someone to act on their behalf if they are unable to act. If EMS clinicians cannot quickly determine the validity of these documents, it is best to begin treatment for these patients.
- You should understand the concepts of abandonment, patient death at the scene, negligence, and confidentiality, as well as the purpose of Good Samaritan laws.
- You must understand the importance of federal and state regulations that govern your performance as an EMR. You must also understand your department's operational regulations. Certain events that involve contagious diseases, abuse, or illegal acts must be reported to the proper authorities. You should know how to deal with these reportable events.
- Crime scene operations are complex environments. Follow proper procedures to ensure that the patient receives proper medical care and that the crime scene is not compromised for the law enforcement investigation.
- Your job is not complete until the patient report is completed. Always document your findings and treatment.
- By understanding and following these legal concepts, you will build the foundation for the skills you need to be an effective EMR.

Vital Vocabulary

abandonment Failure of the emergency medical responder to continue emergency medical treatment until relieved by someone with the same or a higher level of training.

advance directive A legal document that indicates what a person wants done if they are unable to make their own medical decisions. Advance directives include living wills, durable powers of attorney for health care, and do not resuscitate orders.

consent Permission to provide care.

decision-making capacity Ability to understand and process information and make a choice regarding appropriate medical care.

dependent lividity Blood settling to the lowest point of the body after death, causing discoloration of the skin.

do not resuscitate (DNR) order A written request giving permission to medical personnel not to attempt resuscitation in the event of cardiac arrest.

durable power of attorney for health care A legal document that allows a patient to designate another person to make medical decisions on their behalf if they are unable to make their own treatment decisions.

duty to act An emergency medical responder's legal responsibility to respond quickly to an emergency scene and provide medical care (within the limits of training and available equipment).

expressed consent Authorization to provide care or transport that is given explicitly, whether verbally or nonverbally.

Good Samaritan laws Laws that encourage citizens to voluntarily help an injured or suddenly ill person by minimizing the liability for any errors or omissions in providing good faith emergency care.

implied consent Authorization to provide care or transport that is assumed because the individual is unresponsive, underage, or so badly injured or ill that they cannot respond.

informed consent Authorization to provide care or transport that is given by a patient who has decision-making capacity after the potential risks, benefits, and alternatives to treatment have been explained.

living will A legal document that states the types of medical care a person wants, or wants withheld, if they are unable to make their own treatment decisions. Living wills may include do not resuscitate orders.

Prep Kit

negligence Deviation from the accepted standard of care resulting in further injury to the patient.

standard of care The actions expected of a clinician in accordance with their level of education and experience.

standing orders Written documents, signed by the EMS system's medical director, that outline specific directions, permissions, and sometimes prohibitions regarding patient care; also called protocols.

References

American Heart Association (AHA) staff. Advance directives: making crucial health care decisions before an emergency. AHA website. https://www.heart.org/en/health-topics/consumer-healthcare/doctor-appointments-questions-to-ask-your-doctor/advance-directives-making-crucial-healthcare-decisions-before-an-emergency. Reviewed January 17, 2024. Accessed November 19, 2024.

National Association of State EMS Officials. *National EMS Scope of Practice Model 2019.* Washington, DC: National Highway Traffic Safety Administration; February 2019. Report No. DOT HS 812-666. https://www.ems.gov/assets/National_EMS_Scope_of_Practice_Model_2019.pdf. Accessed November 19, 2024.

National Association of State EMS Officials. *National Model EMS Clinical Guidelines: Version 3.0.* https://nasemso.org/wp-content/uploads/National-Model-EMS-Clinical-Guidelines_2022.pdf. Published March 2022. Accessed November 19, 2024.

National Highway Traffic Safety Administration. *National Emergency Medical Services Education Standards.* EMS.gov website. https://www.ems.gov/assets/EMS_Education-Standards_2021_FNL.pdf. Published 2021. Accessed November 19, 2024.

Assessment IN ACTION

On Saturday afternoon, just as you are finishing lunch, you and your partner are dispatched to a local park. When you arrive, you find an 11-year-old girl who was skateboarding and has fallen. She is crying, scared, and in pain. Her right wrist is noticeably deformed, and she has some blood seeping from scrapes on her right arm and right leg. When you ask her about her parents, she says she does not know where they are.

1. What should be your first action?
   - **A.** Send your partner to locate her parents.
   - **B.** Call for help in locating her parents.
   - **C.** Treat the girl to the best of your ability.
   - **D.** Withhold your treatment until her parents have been located.
2. What type of consent, if any, do you have to treat this patient?
   - **A.** Expressed
   - **B.** None
   - **C.** Informed
   - **D.** Implied
3. To what level must you provide care to this patient?
   - **A.** You cannot treat this patient because a parent is not on scene to give you permission.
   - **B.** You must treat the patient to the best of your ability, and provide care that a reasonable, prudent person with similar training would provide under similar circumstances.
   - **C.** You should splint the wrist, bandage the wounds, and let the child return to the park.
   - **D.** You should transport the child to the hospital but should not treat the injuries without parental consent.
4. If you were to treat this patient's injuries and let her 15-year-old brother take her home, you would be guilty of:
   - **A.** libel.
   - **B.** abandonment.
   - **C.** scope of care.
   - **D.** duty to act.
5. Suppose the child's injuries were the result of a crime. In this case, you should:
   - **A.** treat the child immediately without worrying about the scene.
   - **B.** clean up the scene around the patient so it is easier to provide care.
   - **C.** provide emergency care to the patient, write a short report about the incident, and make a sketch of the scene showing how and where you found the patient.
   - **D.** enlist the help of bystanders to help you move the patient from the crime scene.
6. Another person at the park approached the child and began to assist her before you arrived on the scene. The bystander would be covered by what rules in terms of providing aid?
   - **A.** Duty to act
   - **B.** Advance directives
   - **C.** Scope of practice
   - **D.** Good Samaritan laws
7. For negligence to occur, what four conditions must be present?
   - **A.** Duty to act, scope of care, abandonment, proximate cause
   - **B.** Duty to act, breach of duty, resulting injuries, proximate cause
   - **C.** Scope of care, rigor mortis, dependent lividity, standard of care
   - **D.** Abandonment, resulting injuries, implied consent, standard of care
8. When writing your report on the care of the child, your documentation should include all of the following information EXCEPT:
   - **A.** your observations about the scene.
   - **B.** the patient's condition.
   - **C.** the treatment you provided.
   - **D.** a description of the clothing worn by the child.
9. To whom can you give information about the patient's illness or injury?
10. What are some circumstances that could make this situation a reportable event?

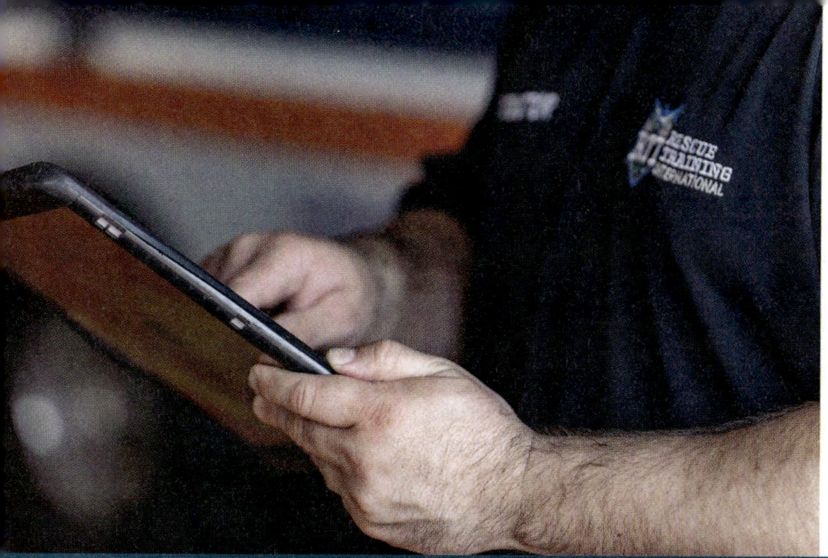

CHAPTER 5

Communications and Documentation

National EMS Education Standard Competencies

Preparatory

Uses knowledge of the emergency medical services (EMS) system, safety/well-being of the emergency medical responder (EMR), medical/legal issues, and ethical issues at the scene of an emergency while awaiting a higher level of care.

Documentation

- Recording patient findings (p 92)

EMS System Communication

- Call for resources (pp 80–92)
- Transfer care of the patient (p 82)
- Interact within the team structure (pp 81–88)

Therapeutic Communication

- Health care literacy (pp 80–92)
- Interviewing techniques (pp 80–92)
- Verbal defusing strategies (pp 80–92)
- Managing communication challenges (pp 86–90)
- Family-centered care (pp 80–92)

Medical Terminology

Uses simple medical and anatomic terms.

Knowledge Objectives

1. Describe the importance of communication and documentation for emergency medical responders (EMRs). (pp 80–92)
2. Describe the different types of equipment used by EMRs in voice, radio, telephone, and data systems. (pp 80–90)
3. Summarize the functions of radio communications during the following phases of a response:
   - Dispatch (p 81)
   - Response to the scene (p 81)
   - Arrival at the scene (p 82)
   - Update of responding emergency medical services (EMS) units (p 82)
   - Transfer of patient care to other EMS personnel (p 82)
   - Postrun activities (p 83)
4. Describe the guidelines for radio communications. (p 83)
5. Discuss the techniques of effective verbal communication. (pp 84–90)
6. Describe the guidelines for effective communication with patients. (pp 84–86)
7. Explain the skills that will help EMRs communicate with:
   - Patients who are hard of hearing or deaf (pp 86–87)
   - Patients who are visually impaired (p 87)
   - Non–English-speaking patients (p 88)
   - Geriatric patients (p 88)
   - Pediatric patients (p 88)
   - Patients with a developmental disability (p 89)
   - Patients displaying disruptive behavior (p 89)
8. Explain the role of medical terminology. (p 90)
9. Describe the legal significance of documentation. (p 92)
10. List the items that EMRs should include in a patient care report to ensure proper documentation. (p 92)

Skills Objectives

1. Demonstrate proper radio communications. (pp 80–83)
2. Demonstrate an understanding of the rules of communication with colleagues, patients, and bystanders as an EMS clinician. (pp 80–90)
3. Demonstrate the techniques of successful cross-cultural communication. (p 88)
4. Demonstrate completion of a patient care report. (p 92)

© Jones & Bartlett Learning

Introduction

A vital part of your role as an emergency medical responder (EMR) involves communication and documentation. **Communication** is the transmission of information to another person. Effective communication is important during every phase of a call. The dispatcher must receive the information from the caller and communicate the location and type of call to designated responders. As an EMR, you need to communicate with patients, bystanders, family members, dispatchers, and other members of the public safety community. After you have completed a call, you must document the condition of the patient and the treatment given. **Documentation** is a recorded description, whether handwritten or electronic, of the emergency situation and the patient care provided. This chapter describes a variety of communications systems and techniques and provides guidelines for creating written documentation for patient care.

Data and Communications Systems

The purpose of a communications system is to send information from one location to another when it is impossible or otherwise not desirable to communicate face to face. The results of using a communications system will be only as accurate as the information that is put into the system. As an EMR, you should have a basic idea of how your department's communications system works. Communications systems can be divided into two categories: those that transmit voice communications and those that transmit data.

Words of Wisdom

It is important for different agencies that are working together to have the ability to communicate with one another. This concept is called *interoperability*.

Voice Systems

Voice communications systems transmit the spoken word from one location to another. The two types of voice systems most commonly used in public safety agencies are radio systems and telephone systems.

Radio Systems

Most EMRs use some type of radio communications system. It is important that you have a working knowledge of the basics of a radio communications system and that you understand how to properly operate the radio system used by your department. Radio communications are regulated by the Federal Communications Commission (FCC). A **channel** is an assigned frequency or frequencies used to carry voice and/or data communications. Frequencies are assigned according to the function of your organization. EMRs who are part of a law enforcement agency are usually assigned different frequencies than EMRs who are part of a fire department.

Many public safety agencies use a **trunked communications system**, a computer-controlled radio system that allows the sharing of a few radio frequencies among a large group of users. Each functional group using the trunked system is assigned to a specific "talk group." Trunked systems permit more efficient use of the limited radio frequencies available to public safety agencies. These systems can transmit voice communications as well as other forms of digital communications. If your agency uses a trunked radio system, then you need to learn how to use it.

Several different types of radios exist. A **base station** is a powerful two-way radio located in a fixed place and attached to one or more antennas. Dispatchers use base stations to send and receive messages to and from the service area. A base station may be attached to several different antennas to reach all parts of a geographic service area. Base stations may be designed to transmit and receive on multiple frequencies. Some systems are designed so that different frequencies are used for different functions of communications.

A **mobile radio** is mounted in a vehicle, such as an ambulance or fire truck, and draws electricity from the electrical system of the vehicle. It has an external antenna, which is usually mounted on the roof or cab of the vehicle. The operating console is mounted so the driver or passenger of the vehicle can conveniently operate the radio. Mobile radios can be used to send and receive voice messages and data.

A **portable radio** is a handheld, self-contained unit that includes a two-way radio with a battery, a built-in microphone, and a built-in antenna (**FIGURE 5-1**). Most portable radios are capable of operating on multiple channels. One drawback of many portable radios is that the controls are small and hard to see in darkness; therefore, emergency medical services (EMS) clinicians who use these radios must become extremely familiar with the controls and operation. Portable radios are low-powered devices and are often used with a repeater system. A **repeater** is a device that receives a weak radio signal, strengthens that signal, and then automatically rebroadcasts it. Repeaters are used to cover geographic areas where radio signals are too weak for effective communications. These geographic areas are sometimes called *dead spots*.

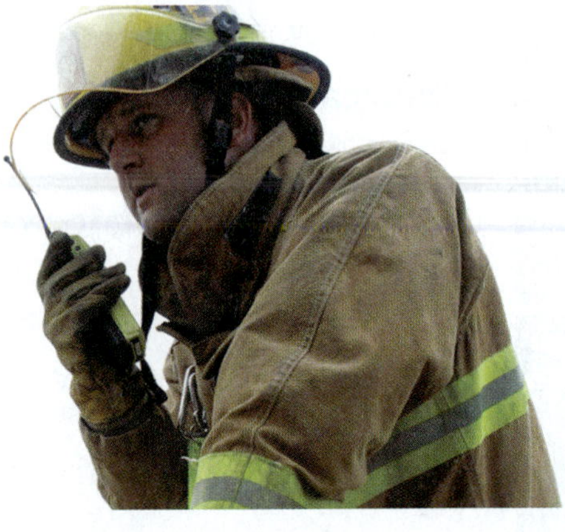

FIGURE 5-1 A portable radio.
© Jones & Bartlett Learning. Courtesy of MIEMSS.

Telephone Systems

Telephone systems primarily send voice communications. Public safety agencies may use cellular phone systems to send dispatch information via text or to handle routine administrative communications. Landline phone systems are tied together through an above-ground or below-ground hardwired system. Mobile phones rely on radio waves between a mobile phone and a cellular tower to create and receive messages. Smartphones use advanced operating systems that combine the features of a cell phone with those of a personal computer and global positioning systems (GPS).

Data Systems

Communications systems are increasingly used to send and receive data through radios, phones, and the Internet. Many different types of data can be sent between EMS personnel and communications centers. **Computer-aided dispatch (CAD)** systems assist 9-1-1 dispatchers to prioritize and record calls, coordinate information that is incoming from multiple streams, and effectively dispatch appropriate responder personnel. When geographic tracking devices are placed on responding vehicles, CAD systems are able to identify the status and location of the unit closest to the emergency and optimize dispatching decisions. Smart dispatching also uses past data to predict future trends; for example, units may be staged closer to areas with high call volumes to decrease the response time.

Paging systems can transmit text messages or voice communications. Pagers are radio receivers that are silent unless activated by a dispatcher. Cell phones can be programmed to operate as part of a paging system. Some departments use paging systems to alert members to emergency incidents.

A **mobile data terminal (MDT)** transmits data messages through a radio system (**FIGURE 5-2**) and is frequently incorporated into a mobile radio system. MDTs reduce the amount of time the radio frequency is in use. CAD systems communicate directly with the MDT and can provide a wealth of knowledge relating to the call without broadcasting it over the radio.

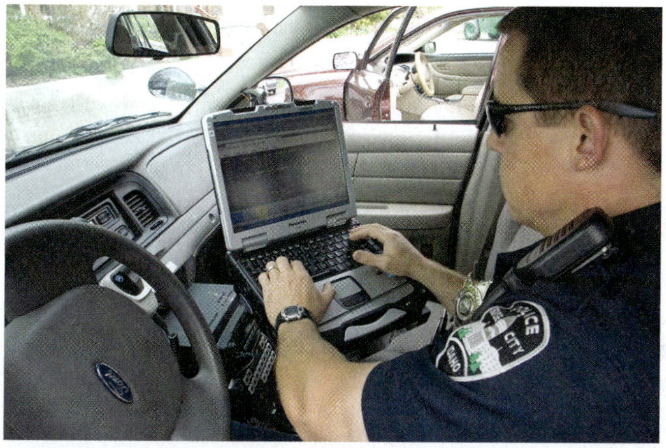

FIGURE 5-2 A mobile data terminal (MDT) can be used to display routing information transmitted from the dispatch center.

© David R. Frazier Photolibrary, Inc./Alamy Stock Photo

Telemetry is a process used by advanced life support clinicians to transmit electrocardiograms and other patient data to online medical control. Telemetry can operate through a phone system or through a radio system.

Digital messaging is technology that includes email, text messages, and social media, which are increasingly used by EMRs to send and receive information within public safety agencies. See your department for policies on the use of digital messaging. Remember, most patient information is confidential. See Chapter 4, *Medical, Legal, and Ethical Issues*, for more information.

As an EMR, you may not use all of these types of communications in your department, but you should understand how various communications devices operate. It is more important for you to understand how to send and receive data than it is to understand how the system is built.

The Functions of Radio Communications

Throughout the different phases of an EMS call, communications systems are used for different functions. Calls for medical assistance can be divided into six phases: dispatch, response to the scene, arrival at the scene, updating responding EMS units, transfer of patient care to other EMS personnel, and postrun activities. During these phases, it is important to communicate certain findings to other members of the EMS or public safety team.

Dispatch

Dispatchers receive information from the caller and determine the best response for the incident. It is your responsibility to keep your equipment ready to receive a call whenever you are on duty. Listen carefully to voice messages to ensure that you receive the information correctly. If you are not sure that you have received all the dispatch information correctly, then ask the dispatcher to repeat it. If you receive dispatch information via an MDT or a text message, then you can refer to the message to verify the location and type of call.

Words of Wisdom

Phases of an EMS call:

1. Dispatch
2. Response to the scene
3. Arrival at the scene
4. Updating responding EMS units
5. Transfer of patient care to other EMS personnel
6. Postrun activities

Response to the Scene

To respond quickly and efficiently to the scene of an emergency, you need to know your response area. Learn how to use maps or GPS devices to help route you to the scene. Listen carefully to your dispatcher, who may be able to give you further information about the location of the call or the condition of the patient while you are en route. If you are delayed in responding to the incident (for example, because you encounter traffic, a blocked railroad crossing, adverse weather conditions, vehicle malfunction, or other unexpected delays), then notify your dispatcher of the situation. Your message will enable the dispatcher to address the problem, such as by sending another unit to the same call or redirecting others traveling the same route (**FIGURE 5-3**).

Words of Wisdom

To ensure you take the fastest route, do not start responding to a call until you know where you are going.

Arrival at the Scene

As you arrive at the scene, perform a scene assessment, which includes a visual survey or an overview of the incident and its surroundings. Your scene assessment of the entire incident gives you an impression of the overall situation, including the number of patients involved and the severity of their injuries. After you have performed this size-up, give the communications center a brief verbal description of the scene. Your report should verify the location of the incident, the type of incident, any hazards present, the number of patients, and any additional assistance required. It is better to request assistance and find you do not need it than to wait and then call for help after determining the need is urgent. Scene assessment is discussed further in Chapter 9, *Patient Assessment*.

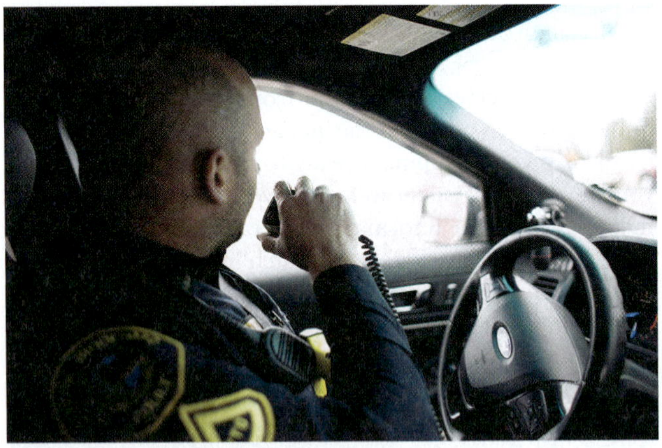

FIGURE 5-3 Notify your dispatcher if you encounter any problems while en route to the scene.

© Derek Davis/Portland Press Herald via Getty Images

Words of Wisdom

Call for any additional resources you may need prior to initiating patient care. You cannot remove your hands from your attempt to control bleeding to use your radio.

Update Responding EMS Units

In some EMS systems, you will be expected to update responding EMS units about the condition of your patient. Your report should include the age and sex of the patient; the chief complaint; the level of responsiveness; and the status of the patient's airway, breathing, and circulation. Let the responding EMS unit know what equipment you need brought in to help treat the patient. By providing this update, you are helping other EMS units know what to expect when they arrive on the scene.

Street Smarts

If unsure of a patient's gender identity or biologic sex, avoid assumptions that may cause you to enter incorrect anatomic information in your report. Sometimes you can simply ask the patient for clarification. You can also refer to the patient using the pronoun "they" in your report to avoid misleading other medical care personnel.

Transfer of Patient Care to Other EMS Personnel

With many EMS incidents, you will be the first trained person to arrive on the scene. You will have performed a primary assessment and started some treatment before emergency medical technicians (EMTs), advanced EMTs, or paramedics arrive. When they arrive, it is important for you to provide them with a handoff report. Describe your findings concisely and accurately.

The easiest way to report your patient assessment results is to use the same systematic approach you follow during patient assessment:

1. Provide the age and sex of the patient.
2. Describe the history of the incident.

YOU are the EMR **CASE 1**

After lunch, you are sent to a single motor vehicle crash. Dispatch reports that police officers are on the scene and only one patient requires medical attention. The driver was outside of the vehicle when police officers arrived. When you arrive on the scene, you park your vehicle in a safe position given the nature of the incident. As you are walking to the location of the crash, a second vehicle traveling down the road passes by you at a high rate of speed and collides with a tree. You see major damage to the front of the vehicle. Both front doors are damaged, and you are not sure if you can open them. Multiple airbags have deployed.

1. What should be your first action?
2. How many additional EMS units should you request?

3. Describe the patient's chief complaint.
4. Describe the patient's level of responsiveness.
5. Describe how you found the patient.
6. Report the status of the patient's vital signs, airway, breathing, and circulation (including any bleeding).
7. Describe the results of the physical examination.
8. Report any pertinent medical conditions using the SAMPLE (Signs and symptoms, Allergies, Medications, Pertinent past medical history, Last oral intake, and Events leading to injury or illness) format.
9. Report the interventions you provided and how the patient responded to them.

Working in a systematic manner as you assess the patient will help ensure that you do not overlook any significant symptoms, signs, or injuries. This process will help to make the handoff report complete and accurate.

EMS clinicians contact online medical control to secure permission to perform certain skills, to get direction regarding patient care, and to give the hospital their patient care reports. As an EMR, you may be present when other EMS clinicians contact online medical control through their radio or cell phone systems. In most EMS systems, EMRs are not required to contact medical control for the basic skills they are permitted to perform. If your EMS system uses online medical control for EMRs, then you will need to learn how and when to contact medical control.

Postrun Activities

After you have turned over the care of the patient to other EMS clinicians, you need to report your status to your communications center. Let the communications center know how long it will take you to get your unit ready for service and when you will be available for another call. Providing a written report of a call is covered later in this chapter in the section on documentation.

The rules, or *protocols*, for communicating with others during each phase of an EMS call may vary from one system to another. Learn and follow the standard procedures and protocols of your department (**TABLE 5-1**).

TABLE 5-1 Guidelines for Effective Radio Communications
Monitor the channel before transmitting to avoid interfering with other radio traffic.
Plan your message before pushing the transmit switch. Keep your transmissions brief and precise. Use a standard format for your transmissions.
Press the push-to-talk (PTT) button on the radio, then wait for 1 second before starting your message. Otherwise, the first part of your message may be cut off before the transmitter is working at full power.
Hold the microphone about 2 to 3 inches (5 to 8 cm) from your mouth. Speak clearly and evenly, but never shout into the microphone. Speak at a moderate, understandable rate, in a clear, even voice.
Identify the person or unit you are calling first, then identify your unit as the sender.
Acknowledge a transmission as soon as you can by saying "Go ahead" and then "Over and out" when you are finished (or whatever terminology is commonly used in your area). If you cannot take a long message, simply say "Stand by" until you are ready.
Use plain English. Avoid meaningless phrases ("Be advised"), slang, or complex codes. Avoid words that are difficult to hear, such as "yes" and "no." Use "affirmative" and "negative."
Be brief. If your message takes more than 30 seconds to send, pause after 30 seconds and say, "Do you copy?" The other party can then ask for clarification if needed. Also, the pause allows other EMS clinicians with emergency traffic to break through if necessary.
Avoid voicing emotions, such as excitement, anger, or irritation, when transmitting. Courtesy is assumed, making it unnecessary to say "please" and "thank you," which wastes air time. Listen to other communications in your system to get a good idea of the common phrases and their uses.
When transmitting a number with two or more digits, say the entire number first and then each digit separately. For example, say "sixty-seven," followed by "six-seven."
Do not use profanity on the radio. Doing so violates Federal Communications Commission rules and can result in substantial fines and even loss of your organization's radio license.
Use EMS frequencies for EMS communications. Do not use these frequencies for any other type of communications.
Reduce background noise as much as possible. Move away from wind, noisy motors, or tools.

© Jones & Bartlett Learning

Verbal Communication

As an EMS clinician, you need to communicate effectively. Verbal communication is an essential part of providing high-quality patient care. Most verbal communication occurs through face-to-face conversations. Effective communication means that the person receiving the message understands exactly what the person who sent the message meant. This process requires feedback; the receiver needs to communicate to the sender that the message has been received and understood.

Both external and internal distractions can negatively affect your ability to communicate. External distractions include noise and the use of electronic devices. Internal distractions include letting yourself think about a personal matter while at the scene. Communication can also be affected if an EMR lacks empathy for a patient or shows prejudice against a certain type or group of people. Effective communication requires you to be patient and to think carefully about your interactions with others. To achieve effective patient communication, always maintain your composure, show empathy, and keep an open mind.

As an EMR, you should master certain communication skills that will enable you to communicate effectively with EMS clinicians and other public safety personnel, as well as the patient and their family. You must be able to determine what the patient needs and then explain this information to others. The following section includes guidelines for effective communication with patients. Most of these guidelines will also promote effective communication with other public safety personnel.

Guidelines for Effective Communication With Patients

Your communication skills will be put to the test when you communicate with patients and/or family members in emergency situations. Remember that someone who is sick or injured is scared and might not understand what you are doing and saying. Therefore, your gestures, body movements, and attitude toward the patient are critically important in gaining the trust of both the patient and family. It cannot be stressed enough that maintaining your composure and showing that you care are a vital part of patient care during stressful situations. The following guidelines for communication will help you calm and reassure your patients.

Introduce Yourself

Introduce yourself by name and title. This gives the patient, family members, and bystanders an idea of who you are and lets them know your qualifications. Many citizens in your community may not understand that trained EMRs arrive in a variety of vehicles, including fire trucks, police vehicles, and private vehicles. Introducing yourself helps put the patient at ease and makes your job of assessing and treating the patient easier (**FIGURE 5-4**).

Ask the Patient's Name and Use It

Ask patients what they wish to be called. Knowing the patient's name helps you to establish rapport. Use the patient's first name only if the patient is a child or the patient asks you to use it. For example, if a young man says his name is "Ron," then he probably wants to be called "Ron." Otherwise, use a courtesy title such as "Mrs. Smith" or "Mr. Jones." Avoid using terms such as "Pops" or "Dear," which may be considered disrespectful or irritating.

Use Appropriate Eye Contact

In the United States, it is typically good practice to make eye contact with the patient as you talk. Doing so helps you establish contact with the individual. Eye contact is also important

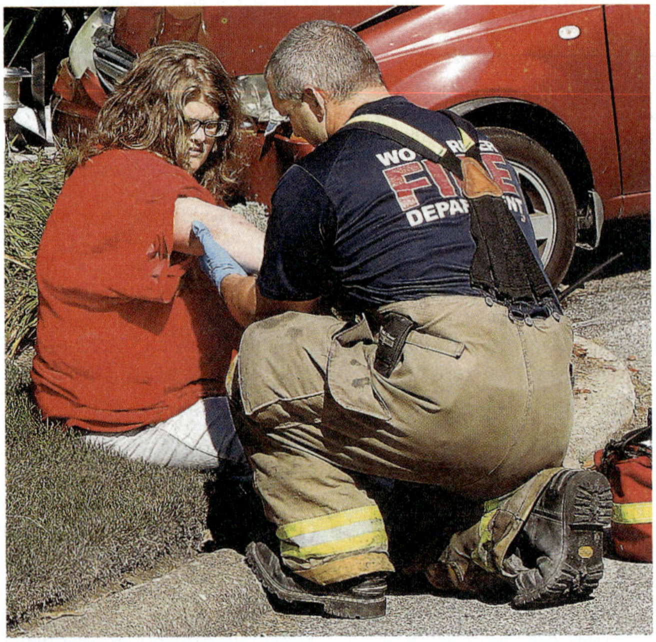

FIGURE 5-4 Introduce yourself by name and title.
© John Badman/The Telegraph/AP Photo

YOU are the EMR **CASE 2**

You are dispatched to a middle school at 1117 hours on a Wednesday morning for a sick 12-year-old girl.

1. What additional information would be useful in helping you to get to the patient quickly?
2. What are some ways that will help you to effectively assess and treat this patient?

as you listen to the patient. Emergency scenes can be noisy and confusing. By maintaining eye contact, you help the patient focus on communicating with you.

Street Smarts

You need to recognize that the concepts of body language and eye contact are often greatly affected by culture. In some cultures, direct eye contact is viewed as impolite, whereas in other cultures it is impolite to look away while speaking. For example, in the United States and most European countries, direct eye contact conveys honesty and respect. Conversely, in Latin American, Asian, and African cultures, direct eye contact conveys confrontation.

Use Language the Patient Can Understand

Use language that is clear and accurate. Avoid using technical medical terms that may frighten or confuse the patient. It is disrespectful to talk down to a patient. Use feedback to determine whether the level of your language is appropriate for the patient.

Words of Wisdom

An EMR's ability to communicate with and care for a patient is highly dependent on the ability of the patient, their family, caregivers, bystanders, and others to understand and process health information. This ability is referred to as health literacy. Because of their work in the field, often as the first points of health care contact, EMRs may be called on to bring health care information and education directly into the patient's home at the time when the patient, and their loved ones and caregivers, most need it. EMRs may bring information to patients, their families, and caregivers from their own knowledge or from printed and Internet resources made available by agency, regional, and state resources. This information may relate to fall prevention, mental health or addiction assistance, awareness of human trafficking, and other topics relevant to EMS.

Speak Slowly and Clearly

In the middle of an emergency call, it is easy for both you and patients to feel rushed. It is important for you to slow down and to speak in a clear voice. By slowing down and speaking clearly, you can avoid having to repeat questions and explanations. This will save you time in the long run and reduce communication errors.

Tell the Truth

It is important to tell patients the truth. Telling the truth helps build trust with a patient. If you fail to tell the truth, then the patient will not believe what you say in the future. There may be times when you do not need to tell the patient all the details in response to a question. There will also be times when you do not know the answer to a patient's question. In these cases, "I don't know" is an acceptable answer.

Allow Time for the Patient to Respond

Rushing a patient can negatively affect communication and delay the exchange of critical information. Because emergency situations can be hectic, use a calm approach. Patients who are sick or injured may be confused and may not be thinking clearly. Some patients may need time to answer even simple questions. Ask one question at a time and allow enough time for the patient to respond to each question.

Limit the Number of People Talking With the Patient

Designate one EMS clinician to talk with the patient. This allows the patient to focus on the questions from one person. It avoids the confusion that results when multiple people are trying to question the patient at the same time. If other EMS clinicians have questions for the patient, then these questions can be addressed to the designated EMS clinician.

Be Aware of Your Body Language

Your body language is a type of nonverbal communication. Do not stand over a patient. If a patient is sitting or lying on the ground, then kneel down or position yourself to get close to the same level as the patient's face. Get close enough to the patient for comfortable conversation. However, avoid getting so close that you invade the patient's personal space. Pay attention to your stance. Crossing your arms in front of you may be interpreted by the patient as an uncaring attitude.

Act and Speak in a Calm, Confident Manner

Remember that although the situation is not an emergency for you, the event taking place is an emergency for the patient. Your role is to give medical care that helps bring the emergency phase of this situation to an end. You need to convey a calm, caring, confident manner to the people present at the scene. Try to make the patient physically comfortable and relaxed.

Respect the Cultural Norms of the Patient

The actions that are considered respectful toward other people vary from one culture to another. Although it is impossible to learn the norms of all cultures, make an effort to learn the respectful actions toward the cultures that are represented within your community. Knowing which actions are acceptable and which are upsetting will enable you to give better care, make your job easier, and create a more positive relationship with these members of your community.

Working with patients and other responders whose backgrounds differ from your own requires **cultural competence**, which is the ability to effectively interact with others regardless of their social, cultural, and linguistic background. A related concept, **cultural humility**, refers to an ongoing process in which a person remains curious about others and continuously reflects on their viewpoints with an open mind. This process allows a person to constantly monitor their attitudes toward others, remain aware of their biases, and adapt their viewpoints if needed.

Use Open-Ended and Closed-Ended Questions Appropriately

When you must question patients to obtain information, structure your questions in one of two formats. The first type of question is an open-ended question, which allows a patient to answer in their own words. It helps you to get a sense of the patient's thoughts. An example of an open-ended question is, "What were you doing before this happened?"

The second type of question is a closed-ended question, which you can use when you are looking for specific information. Often, you will receive a yes or no in response. An example of a closed-ended question is, "Does your arm hurt?"

Treat All Patients as if They Were Members of Your Family

Treat every patient the way you would like a member of your family to be treated. Remember that every patient you treat is someone's mother, father, sister, brother, daughter, or son. This guideline will help you communicate effectively with patients of all ages.

Street Smarts

The role of family-centered care in health care interactions is increasingly understood to benefit not just the patient but also their family and other caregivers. The family-centered care model stresses the importance of treating the patient, family, and all other stakeholders with respect and inclusion while caring for the patient. Encouraging and effectively using the family's assistance during care has been shown to reduce errors and improve the quality of care.

Special Populations

Sensory Changes in Older Adults

Two of the most socializing senses are hearing and sight. Many people experience some loss of hearing as they age, and the ability to see often diminishes as well. For some older people, decreased vision results in the need to wear eyeglasses for reading, and activities such as driving and walking can become more hazardous. Other conditions, such as cataracts (a clouding of the lens of the eye) or macular degeneration (a disease that results in blurred or no vision), may develop.

Impaired vision and confusion often contribute to mistakes in taking medications. Suspect the possibility of medication errors in patients with decreased vision or mental confusion.

Our sense of balance depends on three factors: the semicircular canals in our inner ear, our sense of sight and the sensations we receive from our lower legs and feet. As we age, all three of these mechanisms become less effective. For that reason, older people may have poor balance, be more susceptible to falls, and be more likely to experience dizziness.

Patients Who Present Communication Challenges

Communicating with some patients requires additional considerations. You may need to adjust your usual approach when communicating with patients who are hard of hearing or deaf, patients who are visually impaired, non–English-speaking patients, geriatric patients, pediatric patients, patients with a developmental disability, and patients displaying disruptive behavior.

Communicating With Patients Who Are Hard of Hearing or Deaf

One of the major challenges you will face as an EMR is communicating with a person who is hard of hearing or deaf. Most people have few skills for interacting with people who are hard of hearing and may feel hesitant when asked to do so. A patient of any age may be unable to hear you for a variety of reasons: hereditary deafness; long-term hearing loss caused by illness, ear infections, or injury; or temporary deafness caused by an explosion or other loud noise. Often hearing losses are more pronounced in the higher frequencies, meaning a person may be able to hear a person with a low-pitched voice but not a person with a higher-pitched voice.

A patient with long-term hearing impairment usually develops skills to help compensate for the loss of hearing, such as the ability to read lips. A patient who is temporarily deaf does not have such skills. In either case, your job is to address the medical needs of the patient. Identify yourself by name and title and speak slowly and clearly. Ask, "Can you hear me?" A patient who is deaf may respond by pointing at their ear and shaking their head to suggest deafness. A patient who is temporarily deaf may feel anxious and panicky because they suddenly cannot hear. Help this person focus on the issue by pointing at your ear and shaking your head to show the patient that you are trying to assess whether they can hear. Another option is to write out the question, "Can you hear?" on a piece of paper and show it to the patient. If you think the patient has difficulty hearing you, do not shout. Speak directly into the patient's ear or talk while facing the patient and maintaining eye contact. If you determine that a patient has a hearing aid, ask the patient or caregiver to check to make certain it is in place and is functioning properly.

After you determine the patient is hard of hearing or deaf, do not continue to rely on verbal communication; use other methods. A patient with long-term deafness may try to communicate with you by using sign language (using the hands and fingers to communicate). If you do not know sign language, then consider learning some common medical phrases (**FIGURE 5-5**), or use writing and gestures to communicate.

As you examine the patient for injury, use your own body to show the patient how to inform you whether there is pain in a particular location. Touch a place on your body and make a face to show pain. Then look at the patient and repeat the step on the patient's body. Most people will understand what you are trying to do. Do a complete patient assessment on every patient, whether or not they can communicate with you.

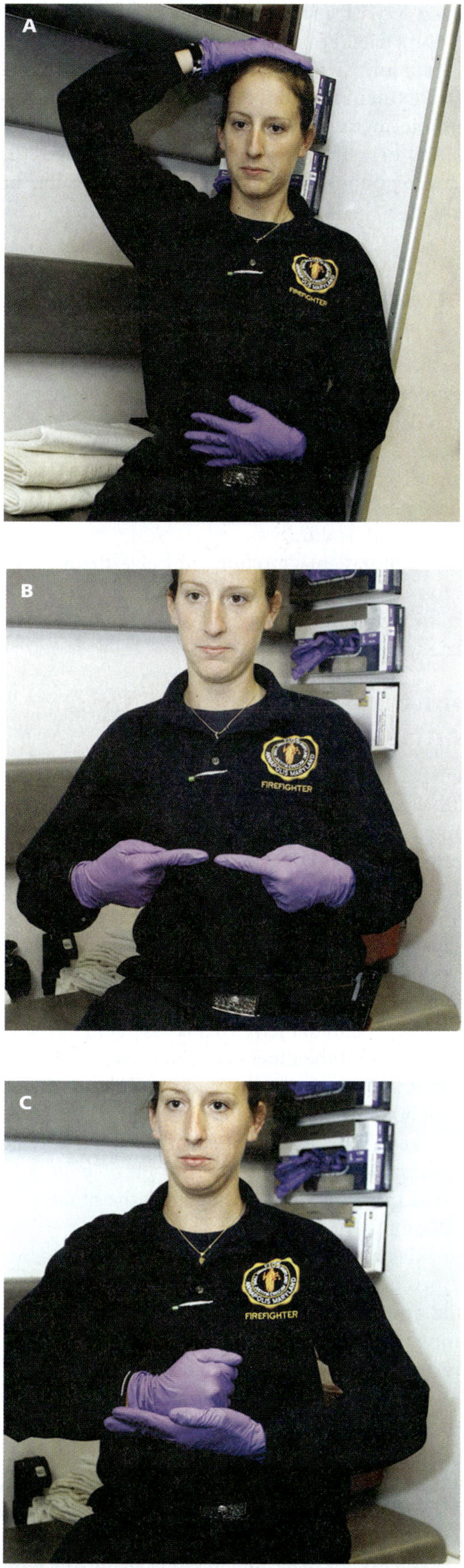

FIGURE 5-5 Simple phrases in sign language. **A.** Sick. **B.** Hurt. **C.** Help.

© Jones & Bartlett Learning. Courtesy of MIEMSS.

Keep the patient informed by making gestures to show that certain things are happening (for example, when the ambulance arrives). Touching is an important part of communication and reassurance for patients who are hard of hearing or deaf, as well as for hearing patients. For example, hold the patient's hand so they know you are there to help.

> **Street Smarts**
>
> When working with patients who are hard of hearing or deaf, use the following techniques:
>
> - Identify yourself by showing the patient your patch or badge.
> - Touch the patient; a patient who is hard of hearing or deaf needs human contact just as much as a hearing patient.
> - Face the patient when you speak so they can see your lips and facial expressions.
> - Speak slowly and clearly; do not shout.
> - Watch the patient's face for expressions of understanding or uncertainty.
> - Repeat or rephrase your comments in clear, simple language.
> - If all of these attempts at communication fail, then write down your questions and offer paper and a pencil to the patient to respond.
> - Some people are both deaf and blind. It may be difficult for you to treat these patients. Take your time, be patient, and use touch as a way of communicating.

If the patient is a hearing child of parents who are deaf, then be sure to communicate with the parents about the child's condition and your actions. Like all parents in similar circumstances, parents who are deaf must consent for you to treat their child. They have a right to know what is being done and are just as upset as hearing parents would be. If the patient is a child who is deaf and has hearing parents, then you need to involve the parents even more than usual. They can assist you in communicating with the child.

If the patient is a parent who is deaf and has a hearing child, then resist the urge to use the child as an interpreter unless the child is obviously mature and capable. Young children cannot understand medical terminology, and misinterpretation can have serious results. Communicate directly with the patient, using whatever methods are most effective.

Communicating With Patients Who Are Visually Impaired

During your initial overview of the scene, look for signs that suggest the patient may be visually impaired. These signs may include the presence of eyeglasses, a cane, or a service animal. As you approach, introduce yourself to the patient. If you think the patient is visually impaired, then ask, "Can you see?"

A patient who is visually impaired may feel vulnerable, especially during the chaos of an emergency scene. Explain what you are doing to the patient. Tell patients when they will feel movement or hear noise and explain any treatments they require. The patient may have learned to use other senses such as hearing, touch, and smell to compensate for the loss of sight. The sounds and smells of the scene may be disorienting. The patient may rely on you to make sense of everything. Tell the patient what is happening, identify noises, and describe the situation and surroundings, particularly if you must move the patient.

Learn the patient's name and use it throughout your examination and treatment, just as you would with a sighted patient. Touch the patient to provide emotional support. If the patient has a service animal such as a dog, then they may initially be more concerned about the dog than about their own injuries. Recognize that the dog and the patient are a unique team who depend on each other. Let the patient direct the dog or tell you how to handle the dog. Restate your question or redirect the patient's attention to the issue at hand. Service dogs are usually not aggressive; avoid separating the patient and the dog if at all possible. If a patient who is visually impaired must be moved and can walk, then ask the patient to hold on to your elbow and stand slightly to your side and rear. Tell the patient about obstructions, steps, and curbs as you lead the way.

If a patient wears eyeglasses, keep them with the patient if at all possible. If the eyeglasses are lost during a medical emergency, make every effort to locate them because your patient may be severely handicapped and anxious without their eyeglasses. Knowing that the eyeglasses are not lost will be a great relief to the patient. If you bring that understanding and empathy to your interactions with patients who are visually impaired, it will help you provide compassionate care.

Do not make the mistake of talking louder when communicating with patients who are visually impaired. Visual impairment and hearing impairment are not related. When caring for a patient who is visually impaired, it may be helpful to maintain physical or verbal contact to let the person know you are still there.

Communicating With Non–English-Speaking Patients

In many communities across the United States, English is not the first or even the most common language. If your patient speaks a language other than English and you cannot understand each other, then you must find ways to communicate so you can meet your responsibility as an EMR to provide the appropriate standard of care. To achieve successful cross-cultural communication, you may be able to adapt some of the techniques recommended for communicating with a patient who is hard of hearing or deaf, such as hand gestures, finger-pointing, and facial expressions. Determine how much English the patient speaks and whether a family member or a friend can act as an interpreter.

If your jurisdiction has a large non–English-speaking population, then memorize common phrases and questions so you can use them when treating these patients. Your community may offer language assistance services that you can access by phone or an electronic device, or through the dispatcher.

> **Special Populations**
>
> **Translators and Translation Apps**
>
> Electronically based translation services can be helpful when trying to communicate with a non–English-speaking patient, particularly if the patient is alone. In some situations, another person on scene may be available to translate, but be mindful of factors that may make this person's assistance inappropriate or unreliable, such as the high emotions often present at emergencies or the sharing of sensitive patient information. Follow the protocols of your local agency regarding this service.

Communicating With Geriatric Patients

Older people tend to require EMS more frequently than younger people. As people age, they are more likely to experience both decreased vision and hearing. When you encounter older people who have hearing or visual impairment, use the same communication skills you would for any other patient with a similar condition. Do not assume all older patients have physical or mental impairments. Many older people are alert and healthy.

Assess all patients carefully and give them time to respond to your questions. Be aware of how older patients respond to you; it may give you clues as to how best to communicate with them.

Communicating With Pediatric Patients

Managing a pediatric emergency can be one of the most stressful situations you face as an EMR. Children are often frightened, anxious, and unable to communicate clearly; their parents or caregivers are usually frightened and anxious as well. Familiar objects and faces can help calm a child. Let a child keep a favorite doll, toy, or blanket to give the child some sense of comfort. Because children often take cues from their parents, use the parents to help you reassure and calm the child. Talk to both the parents and the child as much as possible and explain to them what is happening. Ask a parent to hold the child if the illness or injury permits. If the injury is such that the parent cannot hold the child on their lap, let the parent hold the child's hand or keep the parents where the child can see them. Parents are understandably concerned about their child's condition, especially if they do not clearly understand the situation or if they think the situation is more serious than it is.

Quickly try to develop a rapport with the child by speaking to the child in a professional yet friendly manner. Tell the child your first name, ask their name, and use it when explaining what you are doing. Try to reassure the child that you are there to help in every possible way. Allowing the child to touch the equipment also makes it less frightening. You can allow the child to listen to your (or a parent's) heartbeat with the stethoscope before you listen to theirs.

Avoid standing over the child; instead, squat, kneel, or sit down so that you are on the child's level and establish eye contact (**FIGURE 5-6**). Ask the child simple questions about the pain, and ask for their help in pointing out any painful areas. Giving a child choices helps them to feel more in control. However, make sure you control the choice. For example, you

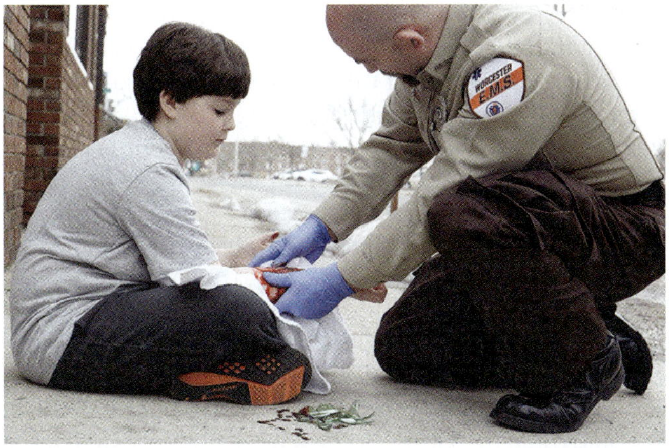

FIGURE 5-6 Squat, kneel, or sit when treating a pediatric patient.
© Jones & Bartlett Learning

can say, "I need to listen to your chest and touch your tummy. Which one would you like for me to do first?" You will do both, but the child has maintained a sense of control over the situation.

Children can see through lies and deception, so be honest with them. You may be surprised at the remarkable level of understanding you can receive from an ill or injured child.

Street Smarts

EMS personnel often have mixed feelings when treating a child. In some situations, the child reminds them of someone they know. Even the most experienced personnel respond emotionally to a seriously ill or injured child. Unless you are prepared, your anxiety and fear may interfere with your ability to deliver proper care. In an atmosphere where everyone involved is tense, you must remain calm and behave in a controlled and professional manner.

Communicating With Patients With a Developmental Disability

You may find it difficult to communicate with patients who have a developmental disability. Ask the family or caregiver about the patient's typical level of communication. Speak slowly, using short sentences and simple words. You may need to repeat statements several times or to rephrase them until the patient understands what you want.

Again, offer emotional support, using reassuring touch if appropriate. Because the chaos surrounding an injury or illness may confuse or frighten these patients, use extra care in dealing with patients with a developmental disability. You may be able to adapt many of the techniques recommended for communicating with children.

Patients Displaying Disruptive Behavior

Disruptive behavior can present a danger to you, the patient, and other people at the scene and can cause delays in treatment. At some time in your career, you will encounter a person who challenges your patience and communication skills.

Patients can become hostile toward EMS clinicians. Signs that a patient may become an aggressor include staring, tone of voice, anxious behavior, mumbling, and pacing. Communication methods to de-escalate a situation (sometimes referred to as defusing) include the following:

- Make sure you have sufficient backup to maintain safety of the patient and your crew.
- Minimize distractions such as bright or flashing lights, loud noise or conversations, or other individuals the patient may see as aggressive or threatening.
- Speak clearly and calmly, in a nonconfrontational manner.
- Use nonthreatening body language when communicating with the patient.
- Attempt to understand the patient's fears and concerns, even if you do not agree with them.
- Be empathetic and professional.
- Set limits on patient behavior that may be destructive or injurious.
- Carefully choose and make clear what you can negotiate with the patient and what is non-negotiable.
- Allow time for the patient to think and respond.
- Do not threaten the patient.

If you are interacting with an angry patient, you must stay calm and try to defuse the situation before it escalates.

YOU are the EMR — CASE 3

Soon after you start your shift at 0700 hours, you hear alert tones from the speaker and hear your dispatcher say, "Unit 433 respond to 85 Norwood Avenue for a 72-year-old woman who is experiencing severe chest pain." You acknowledge the call, verify the location, and begin to respond.

1. Why is it important to know how to operate your radio communications system?
2. Why is it important to use the patient's name, maintain eye contact with the patient, and use language the patient can understand?
3. Why is it important to learn how to communicate effectively with all patients, including those who present communication challenges?

If the patient's behavior presents a threat to you and your crew, take the following steps:

1. Stay between the patient and an exit whenever possible to allow for your escape if the scene becomes violent.
2. Do not take your eyes off the patient or turn your back.
3. If the patient has a weapon, then stay clear and wait for law enforcement personnel—no matter how badly injured the patient seems to be.
4. As soon as your personal safety is ensured, carry out the appropriate emergency medical care.

There may be times when the patient will not allow you to approach, despite all efforts to help. Sometimes family members or friends of the disruptive patient may insist that the person be taken to the hospital, but EMS personnel cannot take a patient with decision-making capacity to the hospital against their expressed wishes. Some frightened, agitated, intoxicated, or disruptive patients can cause serious injury to you, bystanders, or themselves. It is best to wait for assistance from law enforcement in these situations. Note that EMRs who are law enforcement personnel may have additional authority to take a patient to the hospital. Follow the laws and protocols of your local jurisdiction.

Medical Terminology

Medical terminology is a collection of technical terms used by medical personnel to identify anatomic parts of the body, specify illnesses and injuries, and indicate treatments. Medical terminology is intended to clarify language so that one person can communicate clearly to another. Using proper medical terminology allows you to communicate a clear message, avoid errors, and save time.

As an EMR, you are not expected to understand all the medical terminology used by a physician. Your job is to communicate your message to other medical clinicians as clearly as possible. Do not use medical terms if you are unsure of their meaning. It is much better to report that a patient is short of breath, gasping, and breathing at a rate of 32 breaths per minute than to try to remember the correct word for shortness of breath (dyspnea). Using the incorrect word will result in confusion.

As you encounter new terminology, look at the parts of each word. The center of a word contains the *stem* or *root*. There may be a *prefix* at the beginning of the word and a *suffix* at the end of the word. Each of these parts helps you to determine and remember the meaning of the word. By learning a few of these commonly occurring prefixes and suffixes, you will gain some insight into new words you encounter. For example, the prefix *hyper-* means above or excessive. *Hypertension* means excessive tension or pressure. Therefore, *hypertension* is the medical term for what we commonly call high blood pressure.

A list of some of the more commonly encountered prefixes is provided in **TABLE 5-2**. Learning these simple prefixes will help you to understand a significant number of medical terms. When you see a new word, look for the root, the prefix, and the suffix. As you interview patients and relate information to other medical care clinicians, remember to communicate your thoughts as clearly as you can.

TABLE 5-2 Prefixes Commonly Used in Medical Terminology

Prefix	Meaning
brady-	Slow
tachy-	Rapid or swift
therm-	In relation to quantities of heat
hyper-	Above, excessive, or beyond
hypo-	Below, underneath, or deficient
naso-	Denoting the nose
oro-	Denoting the mouth
arterio-	In relation to an artery
cardio-	Heart
hem-, hema-, hemo-	Blood
neuro-	Denoting nerve, nervous system, or nervous tissue
vaso-	Vessel, as in blood vessel

© Jones & Bartlett Learning

YOU are the EMR — CASE 4

You are called to the home of an 85-year-old woman who reports chest pain. You arrive to find her sitting in a chair and leaning forward. She is sweating, is struggling to breathe, and appears uncomfortable. You approach the patient, introduce yourself, and quickly realize she is hard of hearing.

1. What techniques should you use to communicate with the woman?
2. As you gather information about her condition, the woman repeatedly asks, "Am I going to die?" How should you respond?

Voices OF Experience

No matter what the public safety responsibilities are for an EMR, documentation is one of the most important duties. Documentation is particularly important when one responds to medical emergencies and renders patient care and/or transport.

My most humiliating moment in EMS was early in my career (over 30 years ago) when I was subpoenaed to our local state district court for a civil case concerning a motor vehicle crash that had happened several years earlier. Not only did I not remember anything about the incident, but my employer had lost the run report. Our testimony was brief and disappointing. My partner and I testified truthfully that we did not remember the case and that our run report had been lost. We were quickly dismissed from the courtroom, after a serious scolding from the judge about our service's lack of professionalism.

"We were quickly dismissed from the courtroom, after a serious scolding from the judge about our service's lack of professionalism."

The courtroom is not the only place where documentation is important. First and foremost, the caregivers who receive the patient need to know the results of your assessments, your interventions, and how the patient responded. The trending of this information over a period of time is as important as the information itself.

In my current full-time position as EMS Licensing Program Manager for the State of Louisiana, I read a number of patient reports as part of complaint investigations. Every EMS complaint that my agency has investigated has been made or broken by the quality of documentation. Some seemingly insignificant fact is frequently omitted. I can't overemphasize the importance of completeness as well as accuracy and legibility. This is especially important when documenting patient assessments and interventions. If there is some legitimate reason that you deviated from protocol, or the standard of care, then it must be explained.

Therefore, I ask all EMRs to remember to document patient encounters accurately, completely, and legibly.

Steve Erwin, BS, NREMT-I/T, EMSI
Entergy Operations
River Bend Power Station
Louisiana

Adapted from the personal Medical Identification Symbol of the American Medical Association.

Documentation

Documentation is the second major type of communication that you will use in your daily work as an EMR. Documentation is the process of describing the emergency situation and the actions you and other responders took. It may be completed using written or electronic records (**FIGURE 5-7**).

By recording the actions you took at an emergency incident, you provide a record for others and a document you can refer to in the future if necessary. Documentation is helpful to you because you will not be able to remember all the details of every call. It provides a legal record for the actions you took and a basis to evaluate the quality of care you gave. Remember, the call is not over until the paperwork is completed.

Most public safety services have replaced written reporting systems with electronic reporting systems. Electronic reporting systems enable you to transmit patient information directly to a hospital computer system or to other health care clinicians. They also cut down on the time needed to complete a handoff report. It is important that you learn how to use whatever type of reporting system your agency uses.

Proper documentation includes the following:

- The age, race, and sex of the patient
- The history of the incident
- The condition of the patient when found
- The patient's description of the injury or illness
- The patient's chief complaint
- The patient's level of responsiveness
- The status of initial and subsequent vital signs: airway, breathing, and circulation (including severe bleeding)
- The results of the physical examination
- Pertinent medical conditions using the SAMPLE format (discussed in Chapter 9, *Patient Assessment*)
- The treatment you gave the patient
- Any change in the patient's condition after treatment
- The agency and personnel who took over treatment of the patient
- The following times: the time you were dispatched, the time you arrived on the scene, the time other EMS clinicians arrived on the scene, the time you departed the scene
- Other relevant times relating to specific situations, such as time a patient is extricated, time a baby is born, or time CPR is initiated
- Any reportable conditions present
- Any infectious disease exposure
- Anything unusual about the situation
- Any other helpful facts

Include all these details in your handoff report. Complete your patient care report as soon as possible after each call. Your documentation should be clear, concise, and accurate. Follow the standards of your organization. If you make a mistake on a written form, then draw one line through it, place your initials beside it, and make the correction.

Your organization may rely on patient care reports for documenting reportable events. Reportable events include certain infectious diseases and crimes such as knife wounds, gunshot wounds, motor vehicle collisions, suspected child abuse, domestic violence, elder abuse, dog bites, and rape. Learn which crimes are reportable in your area, your agency's procedures for reporting these crimes, and what you are required to do.

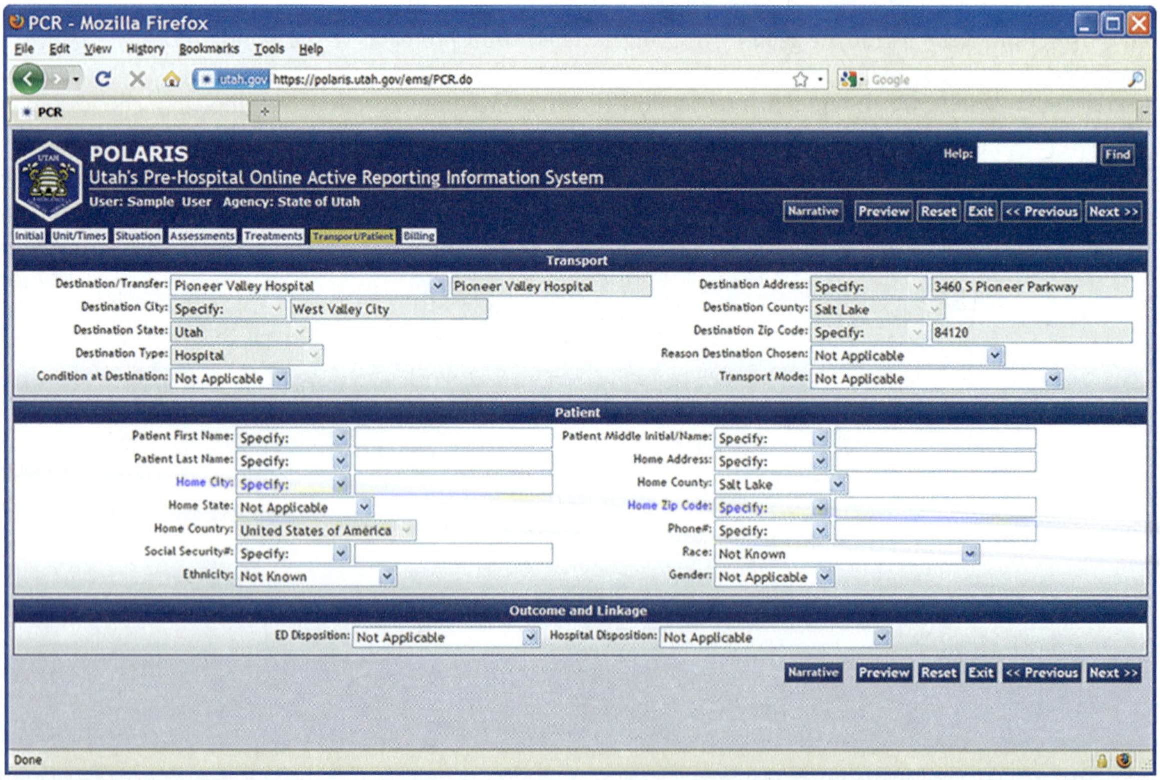

FIGURE 5-7 A patient care report can be completed on an electronic device, such as the one shown here, or on a paper form.
Courtesy of the Utah Department of Health.

YOU are the EMR SUMMARY

You are the EMR: CASE 1

1. What should be your first action?

Your first action should be to call your dispatch center to report your initial assessment of the second collision and request sufficient EMS units to care for the number of patients needing care. In addition, evaluate the need for units to perform extrication, and make sure the scene of both collisions is being secured by law enforcement officers to prevent further accidents.

2. How many additional EMS units should you request?

In the early stages of an emergency, you may not know exactly how many resources will be needed. Therefore, give the dispatch center your best estimate of the number of injured patients and the severity of their injuries. It is better to err on the side of requesting more resources than you need, rather than not having enough emergency responders to treat and transport the patients. Responding units that are not needed can be canceled while en route to the scene.

You are the EMR: CASE 2

1. What additional information would be useful in helping you to get to the patient quickly?

When responding to a large building that contains many rooms, it may be hard to locate a patient without further information. It is helpful to know which entrance to use when driving into a large complex, and you should know which building entrance is closest to the patient. Having someone at the front door to direct you to the patient can save valuable time. If this information is not given to you by the dispatcher, you can request the dispatcher to call back for further information.

2. What are some ways that will help you to effectively assess and treat this patient?

This 12-year-old patient is a child who may think that she is approaching adulthood and may behave maturely for her age, or she may act as if she were a younger child. Remember to introduce yourself, ask the patient's name, and maintain good eye contact. Be sure to use clear language that the child can understand, but do not talk down to her. Let the patient know what you are going to do to prevent frightening her. Gather additional information about her illness from the patient and from the teacher or nurse who has been caring for her. Just as you would do with an adult patient, be aware of your body language and use open- and closed-ended questions appropriately.

You are the EMR: CASE 3

1. Why is it important to know how to operate your radio communications system?

Your radio system is your primary way to communicate with your dispatcher, other public safety clinicians, and hospitals. You use it to direct you to emergency scenes, communicate your status to others, and call for additional help. It is important that you understand the day-to-day operations of your communications system and the special uses that are reserved for unusual circumstances. You cannot be an effective member of the EMS team without an efficient communications system.

2. Why is it important to use the patient's name, maintain eye contact with the patient, and use language the patient can understand?

In emergency situations, patients and family members are experiencing a high level of stress. Emergency scenes are often noisy and confusing and can be dark. These factors make effective communication difficult. Therefore, it is important to work hard to increase the effectiveness of your communication. Use the patient's name, maintain eye contact, and use language the patient can understand to enhance your communication and reduce the stress the patient is feeling.

3. Why is it important to learn how to communicate effectively with all patients, including those who present communication challenges?

EMS personnel provide care to all the citizens of their community. It can be challenging to understand and communicate with some patients, whether because the person has a disability or the environment does not allow easy conversation. It is helpful to learn how to handle these challenges so you can provide the appropriate standard of care.

YOU are the EMR SUMMARY

You are the EMR: CASE 4

1. What techniques should you use to communicate with the woman?

Speak to the patient face to face so she can see your facial expressions and perhaps read your lips. Also, repeat your comments. If you are still having difficulty communicating, then use a sheet of paper to write questions.

2. As you gather information about her condition, the woman repeatedly asks, "Am I going to die?" How should you respond?

Always be honest and share relevant information with the patient. With this type of question, you should tell the woman you are doing everything you can to get her to the hospital safely.

Prep Kit

Ready for Review

- Communications systems allow you to send information from one location to another when it is impossible to communicate face to face. Excellent communication skills are crucial during every phase of a call.
- It is important for you to have a basic idea of how your department's communications system works.
- The two types of voice communications systems are radio systems and telephone systems. As an EMR, you will use two-way radio communications, which include mobile and handheld portable radios. You must know when to use these devices and what type of information you can transmit.
- Throughout the different phases of an EMS call, communications systems are used for different functions. The six phases of an EMS call include dispatch, response to the scene, arrival at the scene, updating responding EMS units, transfer of patient care to other EMS personnel, and postrun activities.
- The protocols for communicating with others during each phase of an EMS call may vary from one system to another. Learn and follow the standard procedures and protocols of your department.
- In addition to radio and telephone communications, you must have excellent person-to-person communication skills. Be able to effectively interact with the patient and any family members, friends, or bystanders. Always maintain your composure, show empathy, and keep an open mind.
- Remember that people who are sick or injured may not understand what you are doing or saying. Therefore, your body language and attitude are important in gaining the trust of both the patient and the family. Take special care of patients such as children, geriatric patients, patients who are hearing impaired, patients who are visually impaired, non–English-speaking patients, patients with a developmental disability, and patients displaying disruptive behavior.
- Medical terminology is used to clarify language so that one clinician can communicate to another the anatomic location of an injury, signs and symptoms of a disease, and treatment given. Do not use medical terms if you are unsure of their meaning.
- Along with your radio report and oral report, you must also complete a formal handoff report that will be given to other EMS clinicians at the scene. Documentation provides a legal record of the actions you took and provides a basis to evaluate the quality of care given. Remember that the call is not over until the paperwork is completed.

Vital Vocabulary

base station A powerful two-way radio that is permanently mounted in a communications center.

channel An assigned frequency or frequencies that are used to carry voice and/or data communications.

communication The transmission of information to another person.

computer-aided dispatch (CAD) A communications system that assists 9-1-1 dispatchers to prioritize and record calls, coordinate information that is incoming from multiple streams, and effectively dispatch appropriate responder personnel.

Prep Kit

cultural competence The ability to effectively interact with others regardless of their social, cultural, and linguistic background.

cultural humility The attribute of being curious about others and keeping an open mind when interacting with people from an unfamiliar culture.

digital messaging Technology that includes email, text messages, and social media, which are increasingly used by EMRs to send and receive various types of information.

documentation A recorded description, whether handwritten or electronic, of the emergency situation and the patient care provided.

mobile data terminal (MDT) A computer terminal mounted in a vehicle that sends and receives data through a radio communications system.

mobile radio A two-way radio that is permanently mounted in an emergency vehicle that draws electricity from the electrical system of the vehicle.

paging systems Communications systems used to send voice or text messages over a radio system to specially designed radio receivers.

portable radio A handheld, battery-operated, two-way radio.

repeater A radio system that automatically retransmits a radio signal on a different frequency.

telemetry A process in which electronic signals are transmitted and received by radio or telephone; commonly used for sending electrocardiogram tracings.

trunked communications system A computer-controlled radio system that allows the sharing of a few radio frequencies among a large group of users.

References

Davies J. Exploring health literacy: improving patient outcomes and reducing resources. EMS.Aware website. https://www.emsaware.org/articlesforthepublic/exploring-health-literacy-improving-patient-outcomes-amp-reducing-resources. Published January 15, 2024. Accessed November 19, 2024.

Dick T. Ease patient's fear for better care. *JEMS*. https://www.jems.com/operations/ease-patient-s-fear-better-car/. Published July 31, 2010. Accessed November 19, 2024.

Dudley N, Ackerman A, Brown KM, et al. Patient- and family-centered care of children in the emergency department. *Pediatrics*. 2015;135(1):e255–e272. doi:10.1542/peds.2014-3424

Johnson Dawkins D, Daum DN. Person-first language in healthcare: the missing link in healthcare simulation training. *Clin Simulat Nurs*. 2022;71:135–140.

Loyacono TR. Family-centered prehospital care. *Emerg Med Serv*. 2001;30(6):64–83.

Respecting patient pronouns and using gender-affirming language in medical care. University of Texas Arlington website. https://academicpartnerships.uta.edu/healthcare-nursing-online-programs/rn-to-bsn/respecting-patient-pronouns-medical-care/. Published July 6, 2022. Accessed November 19, 2024.

The EMS-ED handoff: a critical moment in patient care. NAEMSP National Association of EMS Physicians website. https://naemsp.org/2017-7-27-the-ems-ed-handoff-a-critical-moment-in-patient-care/. Published July 27, 2017. Accessed November 19, 2024.

Assessment IN ACTION

At 2130 hours on a Thursday evening, you are dispatched to a residence for the report of a 2-year-old child who is having a seizure. The mother reports that the child seemed sick all day and is running a high fever. The residence is about 3 minutes from your location.

1. Which phase of an EMS call occurs immediately after an emergency call has been received at the dispatch center?
   - **A.** Arrival at the scene
   - **B.** Response to the scene
   - **C.** Dispatch
   - **D.** Transfer of patient care to other EMS personnel
2. Which of the following techniques will help you to communicate effectively with a pediatric patient?
   - **A.** Stand up straight while talking to the patient.
   - **B.** Use proper medical terminology.
   - **C.** Kneel down to the level of the patient's face.
   - **D.** Turn your back on the child while talking.
3. What should you do if you are unsure of the proper medical term used to describe your patient's illness or injury?
   - **A.** Have the dispatcher look it up for you.
   - **B.** Skip over that part of the transmission.
   - **C.** Describe the illness or injury in plain English.
   - **D.** Use slang terminology.
4. When you send patient information via a portable radio, communications should be:
   - **A.** brief and concise.
   - **B.** coded and scripted.
   - **C.** spoken in a loud voice.
   - **D.** unhurried, with long descriptions.
5. What agency has responsibility for regulating the use of your radio communications?
   - **A.** Your state EMS agency
   - **B.** Your local department
   - **C.** Federal Communications Commission
   - **D.** Department of Homeland Security
6. Your documentation of this call should include all of the following information EXCEPT:
   - **A.** the age of the mother.
   - **B.** the patient's chief complaint.
   - **C.** the patient's level of consciousness.
   - **D.** the results of the patient assessment.
7. Which of the following statements regarding your written documentation is true?
   - **A.** It is a legal document.
   - **B.** It cannot be used in a court of law.
   - **C.** It must be destroyed after 1 year.
   - **D.** It is used only for billing purposes.
8. Why is it important to introduce yourself to the patient using your name and title?
9. What are the six phases of an EMS call?
10. How might your communications change if the patient were a 78-year-old patient who is hard of hearing rather than a 2-year-old child?

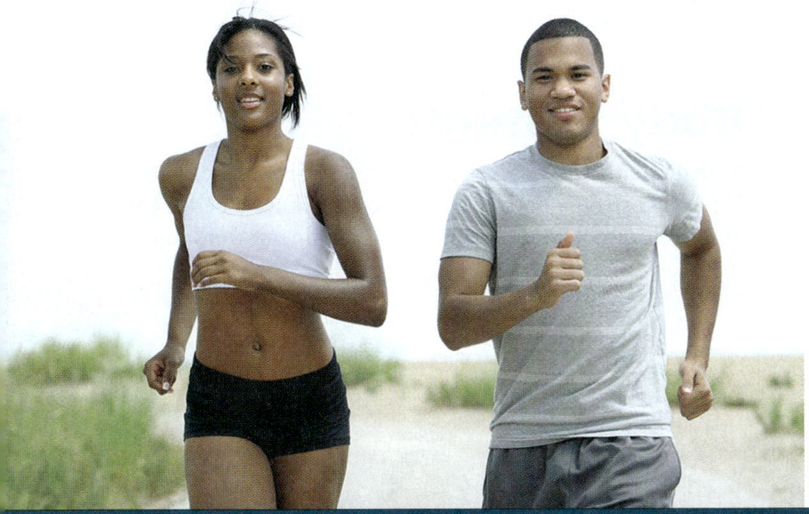

CHAPTER 6

The Human Body

National EMS Education Standard Competencies

Anatomy and Physiology

Uses knowledge of the anatomy and function of the upper airway, heart, vessels, blood, lungs, skin, muscles, and bones as the foundation of emergency care.

Life Span Development

Uses simple knowledge of age-related differences to assess and care for patients.

Knowledge Objectives

1. Know the basic topographic anatomy terms to describe locations on the human body, including the anatomic position and the planes of the body. (pp 98–105)
2. Discuss the anatomy and function of the respiratory system. (p 99)
3. Discuss the anatomy and function of the circulatory system. (pp 100–101)
4. Identify the anatomy and function of the skeletal system. (pp 101–103)
5. Describe the anatomy and function of the muscular system. (p 103)
6. Discuss the anatomy and function of the nervous system. (pp 103–104)
7. Discuss the anatomy and function of the digestive system. (p 104)
8. Describe the anatomy and function of the genitourinary system. (p 104)
9. Name the three major functions of the skin. (p 105)
10. Describe the changes that occur during growth and development at different ages. (pp 105–108)
11. Name the factors that can influence or change vital signs. (pp 106–108)

Skills Objective

1. Identify selected topographic anatomy on a live or simulated patient. (p 98)

© Flashon Studio/Shutterstock

Introduction

To be an effective emergency medical responder (EMR), you must understand the basic structure and functions of the human body. This knowledge helps you better understand the specific location of symptoms the patient is experiencing, perform an adequate patient examination, communicate your findings to the other members of the emergency medical team, and provide proper emergency treatment for the patient's condition. This chapter discusses human anatomy, the relationships among the body systems discussed in this chapter, and how the body changes as it ages.

Topographic Anatomy

The anatomic terms used in this section describe the location of injury or pain. You must know the basic anatomic terms for human body parts because all members of the emergency medical team must be able to speak the same language when treating a patient. However, if you cannot remember the proper anatomic term for a certain body location, you can use lay terms.

Visualize a person standing, facing you, with arms at the sides and thumbs pointing outward (palms toward you). This is the standard anatomic position; keep it in mind when describing a location on the body. **FIGURE 6-1** identifies **topographic anatomy**.

The first terms that should be clarified are left and right. These terms always refer to the patient's left and right, not yours. **Anterior** means front and **posterior** means back. The **midline** refers to an imaginary vertical line drawn from head to toe that divides the body into equal left and right sides.

Two other useful terms are medial and lateral. **Medial** means closer to the midline of the body; **lateral** means farther from the midline. In this context, the eyes are lateral to the nose.

The term **proximal** means close and **distal** means distant. On the body, proximal means close to the point where an arm or leg is attached. Distal means farther from the point of attachment. For example, if the thigh bone (femur) is broken, the break can be either proximal (the end closer to the hip) or distal (the end farther from the hip).

The term **superior** means closer to the head and **inferior** means closer to the feet. For example, the hips are inferior to the chest, and the chest is superior to the hips.

Body Systems

Body systems work together to perform common functions. By studying these body systems, you will have a better background for understanding and treating illnesses and injuries.

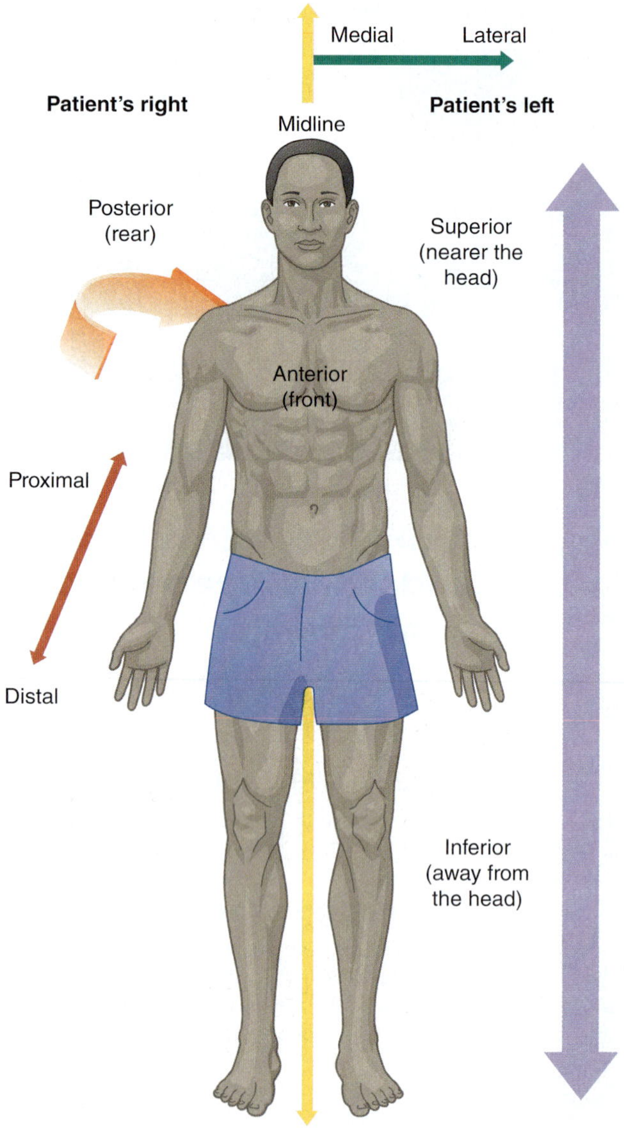

FIGURE 6-1 Topographic anatomy terms for describing a location on the body.
© Jones & Bartlett Learning

YOU are the EMR CASE 1

In the middle of the night, you are dispatched to 114 Foster Center Road for a 69-year-old man reported as sick. As you arrive, the man's wife tells you her husband is having chest pains. As you begin to examine the patient, you notice a long scar down the middle of the man's chest. You ask him if he had a heart operation.

1. Why is some knowledge of anatomy and an understanding of the functions of body systems important in cases like this?

The Respiratory System

Because airway maintenance is one of the most important skills you will learn as an EMR, the **respiratory system** is the first body system we will review.

The respiratory system consists of all the structures of the body that contribute to normal breathing (**FIGURE 6-2**). The function of the respiratory system is to bring oxygen into the body and remove the waste gas, carbon dioxide.

The airway consists of the nose (nasopharynx), mouth (oropharynx), throat (pharynx), **larynx** (voice box), trachea (windpipe), and the passages within the lungs called the bronchi and alveoli (**FIGURE 6-3**).

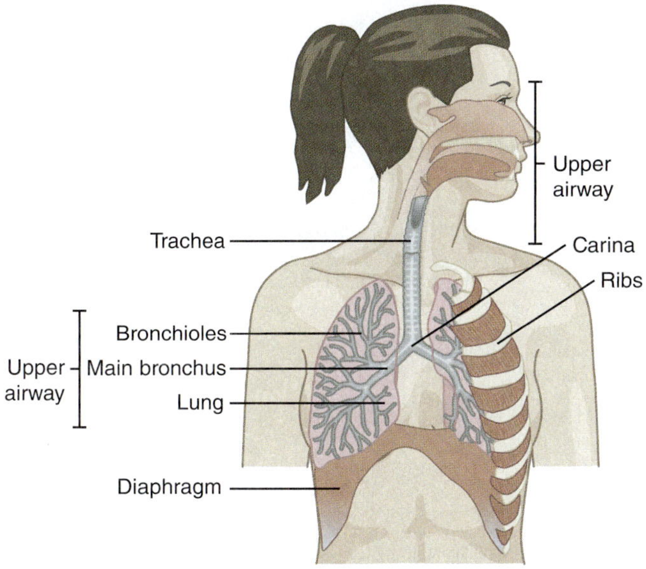

FIGURE 6-2 The respiratory system.
© Jones & Bartlett Learning

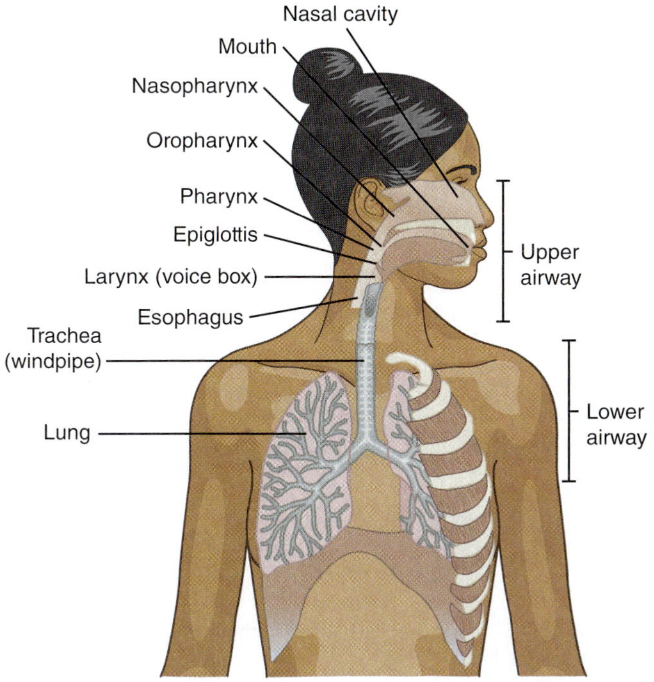

FIGURE 6-3 The airway.
© Jones & Bartlett Learning

At the upper end of the larynx is a small flap of tissue called the **epiglottis**. The epiglottis keeps food from entering the larynx. The larger air passages of the lungs, or bronchi, branch into many narrower passages called bronchioles. The airway ends in tiny air sacs called alveoli. These air sacs are surrounded by tiny blood vessels called capillaries.

Oxygen in the inhaled air passes through the thin walls that separate the air sacs from the blood vessels and is absorbed by the blood. **Carbon dioxide**, a waste product of metabolism, passes from the blood across the same thin walls into the air sacs and is exhaled. This exchange of carbon dioxide for oxygen occurs 12 to 16 times per minute, 24 hours per day, typically without any conscious effort on your part (**FIGURE 6-4**). The rate of breathing increases when the body needs more oxygen or when it generates additional carbon dioxide. Blood transports the inhaled oxygen to all parts of the body through the circulatory system.

Air is inhaled when the **diaphragm**, a large muscle that forms the bottom of the chest cavity, moves downward and

> **Special Populations**
>
> ### Considerations for the Pediatric Respiratory System
>
> Infants and children have somewhat different respiratory systems than adults:
>
> - A child's airway is smaller and more flexible than an adult's. As a result, less pressure is required when performing rescue breathing. Also, the smaller size means it is more easily blocked by a foreign object, secretions, or swelling from illnesses or trauma.
> - A child's tongue is relatively larger than the tongue of an adult (that is, it occupies a greater percentage of the oropharynx). As a result, a child's tongue can more easily block the airway if the child becomes unresponsive.
> - Infants can breathe only through their noses for at least the first 6 months of their lives. Therefore, if an infant's nose becomes blocked by mucus, the infant will show signs of respiratory distress. It is important to clear the nose of an infant to enable breathing.
>
> Airway management procedures are discussed in detail in Chapter 7, *Airway Management*.

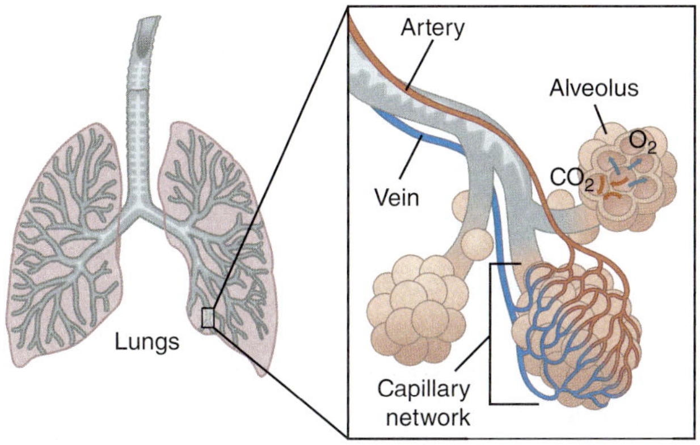

FIGURE 6-4 The exchange of carbon dioxide (CO_2) and oxygen (O_2) in the lungs.
© Jones & Bartlett Learning

the chest muscles contract to expand the size of the chest. Air is exhaled when these muscles relax, thus decreasing the size of the chest (**FIGURE 6-5**).

The Circulatory System

The **circulatory system** is responsible for pumping and circulating blood throughout the body through a network of blood vessels. The circulatory system includes the heart, blood, and blood vessels (**FIGURE 6-6**).

After blood picks up oxygen from the lungs, it travels to the heart, which pumps it to the rest of the body. The cells of the body absorb oxygen and nutrients from the blood and release waste products (including carbon dioxide), which the blood carries back to the lungs and kidneys for removal. In the lungs, the blood exchanges carbon dioxide for more oxygen, and the cycle begins again.

The human heart has four chambers: two on the right side and two on the left side. Each upper chamber is called an atrium. The right atrium receives blood from the veins of the body; the left atrium receives blood from the lungs. The bottom chambers are the right and left ventricles. The right ventricle pumps blood to the lungs; the left ventricle pumps blood throughout the body and is the most muscular chamber of the heart. The four chambers of the heart work together in sequence to pump blood to the lungs and to the rest of the body (**FIGURE 6-7**).

One-way valves in the heart and the veins allow blood to flow in only one direction through the circulatory system. The arteries carry blood away from the heart at high pressure and therefore have thick walls. The arteries closest to the heart are quite large (approximately 1 inch [2 cm] in diameter) but become smaller farther away from the heart.

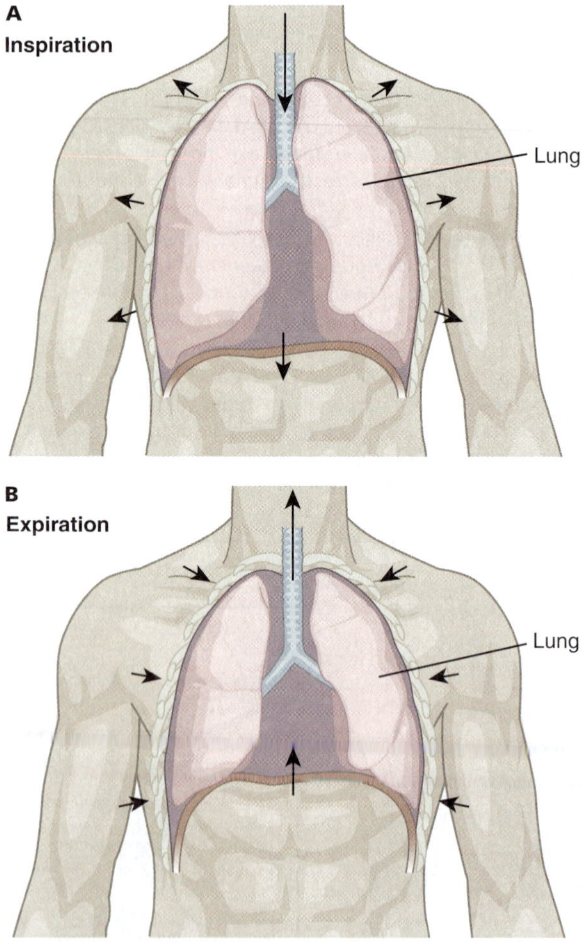

FIGURE 6-5 Mechanism of breathing. **A.** Diaphragm moves downward. **B.** Diaphragm relaxes.

© Jones & Bartlett Learning

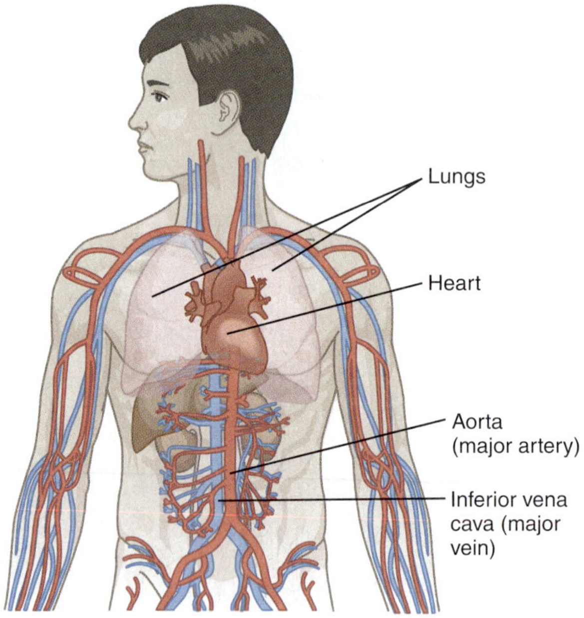

FIGURE 6-6 The circulatory system.

© Jones & Bartlett Learning

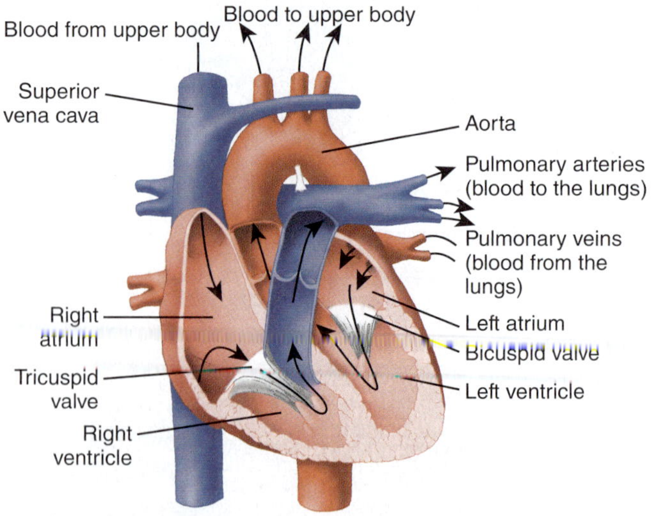

FIGURE 6-7 Schematic representation of the functions of the four chambers of the heart.

© Jones & Bartlett Learning

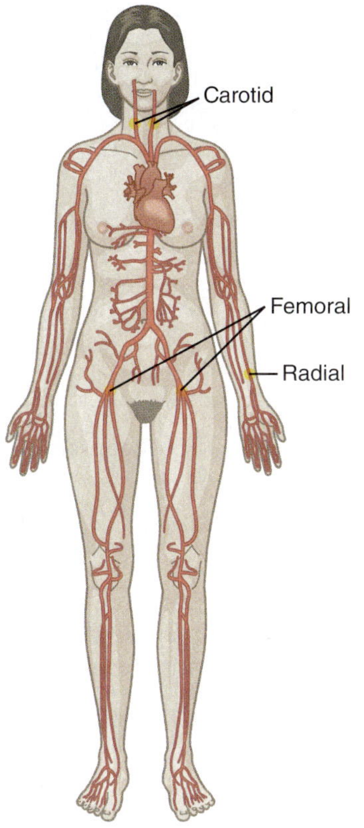

FIGURE 6-8 The locations of the carotid, radial, and femoral pulses.
© Jones & Bartlett Learning

There are three pairs of major arteries: the carotid (located in the neck), the femoral (located on each side of the groin), and the radial (located in the wrists) arteries. The locations of these arteries are shown in **FIGURE 6-8**. Because these arteries lie between a bony structure and the skin, they are used as locations to assess the patient's **pulse**, or the wave of pressure that is created by the heart as it forces blood through the arteries. The pulse is felt (or palpated) by lightly compressing the artery against the adjacent bony structure.

The capillaries are the smallest vessels in the circulatory system. Some capillaries are so small that only one blood cell at a time can go through them. At the capillary level, oxygen and nutrients pass from the blood cells into the cells of body tissues, and carbon dioxide and other waste products pass from the tissue cells to the blood cells, which then return to the lungs.

Veins are the thin-walled vessels of the circulatory system that carry blood back to the heart.

Blood has several components: **plasma**, the clear, yellowish fluid part of the blood; red blood cells; white blood cells; and **platelets**, which are responsible for forming blood clots. Blood gets its red color from the red blood cells that carry oxygen from the lungs to the body tissues and bring carbon dioxide back to the lungs. The white blood cells are known as infection fighters because they attack bacteria and other disease-causing organisms.

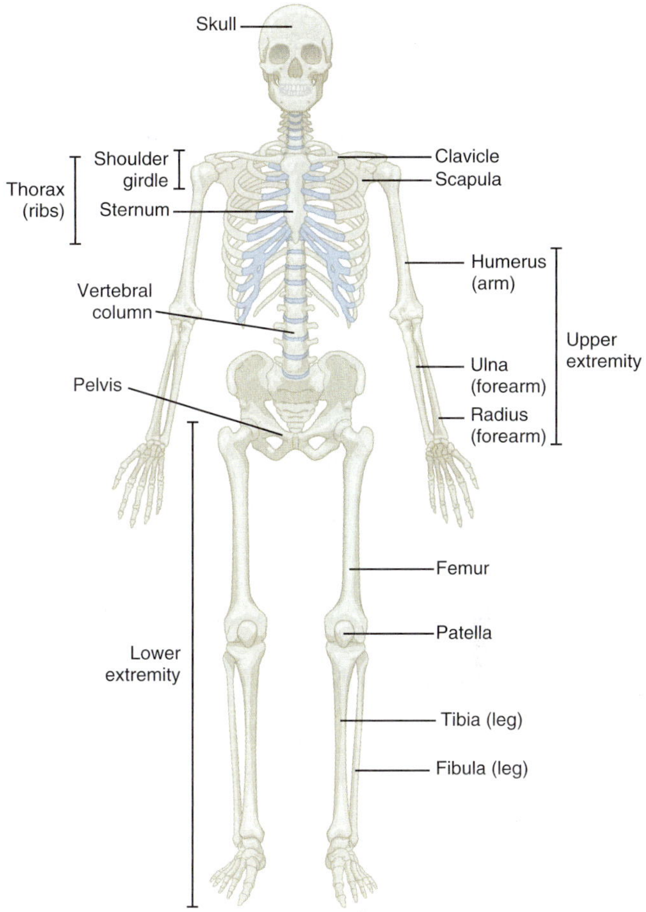

FIGURE 6-9 The human skeleton.
© Jones & Bartlett Learning

The Skeletal System

The skeletal system consists of bones and connective tissues that protect and support the framework for the body. The three main functions of the skeletal system are to:

1. Support the body.
2. Protect vital structures.
3. Produce red blood cells.

The skeletal system is divided into seven areas: the skull, spine, shoulder girdles, upper extremities, rib cage, pelvis, and lower extremities (**FIGURE 6-9**).

The Skull

The bones of the head include the **skull** and the lower jawbone. The skull consists of many bones fused together to form a hollow sphere that contains and protects the brain. The jawbone is the only movable bone and is attached to the skull to complete the structure of the head.

The Spine

The spine consists of a series of 33 separate bones called **vertebrae**. The spinal vertebrae are stacked one on top of

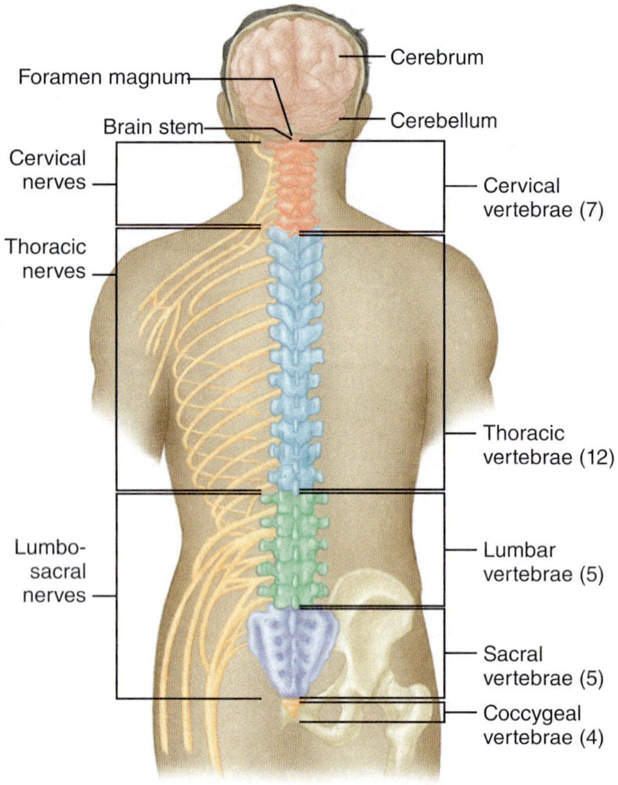

FIGURE 6-10 The five sections of the spine.

© Jones & Bartlett Learning

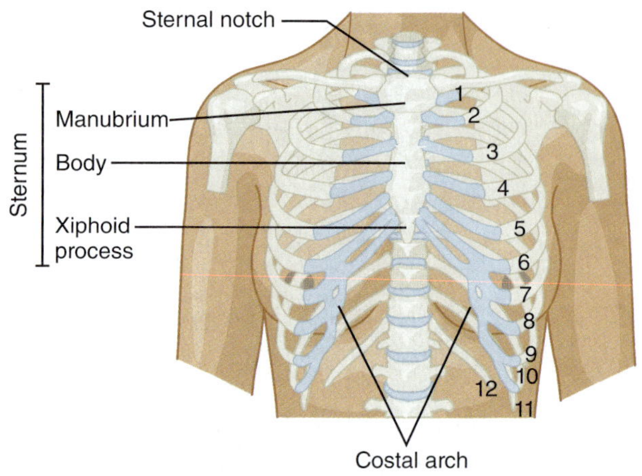

FIGURE 6-11 The rib cage.

© Jones & Bartlett Learning

the other and are held together by muscles, **tendons** (cords that attach muscle to bone), disks, and **ligaments** (fibrous bands that connect bone to bone). The spinal cord, a group of nerves that carry messages to and from the brain, passes through the hole in the center of each spinal vertebra. The vertebrae provide excellent protection for the spinal cord. In addition to protecting the spinal cord, the spine is the primary support structure for the entire body. The spine has five sections (**FIGURE 6-10**):

1. **Cervical spine** (neck)
2. **Thoracic spine** (upper back)
3. **Lumbar spine** (lower back)
4. **Sacrum** (base of spine)
5. **Coccyx** (tailbone)

The Shoulder Girdles

The **shoulder girdles** are the bones that connect the arms to the skeleton. Each shoulder girdle supports an arm and consists of the collarbone (clavicle), the shoulder blade (scapula), and the upper arm bone (humerus).

The Upper Extremity

Each upper extremity consists of three major bones. The upper arm has one bone (the **humerus**), and the forearm has two bones (the **ulna** and the **radius**). The radius is located on the thumb side, or lateral side, of the arm, and the ulna is located on the little-finger or medial side. The wrist and hand are part of the upper extremity and consist of several bones, whose names you do not need to learn at this time. You can consider these bones as one unit for the purposes of emergency medical treatment.

The Rib Cage

The rib cage (chest) is composed of 12 sets of **ribs**. The ribs protect the heart, lungs, liver, and spleen. All of the ribs attach to the spine (**FIGURE 6-11**). The upper five sets of ribs connect directly to the **sternum** (breastbone). The ends of the 6th through 10th rib sets are connected to each other and to the sternum by a bridge of **cartilage**. The 11th and 12th rib sets are attached to the spine but are not attached to the sternum in any way; they are called **floating ribs**.

The sternum is located in the front of the chest. The pointed structure at the bottom of the sternum is called the **xiphoid process**.

The Pelvis

The **pelvis** is a closed bony ring that serves as the link between the body and the lower extremities. It protects the reproductive organs and the other organs located in the lower abdominal cavity.

Words of Wisdom

You can see that a protective bony structure covers each of the essential organs of the body:

- The skull protects the brain.
- The vertebrae protect the spinal cord.
- The ribs protect the heart and lungs.
- The pelvis protects the lower abdominal and reproductive organs.

The Lower Extremity

Each lower extremity consists of the thigh and the lower leg. The thigh bone (**femur**) is the longest and strongest bone in the body. The lower leg has two bones, the **tibia** and **fibula**. The kneecap (patella) is a small, relatively flat bone that protects the front of the knee joint. Like the wrist and hand, the ankle and foot contain many smaller bones that you can consider as one unit.

Words of Wisdom

When you describe the location of an injury or pain, it is more important that other EMS personnel clearly understand the site of the injury or pain than it is that you use exact anatomic terminology. Use the proper names when you can, but strive for accuracy over proper terminology.

Joints

At the point where two bones come in contact, a **joint** is formed. Supporting tissues called tendons and ligaments help to hold the joint together. Most joints are lubricated by a thin fluid that is contained in a sac surrounding the joint.

There are three main types of joints. Fused joints do not permit any movement between the bone ends. The skull is an example of a fused joint. Hinge joints allow movement in only one plane. The knee, elbow, and fingers are examples of hinge joints. Ball-and-socket joints allow movement in more than one plane. The shoulder and the hip are examples of ball-and-socket joints. **FIGURE 6-12** shows different types of joints.

Moveable joints are designed to permit a certain amount of movement. If movement occurs beyond these limits, injury and damage to the joint will occur.

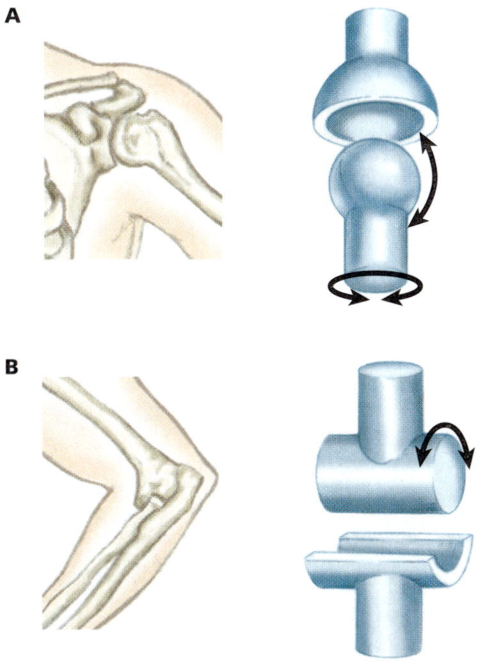

FIGURE 6-12 Different types of joints. **A.** The shoulder is a ball-and-socket joint. **B.** The elbow joint is a hinge joint, which allows motion only in one plane.

© Jones & Bartlett Learning

The Muscular System

The body contains three different types of muscles: skeletal, smooth, and cardiac. Skeletal muscle provides both support and movement. This type of muscle is attached to bone by tendons. These muscles cause movement by alternately contracting (shortening) and relaxing (lengthening). To move bones, skeletal muscles are usually paired in opposition: as one member of the pair contracts, the other relaxes. This mechanical opposition enables you to open and close your hand, turn your head, and bend and straighten your elbow. For example, when the biceps relaxes, an opposing muscle, the triceps, on the back of the arm contracts, straightening the elbow. Because skeletal muscles are under direct, voluntary control of the brain and can be stimulated to contract or relax at will, they are also called voluntary muscle.

Smooth muscle carries out many of the automatic functions of the body, such as propelling food through the digestive system. Because you have no control over smooth muscle, it is also called involuntary muscle.

Cardiac muscle is found only in the heart. This muscle is constantly working. It has a rich blood supply and can live only a few minutes without an adequate supply of oxygen.

The skeletal and muscular systems function together. The two systems combined are referred to as the **musculoskeletal system**.

The Nervous System

The **nervous system** governs the body's functioning. The nervous system consists of the brain, the spinal cord, and the individual **nerves** that extend throughout the body (**FIGURE 6-13**). The brain and spinal cord are called the central nervous system. The cables of nerve fibers outside the central nervous system are called the peripheral nervous system.

The brain is the body's central computer. It controls the functions of thinking, voluntary actions (things you have to

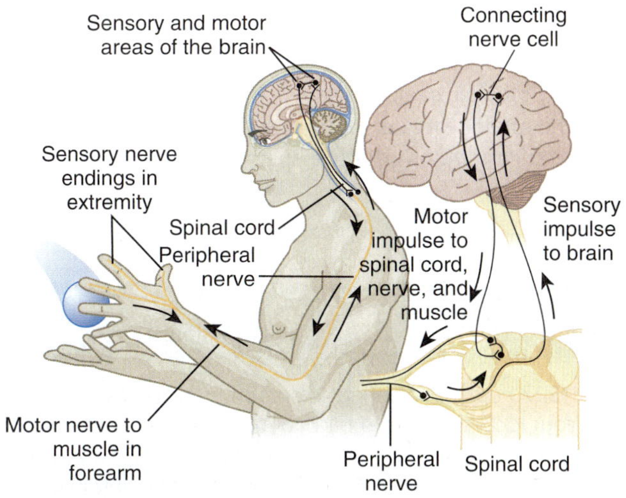

FIGURE 6-13 The nervous system.

© Jones & Bartlett Learning

think about), and involuntary (automatic) functions such as breathing, heartbeat, and digestion.

The spinal cord is a long tubelike structure that extends from the base of the brain. It consists of a complex network of nerves that make up a two-way communication system between the brain and the rest of the body. Nerves branch out from the spinal cord to every part of the body. Some nerves send signals to the brain about the body, such as whether it is feeling heat, cold, pain, or pleasure. Other nerves carry signals to muscles that cause the body to move in response to the sensory signals it has received. Without the nervous system, you would not have these sensations, nor would you be able to control the movement of your muscles.

The Digestive System

The **digestive system** processes and breaks down food. It also absorbs the food's nutrients, which are carried away by the circulatory system to the cells of the body. Food that is not used is eliminated as solid waste from the body.

The major organs of the digestive system are located in the abdomen. The digestive tract is approximately 30 feet (9.1 m) long. It begins at the mouth and continues through the throat, esophagus (tube through which food passes), stomach, small intestine, large intestine, rectum, and anus. Besides the digestive tract, the digestive system also includes the liver, gallbladder, and pancreas (**FIGURE 6-14**).

The liver performs several digestive functions, including the production of bile. Bile is stored in the gallbladder and released into the small intestine to help digest fats. The intestines absorb nutrients, and the circulation returns them to the liver for processing. The liver is one of the most vascular organs in the body.

The pancreas also has several digestive functions. Probably its best-known function is the production of **insulin**. Insulin is released directly into the bloodstream and aids the body in its use of glucose. Diabetes mellitus is caused when insulin production is disrupted.

The Genitourinary System

The **genitourinary system** includes the reproductive organs and the urinary system. It is responsible for sexual reproductive functions and for the removal of waste products from the bloodstream.

The major organs of the male reproductive system are the testes, which produce sperm, and the penis, which delivers sperm to fertilize the female egg. The major organs of the female reproductive system are the ovaries, which produce eggs, and the uterus, which holds the fertilized egg as it develops during pregnancy. The egg released by the ovaries travels to the uterus through the fallopian tubes. The external opening of the female reproductive system is called the birth canal (vagina).

The removal of waste products by the genitourinary system begins in the kidneys, which filter the blood to form urine. The urine flows down from the kidneys through tubes (ureters) into the bladder. The bladder collects and stores the urine before it passes out of the body through the urethra.

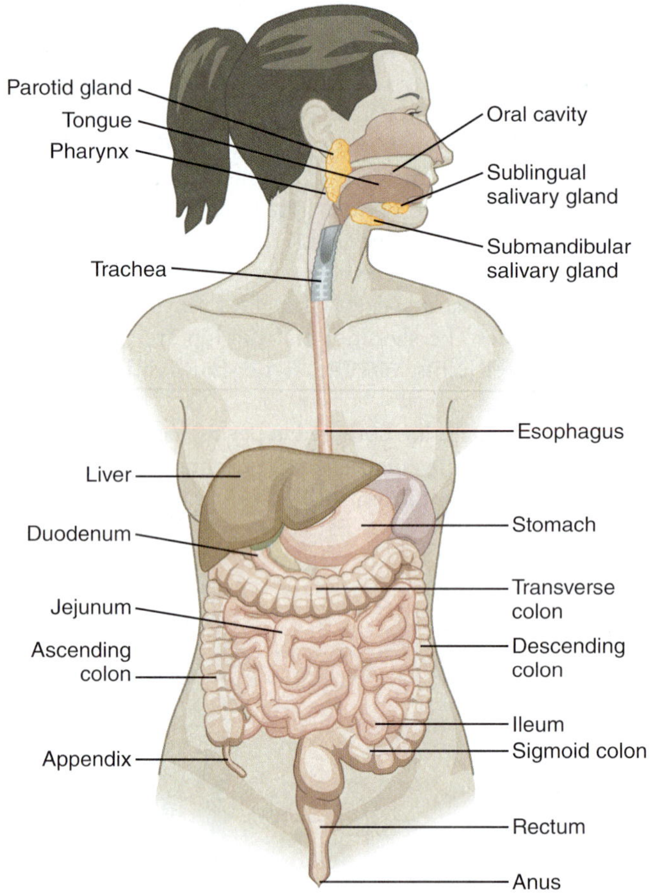

FIGURE 6-14 The digestive system.
© Jones & Bartlett Learning

YOU are the EMR — CASE 2

At 1527 hours on a spring afternoon, you are dispatched to your local skateboard park for the report of an injured skateboarder. As you arrive, you find a 14-year-old boy sitting against a wall, cradling his right arm and moaning in pain. You notice that the lower part of his forearm is bent at an unnatural angle just above his wrist. As you examine the fingers on his right hand, he says they feel numb.

1. Given the location of the young man's injury, what body systems do you think may have been affected?
2. What purpose does the skeletal system serve?

The Skin

Skin is the largest organ of the body. Skin covers all parts of the body and has three major functions:

1. Protects against harmful substances in the environment
2. Regulates body temperature
3. Transmits information from the outside environment to the brain

FIGURE 6-15 identifies the layers of the skin. The dermis is the deeper, or inner, layer of the skin. The prefix *epi-* means "upon." Therefore, the epidermis is the outer layer of skin that is located upon the dermis.

Skin protects the body from the environment. Because skin provides an intact layer of cells that serves as a barrier to most foreign substances, it prevents harmful materials from getting into the body. The skin is an effective barrier to bacteria and viruses as long as it is not broken by injury.

Skin regulates the internal temperature of the body. If the body gets too hot, the small blood vessels close to the skin open up (dilate) and bring more body heat to the surface of the skin, where the heat is transferred to the air. Another source of cooling occurs when sweat released by the skin evaporates on the skin's surface. If the body becomes cold, the blood vessels near the skin surface constrict, transferring more body heat to the inside or core part of the body.

Skin receives information from the environment. The skin can perceive touch, pressure, and pain, and it can sense degrees of heat or cold. These perceptions are picked up by special sensors in the skin and transmitted through the nerves and the spinal cord to the brain. The brain serves as the computer to interpret these sensations.

Stages of Life: Growth and Development

The moment after birth, the body begins an ever-changing journey. As a person grows and develops, the body changes from being a tiny, fragile, totally dependent infant to a full-grown, independent adult. As the body then progresses

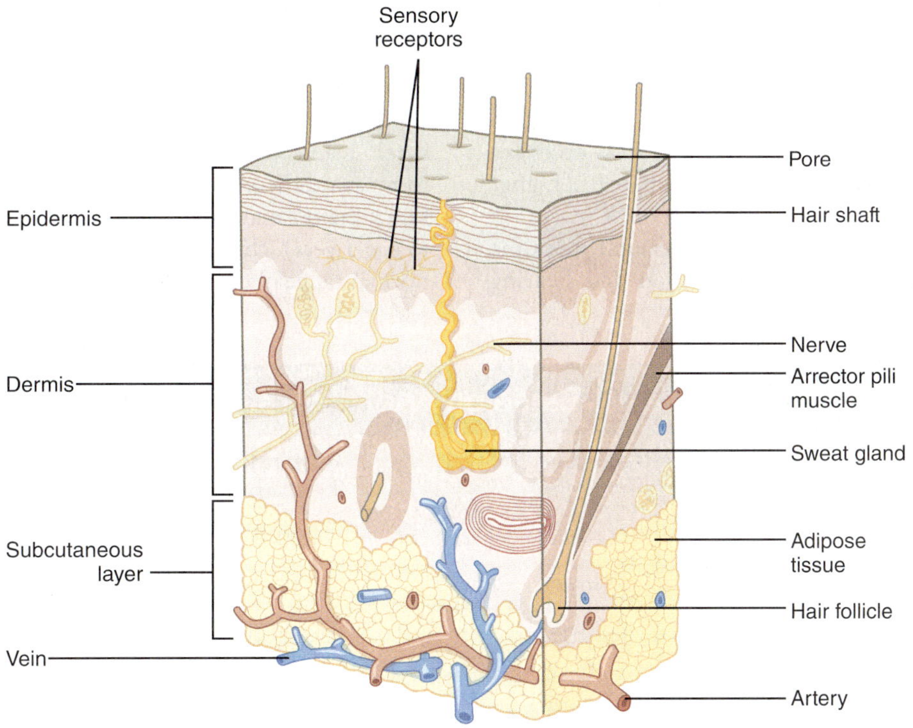

FIGURE 6-15 The skin.

© Jones & Bartlett Learning

YOU are the EMR — CASE 3

Just before 1200 hours on an extremely hot summer day, you are sent to the home of a 74-year-old woman. She called 9-1-1 saying she was feeling weak. She tells you she was working in her garden for a couple of hours this morning, felt tired, and came back into her house about 2 hours ago. She states she has not had much to eat or drink since she came back into her house. Her skin feels cool to your touch.

1. Why is it important to know how a person's body systems change in response to aging?
2. What part of the body helps regulate temperature?

through the natural aging process from adulthood to old age, the functioning of all body systems gradually declines.

Throughout a person's life, the body constantly changes. You need to know how these changes affect the treatment of your patients.

In an infant, the airway is very small and is easily obstructed by swelling or foreign bodies. At birth, infants can breathe only through their noses. Therefore, make sure their noses are not obstructed.

Toddlers (age 1 to 3 years) are unsteady and tend to explore. Their poor coordination and balance put them at a high risk for injuries from falls. Preschool-age children (3 to 6 years) experience rapid changes in growth and development. They are increasingly capable of exploring their environment and are beginning to understand the difference between appropriate and inappropriate behaviors. School-aged children (6 to 12 years) lose their primary teeth, which are then replaced with permanent teeth. They are physically active and susceptible to injuries from bicycle riding and other athletic mishaps. Adolescents (12 to 18 years) test the limits of authority. They see themselves as invincible and do not fully understand the consequences of dangerous actions. During this period, most adolescents get their driving licenses. Inexperience and risk-taking lead to higher incidences of motor vehicle crashes for young drivers.

Early adulthood (18 to 40 years) is the period when most body systems are fully developed. Most people enjoy good health during this period. Lifestyle issues such as excessive alcohol consumption and drug misuse contribute to a higher incidence of injuries and illness.

Middle adulthood (40 to 65 years) is generally the time when body systems start to decline. Vision and hearing become less acute. Cardiovascular and respiratory systems start to weaken. The incidence of a variety of cancers increases during this period. Women experience menopause during their late 40s and early 50s. Weight control becomes more difficult for most people during this period.

During older adulthood (65 years and older), the declines that started in middle adulthood become more pronounced. Respiratory and circulatory systems decline further. Most people in this age group experience some loss of bone strength, which makes them more susceptible to fractures. Many older people experience decreased sensation to heat and cold. Because of this, people in this age group are more likely to sustain burns. Many older adults have poor balance and decreased muscle tone. These factors contribute to a higher incidence of falls. The incidence of mental decline and senility increases in this age group.

Normal physiologic changes throughout a person's life result in an increased occurrence of certain illnesses and injuries at certain stages of life. By understanding these changes, you will be better prepared to provide quality care for your patients.

Vital Signs

Measuring a patient's vital signs allows you to evaluate a variety of bodily functions. The most commonly measured vital signs are pulse (heart rate), respiratory rate, and blood pressure. As an EMR, it is important for you to understand how to measure these vital signs. It is also important for you to know the normal values for vital signs for infants (newborn to age 1 year), children (ages 1 to 12 years), and adults. The normal range of these vital signs is shown in **TABLE 6-1**.

TABLE 6-1 Typical Vital Sign Values Based on Age[a]

Age	Pulse Rate (Heart Rate) (beats/min)[b]	Respirations (breaths/min)	Systolic Blood Pressure (mm Hg)
Infants (newborn to age 1 year)	100–180	30–53	72–104
Children (ages 1 to 12 years)	75–140	18–28	86–115
Older children and adults	60–100	12–20	90–120

[a]Vital signs and age ranges may vary in different sources.
[b]Pulse rate may be slightly slower when children are sleeping.

© Jones & Bartlett Learning

YOU are the EMR — CASE 4

Early Saturday morning, you are dispatched to a local soccer field for a 13-year-old boy injured during a soccer game. You can hear his screams as you are getting out of the ambulance. Family members are surrounding him on the field. You walk up and see that he is cradling his left arm with his right arm. His left shoulder is obviously deformed.

1. What type of joint is involved and how does it work?
2. What effect would the child's injury have on his vital signs?

Voices OF Experience

In 1982, when I completed my first responder course (now EMR), we did not learn a great deal about the human body. What we did learn, I thought was too much. I remember saying to a classmate, "Why do we have to learn all this stuff about the body? Who cares?" I only wanted to learn about how to fix the blood and gut injuries.

Not long after completing the course, my fire department was dispatched to a person who had been shot, and I then realized that everything I had learned about the human body was worth every minute of class time. We arrived to find a 20-something-year-old man on the ground, in a left lateral recumbent position. The patient was awake and alert, complaining of being shot in the leg. As a young EMS clinician eager to save the world, my first reaction was one of disappointment—he was only shot in the leg. We completed our primary assessment and proceeded to our secondary assessment after we confirmed there were no obvious life threats. We were taught to look for entrance wounds and exit wounds when there was a penetrating injury. Our assessment revealed only an entrance wound behind his left upper leg. We thought, "Hey, no big deal," except that this patient was quickly deteriorating and began to complain of left shoulder pain.

> **"As a young EMS provider eager to save the world, my first reaction was one of disappointment—he was only shot in the leg."**

I remembered my instructor telling us that a gunshot entry wound without an exit wound means the bullet can be anywhere. Now we were thinking about the possible path of travel this bullet took and what organs might be affected. From its entrance point, we determined that the popliteal, femoral, or iliac artery may be damaged. If the bullet took an upward path, any organ in the abdominal cavity—especially the left lower and left upper quadrants—could be affected, yet the abdomen was soft and nontender during the assessment. I remembered the diaphragm separated the abdominal and thoracic cavities, so the chest was our next thought. This patient was quickly becoming pale, his pulse was increasing, and his mental state was altered—all signs of shock (hypoperfusion). We decided the bullet could have injured the heart itself, the great vessels, or the lungs. His breathing was rapid but he had equal chest rise.

Although we were unable to locate exactly what was affected, we concluded that the patient was seriously injured, so we placed him supine (flat on his back) and packaged him for transport as soon as the ambulance arrived. While awaiting the ambulance, we administered oxygen and maintained the patient's body temperature. When the ambulance arrived, they were able to leave immediately after our handoff report.

We later learned that the bullet had nicked the pericardial sac that surrounds the heart. The patient was taken into surgery and survived. Our knowledge of the human body, as little as it was, allowed us to quickly realize what the potential injuries might be and prepare this patient for immediate transport.

Guy Peifer, BS, NREMT-P, CIC, RF/PC
Paramedic Program Coordinator, Borough of Manhattan Community College
EMS Education Coordinator, Yonkers Fire Department
Yonkers, New York

Adapted from the personal Medical Identification Symbol of the American Medical Association.

Normal vital signs change with age. The normal pulse rate decreases with age. The normal pulse rate for infants is 100 to 180 beats/min. This rate drops to 60 to 100 beats/min for adults. Respiratory rates also decrease with age. The normal respiratory rate for infants is 25 to 60 breaths/min. This rate drops to 12 to 20 breaths/min for adults. The values for systolic blood pressure increase with age. The normal systolic blood pressure for infants is 50 to 95 mm Hg. In adults, the blood pressure increases to 90 to 140 mm Hg.

Significant variation in normal vital sign values exists within any age group. These variations depend on a person's size, degree of physical conditioning, and medications taken. For example, the normal pulse rate for young adults is 60 to 100 beats/min; however, a long-distance runner or a competitive bicyclist in this age group may have a resting heart rate of 45 beats/min, which is normal and healthy for that person.

Many factors can influence vital signs. Some factors increase certain vital signs and others decrease them. **TABLE 6-2** lists some of the factors you should consider when assessing a patient's condition.

TABLE 6-2 Factors That Can Change Certain Vital Signs

Increase Pulse Rate, Respirations, and/or Systolic Blood Pressure	Decrease Pulse Rate, Respirations, and/or Systolic Blood Pressure
Exercise	Athletic conditioning
Fever	Blood pressure medications
Illness	Use of illegal drugs
Pain	
Stress	
Excess body weight	
Use of illegal drugs	

© Jones & Bartlett Learning

Words of Wisdom

Because it may be hard to remember the normal ranges of vital signs for each age group, many EMS agencies keep a list of these values available electronically or in their jump bags so their personnel can quickly refer to them when needed.

YOU are the EMR SUMMARY

You are the EMR: CASE 1

1. Why is some knowledge of anatomy and an understanding of the functions of body systems important in cases like this?

Having some knowledge of anatomy and the functions of body systems helps you better understand the source of an injury or illness and can improve the care you provide to the patient. Knowing the location of body organs and systems helps you to better determine the types of injuries or illnesses that are more likely to occur. Understanding anatomic terms and medical terminology helps you better communicate with other members of the medical care team. Using proper terminology will also help you avoid misunderstandings when sharing your assessment findings.

You are the EMR: CASE 2

1. Given the location of the young man's injury, what body systems do you think may have been affected?

Given the type of trauma the skateboarder experienced, the location of the injury, and your findings, you should suspect injury to his skeletal system, possible injury to his muscular system, possible injury to the nerves in his right forearm, and possible injury to some of the blood vessels around the injury site, even if there are no signs of external bleeding. In addition, it is important to examine the patient for additional injuries due to the type of trauma he sustained.

2. What purpose does the skeletal system serve?

The skeletal system protects vital structures, such as the spinal cord. It supports the body and produces red blood cells.

You are the EMR: CASE 3

1. Why is it important to know how a person's body systems change in response to aging?

When you are providing care for geriatric patients, it is important for you to know that as the body ages, its ability to sense heat and cold decreases. As a result, older adults tend to have difficulty maintaining a cool body temperature in hot weather, especially when they are exercising or are outside for a long period. In the winter, older adults may have difficulty keeping warm and may wear more clothing than younger people.

2. What part of the body helps regulate temperature?

The skin regulates the internal temperature of the body. If the body gets too hot, blood vessels close to the skin dilate and bring body heat to the surface of the skin. The skin also releases sweat, which evaporates and promotes cooling. If older adults do not drink enough water, their body's cooling mechanism may not be able to keep their bodies cool. If the body becomes cold, blood vessels near the skin surface constrict, keeping heat in the body.

YOU are the EMR **SUMMARY**

You are the EMR: CASE 4

1. What type of joint is involved and how does it work?

Joints are where two bones meet. The shoulder is a ball-and-socket joint, which allows movement in more than one plane. The hip is also a ball-and-socket joint.

2. What effect would the child's injury have on his vital signs?

Pain and stress are among the many factors that can influence a patient's vital signs. On the basis of the child's level of pain indicated by his screams, it would not be surprising if his blood pressure, pulse rate, and respiratory rate were higher than normal.

Prep Kit

Ready for Review

- You need to know basic anatomic terms to understand the location of a patient's specific signs or symptoms and to better communicate with all members of the emergency medical team.
- The respiratory system consists of the lungs and the airway. This system functions to take in air through the airway and transport it to the lungs. In the lungs, red blood cells absorb oxygen and release carbon dioxide so it can be expelled from the body.
- The circulatory system consists of the heart (the pump), the blood vessels (the pipes), and blood (the fluid). Its role is to transport oxygenated blood to all parts of the body and to remove waste products, including carbon dioxide.
- The skeletal system consists of the bones of the body. These bones function to provide support, to protect vital structures, and to produce red blood cells.
- The muscular system consists of three kinds of muscles: voluntary (skeletal) muscle, smooth (involuntary) muscle, and cardiac (heart) muscle. Muscles provide both support and movement. The skeletal system works with the muscular system to provide motion. These two systems together are called the musculoskeletal system.
- The nervous system consists of the brain, the spinal cord, and individual nerves. The brain serves as the central computer, and the nerves transmit messages between the brain and the body.
- The digestive system consists of the mouth, esophagus, stomach, intestines, liver, gallbladder, and pancreas. This system breaks down usable food for use by the body and eliminates solid waste.
- The genitourinary system consists of the organs of reproduction together with the organs involved in the production and excretion of urine.
- Skin covers the entire body. It protects the body from the environment, regulates the internal temperature of the body, and transmits sensations from the skin to the nervous system.
- You need a basic understanding of the body systems to treat the illnesses and injuries you will encounter as an EMR.
- An understanding of some of the changes that occur at different stages within the life cycle helps you to better treat the wide variety of patients you will encounter.
- Vital signs change at different stages of the life cycle. It is important for you to understand these changes so you understand the values you encounter in patients.

Vital Vocabulary

anterior The front surface of the body.

carbon dioxide The gas formed as a waste product of metabolism and excreted through the respiratory system during exhalation.

cartilage A tough, elastic form of connective tissue that covers the ends of most bones to form joints; also found in some specific areas such as the nose and the ears.

cervical spine That section of the spinal column consisting of the seven vertebrae located in the neck.

circulatory system The heart and blood vessels, which together are responsible for the continuous flow of blood throughout the body.

coccyx The tailbone; the small bone at the base of the spinal column.

diaphragm A muscular dome that separates the chest from the abdominal cavity. Contraction of the diaphragm and the chest wall muscles brings air into the lungs; relaxation expels air from the lungs.

Prep Kit

digestive system The gastrointestinal tract (stomach and intestines), mouth, salivary glands, pharynx, esophagus, liver, gallbladder, pancreas, rectum, and anus, which together are responsible for the absorption of food and the elimination of solid waste from the body.

distal Describing structures that are farther from the trunk (or torso) or nearer to the free end of an extremity. Opposite of proximal.

epiglottis The valve located at the upper end of the voice box that prevents food from entering the larynx.

femur The thighbone; the longest and one of the strongest bones in the body.

fibula The smaller of the two bones that form the lower leg, located on the lateral side.

floating ribs The 11th and 12th ribs; they do not connect to the sternum.

genitourinary system The organs of reproduction, together with the organs involved in the production and excretion of urine.

humerus The upper arm bone.

inferior Nearer to the feet than the head.

insulin A hormone produced by the pancreas that enables glucose in the blood to be used by the cells of the body; supplementary insulin is used in the treatment and control of diabetes mellitus.

joint The point where two bones come in contact with each other.

larynx A structure composed of cartilage in the neck that guards the entrance to the windpipe and functions as the organ of voice; also called the voice box.

lateral Away from the midline of the body.

ligaments Fibrous bands that connect bones to bones and support and strengthen joints.

lumbar spine The lower part of the back formed by the lowest five nonfused vertebrae.

medial Closer to the midline of the body.

midline An imaginary vertical line drawn from the head to toe that divides the body into equal left and right sides.

musculoskeletal system The bones and voluntary muscles of the body.

nerves Fiber tracts or pathways that carry messages from the spinal cord and brain to all body parts and back; sensory, motor, or a combination of both.

nervous system The brain, spinal cord, and nerves.

pelvis The closed bony ring, consisting of the sacrum and the pelvic bones, that connects the trunk to the lower extremities.

plasma The clear, yellowish fluid of the blood that carries blood cells, transports nutrients, and removes cellular waste materials.

platelets Microscopic disk-shaped elements in the blood that are essential to the formation of a blood clot, the mechanism that stops bleeding.

posterior The back surface of the body.

proximal Closer to the trunk (or torso). Opposite of distal.

pulse The wave of pressure that is created by the heart when it contracts as a result of forcing the blood out and into the major arteries.

radius The bone on the thumb side of the forearm.

respiratory system All body structures that contribute to normal breathing.

ribs The paired arches of bone, 12 on either side, that extend from the thoracic vertebrae toward the anterior midline of the trunk.

sacrum One of three bones (the others being the two pelvic bones) that makes up the pelvic ring; forms the base of the spine.

shoulder girdles The three bones of the upper extremity; each shoulder supports the clavicle, the scapula, and the humerus.

skull The bones of the head, collectively; the protective structure for the brain.

sternum The breastbone.

superior Closer to the head or above a body part.

tendons Tough, ropelike cords of fibrous tissue that attach muscle to bone.

thoracic spine The 12 vertebrae that attach to the 12 ribs; the upper part of the back.

tibia The shinbone; the larger of the two bones of the lower leg.

topographic anatomy The superficial landmarks on the body that serve as location guides to the structures that lie beneath them.

ulna The bone on the little-finger side of the forearm.

vertebrae The 33 bones of the spinal column: 7 cervical, 12 thoracic, 5 lumbar, 5 sacral, and 4 coccygeal vertebrae.

xiphoid process The flexible cartilage at the lower tip of the sternum.

Assessment IN ACTION

You and your partner are dispatched to a downtown intersection where a 59-year-old woman has been struck by a school bus. As you examine the patient, you find bruising on the right side of her upper back and a small amount of blood coming from her hand. She is having difficulty breathing and reports pain in her abdomen. She also reports pain in her left leg just above her ankle. This area is discolored and appears deformed.

1. All of the following body system(s) may be affected from these injuries EXCEPT the:

A. respiratory system.
B. circulatory system.
C. digestive system.
D. genitourinary system.

2. The blood from the patient's hand is most likely coming from the:

A. arteries.
B. veins.
C. capillaries.
D. aorta.

3. How would you describe the location of the injury to her lower extremity?

A. Distal part of her thigh
B. Proximal part of her thigh
C. Proximal part of her leg
D. Distal part of her leg

4. What part of the skeletal system is designed to protect the heart, lungs, and spleen?

A. Spine
B. Shoulder girdles
C. Rib cage
D. Vertebrae

5. The woman is now reporting numbness in her hands. What system may have been injured?

A. Circulatory system
B. Respiratory system
C. Nervous system
D. Genitourinary system

6. The normal respiratory rate for an adult is how many breaths per minute?

A. 8 to 12
B. 12 to 20
C. 15 to 30
D. 20 to 40

7. On the basis of the woman's injuries, what body system should you address first?

A. Respiratory system
B. Digestive system
C. Nervous system
D. Skeletal system

8. What is the significance of the patient's breathing difficulties?

9. What components make up blood?

10. Why should you measure the patient's vital signs in this situation?

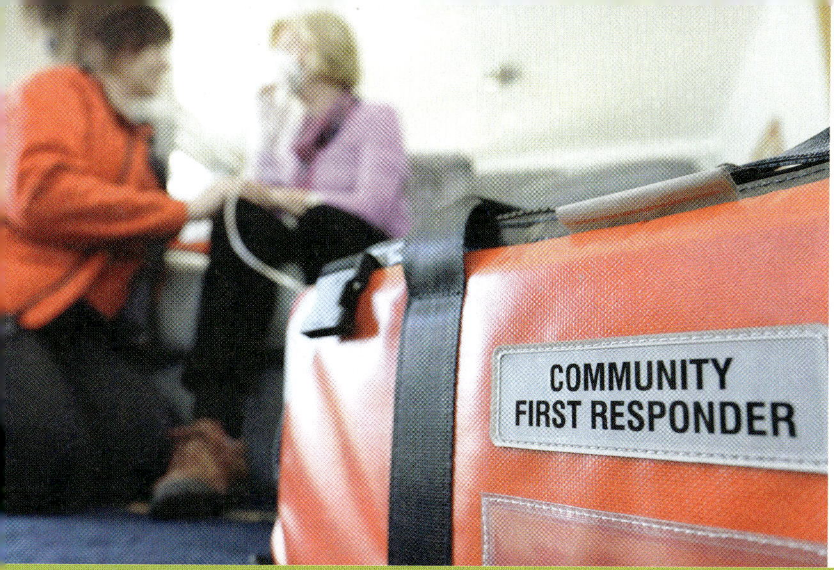

SECTION 2

Airway

7 Airway Management

8 Professional Rescuer CPR

© Peter Cripps/Alamy Stock Photo

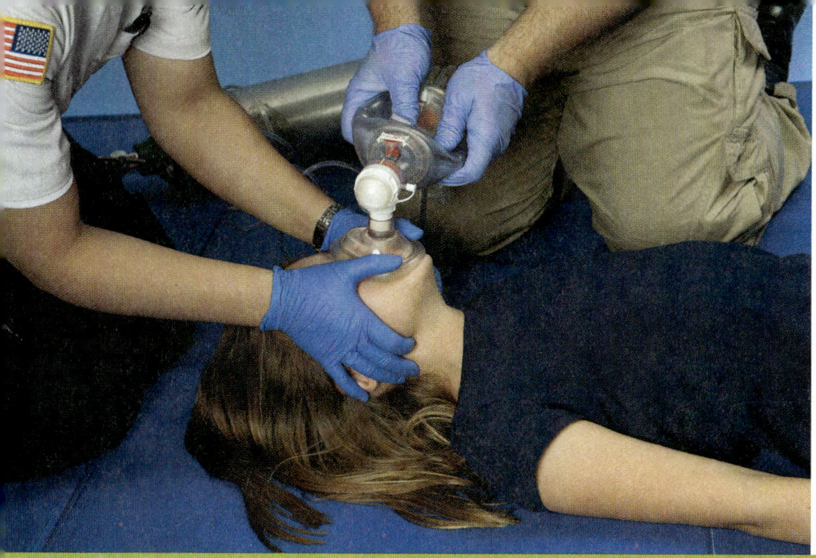

CHAPTER 7

Airway Management

National EMS Education Standard Competencies

Airway Management, Respiration, and Artificial Ventilation

Applies knowledge of anatomy and physiology to ensure a patent airway, adequate mechanical ventilation, and respiration while awaiting additional EMS response for patients of all ages.

Airway Management

- Airway anatomy (pp 117–119)
- Airway assessment (p 120)
- Techniques of ensuring a patent airway (pp 120–133)

Respiration

- Anatomy of the respiratory system (pp 117–119)
- Physiology and pathophysiology of respiration (pp 117–119)
  - Pulmonary ventilation (pp 117–119)
  - Oxygenation (pp 117–119)
  - Respiration (pp 117–119)
    - External (pp 117–119)
    - Internal (pp 117–119)
    - Cellular (pp 117–119)
- Assessment and management of adequate and inadequate respiration (pp 126–129)
- Supplemental oxygen therapy (pp 141–144)

Ventilation

- Assessment and management of adequate and inadequate ventilation (pp 129–133)
- Effect of artificial ventilation on cardiac output (pp 129–133)

Pathophysiology

Uses knowledge of shock and respiratory compromise to respond to life threats.

Medicine

Recognizes and manages life threats based on assessment findings of a patient with a medical emergency while awaiting additional emergency response.

Respiratory

- Respiratory distress/failure/arrest (pp 129–130)
- Upper airway obstruction (pp 136–141)
- Lower airway disease: asthma, bronchiolitis, pneumonia, chronic obstructive pulmonary disease (Chapter 10, *Medical Emergencies*)

Knowledge Objectives

1. Identify the anatomic structures of the respiratory system, including the function of each structure. (pp 117–119)
2. Explain the principles of breathing: ventilation, oxygenation, and respiration. (pp 117–119)
3. State the differences between the respiratory systems of infants, children, and adults. (pp 117–120)
4. Explain how to check a patient's level of responsiveness. (p 120)
5. Describe how to perform the head tilt–chin lift maneuver. (p 121)
6. Describe how to perform the jaw-thrust maneuver. (pp 121–122)
7. Explain how to check for fluids, foreign bodies, or dentures in a patient's mouth. (p 122)
8. List the steps needed to clear a patient's airway using finger sweeps and suction. (pp 122–124)
9. Describe the steps required to maintain a patient's airway using the recovery position, oral airways, and nasal airways. (pp 124–126)
10. Describe the signs of adequate breathing, the signs of inadequate breathing, the causes of respiratory arrest, and the major signs of respiratory arrest. (pp 127–129)

© Jones & Bartlett Learning. Courtesy of Glen Ellman.

11. Describe how to check a patient for the presence of breathing. (pp 126–129)
12. Describe how to perform rescue breathing using a mouth-to-mask device, a mouth-to-barrier device, mouth-to-mouth techniques, and a bag-mask device. (pp 130–133)
13. List the steps for recognizing respiratory arrest and performing rescue breathing in infants, children, and adults. (pp 133–136)
14. Describe the differences between the signs and symptoms of a mild airway obstruction and those of a severe or complete airway obstruction. (pp 136–137)
15. List the steps in managing a foreign body airway obstruction in infants, children, and adults. (pp 137–141)
16. Describe the special considerations of airway care and rescue breathing in children and infants. (pp 137–141)
17. Describe the indications for using supplemental oxygen. (pp 141–144)
18. Describe the equipment used to administer oxygen. (pp 142–143)
19. Describe the safety considerations and hazards of oxygen administration. (p 143)
20. Explain the steps in administering supplemental oxygen to a patient. (pp 143–144)
21. Describe the function and operation of a pulse oximeter. (pp 144–146)
22. List the special considerations needed to perform rescue breathing in patients with stomas. (p 145)
23. Define gastric distention. (p 145)
24. Describe the hazards that dental appliances present during the performance of airway skills. (p 145)
25. Describe the steps in providing airway care to a patient in a vehicle. (pp 145–146)

Skills Objectives

1. Demonstrate how to check a patient's level of responsiveness. (p 120)
2. Demonstrate the head tilt–chin lift maneuver for opening blocked airways. (p 121)
3. Demonstrate the jaw-thrust maneuver for opening blocked airways. (pp 121–122)
4. Demonstrate how to check for fluids, solids, and dentures in a patient's airway. (p 122)
5. Demonstrate how to correct a blocked airway using finger sweeps and suction. (pp 122–123; Skill Drill 7-1)
6. Demonstrate how to place a patient in the recovery position. (p 124)
7. Demonstrate the insertion of oral and nasal airways. (pp 124–127; Skill Drills 7-2, 7-3, and 7-4)
8. Demonstrate how to check for the presence of breathing. (p 128)
9. Demonstrate how to perform rescue breathing using a mouth-to-mask device, a mouth-to-barrier device, mouth-to-mouth techniques, and a bag-mask device. (pp 129–134; Skill Drills 7-5, 7-6, and 7-7)
10. Demonstrate the steps in recognizing respiratory arrest and performing rescue breathing on an adult, a child, and an infant. (pp 135–136; Skill Drill 7-8)
11. Demonstrate the steps needed to remove a foreign body airway obstruction in an infant, a child, and an adult. (pp 137–141; Skill Drill 7-9)
12. Demonstrate administration of supplemental oxygen using a nasal cannula and a nonrebreathing mask. (pp 141–143)
13. Demonstrate the operation of a pulse oximeter. (pp 144–146)
14. Demonstrate rescue breathing on a patient with a stoma. (p 145)
15. Demonstrate airway management on a patient in a vehicle. (pp 145–146)

Introduction

In many emergencies, your ability to open the patient's airway and ensure adequate breathing will be the difference between life and death for the patient. The skills discussed in this chapter are fundamental to your role as an emergency medical responder (EMR). The ABC (Airway, Breathing, and Circulation) mnemonic, paired with the "check and correct" concept, represents a vital principle of emergency medicine: You must check and correct the airway (*A*) before you turn your attention to the patient's breathing status (*B*), and you must check and correct breathing before you attend to circulatory problems (*C*), such as bleeding. While some emergencies, such as life-threatening external bleeding or cardiac arrest, may require an initial change to this sequence, for most calls, your care will be guided by the ABC sequence.

Words of Wisdom

The airway and breathing skills presented in this chapter can be performed in conjunction with circulation skills, thus enabling you to provide **cardiopulmonary resuscitation (CPR)**. CPR is used to save the lives of people who are experiencing cardiac arrest (stoppage of the heart). Chapter 8, *Professional Rescuer CPR*, discusses circulation skills further.

This chapter focuses on the airway and breathing components of the ABC mnemonic. Airway skills include the following:

- Checking a patient's level of consciousness (responsiveness) and manually correcting a blocked airway by using the head tilt–chin lift or jaw-thrust maneuvers

- Checking the patient's airway for foreign objects and removing anything found
- Using oral and nasal airways to keep the patient's airway open

Breathing skills include the following:

- Checking patients to determine whether they are breathing adequately and correcting breathing problems by using the appropriate rescue breathing technique
- Determining the need for supplemental oxygen and administering it using a nasal cannula and a nonrebreathing mask

Patients with airway problems will likely be extremely anxious during the episode. It is your responsibility as an EMR to treat these patients and their families with compassion while providing care.

This chapter begins with a review of the major structures of the respiratory system. You must understand how this system is supposed to work before you will be able to recognize and address problems.

Anatomy and Function of the Respiratory System

To maintain life, all organisms must receive a constant supply of certain substances. In humans, these basic life-sustaining substances are food, water, and **oxygen**. A person can live several weeks without food because the body can use nutrients it has stored. Although the body does not store as much water, it is possible to live several days without fluid intake. However, lack of oxygen, even for a few minutes, can result in irreversible damage and death.

The most sensitive cells in the human body are located in the brain. If brain cells are deprived of oxygen and nutrients for 4 to 6 minutes, they begin to die. Brain death is followed by the death of the entire body. Brain cells cannot be replaced once they are destroyed, which is why it is important for you to understand the anatomy and function of the respiratory system and the critical role it plays in supporting life.

The main purpose of the respiratory system is to provide oxygen and to remove carbon dioxide from the red blood cells as they pass through the lungs. At its broadest level, breathing can be understood as a function of ventilation, oxygenation, and respiration (**TABLE 7-1**).

The parts of the body used in breathing are shown in **FIGURE 7-1** and include the mouth (**oropharynx**), the nose (**nasopharynx**), the throat (**pharynx**), the windpipe (**trachea**), the lungs, the diaphragm (the muscle between the chest and the abdomen), and numerous chest muscles (including the intercostal muscles found between the ribs). Air enters the body through the nose and mouth. In an unresponsive patient lying on their back, the passage of air through both the nose and mouth may be blocked by the tongue (**FIGURE 7-2**).

TABLE 7-1 Physiology of Breathing

Function	Definition
Ventilation	The physical act of moving air into and out of the lungs. Also referred to as pulmonary ventilation.
Oxygenation	The process of loading oxygen molecules onto hemoglobin molecules in the bloodstream.
Respiration	The actual exchange of oxygen and carbon dioxide in the alveoli as well as the tissues of the body. It can be further classified by the following three processes: • **External respiration**: exchange of gases between the lungs and blood • **Internal respiration**: exchange of gases between the blood and tissue cells • **Cellular respiration** (or cellular metabolism): use of oxygen by the cells to carry out their specific activities

© Jones & Bartlett Learning

The tongue is attached to the lower jaw (**mandible**). When a person has a loss of consciousness, the jaw relaxes and the tongue falls backward into the rear of the mouth, effectively blocking the passage of air from both the nose and the mouth to the lungs. A partially blocked airway often produces a snoring sound. At the back of the throat are two passages: the **esophagus** (the tube through which food passes) and the trachea. The epiglottis is a thin flapper valve that allows air to enter the trachea but helps prevent food or water from entering the airway. Air passes from the throat to the larynx (voice box), which can be seen externally as the Adam's apple in the front of the neck. Below the trachea, the **airway** divides into the **bronchi** (two large tubes supported by cartilage). The bronchi branch into smaller and smaller airways in the **lungs**. The lungs are located on either side of the heart and are protected by the sternum at the front of the body and by the rib cage at the sides and back.

The smaller airways that branch from the bronchi are called bronchioles. The bronchioles end as tiny air sacs called **alveoli**. The alveoli are surrounded by extremely small blood vessels, the **capillaries**. The actual exchange of gases takes place across a thin membrane that separates the capillaries of the circulatory system from the alveoli of the lungs (**FIGURE 7-3**). The incoming oxygen passes from the alveoli into the blood, and the outgoing carbon dioxide passes from the blood into the alveoli. The exchange of oxygen and carbon dioxide that occurs in the alveoli is called **alveolar ventilation**. The amount of air pulled into the lungs and removed from the lungs in 1 minute is called **minute ventilation**.

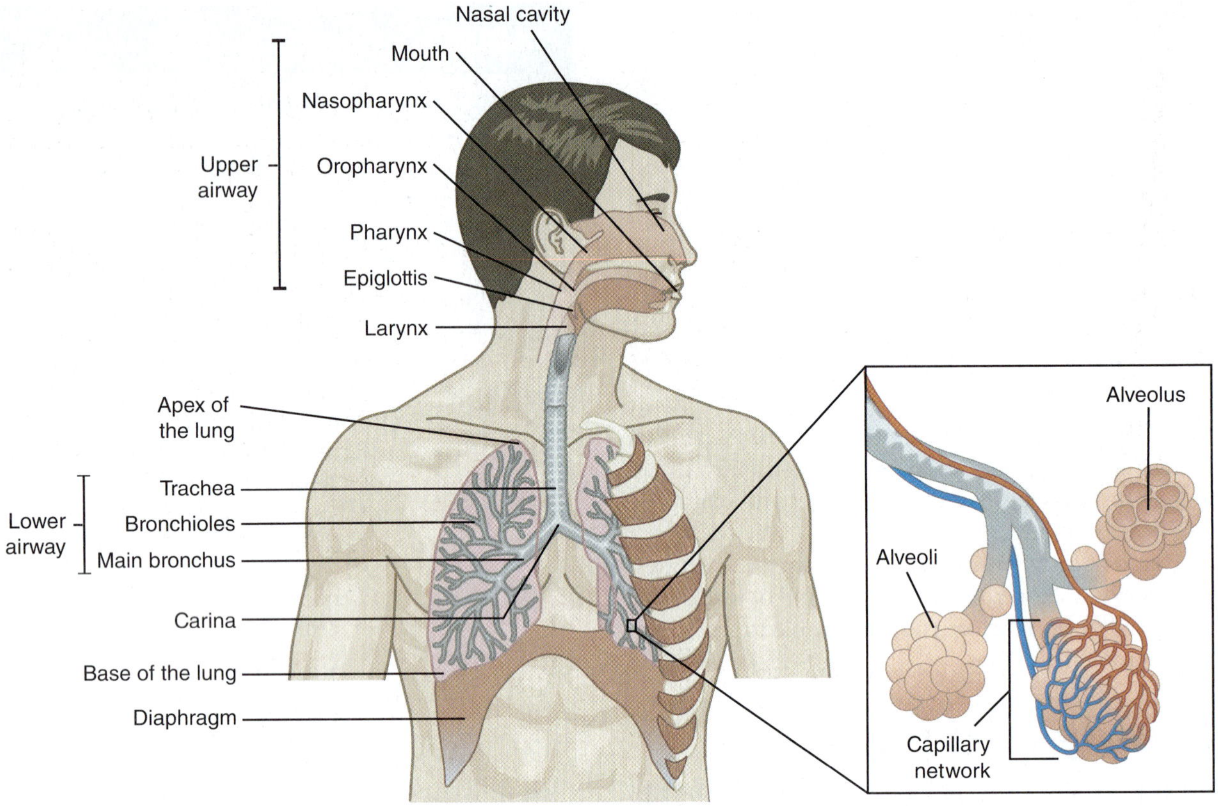

FIGURE 7-1 Anatomy of the respiratory system.

© Jones & Bartlett Learning

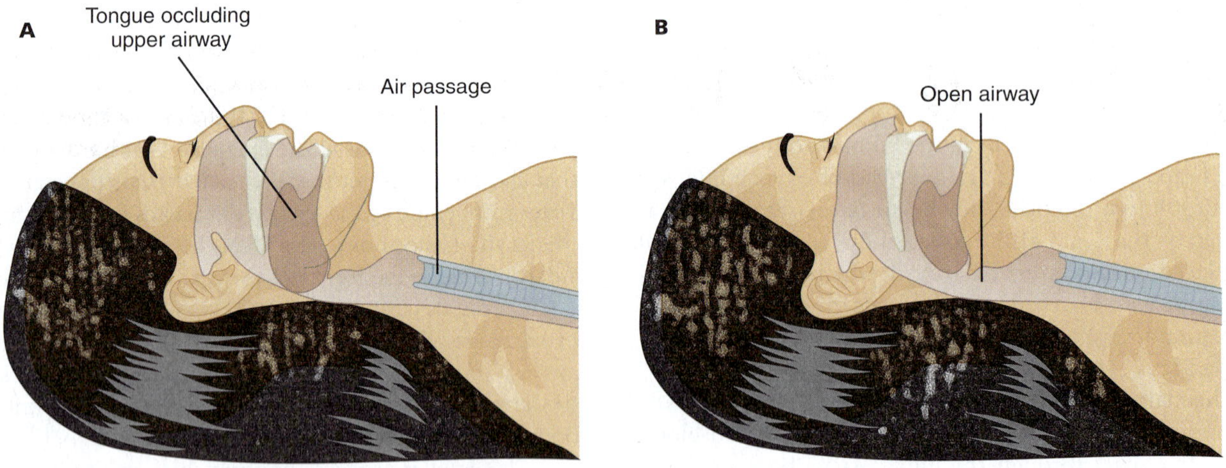

FIGURE 7-2 **A.** Airway obstructed by the tongue in an unresponsive patient. **B.** Open airway.

© Jones & Bartlett Learning

When a patient is not breathing, artificial ventilation is necessary to supply oxygen to the brain, the heart, and the rest of the body. During CPR, the blood being pushed out of the heart (cardiac output) depends on the oxygen supplied by artificial ventilation.

The lungs consist of soft, spongy tissue with no muscles. Therefore, movement of air into the lungs depends on movement of the rib cage and the diaphragm. As the rib cage expands, air is drawn into the lungs through the trachea. The diaphragm, a muscle that separates the abdominal cavity from the chest, is dome shaped when it is relaxed. When the diaphragm contracts during inhalation, it flattens and moves downward. This action increases the size of the chest cavity and helps draw air into the lungs through the trachea. On exhalation, the diaphragm relaxes and once again becomes dome shaped. In normal breathing, the combined actions of the diaphragm and the rib cage automatically produce adequate inhalation and exhalation (**FIGURE 7-4**).

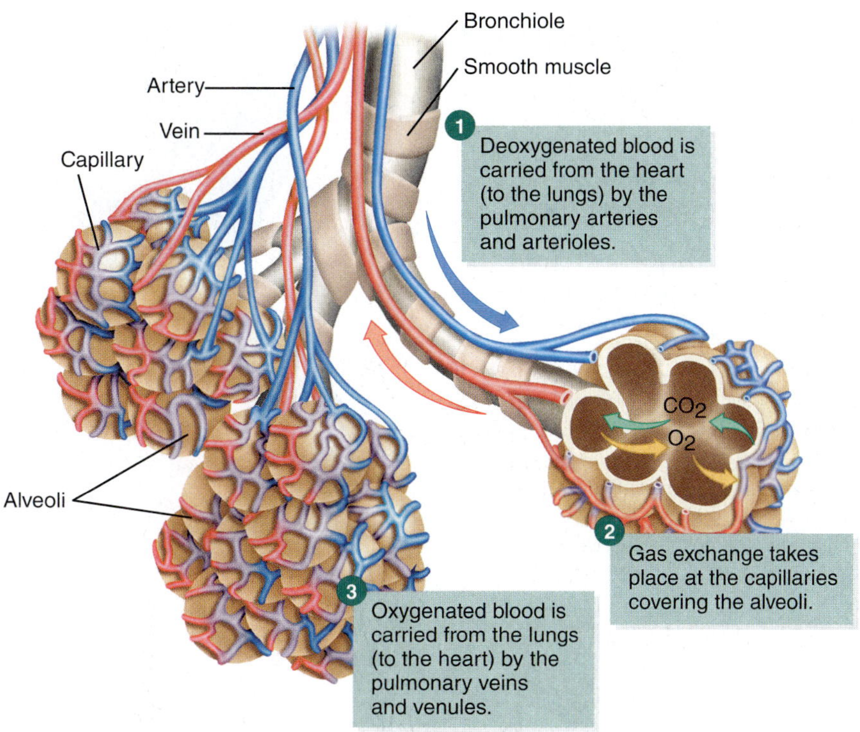

FIGURE 7-3 The exchange of gases occurs in the alveoli of the lungs.
© Jones & Bartlett Learning

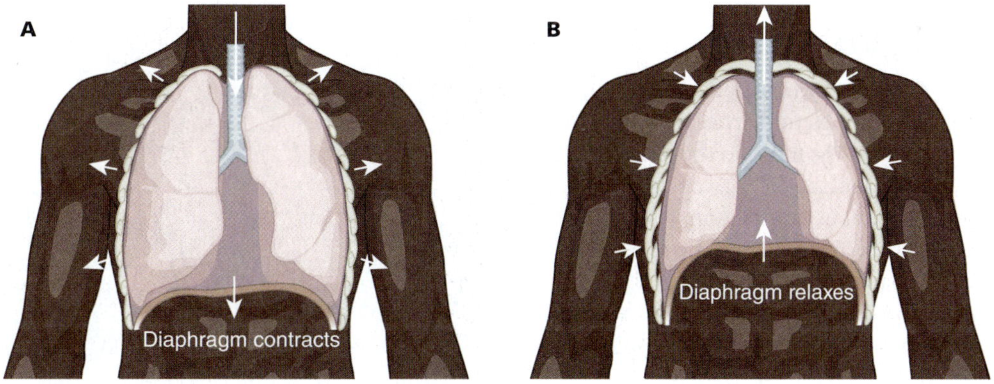

FIGURE 7-4 Normal mechanical act of breathing. **A.** Inhalation. **B.** Exhalation.
© Jones & Bartlett Learning

YOU are the EMR — CASE 1

At 1943 hours you are dispatched to an apartment complex for a report of a 67-year-old woman who is sick. While you are responding to the scene, your dispatcher informs you that the patient's husband states the woman is now unresponsive. When you arrive at the apartment, the patient's husband tells you his wife became dizzy shortly after taking a new medicine ordered by her physician. You approach the woman and ask if she can hear you. She does not respond. You gently shake the patient's shoulder and get no response.

1. What is the next step you should take to assess and treat this patient?
2. How would your method of opening the patient's airway change if the patient had fallen or blacked out?
3. What techniques can you use to maintain an open airway?

Special Populations

Understanding the Pediatric Patient's Respiratory System

- The structures of the respiratory system in children and infants are smaller than they are in adults. Therefore, the air passages of children and infants may be more easily blocked by secretions or by foreign objects.
- In children and infants, the tongue is proportionally larger than it is in adults (**FIGURE 7-5**). Therefore, the tongue of these smaller patients is more likely to block the airway than it would in an adult patient.
- Because the trachea of an infant or child is more flexible than that of an adult, it is more likely to become narrowed or blocked than that of an adult.
- The head of a child or an infant is proportionally larger than the head of an adult. You will learn slightly different techniques for opening the airways of children.
- Children and infants have smaller lungs than adults. You need to give them smaller breaths when you perform rescue breathing.
- Most children and infants have healthy hearts. When a child or infant experiences cardiac arrest, it is usually because the patient has a blocked airway or has stopped breathing, not because there is a problem with the heart.
- From birth to about 6 months of age, children are "nose breathers." They are not yet able to breathe through their mouths.

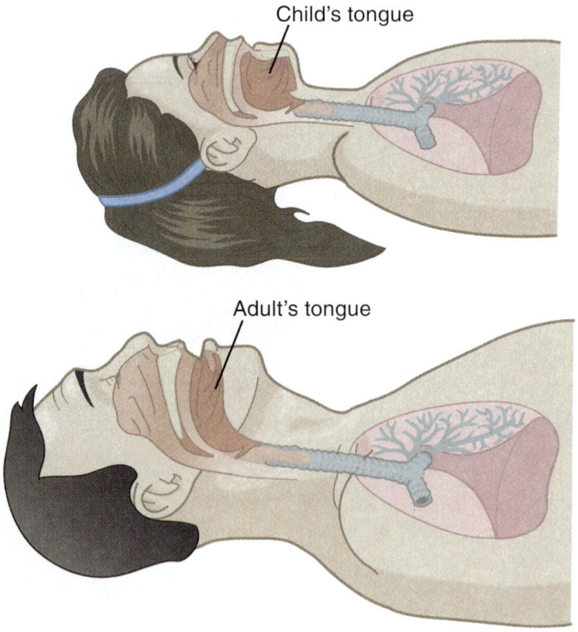

FIGURE 7-5 The anatomy of a child's airway differs from that of an adult. The tongue is proportionally larger (occupies a greater percentage of the oropharynx) and can more easily block the airway. Also, the back of the child's head is larger, so head positioning requires more care.
© Jones & Bartlett Learning

A Is for Airway

The patient's airway is the pipeline that transports life-giving oxygen from the air to the lungs and transports the waste product, carbon dioxide, from the lungs to the air. In healthy people who are alert and oriented, the airway automatically stays open. An injured or seriously ill person, however, may not be able to protect the airway, and it may become blocked by foreign objects or the patient's own tongue.

If a patient cannot protect their airway, you must take certain steps to check the condition of the patient's airway and correct the problem to keep the patient alive.

Check for Responsiveness

The first step in assessing a patient's airway is to check the patient's level of responsiveness. When you first approach a patient, you can immediately determine whether the patient is responsive or unresponsive by asking, "Are you okay? Can you hear me?" (**FIGURE 7-6**). If you get a response, you can assume the patient is alert and has an open airway.

If you do not get a response, grasp the patient's shoulder and gently shake the patient. Then repeat your questions. If the patient still does not respond, assume you will need more help. Before doing anything for the patient, call 9-1-1 if the emergency medical services (EMS) system has not already been activated, especially if you are the only rescuer. Position the patient by supporting the patient's head and neck and placing the patient on their back.

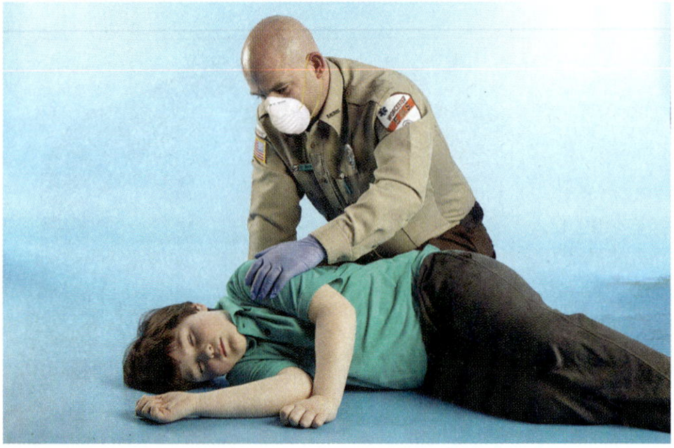

FIGURE 7-6 Establish the level of consciousness.
© Jones & Bartlett Learning. Courtesy of MIEMSS.

Treatment

The steps in airway assessment are as follows:

1. Check for responsiveness.
2. Correct the blocked airway using the head tilt–chin lift or jaw-thrust maneuver.
3. Check the airway for fluids, foreign bodies, or dentures.
4. Correct the airway using finger sweeps or suction if a foreign body is seen.
5. Manually maintain the airway with an oral or nasal airway, or place the patient in the recovery position (explained later in this chapter).

Correct the Blocked Airway

An unresponsive patient will not be able to keep their airway open. An unresponsive patient's airway is often blocked (occluded) because the tongue has dropped back and is obstructing it. In this case, simply opening the airway with the head tilt–chin lift or jaw-thrust maneuver may enable the patient to breathe spontaneously.

Head Tilt–Chin Lift Maneuver

To open a patient's airway using the **head tilt–chin lift maneuver**, place one hand on the patient's forehead and place the fingers of your other hand under the bony part of the lower jaw near the chin. Push down on the forehead and lift up and forward on the chin (**FIGURE 7-7**). Be certain you are not merely pushing the mouth closed when you use this maneuver.

Follow these steps to perform the head tilt–chin lift maneuver:

1. Place the patient on their back and kneel beside the patient.
2. Place one hand on the patient's forehead and apply firm pressure backward with your palm. Move the patient's head back as far as possible.
3. Place the tips of the fingers of your other hand under the bony part of the lower jaw near the chin.
4. Lift the chin forward to help tilt back the head.

Jaw-Thrust Maneuver

The **jaw-thrust maneuver** is another way to open a patient's airway. If a patient was injured in a fall, diving mishap, or motor vehicle crash and has a suspected neck injury, tilting the head may cause permanent paralysis. If you suspect a neck injury, first try to open the airway using the jaw-thrust maneuver. Open the airway by placing your fingers under the angles of the jaw and pushing upward. At the same time, use your thumbs to open the mouth slightly. The jaw-thrust maneuver should open the airway without extending the neck (**FIGURE 7-8**).

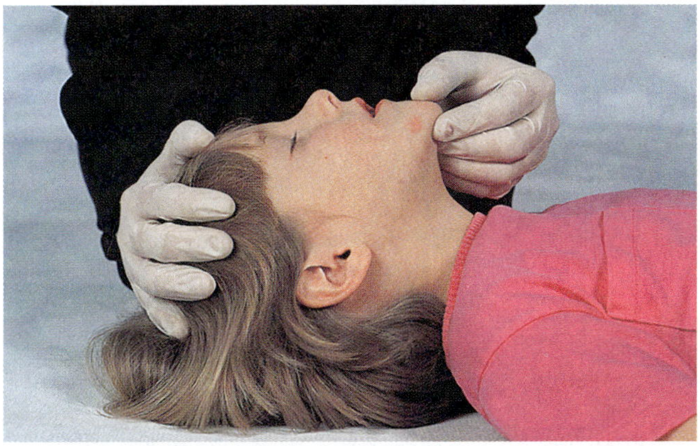

FIGURE 7-7 Open the patient's airway using the head tilt–chin lift maneuver.

© Jones & Bartlett Learning. Courtesy of MIEMSS.

> **Special Populations**
>
> **Opening the Airway of a Child or Infant**
>
> When opening the airway of a child or an infant, use the same general techniques that you use for an adult patient. The head tilt–chin lift maneuver can be used for children or infants who have not sustained an injury to the neck or head. When using the head tilt–chin lift maneuver on a child or infant, be sure that you do not hyperextend the neck when you tilt the head back. In infants and some small children, the overextension may obstruct the airway because of the flexibility of the child's neck. Smaller children may breathe easier if the neck is held in a neutral position rather than overextended. The ideal position is achieved when the patient's ear canal is on the same horizontal plane as the sternal notch, known as the sniffing position. The sniffing position can be achieved by placing a hand under the back of the patient's head and lifting until the ears and sternal notch are in line with one another, being careful to avoid flexing or extending the head. You can place a folded towel under the patient's shoulders to help maintain this position. If the possibility of injury to the head or neck exists, use the jaw-thrust maneuver to open the airway. If the jaw-thrust maneuver does not open the airway, use the head tilt–chin lift maneuver because opening the airway is a top priority for an unresponsive patient.

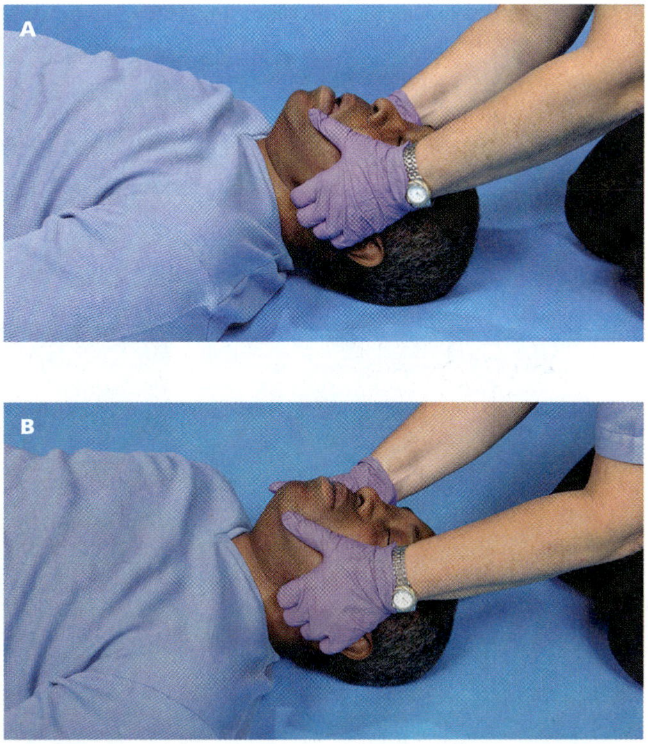

FIGURE 7-8 The jaw-thrust maneuver should open the patient's airway without extending the neck. **A.** Kneeling above the patient's head, place your fingers behind the angles of the lower jaw and move the jaw upward. Use your thumbs to help position the lower jaw. **B.** The completed maneuver should look like this.

© Jones & Bartlett Learning. Courtesy of MIEMSS.

Follow these steps to perform the jaw-thrust maneuver:

1. Place the patient on their back and kneel at the top of the patient's head. Place your fingers behind the angles of the patient's lower jaw and move the jaw forward with firm pressure.
2. Tilt the head backward to a neutral or slight sniffing position. Do not extend the cervical spine in a patient who has sustained an injury to the head or neck.
3. Use your thumbs to pull down the patient's lower jaw, opening the mouth enough to allow breathing through the mouth and nose.

If you are unable to open the patient's airway using the jaw-thrust maneuver, try the head tilt–chin lift maneuver as a secondary attempt to open the patient's airway.

Safety

Take standard precautions whenever you may come in contact with body fluids.

Check for Fluids, Foreign Bodies, or Dentures

After you have opened the patient's airway by using either the head tilt–chin lift or the jaw-thrust maneuver, look in the patient's mouth to see if anything is blocking the patient's airway. Potential blocks include secretions, such as vomitus, mucus, or blood; foreign objects, such as candy, food, or dirt; and dentures or false teeth that may have become dislodged and are blocking the patient's airway. If you find anything in the patient's mouth, remove it by using one of the techniques noted in the following sections. If the patient's mouth is clear, consider using one of the devices described in the section on airway devices.

Correct the Airway Using Finger Sweeps or Suction

You must immediately clear vomitus, mucus, blood, and foreign objects from the patient's airway.

Finger Sweeps

Finger sweeps can be done quickly and require no special equipment except a set of medical gloves. Finger sweeps are sometimes necessary even when you have a suction device available. Never use a finger sweep unless you can see the object. If you must perform a finger sweep, ensure that the patient is unresponsive with no gag reflex so that they do not bite down on your fingers.

To perform a finger sweep, follow the steps in **SKILL DRILL 7-1**.

Suctioning

Sometimes a finger sweep is not enough to clear the materials completely from the patient's mouth and upper airway. Suction machines can help remove secretions such as

SKILL DRILL 7-1

Clearing the Airway Using Finger Sweeps

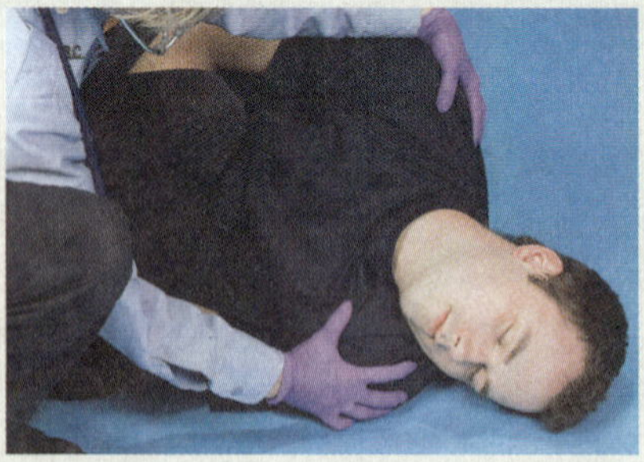

STEP 1 Turn the patient onto their side.

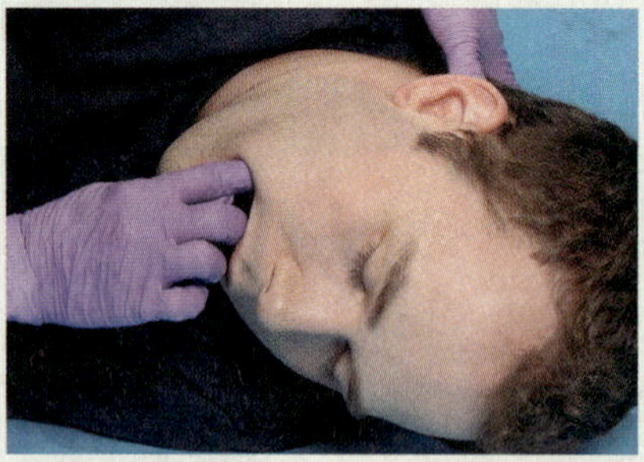

STEP 2 Insert your fingers into the patient's mouth.

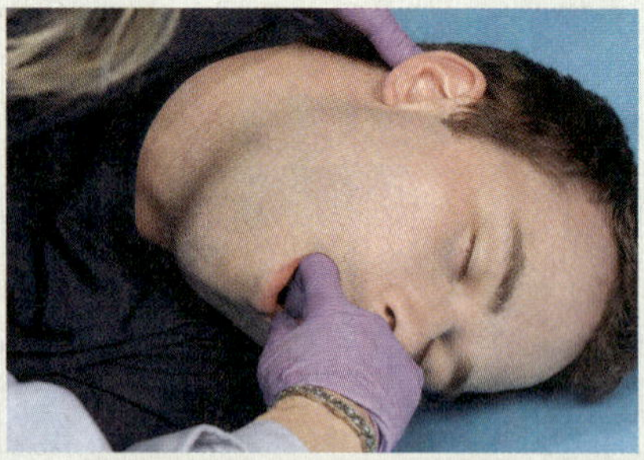

STEP 3 Curve your fingers into a C-shape and sweep them from one side of the back of the mouth to the other side. Scoop out as much of the foreign material as possible. A gauze pad wrapped around your gloved fingers may help remove the obstructing materials. Repeat the finger sweeps until you have removed all foreign material from the patient's mouth.

© Jones & Bartlett Learning. Courtesy of MIEMSS.

vomitus, blood, and mucus from the patient's mouth. Two types of suction devices are available: manual and mechanical. **Suctioning** the airway (either manually or mechanically) is a lifesaving technique. Although a gauze pad and your gloved fingers can do most of the work, the use of supplementary suction devices enables you to remove a greater amount of obstructing material from the patient's airway.

Safety

If the possibility of a spinal cord injury exists, log roll the patient onto the side and keep the head, neck, and spine aligned. Open the mouth and use your gloved fingers in the same manner to clean out the mouth.

Manual Suction Devices. A **manual suction device** is relatively inexpensive and compact enough to fit into the EMR's life support kit (**FIGURE 7-9**). These devices can come in various forms. With most manual suction devices, you insert the end of the suction tip into the patient's mouth and squeeze or pump the hand-powered pump. Be sure that you do not insert the tip of the suction device farther than you can see. Manual suction devices are used in the same way as the mechanical suction devices described in the following section. The only difference is the power source. Follow local medical protocols regarding authorization to use suction devices in the field.

Mechanical Suction Devices. A **mechanical suction device** uses either a battery-powered pump or an oxygen-powered **aspirator** to create a vacuum that will draw the obstructing materials from the patient's airway (**FIGURE 7-10**). Usually, both a rigid suction tip and a flexible whistle-tip catheter can be used with mechanical suction devices. To use this type of suction machine, you must first learn how to operate the device and control the force of the suction. When using mechanical suction, first clear the patient's mouth of large pieces of material with your gloved fingers. After the mouth is clear, turn on the suction device and use the rigid tip to remove most of the remaining material (**FIGURE 7-11**). Do not suction for more than 10 seconds at a time because the suction draws air, in addition to the obstructing material, out of the patient's airway. If the rigid tip has a suction control port (a small hole located close to the tip's handle), place a finger over the hole to create the suction. Do not keep your finger over this control port for longer than the allotted time because you may rob the patient of oxygen.

Safety

Do not suction any deeper than you can see into the patient's mouth.

After you have cleared most of the obstructing material from the patient's mouth and upper airway with the rigid tip, change to the flexible tip and clear material from the deeper parts of the patient's throat (**FIGURE 7-12**). Flexible whistle-tip catheters also have suction control ports, which are located close to the end of the catheter that attaches to the suction machine. Again, place a finger over the control port to achieve suction.

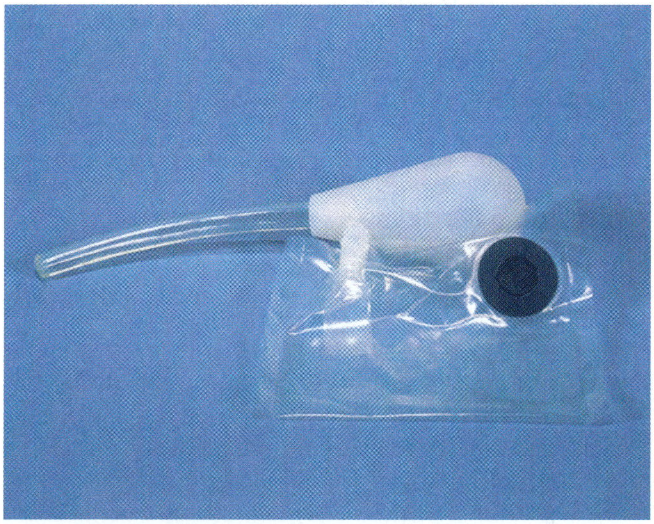

FIGURE 7-9 Manual suction device.
© Jones & Bartlett Learning. Courtesy of MIEMSS.

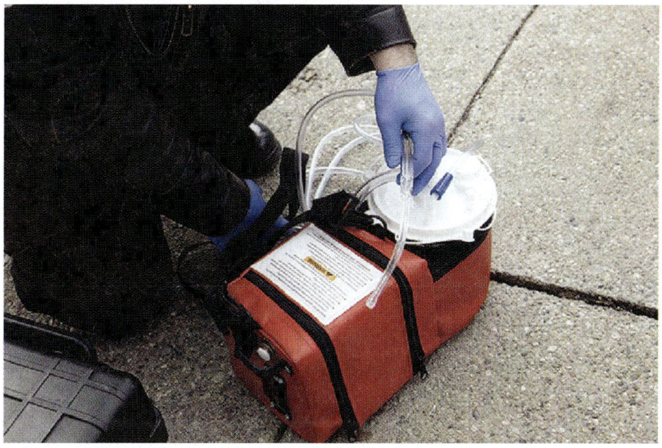

FIGURE 7-10 Battery-powered suction device.
© Jones & Bartlett Learning

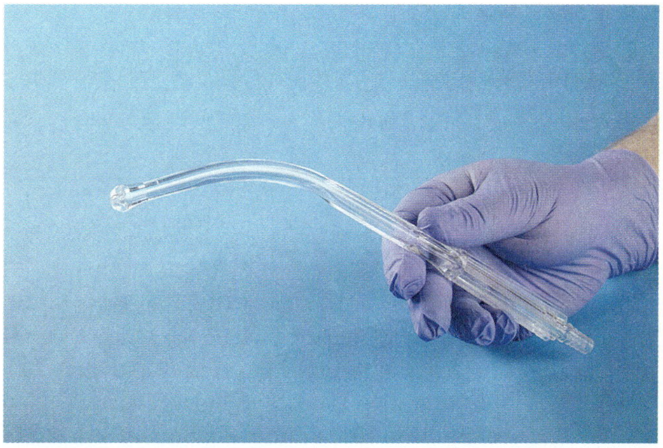

FIGURE 7-11 Rigid suction tip.
© Jones & Bartlett Learning

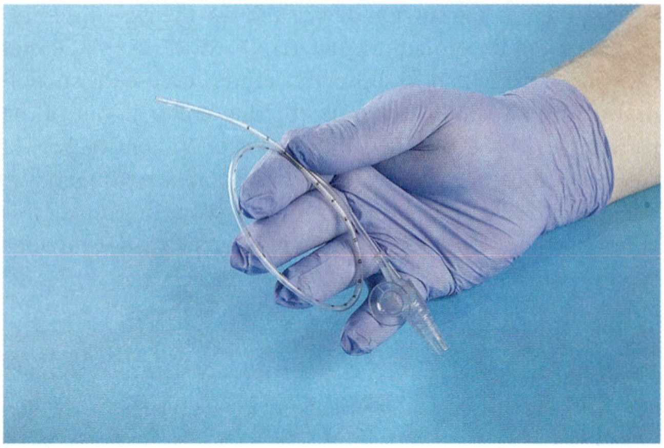

FIGURE 7-12 Flexible suction catheter.
© Jones & Bartlett Learning

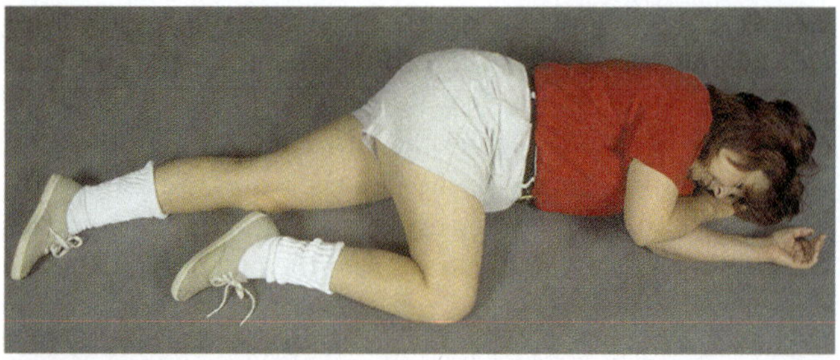

FIGURE 7-13 Recovery position for an unresponsive patient.
© Jones & Bartlett Learning. Courtesy of MIEMSS.

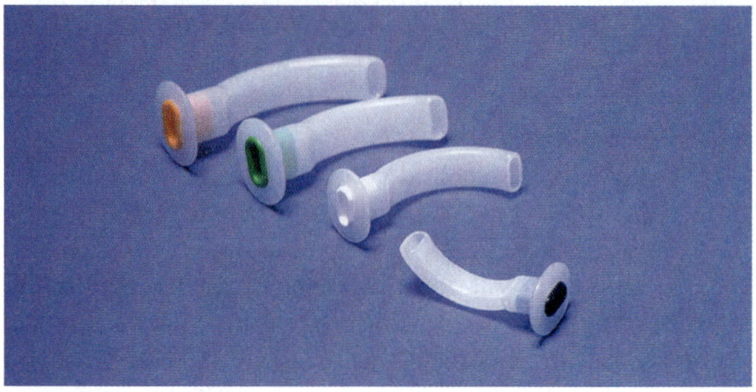

FIGURE 7-14 Oral airways.
© Jones & Bartlett Learning

Special Populations

Suctioning the Airway of a Child or Infant

The procedure for suctioning the airways of infants and children is generally the same as for adults, with the following exceptions:

- Use a tonsil tip or rigid tip to suction the mouth. Do not insert the tip any farther than you can see.
- Use a flexible catheter to suction the nose of a child; set the suction on low or medium power.
- Use a bulb syringe to suction the nose of an infant. Remember that an infant can breathe only through the nose.
- Do not suction the airway for longer than 10 seconds at a time. Try to ventilate and reoxygenate the patient before repeating the suctioning.

Maintain the Airway

Some patients will not be able to maintain an open airway without assistance. After you open the airway manually by using the head tilt–chin lift or jaw-thrust maneuver, you can continue holding the patient's head in this position to keep the airway open. In some cases, it may be necessary to insert an oral or nasal airway adjunct to maintain the patient's airway after you have opened it manually.

Treatment

Do not forget to ventilate all patients who are not breathing adequately.

Recovery Position

If the patient is breathing adequately without assistance and has not sustained trauma, one way to keep the airway open is to place the patient in the recovery position (**FIGURE 7-13**). The recovery position helps keep the patient's airway open by allowing secretions to drain out of the mouth instead of draining into the trachea. It also uses gravity to help keep the patient's tongue and lower jaw from blocking the airway.

Although the recovery position does allow for secretions to drain naturally out of the airway, when the patient begins to vomit, you must pay close attention to the airway. Try to sweep large pieces out of the mouth while the patient is still on their side, and be particularly attentive when continuous vomiting occurs. Suction equipment may be needed to help keep the airway open (**patent**) in these patients.

To place a patient in the recovery position, carefully roll the patient onto one side while you support the patient's head. Roll the patient as a unit without twisting the body. You can use the patient's hand to help hold their head in the proper position. Place the patient's face on its side so any secretions drain out of the mouth. The head should be in a position similar to the tilted-back position of the head tilt–chin lift maneuver.

When placing the patient in a recovery position, be sure you can still monitor their breathing. If, at any time, you see a change in the patient's breathing pattern or believe the airway is compromised, take corrective measures to open the airway.

Airway Adjuncts

This section discusses the indications for the use of oral airways and nasal airways and the steps required for the proper insertion of each.

Oral Airway. An **oral airway**, also called an oropharyngeal airway, has two primary purposes: It maintains the patient's airway after you have manually opened the airway, and it functions as a pathway through which you can suction the patient (**FIGURE 7-14**). You can use oral airways for unresponsive patients who are breathing or who are in **respiratory arrest** (sudden stoppage of breathing). You can use an oral airway in any unresponsive or pain-responsive patient who does not have a **gag reflex**. You cannot use oral airways in alert patients because they have a gag reflex. These airways can be used with mechanical breathing devices such as the **pocket mask** or a **bag-mask device**.

> **Signs and Symptoms**
>
> The signs and symptoms of respiratory arrest include the following:
>
> - No chest movement
> - No breath sounds
> - No air movement
> - Cyanosis (insufficient air exchange and low levels of oxygen in the blood, causing the blood and vessels to appear blue, and the lips, mucous membranes, nail beds, and skin over the blood vessels appear blue or gray)
> - Slow, gasping respirations

Two styles of oral airways are available: One style has an opening down the center, and the other has a slot (or opening) along each side. The slot permits the free flow of air and allows you to suction through the airway. Before you insert the oral airway, you need to select the proper size. Choose the proper size by measuring from the earlobe to the corner of the patient's mouth. When properly inserted, the airway will rest inside the mouth. The curve of the airway should follow the contour of the tongue. The flange should rest against the lips. The other end should be resting in the back of the throat.

SKILL DRILL 7-2 explains how to insert an oral airway.

Be especially careful when you insert the airway. You could injure the roof of the patient's mouth by the rough insertion of an oral airway. When placing the oral airway, be sure that you do not force the tongue into the back (posterior) of the throat. Remember, an oral airway does not open the patient's airway. It will maintain the open airway after you have opened it with a manual technique.

The roof of a child's mouth is more fragile than that of an adult, so be especially careful to avoid injuring it as you insert the oral airway. The technique for inserting an oral airway in a child involves using a tongue blade to depress the tongue. This method will press the tongue forward and away from the roof of the mouth so you can insert the airway in straight, without rotating it and damaging the soft tissue. Use the steps in **SKILL DRILL 7-3** to insert an oral airway in a child or an infant.

Nasal Airway. A second type of device you can use to keep the patient's airway open is a **nasal airway**, also called a nasopharyngeal airway (**FIGURE 7-15**). This device is inserted into the patient's nose. You can use nasal airways in both unresponsive and alert patients who are unable to maintain an open airway. Usually, a patient will tolerate a nasal airway better than an oral airway. A nasal airway is less likely to cause vomiting. One disadvantage of a nasal airway is that you cannot suction through it because the inside diameter of the airway is too small for the standard whistle-tip catheter suction tip.

EMRs usually do not use nasal airways for children. If you have questions about using nasal airways in pediatric patients, check with your medical director.

SKILL DRILL 7-2

Inserting an Oral Airway

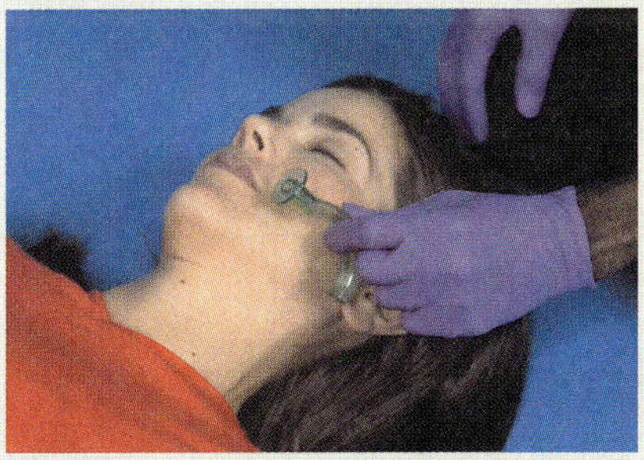

STEP 1 Select the proper size airway by measuring from the patient's earlobe to the corner of the mouth.

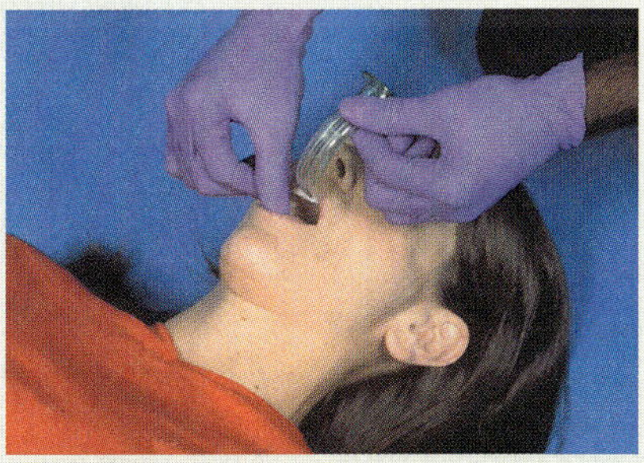

STEP 2 Open the patient's mouth with one hand after manually opening the patient's airway with either a head tilt–chin lift or jaw-thrust maneuver. Hold the airway upside down with your other hand. Insert the airway into the patient's mouth and guide the tip of the airway along the roof of the patient's mouth, advancing it until you feel resistance.

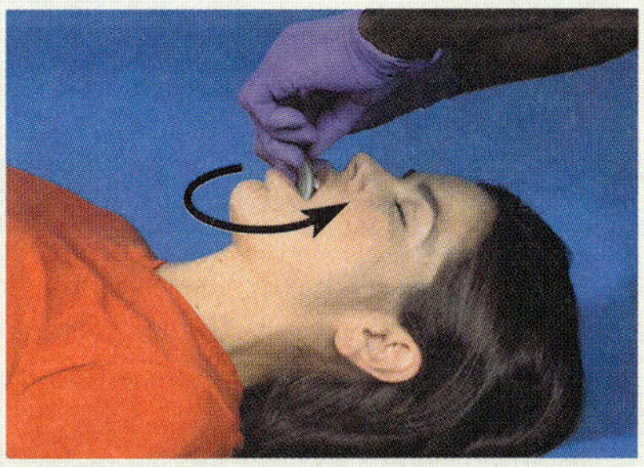

STEP 3 Rotate the airway 180° until the flange comes to rest on the patient's lips and teeth.

© Jones & Bartlett Learning. Courtesy of MIEMSS.

SKILL DRILL 7-3

Inserting an Oral Airway in a Child

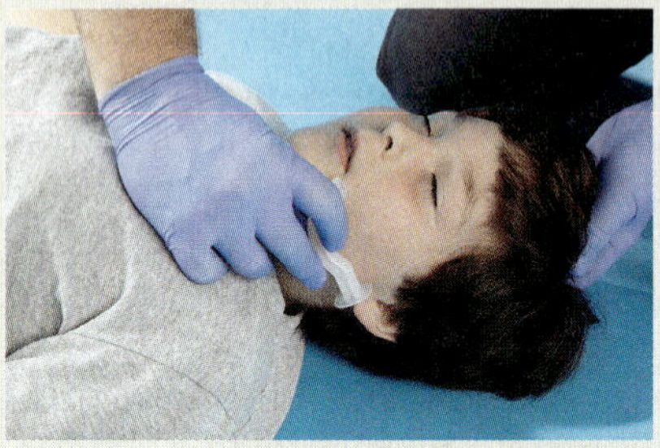

STEP 1 Select the proper size oral airway by measuring from the patient's earlobe to the corner of the mouth.

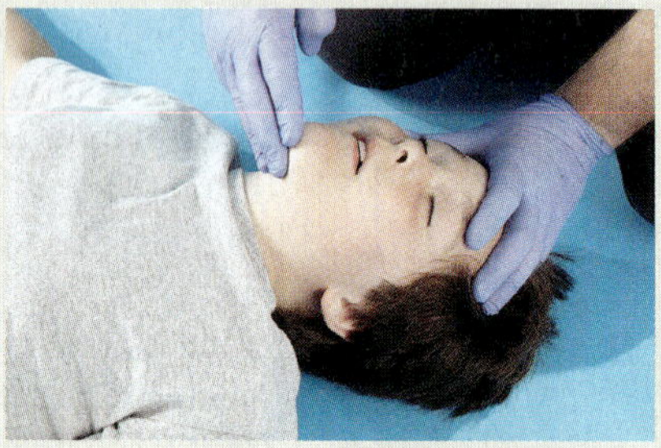

STEP 2 Position the patient's airway. If the emergency is medical, use the head tilt–chin lift maneuver, avoiding hyperextension. If the patient has a traumatic injury, use the jaw-thrust maneuver.

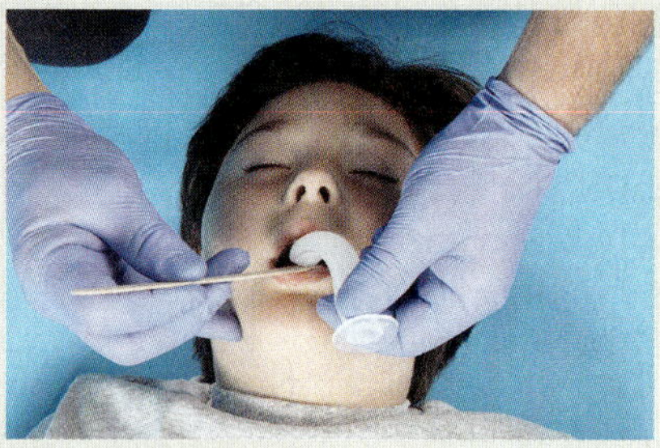

STEP 3 Depress the patient's tongue with a tongue blade. Press the tongue forward and away from the roof of the mouth. Follow the anatomic curve of the roof of the patient's mouth to slide the airway into place. Be gentle. The mouths of children and infants are fragile.

© Jones & Bartlett Learning

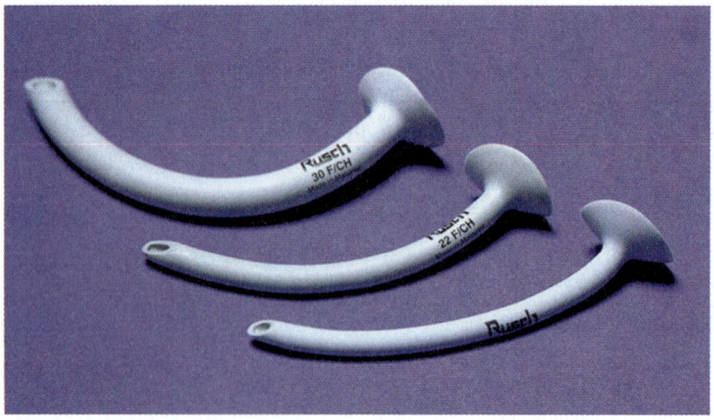

FIGURE 7-15 Nasal airways.
© Jones & Bartlett Learning. Courtesy of MIEMSS.

Treatment

If a patient has sustained severe head trauma, it is possible that the insertion of a nasal airway may further damage the brain. Do not attempt to insert a nasal airway in patients with suspected head trauma.

You will have to select the proper size nasal airway for the patient. Measure from the earlobe to the tip of the patient's nose. Coat the airway with a water-soluble lubricant before inserting it. This step makes it easier for you to insert the airway and reduces the chance of causing trauma to the patient's airway. Insert the airway in the larger nostril with the bevel against the septum. As you insert the airway, follow the curvature of the floor of the nose. The airway is fully inserted when the flange, or trumpet, rests against the patient's nostril. At this point, the other end of the airway will reach the back of the patient's throat and it will maintain an open airway for the patient.

SKILL DRILL 7-4 describes the steps to insert a nasal airway.

Treatment

To open the patient's airway:

1. Perform the head tilt–chin lift maneuver or the jaw-thrust maneuver.
2. Maintain the patient's airway by continuing to apply the head tilt–chin lift or jaw-thrust maneuver and then insert an oral airway or a nasal airway.
3. Place the patient in the recovery position.

After you open and maintain the patient's airway, continue to monitor the status of the patient's breathing.

B Is for Breathing

After you have checked and corrected the patient's airway, you will next check and correct the patient's breathing. To do this, you must understand the signs of adequate breathing, the signs of inadequate breathing, and the signs and causes of respiratory arrest.

Check Breathing

As discussed previously, your assessment of any motionless patient begins by checking for responsiveness and assessing for breathing. You will use the look, listen, and feel technique to assess if an unresponsive patient is breathing adequately.

SKILL DRILL 7-4

Inserting a Nasal Airway

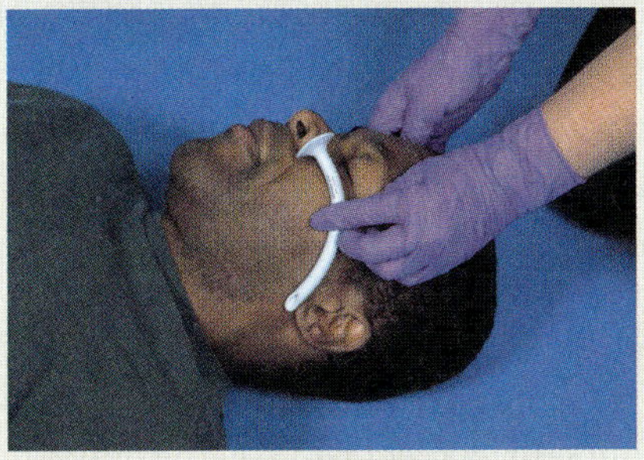

STEP 1 Select the proper size airway by measuring from the earlobe to the tip of the patient's nose.

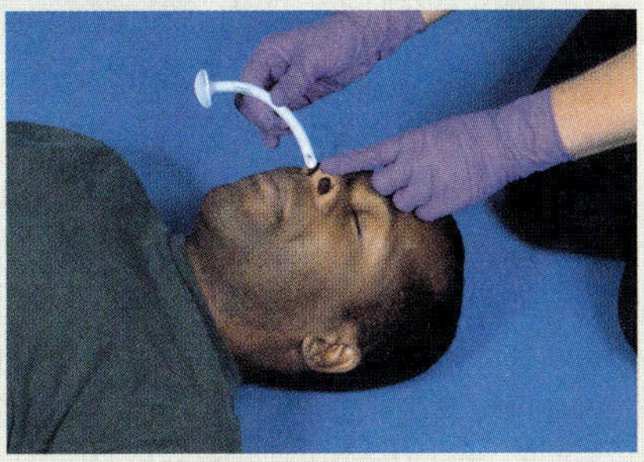

STEP 2 Coat the airway with a water-soluble lubricant. Select the larger nostril, and gently stretch the nostril open by using your thumb. Insert the lubricated airway into the larger nostril with the bevel against the septum.

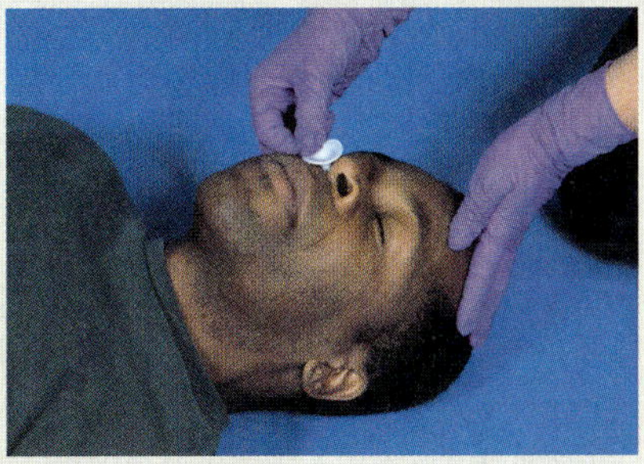

STEP 3 Advance the airway until the flange rests against the nose. Do not force the airway. If you feel any resistance, remove the airway and try to insert it in the other nostril.

© Jones & Bartlett Learning. Courtesy of MIEMSS.

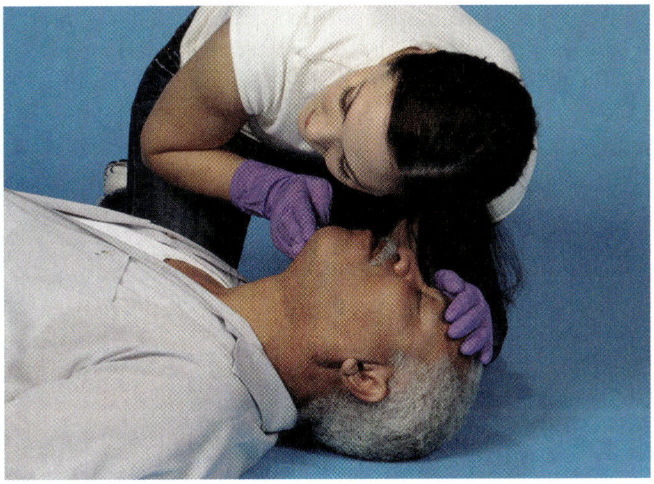

FIGURE 7-16 Determine responsiveness and check for breathing.

© Jones & Bartlett Learning. Courtesy of MIEMSS.

TABLE 7-2 Normal Respiratory Rate Ranges

Adults (and children older than 15 years)	12 to 20 breaths/min
Children 12 to 15 years	15 to 20 breaths/min
Children 6 to 12 years	18 to 30 breaths/min
Children 4 to 6 years	22 to 34 breaths/min
Children 1 to 4 years	24 to 40 breaths/min
Infants 1 month to 1 year	30 to 53 breaths/min
Newborns to 1 month (includes term and preterm infants)	30 to 60 breaths/min

Data from American Heart Association (AHA). *Pediatric Advanced Life Support Provider Manual*. Dallas, TX: AHA; 2020; National Association of State EMS Officials. *National Model EMS Clinical Guidelines*. Version 3.0. https://nasemso.org/wp-content/uploads/National-Model-EMS-Clinical-Guidelines_2022.pdf. Updated March 2022. Accessed November 27, 2024; Van de Voorde P, Turner NM, Djakow J, et al. European Resuscitation Council Guidelines 2021: Paediatric Life Support. *Resuscitation*. 2021;161:327–387.

To do so, place the side of your face close to the patient's nose and mouth and watch the patient's chest (**FIGURE 7-16**). By positioning yourself in this way, you can look for the rise and fall of the patient's chest, listen for the sounds of air passing into or out of the patient's nose and mouth, and feel the air moving on the side of your face.

Signs of Adequate Breathing

The respiratory rate in newborns is normally in the range of 30 to 60 breaths/min. The rate decreases with age until reaching a normal range of 12 to 20 breaths/min in adulthood (**TABLE 7-2**). Remember, one breath includes both an inhalation and an exhalation.

If the patient is breathing adequately, you can continue to maintain the airway and monitor the rate and depth of respirations to ensure that adequate breathing continues.

Signs of Inadequate Breathing

If a patient is breathing inadequately, you will detect signs of abnormal respirations. Sounds such as noisy respirations, wheezing, or gurgling indicate a partial blockage or constriction somewhere along the respiratory tract. Rapid or gasping respirations may indicate that the patient is not receiving an

Voices of Experience

Many years ago, when I was a brand new paramedic at an all-volunteer suburban ambulance agency, I often responded in a fly-car and then a BLS crew would respond to meet me. One Saturday morning, I received a call for a man who had collapsed in a grocery store. I was the first responder on scene and was met by the store manager, who led me to the pharmacy's waiting area at the front of the store, near the busy checkout lines. I found the patient lying on the floor on his back. He was unresponsive and had gasping respirations. As I was opening his airway, the fire department arrived. One EMR immediately took over airway management and a second EMR confirmed that there were no pulses and started chest compressions. The other firefighters set up some shopping carts to block curious observers from crowding around and took turns giving compressions.

> **"I truly believe that without the excellent airway management by the EMRs, the patient would not have regained pulses."**

With the firefighters providing BLS, I applied the cardiac monitor. It showed a slow irregular rhythm, but with no pulses felt, I started treatment for PEA (pulseless electrical activity). The EMR who was managing the airway noted that it was difficult to ventilate the patient with a bag-mask device. He repositioned the head and inserted an oropharyngeal airway. He also noted that there was a small amount of blood in the mouth, which he suctioned. Following these actions, the EMR reported that ventilations were much improved, which was confirmed by good equal chest expansion and air movement on auscultation. After medications I administered and the much-improved oxygenation and ventilation restored palpable carotid pulses, compressions were discontinued. However, the patient was still unresponsive and had not resumed breathing, so airway management remained critical.

By this time, the ambulance had arrived. Working as a team, we logrolled the patient onto a backboard, in case we might need to resume CPR, and moved to the ambulance, with the EMR maintaining ventilations during the move. Once on the ambulance, I was able to intubate the patient and ventilation continued through the tube.

Additionally, knowing that the EMR was competently managing the airway allowed me to concentrate on other aspects of patient care so that we could deliver a patient with adequate pulses and improved oxygenation levels to the emergency department.

Sharon F Chiumento, BSN, EMTP
Monroe Community College
Rochester, New York

Adapted from the personal Medical Identification Symbol of the American Medical Association.

adequate amount of oxygen as a result of illness or injury. The patient's skin may be pale or even cyanotic, especially around the lips or fingernail beds.

The most critical sign of inadequate breathing is respiratory arrest (total lack of respirations). As discussed previously, this critical state is characterized by a lack of chest movements, lack of breath sounds, and lack of air against the side of your face. In patients with severe hypothermia, respirations can be slowed (and/or shallow) to the point that the patient does not appear to be breathing.

Special Populations

Respiratory Compromise in Pediatric Patients

Respiratory emergencies can progress rapidly in children. It is important for the EMR to recognize the signs and symptoms of respiratory distress, respiratory failure, and respiratory arrest, and to intervene promptly before the child's condition deteriorates.

- **Respiratory distress** refers to difficulty breathing and involves an abnormal respiratory rate or effort. It can range from mild to severe and can progress to respiratory failure. It is indicated by the following:
  - A breathing rate of more than 60 breaths/min in infants
  - A breathing rate of more than 30 to 40 breaths/min in children
  - Nasal flaring on each breath
  - Retraction of the skin between the ribs and around the neck muscles
  - **Stridor** (a high-pitched sound during inhalation)
  - Cyanosis of the skin
  - Altered mental status
  - Combativeness or restlessness

  If you see that any of the listed signs are present, try to determine the cause. Support the child's respirations by placing the child in a comfortable position, usually sitting. Keep the child as calm as possible by letting a parent hold the child if practical. Prepare to administer oxygen if it is available and you are trained in its use. Monitor the child's vital signs and arrange for prompt transport to an appropriate medical facility.
- **Respiratory failure** occurs when oxygen levels are too low to meet the body's needs and ventilation is impaired, leading to high carbon dioxide levels. Respiratory failure is accompanied by serious signs and symptoms and must be corrected quickly. Be alert for the following signs:
  - A breathing rate of fewer than 20 breaths/min in an infant
  - A breathing rate of fewer than 10 breaths/min in a child
  - Limp muscle tone
  - Unresponsiveness
  - Decreased or absent heart rate
  - Weak or absent distal pulses

  A child in respiratory failure is on the verge of experiencing respiratory and cardiac arrest. Immediately assess the child and take whatever steps are appropriate to support the patient. Support respirations by performing mouth-to-mask or bag-mask ventilations. Administer oxygen if it is available and you have been trained to use it. Begin chest compressions if the heart rate is absent or less than 60 beats/min. Arrange for prompt transport to an appropriate medical facility. Continue to monitor the patient's vital signs and support the ABCs as well as you can.
- Respiratory arrest refers to complete cessation of breathing (apnea) or agonal gasps that will lead to cardiac arrest if the EMR does not intervene immediately.

Many causes of respiratory arrest exist. One common cause is heart disease, which claimed 702,880 lives in 2022 in the United States according to the Centers for Disease Control and Prevention. Other major causes of respiratory arrest include the following:

- Mechanical blockage or obstruction caused by the tongue
- Vomitus, particularly in a patient weakened by a condition such as a stroke
- Foreign objects such as broken teeth, dentures, balloons, marbles, pieces of food, or pieces of hard candy (especially in small children)
- Illness or disease
- Drug overdose
- Poisoning
- Severe loss of blood
- Electrocution by electrical current or lightning

Correct the Breathing

You must breathe for any patient who is not breathing adequately. As you perform **rescue breathing**, keep the patient's airway open by using the head tilt–chin lift maneuver (or the jaw-thrust maneuver for patients with suspected head or spinal injuries). To perform rescue breathing, pinch the patient's nose with your thumb and forefinger, take a deep breath, and blow slowly into the patient's mouth for 1 second (**FIGURE 7-17**). Use slow, gentle, sustained breathing and just enough breath to make the patient's chest rise to minimize the amount of air blown into the stomach. Remove your mouth and allow the patient's lungs to deflate. Breathe for the patient a second time. After these first two breaths, breathe once into the patient's mouth every 6 seconds (10 breaths/min) for an adult. For children, deliver one breath every 2 to 3 seconds (20 to 30 breaths/min). With an unresponsive patient, recall that you need to check for the presence of circulation before you correct the patient's

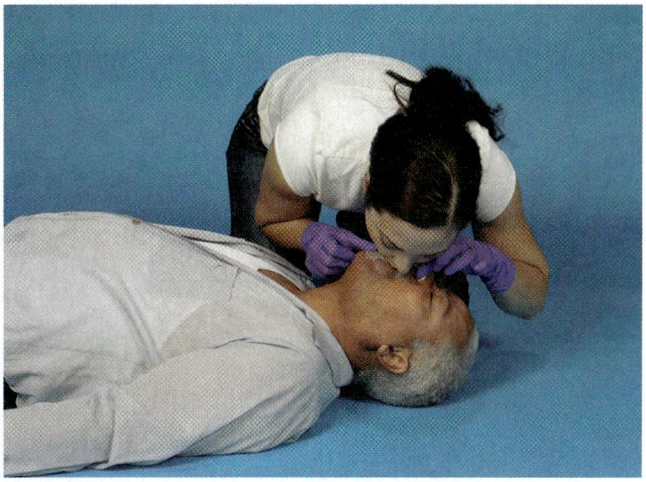

FIGURE 7-17 To perform rescue breathing, pinch the patient's nose with your thumb and forefinger, then blow slowly into the patient's mouth. As shown here, use a barrier device if available.

© Jones & Bartlett Learning. Courtesy of MIEMSS.

breathing. These situations are described in Chapter 8, *Professional Rescuer CPR*.

You can perform rescue breathing by using a mouth-to-mask device, a barrier device, a bag-mask device, or just your mouth. The skill of performing mouth-to-mouth ventilation is no longer recommended as a primary means of performing CPR but is presented here as a fallback method of performing ventilation if you have no equipment for performing other means of ventilation. Mouth-to-mask devices, barrier devices, and bag-mask devices prevent you from putting your mouth directly on the patient's mouth. These devices should be available to you as an EMR. If a rescue breathing device is unavailable, you must weigh the potential good to the patient against the possibility that you will contract an infectious disease if you perform mouth-to-mouth rescue breathing.

Mouth-to-Mask Rescue Breathing

Your EMR life support kit should contain an artificial ventilation (breathing) device that enables you to perform rescue breathing without mouth-to-mouth contact with the patient. This simple piece of equipment is a mouth-to-mask ventilation device. A mouth-to-mask ventilation device consists of a mask that fits over the patient's mouth and nose, a one-way valve, and a mouthpiece through which the rescuer breathes (**FIGURE 7-18**). It may also have an inlet port for supplemental oxygen and a tube between the mouthpiece and the mask. Because mouth-to-mask devices prevent direct contact between you and the patient, they reduce, but do not eliminate, the risk of transmitting infectious diseases.

To use a **mouth-to-mask ventilation device** for rescue breathing, follow the steps in **SKILL DRILL 7-5**. Practice this technique frequently on a manikin until you can do it well. These devices provide relatively limited protection against viral diseases transmitted by respiratory secretions, such as coronavirus disease 2019 (COVID-19).

Mouth-to-Barrier Rescue Breathing

Mouth-to-barrier devices also provide a barrier between the rescuer and the patient (**FIGURE 7-19**). A wide variety of devices is available. Some of them are small enough to carry in your pocket. Most consist of a port or hole that you breathe into and a mask or plastic film that covers the patient's face. Some also have a one-way valve that prevents backflow of secretions and gases. These devices provide variable degrees of infection control but are not designed to prevent transmission of COVID-19.

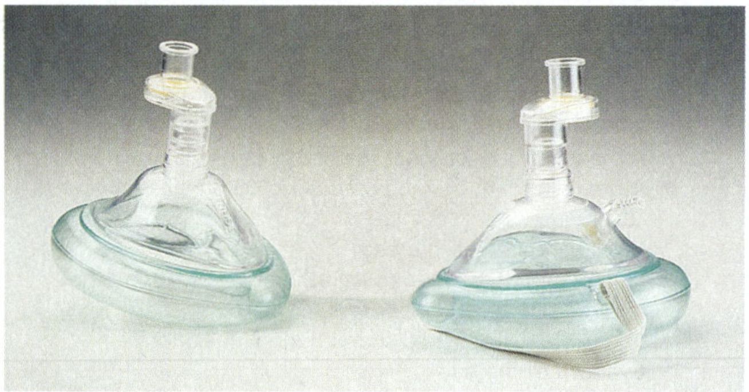

FIGURE 7-18 Mouth-to-mask ventilation devices.
© Jones & Bartlett Learning. Courtesy of MIEMSS.

SKILL DRILL 7-5

Performing Mouth-to-Mask Rescue Breathing

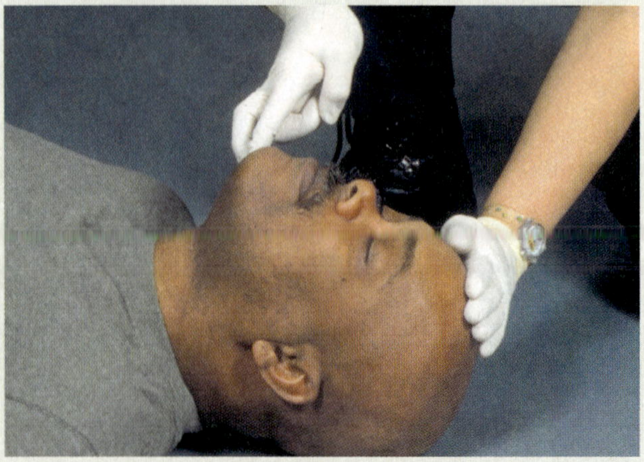

STEP 1 Position yourself at the patient's head. Open the airway using the head tilt–chin lift maneuver.

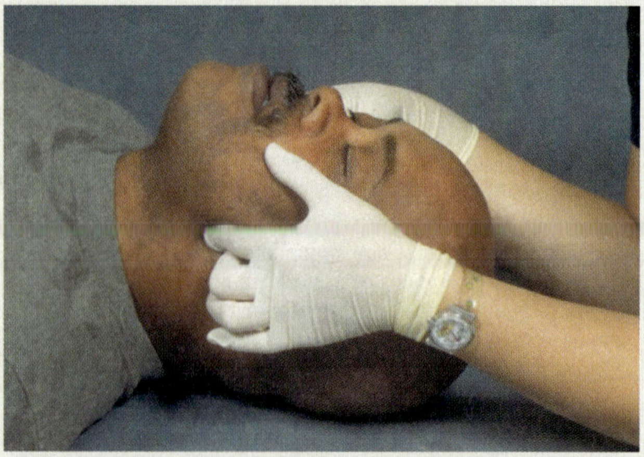

STEP 2 Alternatively, use the jaw-thrust maneuver for a patient with suspected head or spinal injuries.

SKILL DRILL 7-5 (continued)

Performing Mouth-to-Mask Rescue Breathing

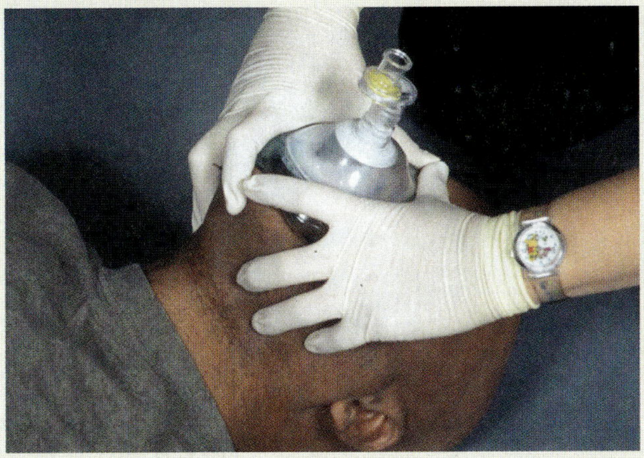

STEP 3 Grasp the mask and the patient's jaw, using both hands. Use the thumb and forefinger of each hand to hold the mask tightly against the face. Hook the other three fingers of each hand under the patient's face.

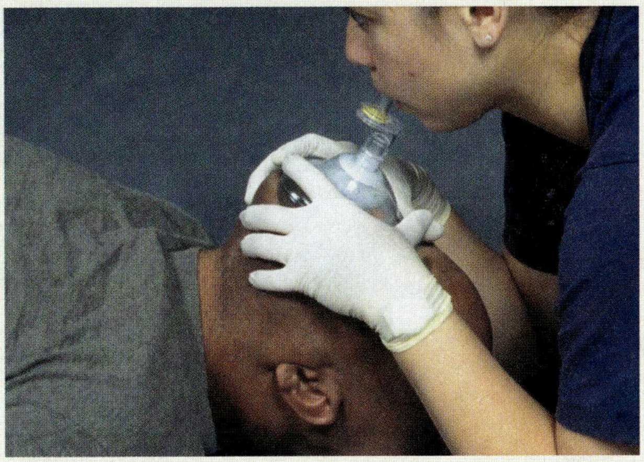

STEP 4 Maintain an airtight seal as you pull up on the jaw to maintain the proper head position. Take a deep breath and then seal your mouth over the mouthpiece. Breathe slowly into the mouthpiece for 1 second until the patient's chest rises. Monitor the patient for proper head position, air exchange, and vomiting.

© Jones & Bartlett Learning. Courtesy of MIEMSS.

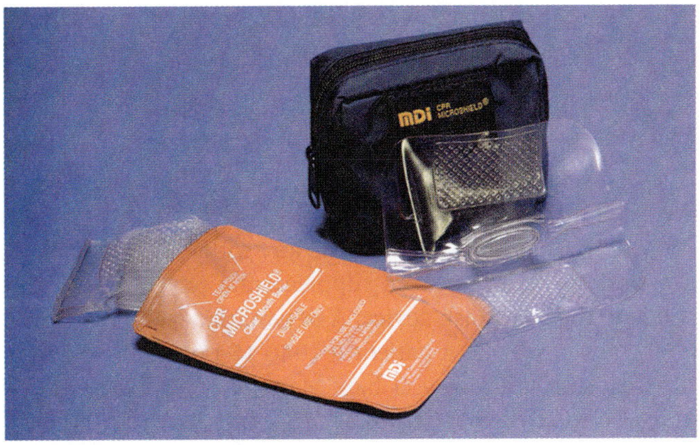

FIGURE 7-19 Barrier devices.
© Jones & Bartlett Learning. Courtesy of MIEMSS.

Safety

Mouth-to-barrier rescue breathing and mouth-to-mouth rescue breathing are not safe in the context of active community transmission of aerosolized viral disease, such as that seen during the COVID-19 pandemic. EMRs should use a bag-mask device in these scenarios when possible. Although droplet transmission is possible even when using a bag-mask device, the likelihood is far less.

To perform mouth-to-barrier rescue breathing, follow the steps in **SKILL DRILL 7-6**.

Bag-Mask Device

The bag-mask device has three parts: a self-inflating bag, one-way valves, and a face mask (**FIGURE 7-20**). To use

YOU are the EMR — CASE 2

At 0137 hours on a Saturday, you are dispatched to a local university dormitory for a report of a sick person. As you arrive at the student's room, you are met by a shocked-looking group of students. A young man is lying on his bed. He does not respond to verbal stimuli or to your shaking of his shoulder. He appears to be turning blue. One of the students says, "Dan may have overdosed on drugs." He has a carotid pulse, so you look, listen, and feel for respirations. The patient has gurgling respirations only two to three times per minute.

1. What is the first action you should take?
2. How can you provide oxygen to this patient?
3. What methods do you have to keep his airway open?

SKILL DRILL 7-6

Performing Mouth-to-Barrier Rescue Breathing

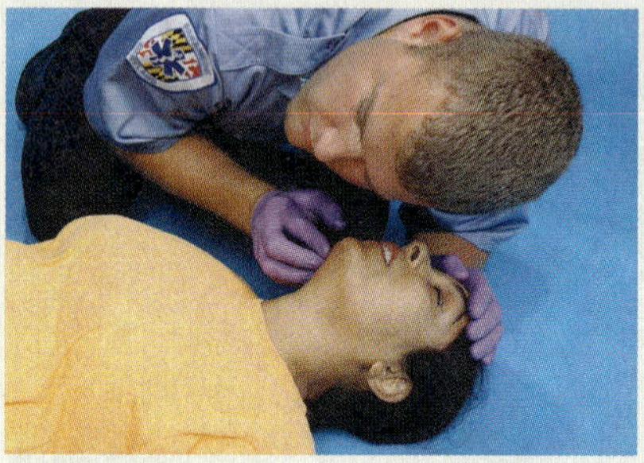

STEP 1 Open the airway using the head tilt–chin lift maneuver. Press on the forehead to maintain the backward tilt of the head.

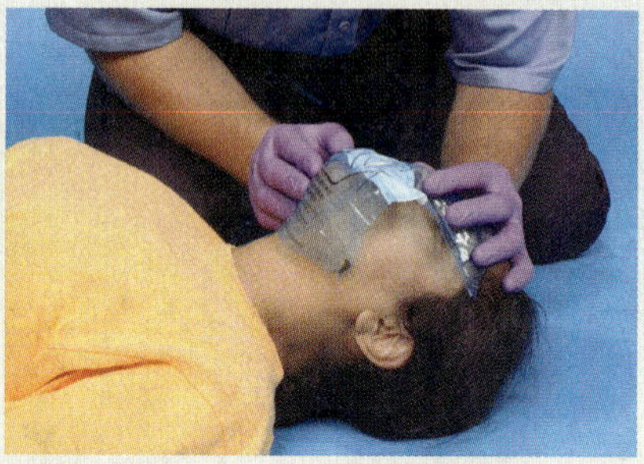

STEP 2 Keep the patient's mouth open with the thumb of whichever hand you are using to lift the patient's chin. Place the barrier device over the patient's mouth.

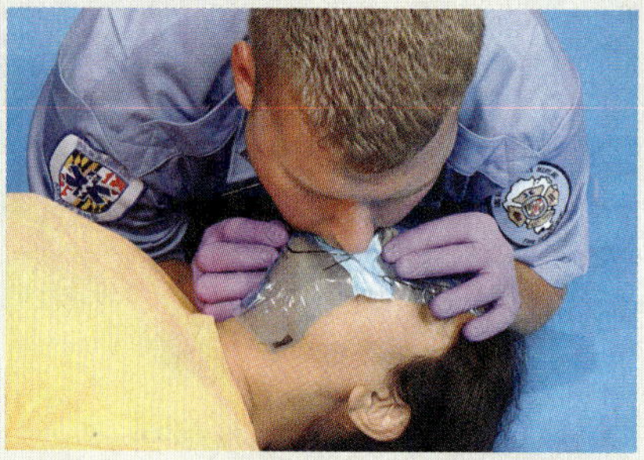

STEP 3 Pinch the patient's nostrils together with your thumb and forefinger. Take a deep breath and then make a tight seal by placing your mouth on the barrier device around the patient's mouth. Breathe slowly into the patient's mouth for 1 second. Breathe until the patient's chest rises.

Remove your mouth and allow the patient to exhale passively. Check to see that the patient's chest falls after each exhalation.

Repeat this rescue breathing sequence every 6 seconds (10 breaths/min) for an adult. For children, deliver one breath every 2 to 3 seconds (20 to 30 breaths/min).

© Jones & Bartlett Learning. Courtesy of MIEMSS.

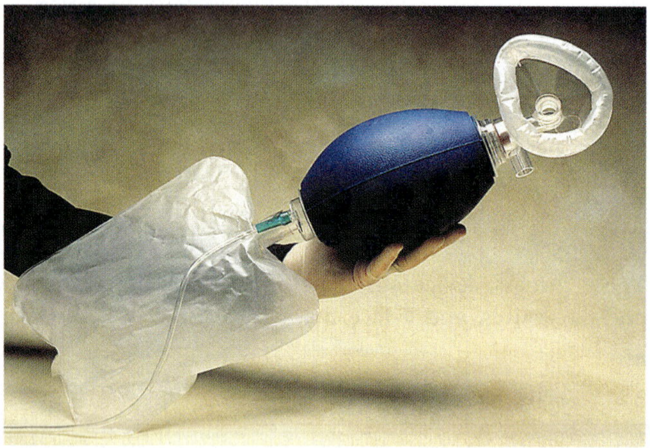

FIGURE 7-20 A bag-mask device.
© Jones & Bartlett Learning. Courtesy of MIEMSS.

this device, you place the mask over the face of the patient and make a tight seal. Squeezing the bag pushes air through a one-way valve, through the mask, and into the patient's mouth and nose. As the patient passively exhales, a second one-way valve near the mask releases the air.

The self-inflating bag refills with air when you release the pressure on it. The bag-mask device delivers 21% oxygen (the percentage of oxygen in room air) without supplemental oxygen attached. However, supplemental oxygen is usually added to the bag-mask device. A bag-mask device can deliver up to 90% oxygen to a patient if 10 to 15 L/min of oxygen is supplied into the reservoir bag. Many bag-mask devices are designed to be discarded after a single use.

The bag-mask device is used for the same purpose as a mouth-to-mask device: to ventilate a nonbreathing patient. Although the bag-mask device can administer up to 90% oxygen when used with supplemental oxygen, there are disadvantages to its use. First, as a single rescuer, you may find it difficult to maintain a seal between the patient's face and the mask with one hand. Second, the bag-mask device may be difficult to use if you have small hands because you may not be able to squeeze the bag hard enough to get an adequate volume of air into the patient.

Bag-Mask Device Technique. To use a bag-mask device, follow the same steps you use to perform rescue breathing. Determine whether the patient is unresponsive. Kneel above the patient's head. This position will enable you to keep the airway open, make a tight seal on the mask, and squeeze the bag. Maintain the patient's neck in an extended position. The bag-mask device does not maintain the patient's airway in an open position. You must continue to stabilize the head and maintain the head either in an extended position for the head tilt–chin lift maneuver or in a neutral position for the jaw-thrust maneuver.

Open the patient's airway using the head tilt–chin lift maneuver or the jaw-thrust maneuver for patients with suspected head or spinal injuries. Check to see if the patient is breathing by looking at the patient's chest, listening for the sound of air movement, and feeling for the movement of air on the side of your face and ear. If the patient is not breathing, consider using an oral or nasal airway.

Treatment

The three methods for performing rescue breathing are all potentially lifesaving. Use a mouth-to-mask device, a mouth-to-barrier device, or a bag-mask device whenever possible. If a rescue breathing device is not available, you must weigh the potential good to the patient against the limited chance that you will contract an infectious disease from mouth-to-mouth breathing.

The specific steps for using a bag-mask device are shown in **SKILL DRILL 7-7**.

Street Smarts

If you are alone and need to ventilate a patient with a bag-mask device, kneel at the top of the patient's head and use your knees to hold the head in the correct position. You can then use both hands to ventilate the patient without trying to hold the bag, create a seal with the mask, and keep the head in the proper position.

With sufficient training and practice, a single rescuer can ventilate a patient using a bag-mask device; however, it can be difficult to maintain a good seal and squeeze the bag. Use of a bag-mask device is best accomplished as a two-person operation if additional rescuers are present (**FIGURE 7-21**). With two rescuers, one person squeezes the bag and the other person uses both hands (using the E-C technique) to seal the mask to the patient. Most people can seal the mask much more easily using both hands.

Using the bag-mask device requires proper training and practice. The device can be a lifesaving tool. Your EMS agency may use bag-mask devices for nonbreathing patients, or you may be asked to assist emergency medical technicians or paramedics in ventilating nonbreathing patients so they can perform other needed skills. Check with your supervisor or medical director to learn the protocols for your service.

Treatment

If paramedics have inserted an endotracheal tube down the patient's windpipe (trachea), the bag-mask device is connected directly to the end of the endotracheal tube. In this case, no face mask is needed. When you squeeze the bag-mask device, you force air directly into the patient's lungs. You should receive instruction in this type of ventilation if you will be performing it.

Airway and Breathing Review

Assume that all unresponsive patients may be in respiratory arrest until you can assess them and determine whether they are breathing adequately.

Performing Rescue Breathing on Adults

A summary of the steps required to recognize respiratory arrest and perform rescue breathing in adults follows. Begin by checking the airway and correcting any problems:

1. Check for responsiveness by shouting, "Are you okay?" and gently shaking the patient's shoulder. If the patient is unresponsive and has no pulse, place the patient on their back, activate the EMS system, and begin CPR. If the patient has a pulse, continue with Step 2.
2. Correct a blocked airway by using the head tilt–chin lift maneuver or, if the patient has sustained any injury to the head or neck, the jaw-thrust maneuver.
3. Check the mouth for any secretions, vomitus, or solid objects. If found, clear the mouth.
4. Correct a blocked airway, if needed, by using finger sweeps or suction to remove foreign substances.
5. Maintain the airway by manually holding it open or by using an oral or nasal airway.

Next check the patient's breathing and correct any problems:

1. Check that the patient is breathing adequately by looking for the rise and fall of the patient's chest and listening for the sound of air moving in and out of the patient's nose and mouth. If the patient is breathing adequately, place the patient in the recovery position. If the patient is not breathing, go to Step 2.
2. Correct the lack of breathing by performing rescue breathing using a mouth-to-mask or mouth-to-barrier device, if available. Blow slowly into the patient's mouth for 1 second, using slow, gentle, sustained breaths with enough force to make the chest rise. Remove your mouth and allow the lungs to deflate. Breathe for the patient a second time. After these first two breaths, breathe once into the patient's mouth approximately every 6 seconds, or 10 times per minute.

Often, when rescue breathing is necessary, cardiac compressions are also required. External cardiac compressions are explained in Chapter 8, *Professional Rescuer CPR*.

SKILL DRILL 7-7

Using a Bag-Mask Device With One Rescuer

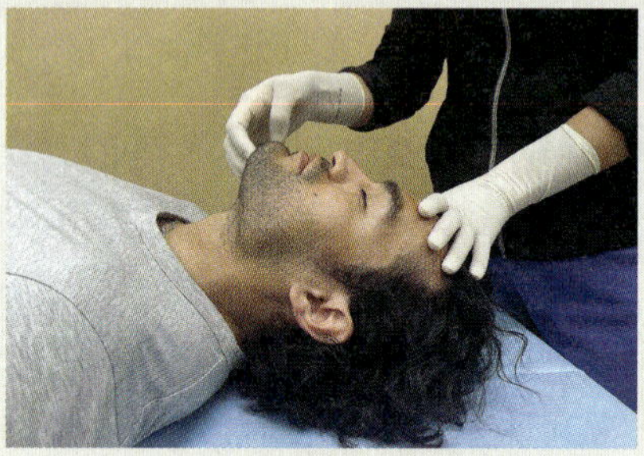

STEP 1 Position yourself above the patient's head. Open the airway and continue to stabilize the head and maintain the head either in an extended position for the head tilt–chin lift maneuver or in a neutral position for the jaw-thrust maneuver. Check for fluids, foreign bodies, or dentures. Suction, if needed. Consider the use of an oral or nasal airway.

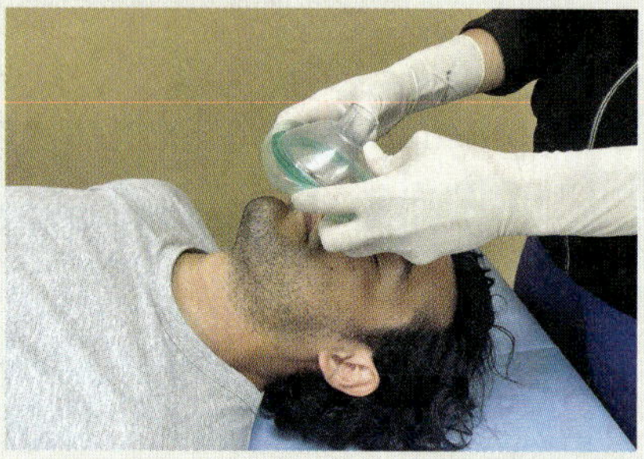

STEP 2 Select the proper mask size. The mask should be large enough to seal over the bridge of the patient's nose and fit in the groove between the lower lip and the chin. A mask that is too small or too large may make it impossible to maintain a seal.

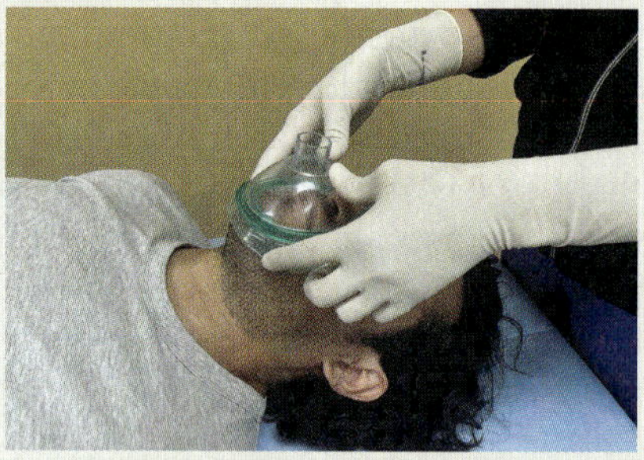

STEP 3 Place the mask over the patient's face. Start by putting the angled or grooved end of the mask over the bridge of the nose. Then bring the bottom of the mask against the groove between the lower lip and the chin.

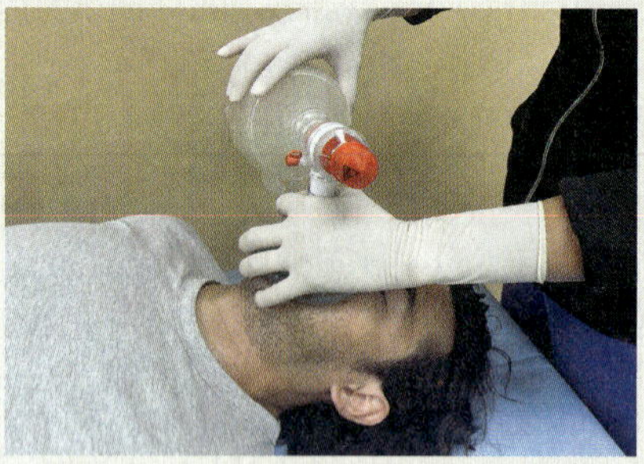

STEP 4 Attach the bag to the mask. Seal the mask using an EO-clamp technique. Use your middle, ring, and little fingers to form an "E." Place these three fingers of one hand under the angle of the jaw. Lift up on the jaw. Make an "O" by placing your thumb and index finger on top of the mask, encircling the neck of the mask. Clamp the mask by lifting the jaw and bringing the mask in contact with the jaw. Continue to hold the mask in position.

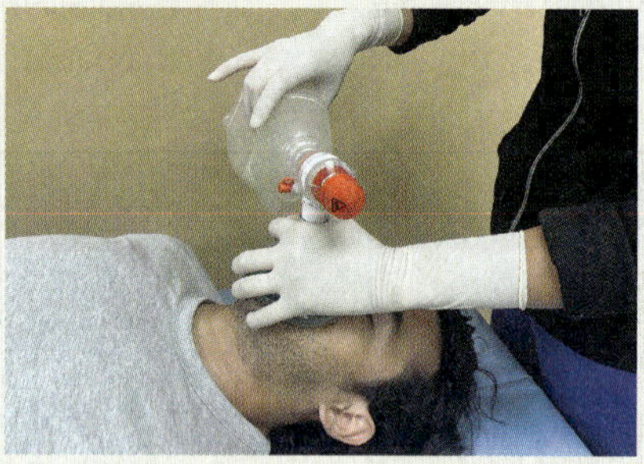

STEP 5 Squeeze the bag until you see the chest rise. Repeat every 6 seconds for adults and every 2 to 3 seconds for infants and children. Avoid overinflating the lungs. If you do not see the chest rise, check for air leaking around the mask or for an airway obstruction.

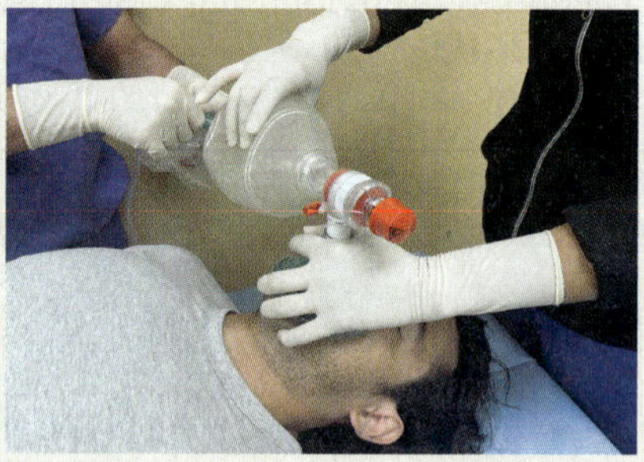

STEP 6 Add supplemental oxygen if it is available. Adjust the oxygen regulator to deliver 10 to 15 L/min. Connect the oxygen tubing to the flowmeter outlet. Continue ventilating the patient at the recommended rate. The specific steps for using supplemental oxygen are explained later in this chapter.

Courtesy of Stephen J. Rahm, NRP, FcEHS.

Performing Rescue Breathing on Children and Infants

The steps required to determine responsiveness and check and correct the patient's airway and breathing are similar for adults, children, and infants. However, some differences exist. You must learn and practice the different airway and breathing sequences for children and infants.

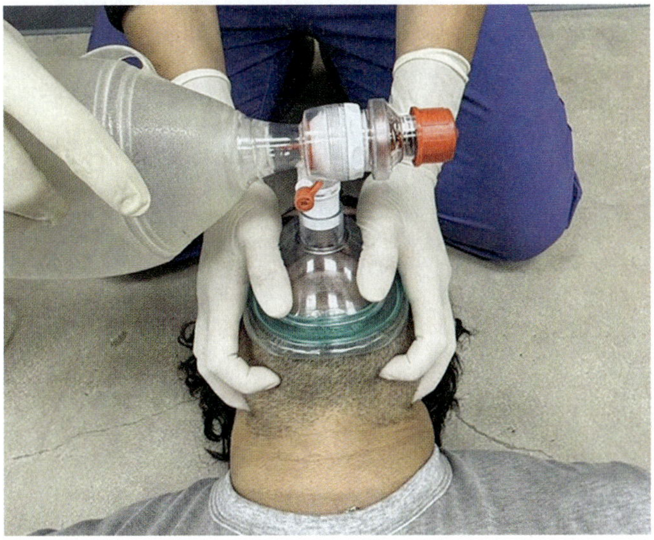

FIGURE 7-21 With two-person bag-mask ventilation, you hold the mask in place while your partner squeezes the bag with a few fingers of one hand until the patient's chest rises adequately.
Courtesy of Stephen J. Rahm, NRP, FcEHS.

Rescue Breathing for Children

For the purposes of performing rescue breathing, a child is a person between age 1 year and the beginning of puberty (age 12 to 14 years). Keep the following differences between adult patients and children in mind:

1. Children are smaller than adults. You will not have to use as much force to open their airways and tilt their heads.
2. The rate of rescue breathing is slightly faster for children. Give 1 rescue breath every 2 to 3 seconds (approximately 20 to 30 rescue breaths/min) instead of the adult rate of 1 rescue breath every 6 seconds (10 rescue breaths/min).

Rescue Breathing for Infants

If the patient is an infant (younger than 1 year), you must vary rescue breathing techniques slightly. Remember, an infant is tiny and must be treated extremely gently.

The steps in rescue breathing for an infant are shown in **SKILL DRILL 7-8**.

The rate of rescue breathing for infants is the same as that for children. If the patient is breathing adequately, place the patient in the recovery position. Often when rescue breathing is necessary, external cardiac compressions are also required.

SKILL DRILL 7-8

Performing Infant Rescue Breathing

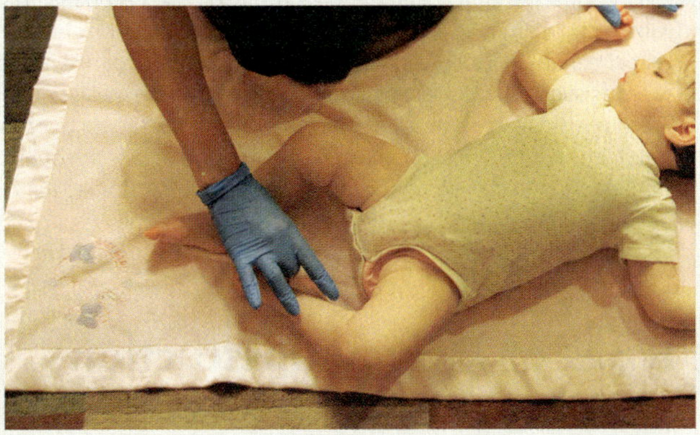

STEP 1 Check for responsiveness by gently shaking the infant's shoulder or tapping the bottom of the foot. If the infant is unresponsive, place the infant on their back and shout for help or activate the EMS system.

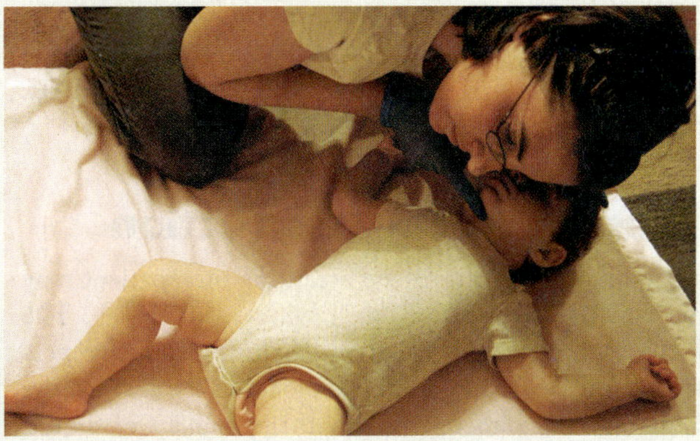

STEP 2 Check the brachial pulse (located inside of the upper arm). Simultaneously check for the absence of breathing or only gasping breaths by looking for the rise and fall of the infant's chest and listening for the sound of air moving in and out of the infant's mouth and nose. If the patient is not breathing and a pulse is present, proceed to Step 3.

(continues)

SKILL DRILL 7-8 (continued)

Performing Infant Rescue Breathing

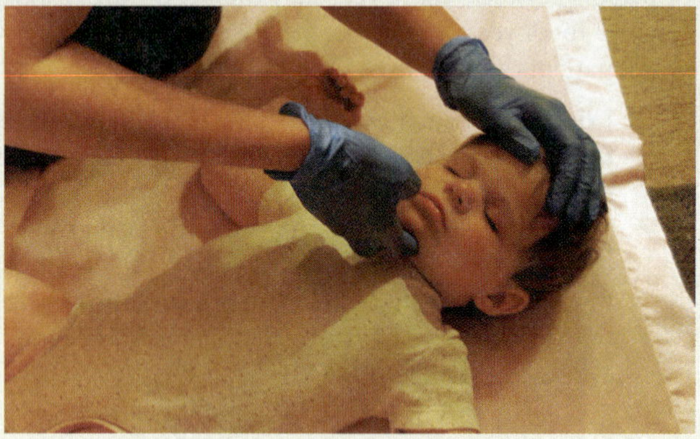

STEP 3 Check the airway and open it by using the head tilt–chin lift maneuver. Do not tip the infant's head back too far because this may block the infant's airway. Tilt it only enough to open the airway.

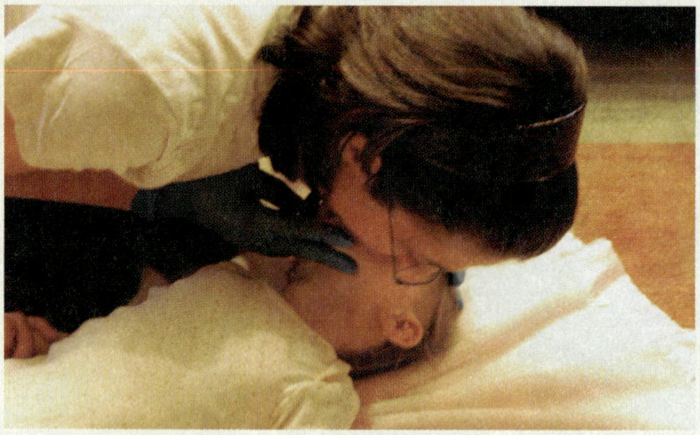

STEP 4 Begin rescue breathing. Cover the infant's mouth and nose with your mouth. Breathe gently into the infant's mouth and nose for 1 second. Watch the chest rise with each breath. Remove your mouth and allow the lungs to deflate.

Do not overinflate an infant's lungs. Use small puffs of air, enough to make the chest rise with each breath. After these first two breaths, give 1 rescue breath every 2 to 3 seconds, or 20 to 30 rescue breaths/min.

Courtesy of Jennifer and Marc Lemaire.

Foreign Body Airway Obstruction

The first part of this section discusses the causes and recognition of mild airway obstruction and severe airway obstruction. The second part of this section discusses the management of foreign body airway obstruction in adults, children, and infants.

Causes of Airway Obstruction

Your attempt to perform rescue breathing on a patient may not be effective because of an **airway obstruction**. The most common airway obstruction in an unresponsive person is the tongue. If the tongue is blocking the airway, the head tilt–chin lift maneuver or jaw-thrust maneuver should open the airway. However, if a foreign body is lodged in the air passage, you must use other techniques.

Food is the most common foreign object that causes an airway obstruction. An adult may choke on a large piece of meat; a child may choke on candy, a peanut, or a piece of a hot dog. Children may put small objects in their mouths and inhale such things as tiny toys or balloons. Vomitus may obstruct the airway of a child or an adult (**FIGURE 7-22**).

Special Populations

Airway Obstruction in Pediatric Patients

Children often swallow small, round objects such as marbles, beads, buttons, and coins. If these objects do not become airway obstructions, they usually pass uneventfully through the child and are eliminated in a bowel movement. However, sharp or straight objects such as open safety pins, bobby pins, and bones are dangerous if swallowed. Arrange for prompt transport to an appropriate medical facility because special instruments and techniques are required to locate and remove the object from the stomach and intestinal tract.

Types of Airway Obstruction

Airway obstruction may be partial (a mild obstruction) or complete (a severe obstruction). The first step in caring for an alert person who may have an obstructed airway is to ask, "Are you choking?" If the patient can reply to your question, the airway is not completely blocked. If the patient is unable to speak or cough, the airway is completely blocked.

Mild Airway Obstruction

In partial or mild airway obstruction, the patient coughs and gags. This indicates that some air is passing around the

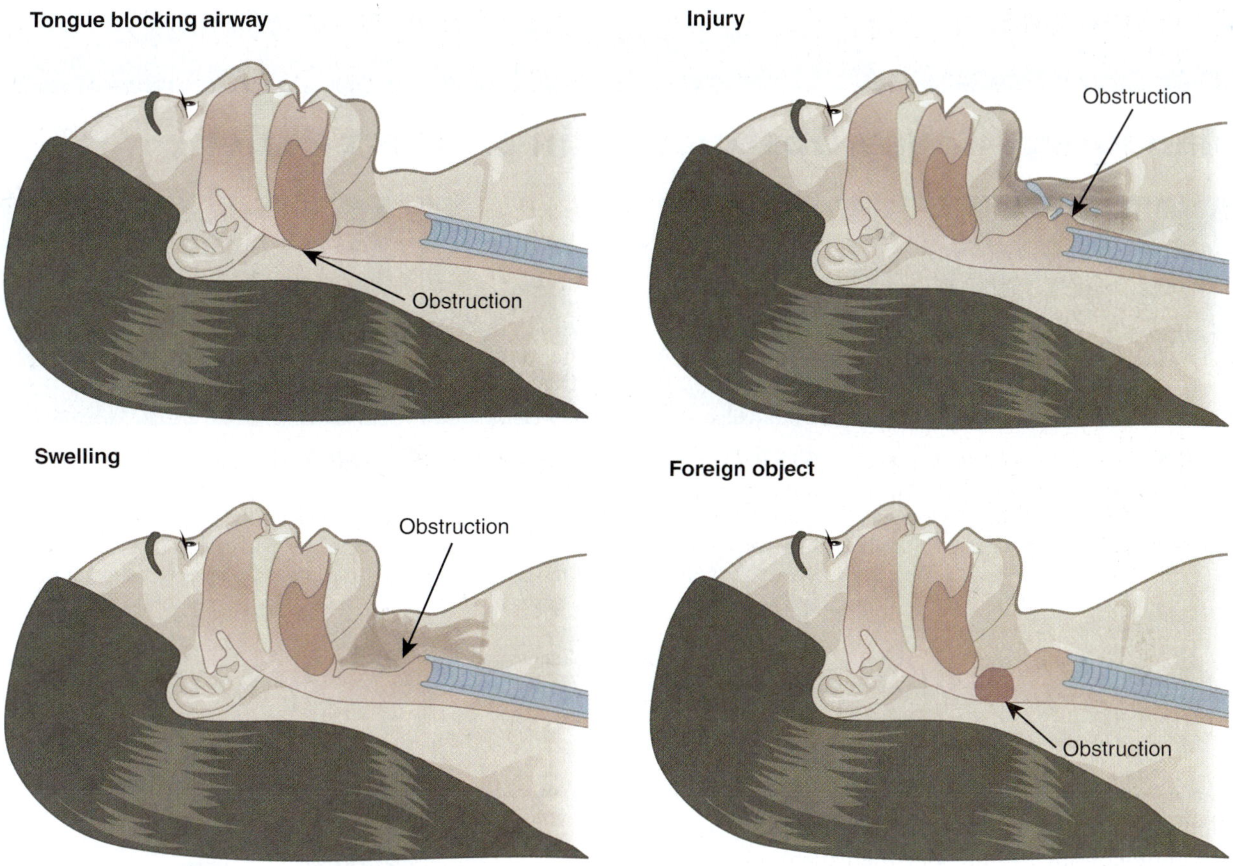

FIGURE 7-22 Common causes of airway obstruction.

© Jones & Bartlett Learning

obstruction. The patient may even be able to speak, although with difficulty.

To treat a mildly obstructed airway, encourage the patient to cough. Coughing is the most effective way of expelling a foreign object. If the patient is unable to expel the object by coughing (if, for example, a bone is stuck in the throat), arrange for the patient's *prompt transport* to an appropriate medical facility. Such a patient must be monitored carefully while awaiting transport and during transport because a mild obstruction can become a severe (complete) obstruction at any moment.

Severe Airway Obstruction

A patient with a severe (complete) airway obstruction will have different signs and symptoms than a patient with a mild airway obstruction. With no fresh oxygen entering the lungs, the body quickly uses all the oxygen breathed in with the last breath. The patient is unable to breathe in or out and, because they cannot exhale air, speech is impossible. Other symptoms of a severe airway obstruction may include poor air exchange, increased breathing difficulty, and a silent cough. If the airway is completely obstructed, the patient will become unresponsive in 3 to 4 minutes.

In patients older than 1 year, your initial effort should be to dislodge the object by administering back slaps. If back slaps fail, you should perform abdominal thrusts, also called the **Heimlich maneuver**. Abdominal thrusts compress the air that remains in the lungs, pushing it upward through the airway so that it exerts pressure against the foreign object. The pressure pops the object out, in much the same way that a cork pops out of a bottle after the bottle has been shaken to increase the pressure. Many rescuers report that abdominal thrusts can cause an obstructing piece of food to fly across the room. A person who has had an obstruction removed from the airway by abdominal thrusts should be transported to a hospital for examination by a physician.

Management of Foreign Body Airway Obstructions

Relieving a foreign body airway obstruction requires no special equipment. The following sections describe the steps that you need to learn to relieve foreign body airway obstructions in adults, children, and infants. Performing these steps can make the difference between life and death for these patients.

Airway Obstruction in an Adult

The steps to treat severe airway obstruction vary, depending on whether the patient is alert or unresponsive. For most adults and children older than 1 year, if the patient is alert, stand behind and toward the side of the patient, place an arm across their chest for support, and give five back slaps by striking the person between the shoulder blades with the heel of your open hand. If the object is not dislodged, give five abdominal thrusts, described as follows.

Locate the xiphoid process (the bottom of the sternum) and the navel. Place one fist above the navel and well below the xiphoid process, thumb side against the patient's

SKILL DRILL 7-9

Managing Airway Obstruction in an Alert Patient

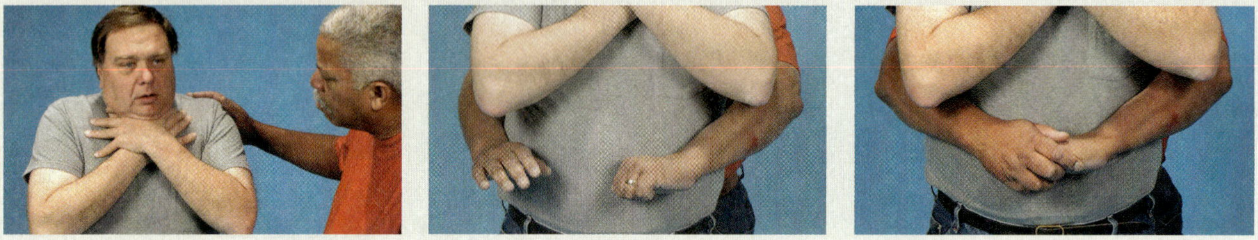

STEP 1 Look for signs of choking. Ask, "Are you choking? Can you speak? Can I help you?" If there is no verbal response, assume the airway obstruction is complete.

STEP 2 Stand behind the patient and first attempt to dislodge the object by giving five back slaps (striking the person between the shoulder blades with the heel of your open hand). If the back slaps do not dislodge the object, position the thumb side of your fist against the patient's abdomen, just above the patient's navel.

STEP 3 Press into the patient's abdomen with a quick, upward thrust. Repeat the abdominal thrusts five times. Continue this cycle of five back slaps and five abdominal thrusts until the airway is cleared or the person becomes unresponsive.

© Jones & Bartlett Learning. Courtesy of MIEMSS.

abdomen. Grasp your fist with your other hand. Then apply abdominal thrusts sharply and firmly, bringing your fist in and slightly upward. Do not give the patient a bear hug; rather, apply pressure at the point where your fist contacts the patient's abdomen. Each thrust should be distinct and forceful. Repeat these abdominal thrusts five times. Continue this cycle of five back slaps and five abdominal thrusts until the airway is cleared or the patient becomes unresponsive, in which case you should then begin CPR.

SKILL DRILL 7-9 describes the steps to assist an alert patient with a complete airway obstruction. Review the steps until you can carry them out automatically.

If the patient has obesity that prevents you from reaching your arms around the abdomen or is in the late stages of pregnancy, use chest thrusts instead of abdominal thrusts (**FIGURE 7-23**). Chest thrusts are done by standing behind the patient and placing your arms under the patient's armpits to encircle the patient's chest. Press with quick, backward thrusts.

If the patient becomes unresponsive, perform the following steps:

1. Ensure that the EMS system has been activated.
2. Begin CPR:
   a. Perform chest compressions. (This part of the CPR sequence is covered in Chapter 8, *Professional Rescuer CPR*).
   b. Open the airway and look in the mouth when it becomes time for the breathing portion of the CPR cycle. Remove the foreign body only if you can see it.
   c. Attempt to ventilate. If you are unable to ventilate, reposition the patient's head and reattempt ventilation. If both breaths do not produce visible chest rise, continue chest compressions.
3. Continue these steps of CPR until more advanced EMS personnel arrive.

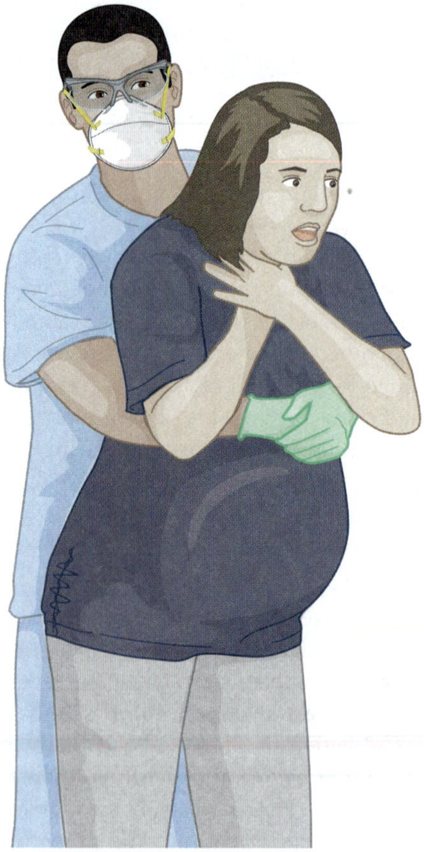

FIGURE 7-23 For a patient in the late stages of pregnancy, perform chest thrusts, not abdominal thrusts.

© Jones & Bartlett Learning

Recent studies have shown that performing chest compressions on an unresponsive patient increases the pressure in the chest similar to performing abdominal thrusts and may relieve an airway obstruction. Therefore, performing CPR on

Foreign Body Airway Obstruction in an Adult	
Steps	**Adequately Performed**
1. Ask: "Are you choking?"	
2. Give five back slaps then five abdominal thrusts (chest thrusts for pregnant patient or patient with obesity).	
3. Repeat this cycle until foreign body is dislodged or patient becomes unresponsive.	
If the patient becomes unresponsive:	
4. Ensure the EMS system has been activated.	
5. Perform chest compressions.	
6. Open the airway and look in the mouth. Remove the foreign body only if you can see it.	
7. Attempt to ventilate. If you are unable to ventilate, reposition the patient's head and reattempt ventilation. If both breaths do not produce visible chest rise, continue chest compressions.	
8. Continue these steps until more advanced EMS personnel arrive.	

FIGURE 7-24 Skill performance sheet: Foreign Body Airway Obstruction in an Adult.

© Jones & Bartlett Learning

a patient who has become unresponsive has the same effect as performing abdominal thrusts on an alert patient.

A skill performance sheet is shown in **FIGURE 7-24** for your review and practice.

Airway Obstruction in a Child

A severe airway obstruction exists when the child has poor air exchange, increased breathing difficulty, a silent cough, the inability to speak, or no air movement because of an obstruction. You have only a few minutes to act before permanent brain damage occurs. Use abdominal thrusts. Abdominal thrusts provide enough energy to expel most foreign objects that could completely block a child's airway (**FIGURE 7-25**).

The steps for relieving an airway obstruction in an unresponsive child (age 1 year to the onset of puberty) are the same as for an adult patient. When opening the airway of a child or infant, tilt the head back just past the neutral position. Tilting the head too far back (hyperextending the neck) can obstruct the airway of a child or infant. If you are by yourself and an alert child with an airway obstruction becomes unresponsive, perform CPR for five cycles (approximately 2 minutes) before activating the EMS system.

A skill performance sheet is shown in **FIGURE 7-26** for your review and practice.

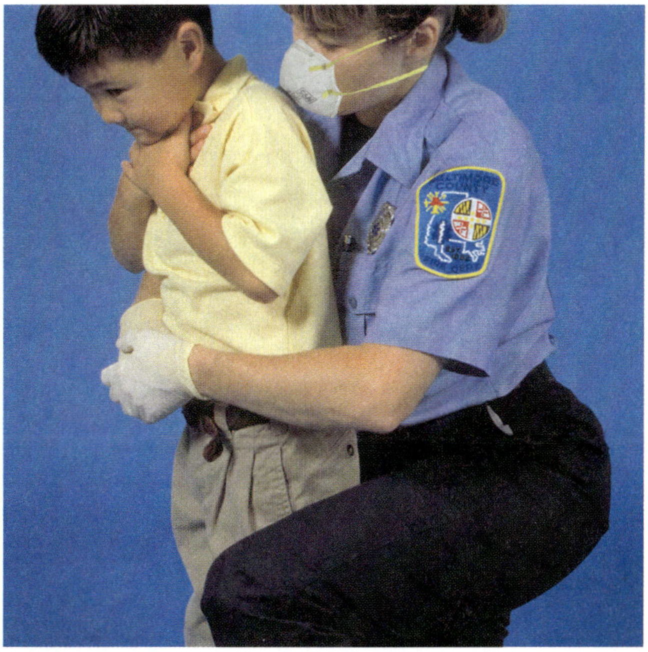

FIGURE 7-25 Performing abdominal thrusts on a child.

© Jones & Bartlett Learning. Courtesy of MIEMSS.

Airway Obstruction in an Infant

The process for relieving an airway obstruction in an infant (younger than 1 year) must take into consideration that an infant is extremely fragile. An infant's airway structures are extremely small, and they are more easily injured than those of an adult. If you suspect an airway obstruction, assess the infant to determine whether there is any air exchange. If the infant has an audible cry, the airway is not completely obstructed. Ask the person who was with the infant what was happening when the episode began. This person may have seen the infant put a foreign body into their mouth.

Suspect a severe airway obstruction if you observe no movement of air from the infant's mouth and nose, a sudden onset of severe breathing difficulty, a silent cough, or a silent cry. To relieve an airway obstruction in an infant, use a combination of back slaps and chest thrusts (**FIGURE 7-27**). You must have a good grasp of the infant to alternate the back

Foreign Body Airway Obstruction in a Child	
Steps	**Adequately Performed**
1. Ask: "Are you choking?"	
2. Give five back slaps then five abdominal thrusts.	
3. Repeat this cycle until foreign body is dislodged or patient becomes unresponsive.	
If the patient becomes unresponsive:	
4. If a second rescuer is available, have him or her activate the EMS system.	
5. Perform chest compressions.	
6. Open the airway and look in the mouth. Remove the foreign body only if you can see it.	
7. Attempt to ventilate. If you are unable to ventilate, reposition the patient's head and reattempt ventilation. If both breaths do not produce visible chest rise, continue chest compressions.	
8. Continue these steps until more advanced EMS personnel arrive.	
NOTE: If you are by yourself, perform CPR for five cycles (about 2 minutes) and then activate the EMS system.	

FIGURE 7-26 Skill performance sheet: Foreign Body Airway Obstruction in a Child.
© Jones & Bartlett Learning

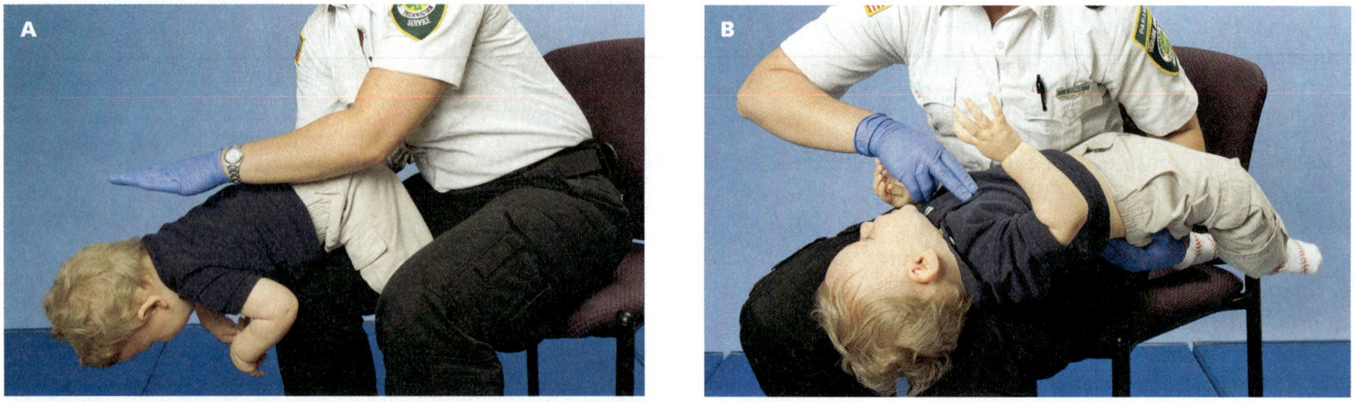

FIGURE 7-27 Administering back slaps and chest thrusts in an infant. **A.** Hold the infant facedown with the body resting on your forearm. Support the jaw and face with your hand without blocking the airway and keep the head lower than the rest of the body. Give the infant five back slaps between the shoulder blades, using the heel of your hand. **B.** Sandwich the infant between your hands, turn the infant over, and give the infant five quick chest thrusts, using two fingers placed on the lower half of the sternum (finger position should be the same as that for CPR for infants).
© Jones & Bartlett Learning

slaps and the chest thrusts. Review the following sequence until you can carry it out automatically. To assist an alert infant with a severe airway obstruction, you must:

1. Assess the infant's airway and breathing status. Determine that there is no air exchange.
2. Place the infant in a facedown position over one arm so you can deliver five back slaps. Support the infant's head and neck with one hand and place the infant facedown with the head lower than the trunk. Rest the infant on your forearm and support your forearm on your thigh. Use the heel of your hand and deliver up to five back slaps forcefully between the infant's shoulder blades.
3. Support the head and turn the infant faceup by sandwiching the infant between your hands and arms. Rest the infant on their back with the head lower than the trunk.
4. Deliver five chest thrusts in the middle of the sternum. Use two fingers to deliver the chest thrusts in a firm manner.
5. Repeat the series of back slaps and chest thrusts until the foreign object is expelled or until the infant becomes unresponsive.

If the infant becomes unresponsive, continue with the following steps:

1. Ensure that the EMS system has been activated.
2. Begin CPR:
   a. Perform chest compressions.
   b. Open the airway and look in the mouth. Remove the foreign body only if you can see it.
   c. Attempt to ventilate. If you are unable to ventilate, reposition the patient's head and reattempt ventilation. If both breaths do not produce visible chest rise, continue chest compressions.
3. Continue these CPR steps until more advanced EMS personnel arrive.

NOTE: If you are by yourself, perform CPR for five cycles (approximately 2 minutes) and then activate the EMS system.

Recent studies have shown that performing chest compressions on an unresponsive patient increases the pressure in the chest similar to performing chest thrusts and may relieve an airway obstruction. Therefore, performing CPR on an infant who has become unresponsive has the same effect as performing the chest thrusts on an alert patient.

A skill performance sheet is shown in **FIGURE 7-28** for your review and practice.

Oxygen Administration

Under normal conditions, the body can operate efficiently using normal air (also known as room air), even though it contains only 21% oxygen. Because blood is the vehicle that delivers oxygen to the cells, when there is less blood, less oxygen is delivered. The amount of blood loss that occurs after a traumatic injury could mean that insufficient oxygen is delivered to the cells of the body. This results in shock. Administering supplemental oxygen to a patient showing signs and

Foreign Body Airway Obstruction in an Infant	
Steps	**Adequately Performed**
1. Confirm severity of airway obstruction. Check for sudden onset of serious breathing difficulty, ineffective cough, silent cough, or cry.	
2. Give up to five back slaps and up to five chest thrusts.	
3. Repeat Step 2 until the foreign body is dislodged or until the infant becomes unresponsive.	
If the infant becomes unresponsive:	
4. If a second rescuer is available, have him or her activate the EMS system.	
5. Perform chest compressions.	
6. Open the airway and look in the mouth. Remove the foreign body only if you can see it.	
7. Attempt to ventilate. If you are unable to ventilate, reposition the patient's head and reattempt ventilation. If both breaths do not produce visible chest rise, continue chest compressions.	
8. Continue these steps until more advanced EMS personnel arrive.	
NOTE: If you are by yourself, perform CPR for five cycles (about 2 minutes) and then activate the EMS system.	

FIGURE 7-28 Skill performance sheet: Foreign Body Airway Obstruction in an Infant.

© Jones & Bartlett Learning

YOU are the EMR — CASE 3

You are enjoying a well-deserved day off. It is a mild and sunny day in spring, so you decide to go for a run in a local park. After a tiring but refreshing run, you are heading back to your vehicle when you notice an energetic group of young children from a daycare center. They seem to be enjoying an afternoon snack on the lawn. As you pass by, one of the caregivers begins to yell for help. You look over and see a boy, about 9 years old, who is holding his neck and has a panicked look in his eyes. You run over and introduce yourself to the caregiver. She tells you the children were enjoying a snack and she thinks that Matt may have gotten something caught in his throat.

1. What is the first step you should take?
2. What else should you do for this patient?
3. How long should you continue your treatment?

symptoms of shock increases the amount of oxygen delivered to the cells of the body and often makes a positive difference in the patient's outcome.

Patients who have experienced a heart attack or stroke, or patients who have a chronic heart or lung disease, may be unable to get sufficient oxygen from room air. These patients may also benefit from receiving supplemental oxygen.

Not all EMRs are approved to administer oxygen; however, knowing this skill can help you when you are in a situation where EMS response may be delayed. By learning this skill, you will be able to assist other members of the EMS team. Administer oxygen only after receiving proper training and with the approval of your medical director.

Oxygen Equipment

Several pieces of equipment are required to administer supplemental oxygen, including an oxygen cylinder, a pressure regulator/flowmeter, and a nasal cannula or face mask. The characteristics and operation of each piece of equipment are described in the following sections.

Oxygen Cylinders

Oxygen cylinders used in the United States must be marked with a green color and labeled as medical oxygen (**FIGURE 7-29**). Medical oxygen is compressed to approximately 2,000 pounds per square inch (psi). The portable oxygen cylinders used by most EMS systems are either size D or E. D cylinders hold approximately 350 L of oxygen, and E cylinders hold approximately 680 L of oxygen. The exact capacity of a cylinder depends on the metal used in the construction and the individual manufacturer. The amount of time an oxygen tank will last depends on the flow rate (liters per minute) at which the oxygen is being delivered to the patient. At 2 L/min, a full D cylinder will last approximately 170 minutes. At 10 L/min a full D cylinder will last approximately 30 minutes. A valve at the top of the oxygen cylinder allows you to control the flow of oxygen from the cylinder.

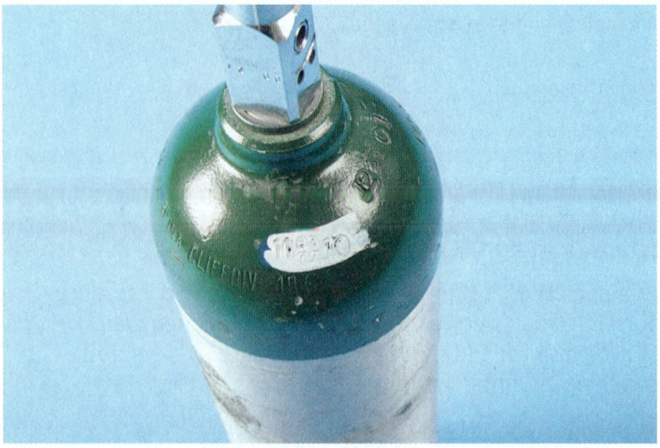

FIGURE 7-29 Oxygen tanks for medical use have a series of letters and numbers stamped into the metal on the collar of the cylinder.
© Jones & Bartlett Learning

Pressure Regulator/Flowmeter

Oxygen in the cylinder is stored at 2,000 psi. Oxygen can be used only when that pressure is regulated down to approximately 50 psi, which is done by using a pressure regulator. The pressure regulator and the **flowmeter** are a single unit attached to the outlet of the oxygen cylinder (**FIGURE 7-30**). After the pressure has been reduced, you can adjust the flowmeter to deliver oxygen at a rate of 1 to 15 L/min. Because patients with different medical conditions require different amounts of oxygen, the flowmeter lets you select the proper amount of oxygen to administer. A gasket between the cylinder and the pressure regulator/flowmeter ensures a tight seal and maintains the high pressure inside the cylinder. Always check for this gasket before attaching the regulator.

Nasal Cannulas and Face Masks

The third part of an oxygen-delivery system is a device that ensures the oxygen is delivered to the patient and is not lost in the air. A **nasal cannula** is a simple oxygen-delivery device that has two small prongs that fit into the patient's nostrils (**FIGURE 7-31**). A cannula delivers low-flow oxygen at

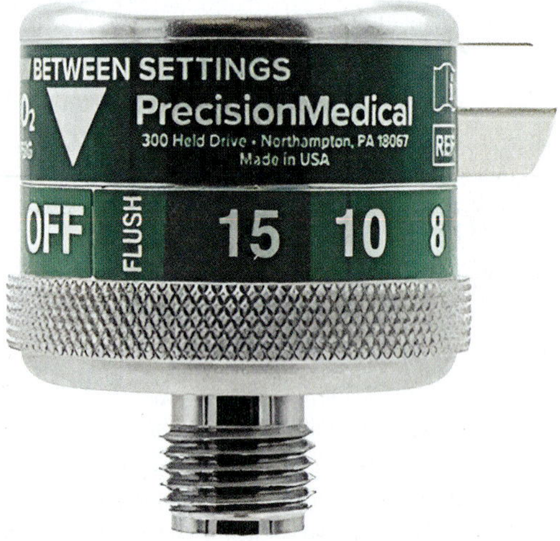

FIGURE 7-30 The regulator/flowmeter attaches to the outlet of the oxygen cylinder.
Used with permission from Precision Medical, Inc.

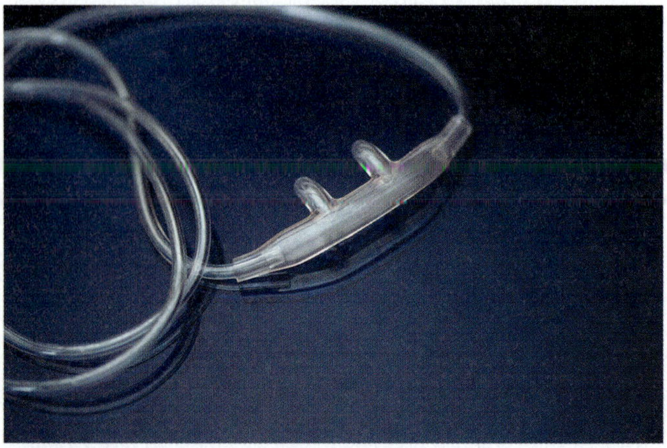

FIGURE 7-31 A nasal cannula.
© MedStockPhotos/Alamy Stock Photo

1 to 6 L/min. Each liter per minute of oxygen provides approximately 4% additional oxygen to the patient. For example, an oxygen flow of 4 L/min would add 16% oxygen to the 21% in room air for a total of 37% oxygen flow to the patient. Low-flow oxygen can be used for fairly stable patients, such as those with slight chest pain or mild shortness of breath.

A **face mask** is placed over the patient's nose and mouth to deliver oxygen through the patient's mouth and nostrils. Nonrebreathing masks are most commonly used by EMRs. A nonrebreathing mask consists of connecting tubing, a reservoir bag, one-way valves, and a face piece (**FIGURE 7-32**). It is used to deliver a high flow of oxygen at 10 to 15 L/min. A nonrebreathing face mask can deliver concentrations of oxygen as high as 90%. The mask works by storing oxygen in the reservoir bag. When the patient inhales, oxygen is drawn from the reservoir bag. When the patient exhales, the air is exhausted through the one-way valves on the side of the mask.

Use nonrebreathing face masks for patients who require higher flows of oxygen. These include patients experiencing serious shortness of breath, severe chest pain, carbon monoxide poisoning, and congestive heart failure. Patients who show signs and symptoms of shock should also be treated with high-flow oxygen from a nonrebreathing face mask.

Safety Considerations

Oxygen does not burn or explode by itself. However, it actively supports combustion and can quickly turn a small spark or flame into a serious fire. Therefore, keep all sparks, heat, flames, and oily substances away from oxygen equipment. Smoking is never safe around oxygen equipment.

The pressurized cylinders are also hazardous because the high pressure in an oxygen cylinder can cause an explosion if the cylinder is damaged. Secure the oxygen cylinder so that it will not fall. If the shut-off valve at the top of the cylinder is damaged, the cylinder can take off like a rocket. Oxygen cylinders should be kept inside sturdy carrying cases that protect the cylinder and regulator/flowmeter. Handle the cylinder carefully to guard against damage.

Administering Supplemental Oxygen

To administer supplemental oxygen, place the regulator/flowmeter over the stem of the oxygen cylinder and line up the pins on the pin-indexing system correctly (**FIGURE 7-33**). Check for the mandatory gasket. Tighten the securing screw firmly by hand. With the special key or wrench provided, turn the cylinder valve counterclockwise to allow oxygen from the cylinder to enter the regulator/flowmeter.

Check the gauge on the pressure regulator/flowmeter to see how much oxygen pressure remains in the cylinder. If the cylinder contains less than 500 psi, the cylinder does not contain sufficient oxygen for emergency use and should be replaced with a full cylinder (2,000 psi).

To administer oxygen, you will need to adjust the flowmeter to deliver the desired liter-per-minute flow of oxygen. The patient's condition and the type of oxygen delivery device you use (a mask or a nasal cannula) dictate the proper flow. When the oxygen flow begins, place the face mask or

Treatment

As an EMR, you may administer oxygen and should understand its medication properties.

Oxygen (O_2)

Effects. Increases the level of oxygen saturation in the bloodstream

Indications. Shortness of breath, decreased levels of oxygen saturation, chest pain with shortness of breath, suspected carbon monoxide poisoning, shock, decreased levels of consciousness

Contraindications: Should not be used for patients who are hyperventilating unless they have diabetes

Side effects. May reduce the respiratory drive in patients with COPD. However, do not withhold oxygen from a patient with COPD. Continue to monitor their breathing status after you begin to administer oxygen.

Route of administration. Inhalation

Dosages. 1 to 6 L/min by nasal cannula; 10 to 15 L/min by face mask

For more information about medication properties, see Chapter 10, *Medical Emergencies*.

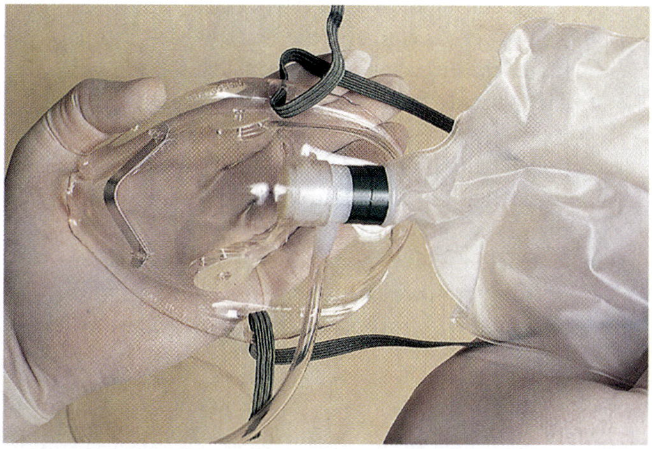

FIGURE 7-32 A nonrebreathing oxygen mask.

© Jones & Bartlett Learning. Courtesy of MIEMSS.

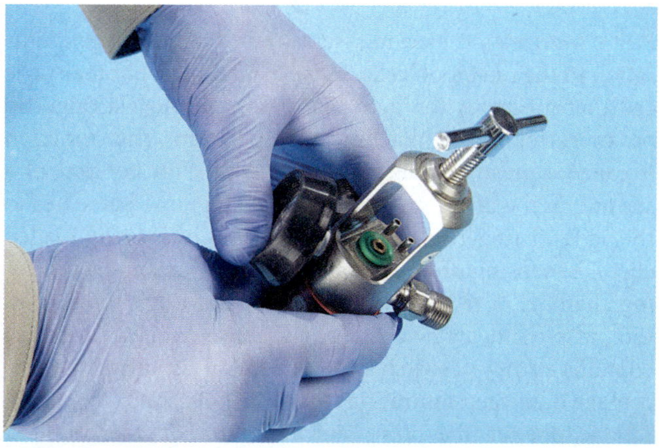

FIGURE 7-33 A valve stem with pin-index holes.

© Jones & Bartlett Learning

nasal cannula onto the patient's face. Never place a mask over a patient's face until the oxygen is flowing and the reservoir bag on a nonrebreather is inflated.

To use a nasal cannula, first adjust the flow to 1 to 6 L/min and then apply the cannula to the patient. The cannula should fit snugly but should not be tight. To use a nonrebreathing mask, first adjust the oxygen flow to 12 to 15 L/min to inflate the reservoir bag before putting it on the patient. After the bag inflates, place the mask over the patient's face. Adjust the straps to secure a snug fit. Adjust the liter flow to keep the bag at least partially inflated while the patient inhales.

Hazards of Supplemental Oxygen

Supplemental oxygen can be lifesaving, but you must use it carefully so that you, your team, and the patient remain safe. Although this chapter provides you with a basic outline on setting up oxygen equipment, you will need additional class work and practical training before you administer oxygen in emergency situations.

Safety

Avoid using oxygen around fire or flames. Secure oxygen cylinders to minimize the danger of explosion.

Words of Wisdom

Some patients who have respiratory conditions such as asthma or emphysema may use a **metered-dose inhaler (MDI)** to administer medications to help them breathe. An MDI is a miniature spray container used to direct medications through the mouth and into the lungs. MDIs deliver the same amount of medication each time they are used. MDIs should be shaken before they are administered to ensure that the patient receives a uniform amount of medicine each time they use the inhaler. Many patients will use their inhaler before they call for EMS assistance. If your local protocols permit you to assist patients with using their MDIs, you need to have special training in the proper use of these devices.

Pulse Oximetry

Pulse oximetry is used to assess the amount of oxygen saturation in the red blood cells. It does this using a photoelectric cell that measures the light that passes through a fingertip or an earlobe. The machine that performs this function is called a pulse oximeter. A **pulse oximeter** consists of a sensing probe and a monitor. The sensing probe attaches to the patient's fingertip or earlobe by means of a spring-loaded clip. The sensing probe contains a light source and a receiving chamber. The sensing probe attaches to the monitor of the pulse oximeter by a cable. The pulse oximeter monitor contains an on–off switch and a screen for displaying the percentage of oxygen saturation (**FIGURE 7-34**).

To operate the pulse oximeter, turn on the monitor. Most pulse oximeters perform a self-check to ensure that the machine is operating correctly. This self-check will vary

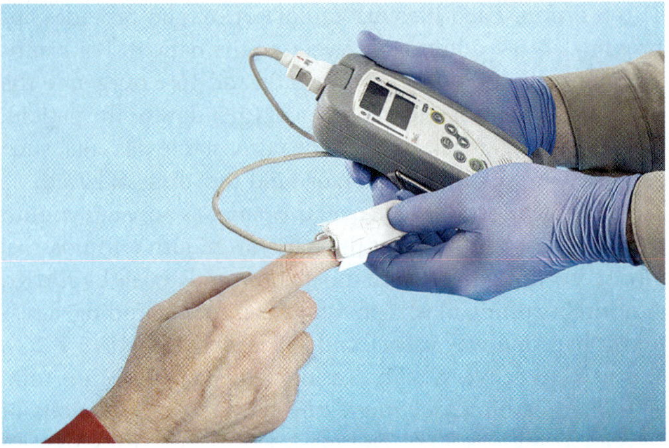

FIGURE 7-34 A pulse oximeter, which consists of a sensing probe and a monitor, is used to measure the percentage of oxygen saturation in the blood.
© Jones & Bartlett Learning

depending on the brand of the oximeter. After you confirm that the monitor is operating correctly, place the sensing probe over the patient's fingertip or earlobe. The monitor should then display the percentage of saturation of the patient's blood. In a healthy patient, the oxygen saturation should be 94% or greater when breathing room air.

If a patient has difficulty breathing as a result of injury or a disease process, the oxygen saturation level may be much lower than 90%. The pulse oximeter cannot tell you what is wrong with the patient. You must perform a thorough patient assessment, including obtaining a good medical history. The pulse oximeter can help you to recognize that the patient is having a problem. It can also help you to determine whether your treatment is helping the patient. If the steps you are taking to treat the patient coincide with an increased percentage of oxygen saturation, you can take that as a positive sign.

Like any other device, a pulse oximeter has certain limitations. An inaccurate pulse oximetry reading may be caused by the following situations:

- The patient has sustained considerable blood loss (hypovolemia).
- The patient is experiencing anemia (decreased level of circulating red blood cells).
- The patient is cold and the blood vessels in the fingertips or earlobes are constricted.
- The patient's fingers are very dirty, or the patient is wearing certain types of nail polish, such as gel nail polish (though research has suggested its effect is not clinically significant and may not justify removal in the prehospital setting)
- The patient has experienced carbon monoxide poisoning, in which case the red blood cells are saturated with carbon monoxide instead of with oxygen.

Remember, no machine can replace a careful patient assessment, including a good medical history. Pulse oximetry should not be the only way of evaluating your treatment. Evaluating the patient's skin color, work and rate of breathing, and overall chief complaint should always be the primary methods of gauging patient treatment.

Special Considerations

As an EMR, you will encounter some situations that require a slight modification in your ventilation technique. These situations include rescue breathing for patients with stomas, gastric distention, patients with dental appliances, and airway management in a vehicle. By adapting to these situations, you can ensure effective ventilation for these patients.

Rescue Breathing for Patients With Stomas

Some people have had surgery that removed part or all of the larynx. In these patients, the upper airway has been rerouted to open through a **stoma** (hole) in the neck. These patients are sometimes referred to as neck breathers. Therefore, you must give rescue breathing through the stoma in the patient's neck. The technique is called **mask-to-stoma breathing**.

The steps in performing mask-to-stoma breathing are as follows:

1. Check every patient for the presence of a stoma.
2. If you locate a stoma, keep the patient's neck straight; do not hyperextend the patient's head and neck.
3. Examine the stoma and clean away any mucus in it.
4. If you observe a breathing tube in the opening, remove it to be sure the opening is clear. Clean the breathing tube rapidly and replace it into the stoma. Moistening the tube will make it easier to insert the tube.
5. Place the mask directly over the stoma and use the same procedures as in mouth-to-mask breathing. It is not necessary to seal the mouth and nose of most people who have a stoma.
6. If the patient's chest does not rise, they may be a partial neck breather. In these patients, seal the mouth and nose with one hand and then breathe through the stoma. You can also use a bag-mask or pocket-mask device to ventilate a patient with a stoma (**FIGURE 7-35**).

Words of Wisdom

The mask from a pediatric bag-mask device is the best size to use when ventilating through a stoma.

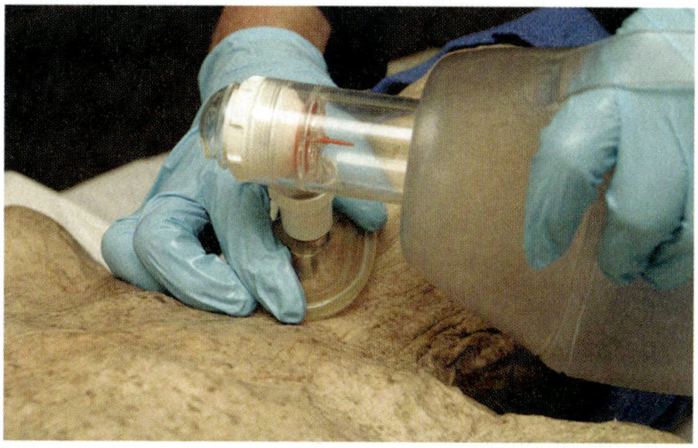

FIGURE 7-35 You can use a bag-mask device to ventilate a patient with a stoma.

© Jones & Bartlett Learning. Courtesy of MIEMSS.

Gastric Distention

Gastric distention occurs when air is forced into the stomach instead of the lungs. This condition makes it harder to get an adequate amount of air into the patient's lungs, and it increases the chance that the patient will vomit. Deliver rescue breaths slowly, just enough to make the chest rise.

Remember, the lungs of children and infants are smaller and require smaller, gentler breaths during rescue breathing. The excess air may enter the stomach and cause gastric distention. Preventing gastric distention is much better than trying to correct it after it has occurred.

Dental Appliances

Do not remove dental appliances that are firmly attached. They may help keep the patient's mouth full so you can make a better seal between the patient's mouth and a breathing device. Loose dental appliances, however, may cause difficulties. Partial dentures may become dislodged during trauma or while you perform airway care and rescue breathing. If you discover loose dental appliances during your exam of the patient's airway, remove the dentures to prevent them from occluding the airway. Put them in a safe place so they will not get damaged or lost.

Airway Management in a Vehicle

Airway management at the scene of a motor vehicle crash may require special considerations and modifications. If the patient is lying on the seat or floor of the vehicle, you can apply the head tilt–chin lift maneuver. Use the jaw-thrust

YOU are the EMR — **CASE 4**

It is 2300 hours and you are dispatched to an unknown medical emergency at the home of a 54-year-old man. As you enter the home, the man's wife says he woke up out of a sound sleep reporting crushing chest pain. The patient is in bed. He has difficulty speaking in full sentences and is gasping. Your partner returns to the ambulance to get the stretcher. Your primary assessment shows a pulse oximetry reading of 80%.

1. What would be the most effective way to deliver oxygen to the man?
2. Suddenly the man starts vomiting. What should you do?

maneuver if you suspect the crash could have caused a head or spine injury.

A patient who is in a sitting or semireclining position should be approached from the side by leaning in through the window or across the front seat. Grasp the patient's head with both hands. Put one hand under the patient's chin and the other hand on the back of the patient's head just above the neck. Maintain a slight upward pressure to support the head and cervical spine and to ensure that the airway remains open. This technique will often enable you to maintain an open airway without moving the patient. This technique has several advantages:

1. You do not have to enter the vehicle.
2. You can easily monitor the patient's carotid pulse and breathing patterns by using your fingers.
3. It stabilizes the patient's cervical spine.
4. It opens the patient's airway.

See Chapter 18, *Vehicle Extrication and Special Rescue*, for further discussion of providing airway management to a patient who is trapped in a vehicle

Safety

Whenever you are working around motor vehicles, be aware of the possibility of undeployed airbags. Do not put yourself in front of an undeployed airbag.

YOU are the EMR — SUMMARY

You are the EMR: CASE 1

1. What is the next step you should take to assess and treat this patient?

By asking the woman if she can hear you and by gently shaking her shoulder, you have checked for responsiveness. Because she is unresponsive, your next step is to open the woman's airway by using the head tilt–chin lift maneuver or the jaw-thrust maneuver.

2. How would your method of opening the patient's airway change if the patient had fallen or blacked out?

The method for opening the patient's airway depends on the patient's condition. If the patient has fallen or may have sustained an injury to the head or spine, first use the jaw-thrust maneuver to try to open the airway. For patients who have not been injured, use the head tilt–chin lift maneuver to open the airway.

3. What techniques can you use to maintain an open airway?

After opening a patient's airway, you can use the head tilt–chin lift maneuver or the jaw-thrust maneuver to maintain the airway. Other ways of maintaining the patient's airway include inserting an oral airway, inserting a nasal airway, or placing the patient in the recovery position.

You are the EMR: CASE 2

1. What is the first action you should take?

First, open the patient's airway by performing either the head tilt–chin lift maneuver or the jaw-thrust maneuver. This step may enable the patient to start breathing again. Once breathing resumes, ensure that the patient is breathing at a rate of 12 to 20 times a minute. If the patient does not begin to breathe adequately, then perform rescue breathing.

2. How can you provide oxygen to this patient?

To provide oxygen to this patient, begin rescue breathing. You can use a mouth-to-mask device, a mouth-to-barrier device, or a bag-mask device. Ensure adequate chest rise with each rescue breath, and provide one breath every 6 seconds, or approximately 10 breaths/min.

3. What methods do you have to keep his airway open?

You can maintain the airway in several different ways. One method to keep the airway open is to continue to apply the head tilt–chin lift maneuver. Another method is to insert either an oral airway or a nasal airway. A third method is to place the patient in the recovery position if he is breathing adequately.

You are the EMR: CASE 3

1. What is the first step you should take?

First, ask the boy whether he is choking. If he nods yes and cannot talk, assume he has a severe (complete) airway obstruction. At the same time, if a second person is present on the scene, instruct them to call 9-1-1. Patients who have sustained a severe airway obstruction must be evaluated by a physician.

2. What else should you do for this patient?

After you have determined that Matt has a severe airway obstruction, provide five back slaps. If the obstruction is not dislodged, give five abdominal thrusts. Stand behind the patient and position the thumb side of your fist just above the patient's navel. Press into the patient's abdomen with quick, upward thrusts.

YOU are the EMR SUMMARY

3. How long should you continue your treatment?

Repeat cycle of back slaps and abdominal thrusts until either the foreign body is expelled or the patient becomes unresponsive, in which case you should then begin CPR.

You are the EMR: CASE 4

1. What would be the most effective way to deliver oxygen to the man?

Given the man's inability to speak in full sentences and obvious difficulty breathing, your best choice is to use a nonrebreathing mask. A nonrebreathing face mask can deliver oxygen concentrations as high as 90%.

2. Suddenly the man starts vomiting. What should you do?

Remove the nonrebreathing mask and use either a manual or mechanical suctioning device to clear out the man's mouth, being careful not to suction for more than 10 seconds at a time.

Prep Kit

Ready for Review

- The main purpose of the respiratory system is to provide oxygen and to remove carbon dioxide from the red blood cells as they pass through the lungs. The structures of the respiratory system in children and infants are smaller than they are in adults. Thus, the air passages of children and infants may be more easily blocked by secretions or by foreign objects.
- When a patient experiences possible respiratory arrest, check for responsiveness; open the blocked airway using either the head tilt–chin lift or jaw-thrust maneuver; check for fluids, solids, or dentures in the mouth; and correct the airway, if needed, using finger sweeps or suction.
- Maintain the airway by continuing to manually hold the airway open, by placing the patient in the recovery position, or by inserting an oral or a nasal airway. Check the chest for signs of breathing and correct any problems by using a bag-mask device. If such a device is not available, consider using a mouth-to-mask device, mouth-to-barrier device, or mouth-to-mouth rescue breathing. Remember that the risk of disease transmission is higher with these devices but that danger exists with the bag-mask device also. It is important to use the correct sequence for adults, children, and infants.
- If the airway is obstructed in an alert adult or child, kneel or stand behind the patient and provide five back slaps. If the airway is not cleared, provide five abdominal thrusts. Repeat this cycle until the obstruction is relieved or the patient becomes unresponsive. For an unresponsive adult or child with an airway obstruction, perform chest compressions. Move to the head, open the airway, and look in the patient's mouth. Do not perform a finger sweep, regardless of the patient's age, unless you can see the object. Attempt rescue breathing again. If the airway is still obstructed, repeat chest compressions, visualization of the mouth, and ventilation attempts until the obstruction is relieved.
- Administering supplemental oxygen to patients showing signs and symptoms of shock increases the amount of oxygen delivered to the cells of the body and often improves the patient's outcome. Patients who have experienced a heart attack or stroke or patients who have chronic heart or lung disease may also benefit from receiving supplemental oxygen.
- Use pulse oximetry to assess the amount of oxygen saturation in the red blood cells.

Vital Vocabulary

airway The passages from the openings of the mouth and nose to the air sacs in the lungs through which air enters and leaves the lungs.

airway obstruction Partial (mild) or complete (severe) obstruction of the respiratory passages resulting from blockage by food, small objects, or vomitus.

Prep Kit

alveolar ventilation The exchange of oxygen and carbon dioxide that occurs in the alveoli.

alveoli The air sacs of the lungs where the exchange of oxygen and carbon dioxide takes place.

aspirator A suction device.

bag-mask device A patient ventilation device that consists of a bag, one-way valves, and a face mask.

bronchi The two main branches of the trachea that lead into the right and left lungs. Within the lungs, they branch into smaller airways.

capillaries The smallest blood vessels that connect small arteries and small veins. Capillary walls serve as the membrane to exchange oxygen and carbon dioxide.

cardiopulmonary resuscitation (CPR) The combination of chest compressions and rescue breathing used to establish adequate ventilation and circulation in a pulseless, nonbreathing patient.

cellular respiration The use of oxygen by the cells to carry out their specific activities; also called cellular metabolism.

esophagus The tube through which food passes. It starts at the throat and ends at the stomach.

external respiration The exchange of gases between the lungs and blood.

face mask A clear plastic mask used for oxygen administration that covers the mouth and nose.

flowmeter A device on oxygen cylinders used to control and measure the flow of oxygen.

gag reflex A strong involuntary effort to vomit caused by something being placed or caught in the throat.

gastric distention Inflation of the stomach caused when excessive pressures are used during artificial ventilation and air is directed into the stomach rather than the lungs.

head tilt–chin lift maneuver A method of opening the airway by tilting the patient's head backward and lifting the chin forward, bringing the entire lower jaw with it.

Heimlich maneuver A method of relieving an upper airway obstruction by delivering a series of manual thrusts to the abdomen.

internal respiration The exchange of gases between the blood and tissue cells.

jaw-thrust maneuver A method of opening the airway by bringing the patient's jaw forward without extending the neck.

lungs The organs that supply the body with oxygen and eliminate carbon dioxide from the blood.

mandible The lower jaw.

manual suction device A hand-powered device used for clearing the upper airway of mucus, blood, or vomitus.

mask-to-stoma breathing A means of providing rescue breathing to patients who, because of surgical removal of the larynx, have a stoma.

mechanical suction device A battery-powered pump or an oxygen-powered aspirator used for clearing the upper airway of mucus, blood, or vomitus.

metered-dose inhaler (MDI) A miniature spray container used to direct medications through the mouth and into the lungs.

minute ventilation The amount of air pulled into the lungs and removed from the lungs in 1 minute.

mouth-to-mask ventilation device A piece of equipment that consists of a mask, a one-way valve, and a mouthpiece. Rescue breathing is performed by breathing into the mouthpiece after placing the mask over the patient's mouth and nose.

nasal airway An airway adjunct that is inserted into the nostril of a patient who is unable to maintain a natural airway; also called a nasopharyngeal airway.

nasal cannula A clear plastic tube, used to deliver oxygen, that fits onto the patient's nose.

nasopharynx The posterior part of the nose.

oral airway An airway adjunct that is inserted into the mouth to keep the tongue from blocking the upper airway; also called an oropharyngeal airway.

oropharynx The posterior part of the mouth.

oxygen A colorless, odorless gas that is essential for life.

oxygenation The process of loading oxygen molecules onto hemoglobin molecules in the bloodstream.

patent Open, clear of obstruction.

pharynx The throat.

pocket mask A mechanical breathing device used to administer mouth-to-mask rescue breathing.

pulse oximeter A machine that consists of a monitor and a sensing probe that measures the oxygen saturation in the capillary beds.

pulse oximetry An assessment tool that measures oxygen saturation in the capillary beds.

rescue breathing An artificial means of breathing for a patient.

Prep Kit

respiration The exchange of oxygen and carbon dioxide in the alveoli as well as the tissues of the body; classified as external, internal, or cellular.

respiratory arrest Sudden stoppage of breathing.

respiratory distress A condition marked by difficulty breathing and an abnormal respiratory rate or effort; can range from mild to severe and can progress to respiratory failure.

respiratory failure A condition in which oxygen levels are too low to meet the body's needs and ventilation is impaired, leading to high carbon dioxide levels; accompanied by serious signs and symptoms and must be corrected quickly.

stoma A surgical opening in the neck that connects the windpipe (trachea) to the skin.

stridor A harsh, high-pitched respiratory sound, generally heard during inhalation, that is caused by partial blockage or narrowing of the upper airway.

suctioning Aspirating (sucking out) fluid in the mouth or airway by mechanical means.

trachea The windpipe.

ventilation The physical act of moving air into and out of the lungs; also called pulmonary ventilation.

References

Al-Halawani R, Charlton PH, Qassem M, Kyriacou PA. A review of the effect of skin pigmentation on pulse oximeter accuracy. *Physiol Meas.* 2023;44(5):05TR01. doi:10.1088/1361-6579/acd51a

Heart disease facts. Centers for Disease Control and Prevention website. https://www.cdc.gov/heart-disease/data-research/facts-stats/index.html. Published October 24, 2024. Accessed November 27, 2024.

Yeganehkhah M, Dadkhahtehrani T, Bagheri A, Kachoie A. Effect of glittered nail polish on pulse oximetry measurements in healthy subjects. *Iran J Nurs Midwifery Res.* 2019;24(1):25–29.

Yek JLJ, Abdullah HR, Goh JPS, Chan YW. The effects of gel-based manicure on pulse oximetry. *Singapore Med J.* 2019;60(8):432–435.

Assessment IN ACTION

You are dispatched to a local park for a report of a woman who ran into a tree while roller skating. She was wearing a helmet. You can see she is bleeding heavily from a laceration on her knee. She is unresponsive. A friend skating with her says she tried to rouse the woman but was unable.

1. Your first step in assessing this patient should be to:
   A. shake her shoulder.
   B. check her pulse.
   C. check for breathing.
   D. establish her level of responsiveness.
2. If you are unable to get oxygen into the patient with your first attempt, what should be your next step?
   A. Log roll her onto her side.
   B. Attempt the jaw-thrust maneuver again and try to ventilate.
   C. Give a bigger rescue breath.
   D. Give abdominal thrusts.
3. From what you have learned about the respiratory system, what is the normal breathing rate for an adult?
   A. 4 to 10 breaths/min
   B. 12 to 20 breaths/min
   C. 22 to 30 breaths/min
   D. 31 to 50 breaths/min
4. The woman starts to vomit. You need to place her on her side to ensure she does not choke. How should you do that?
   A. Grab her arms and pull her over.
   B. Log roll her onto her side while making sure her head, neck, and spine are aligned.
   C. Turn her head to the side.
   D. Lift her to a semireclining position and start suctioning.
5. Supplemental oxygen is kept in cylinders and stored at 2,000 psi. Which device reduces the pressure for emergency use in the field?
   A. Gas gauge
   B. Nasopharynx airway
   C. Pressure regulator/flowmeter
   D. Nasal cannula
6. How do you open the airway in a patient who has sustained significant trauma?
7. The woman is breathing at a rate of 3 to 4 breaths/min. What should you do next?
8. Which parts of the body are used in breathing?
9. The recovery position is used for:
   A. patients who need an open airway while rescue breathing is performed.
   B. patients who are breathing but unresponsive.
   C. patients who are not breathing at least 10 to 12 times per minute.
   D. patients who require simultaneous chest compressions and airway suctioning.
10. What is a stoma?

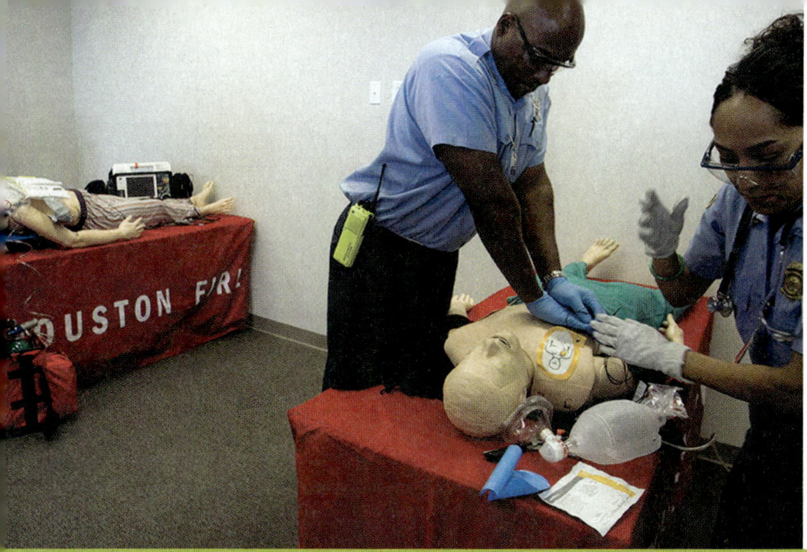

CHAPTER 8

Professional Rescuer CPR

National EMS Education Standard Competencies

Shock and Resuscitation

Uses assessment information to recognize shock, respiratory failure or arrest, and cardiac arrest based on assessment findings and manages the emergency while awaiting additional emergency response.

Resuscitation From Cardiac Arrest

- Ethical issues in resuscitation (pp 154–156)
- CPR physiology (pp 155–156)
- CPR system components (pp 156–164)
- Special arrest and peri-arrest situations (pp 158–170)

Assessment

Uses scene information and patient assessment findings to identify and manage immediate life threats and injuries within the scope of practice of the EMR.

Primary Assessment

- Primary assessment (pp 168–170)
- Begin interventions needed to preserve life (pp 164–170)

Anatomy and Physiology

Uses knowledge of the anatomy and function of the upper airway, heart, vessels, blood, lungs, skin, muscles, and bones as the foundation of emergency care.

Pathophysiology

Uses knowledge of shock and respiratory compromise to respond to life threats.

Knowledge Objectives

1. Describe the anatomy and function of the circulatory system. (pp 152–154)
2. Describe some of the causes of cardiac arrest. (p 154)
3. Describe the components of cardiopulmonary resuscitation (CPR). (pp 154–155)
4. List the six links in the cardiac chain of survival. (p 155)
5. Describe the conditions under which emergency medical responders (EMRs) should start and stop CPR. (pp 155–156)
6. Describe how to perform chest compressions on the following patients:
   - Adults (pp 156–157)
   - Infants (pp 157–158)
   - Children (p 158)
7. Explain the steps in performing one-rescuer adult CPR. (pp 158–159)
8. Explain the steps in performing two-rescuer adult CPR. (pp 159–160)
9. Describe how to switch rescuer positions during two-rescuer adult CPR. (pp 160–162)
10. Explain the steps in performing one-rescuer infant CPR. (p 162)
11. Explain the steps in performing two-rescuer infant CPR. (pp 162–163)
12. Explain the steps of child CPR. (pp 163–164)
13. List the four signs of effective CPR. (p 164)
14. Describe the complications of performing CPR. (p 164)
15. Explain the importance of creating sufficient space to perform CPR. (p 166)
16. Describe the indications for the use of automated external defibrillation by EMRs. (p 166)
17. Explain the steps in performing automated external defibrillation. (pp 168–170)
18. Explain the importance of CPR training. (p 170)
19. Discuss the legal implications of performing CPR. (p 170)

Skills Objectives

1. Demonstrate chest compressions on an adult. (pp 156–158; Skill Drill 8-1)
2. Demonstrate chest compressions on an infant. (pp 157–158)
3. Demonstrate chest compressions on a child. (p 158)

© Brett Coomer/Houston Chronicle/Hearst Newspapers/Getty Images

4. Demonstrate one-rescuer adult CPR. (pp 158–159; Skill Drill 8-2)
5. Demonstrate two-rescuer adult CPR. (pp 159–161; Skill Drill 8-3)
6. Demonstrate how to switch rescuer positions during two-rescuer adult CPR. (p 162)
7. Demonstrate one-rescuer infant CPR. (p 162)
8. Demonstrate two-rescuer infant CPR. (p 163)
9. Demonstrate child CPR. (pp 163–164)
10. Demonstrate creating sufficient space to perform CPR. (p 166)
11. Demonstrate automated external defibrillation. (pp 166–169; Skill Drill 8-4)

Introduction

Cardiopulmonary resuscitation (CPR) consists of three major sets of skills: the *C* (circulation) skills, the *A* (airway) skills, and the *B* (breathing) skills. Airway and breathing procedures may be lifesaving for a patient who has stopped breathing and whose heart is still beating. In most cases, however, by the time you arrive on the scene, the patient has not only stopped breathing, but the heart has stopped beating as well. If the patient has no heartbeat and is not breathing or only gasping, rescue breathing alone will not save the patient's life. Forcing air into the lungs is useless unless the circulatory system can carry the oxygen in the lungs to all parts of the body. Chapter 7, *Airway Management*, discusses the airway and breathing skills.

If the patient's heart has stopped, you can maintain or restore circulation manually via **chest compressions**. According to recent studies, it is important to restore circulation before starting rescue breathing. Therefore, in this chapter, you will learn to perform the circulation skills before you perform the airway and breathing skills (a CAB sequence). To maintain both a heartbeat and **ventilation**, chest compressions and rescue breathing must be done together. By combining the circulation, airway, and breathing skills, you will be able to perform CPR. Statistics show that approximately 70% of patients who experience cardiac arrest are in a state of ventricular fibrillation, a condition in which the heart muscle is quivering and not effectively pumping blood. Therefore, this chapter covers the theory and the steps you need to learn to use an automated external defibrillator (AED) to defibrillate these patients.

Anatomy and Function of the Circulatory System

The **circulatory system** consists of a pump (the heart), a network of pipes (the blood vessels), and fluid (blood). After blood picks up oxygen in the lungs, it travels to the heart, which, in turn, pumps the oxygenated blood to the rest of the body.

The heart, which is about the size of your fist, is located in the chest between the lungs. The cells of the body absorb oxygen and nutrients (including glucose) from the blood and produce waste products (including carbon dioxide) that the blood carries back to the lungs. In the lungs, the blood exchanges the carbon dioxide for more oxygen. Blood then returns to the heart to be pumped out again. Other metabolic waste products are removed by the kidneys and liver.

The human heart consists of four chambers, two on the right side of the heart and two on the left side. Each upper chamber is called an atrium. The right atrium receives blood from the veins of the body; the left atrium receives highly oxygenated blood from the lungs. The bottom chambers are known as the ventricles. The right ventricle pumps deoxygenated blood to the lungs; the left ventricle pumps highly oxygenated blood to the heart muscle and throughout the body. The most muscular chamber of the heart is the left ventricle, which needs the most power because it must force blood to all parts of the body. The four chambers of the heart work together in a well-ordered sequence to pump blood to the lungs and to the rest of the body (**FIGURE 8-1**).

One-way valves in the heart and veins allow the blood to flow in only one direction through the circulatory system. The arteries carry blood away from the heart at high pressure; therefore, the walls of arteries are thick. The main artery carrying blood away from the heart, the aorta, is quite large (approximately 1 inch [2.5 cm] in diameter), but arteries become smaller in diameter farther away from the heart. These smaller arteries eventually branch into the capillaries, the smallest pipes in the circulatory system. Some capillaries are so small that only one blood cell at a time can go through them. At the capillary level, oxygen passes from the blood cells into the cells of body tissues, and carbon dioxide and other waste products pass from the tissue cells to the blood cells, which then return to the lungs. Veins are the thin-walled pipes of the circulatory system that carry blood back to the heart.

The four major artery locations are as follows: the neck (carotid arteries); the wrist (radial arteries); the arm (brachial arteries); and the groin (femoral arteries). The locations of these arteries are shown in **FIGURE 8-2**. Because these arteries lie between a bony structure and the skin, you can use them to palpate the patient's **pulse**. A pulse is generated when the heart contracts and sends a pressure wave through the artery. The **carotid pulse** is assessed on either side of the neck, the **radial pulse** is assessed at the thumb side of the

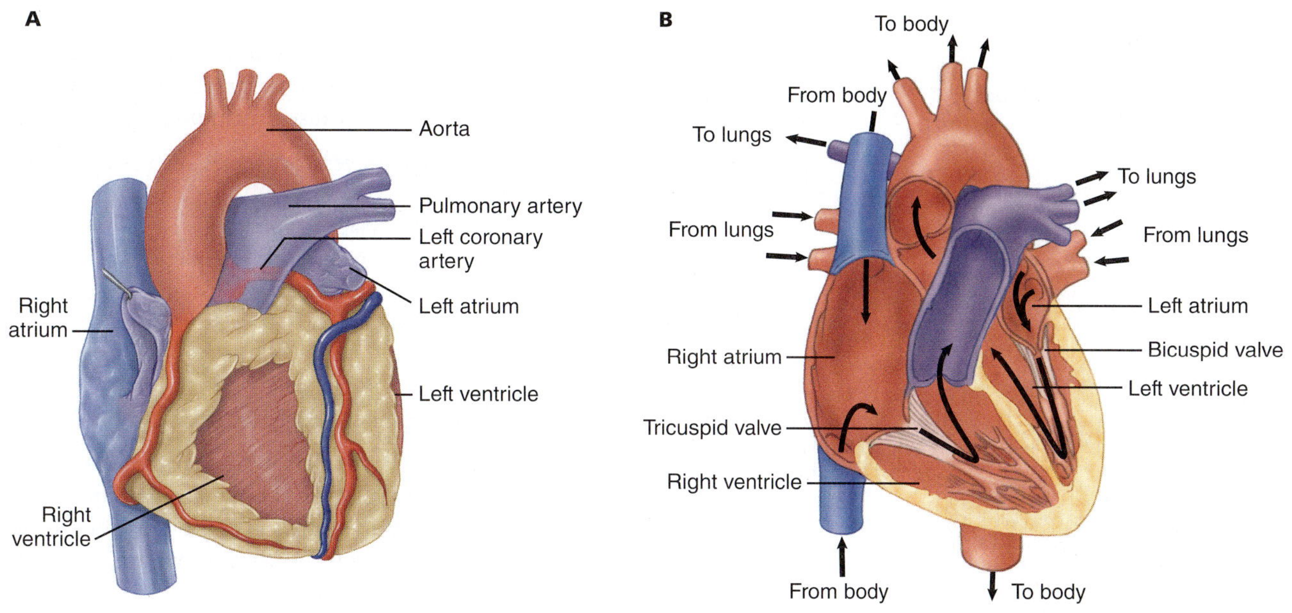

FIGURE 8-1 The heart functions as the pump of the human circulatory system. **A.** External view. **B.** Cross-sectional view.
© Jones & Bartlett Learning

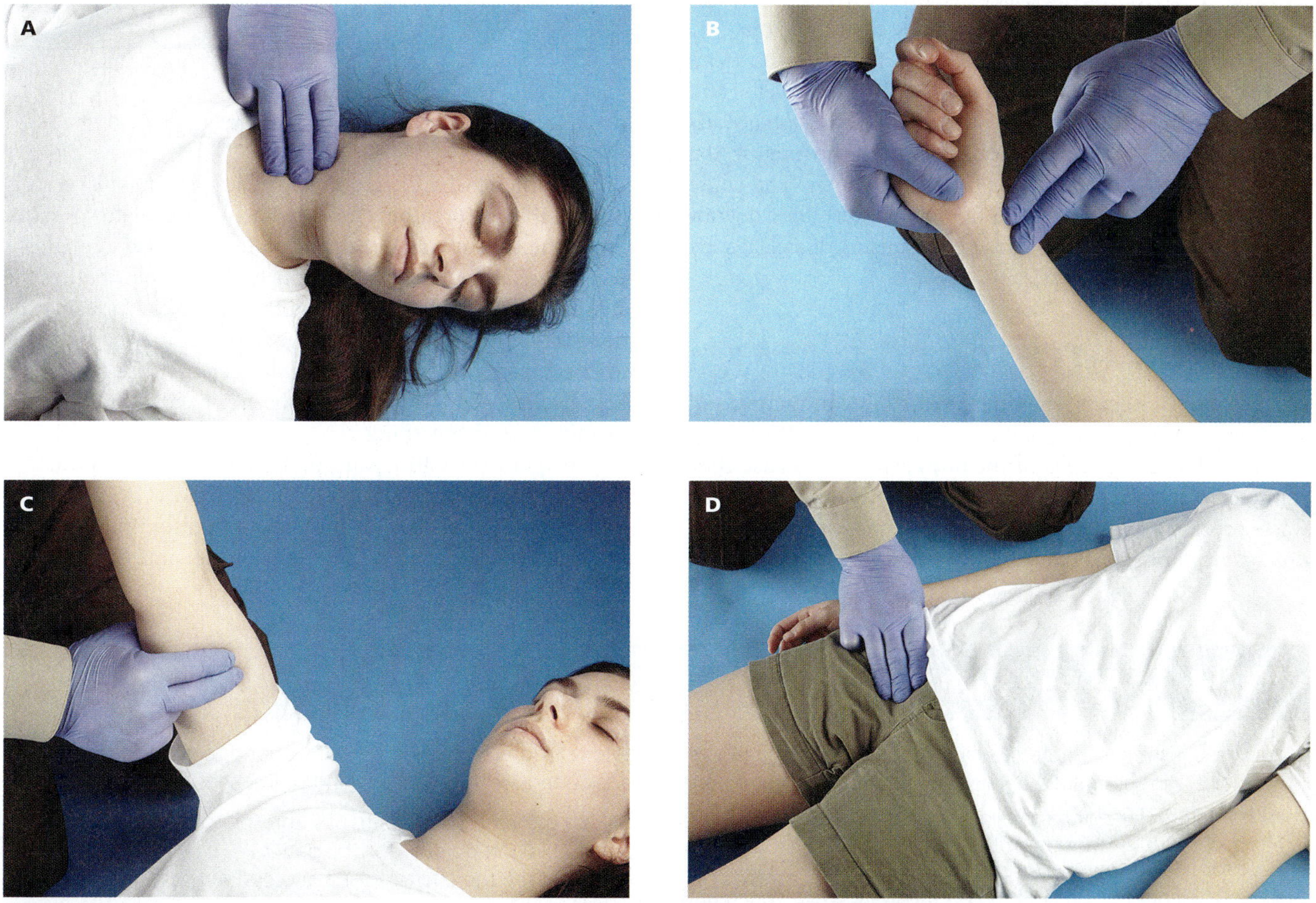

FIGURE 8-2 Locations for assessing the patient's pulse. **A.** Neck (carotid pulse). **B.** Wrist (radial pulse). **C.** Arm (brachial pulse). **D.** Groin (femoral pulse).
© Jones & Bartlett Learning

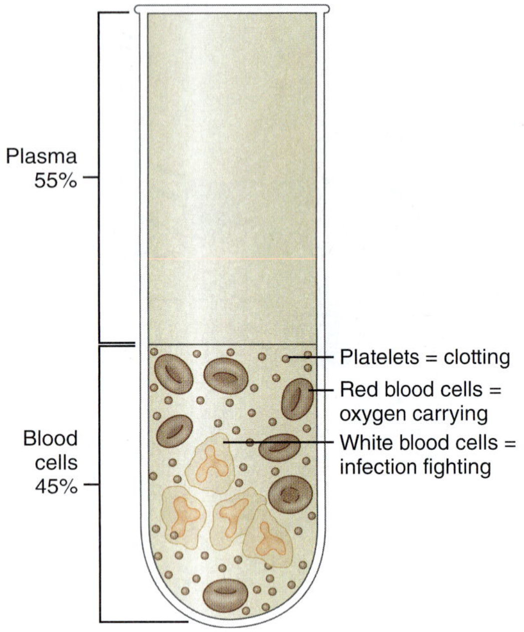

FIGURE 8-3 The components of blood.
© Jones & Bartlett Learning

wrist, the **brachial pulse** is assessed on the inside of the upper arm, and the **femoral pulse** is assessed at the groin.

Blood has several components: **plasma** (a clear, straw-colored fluid), red blood cells, white blood cells, and **platelets** (**FIGURE 8-3**). The red blood cells give blood its red color. Red blood cells carry oxygen from the lungs to the body and bring carbon dioxide back to the lungs. The white blood cells are called infection fighters because they devour bacteria and other disease-causing organisms. Platelets start the blood-clotting process.

Cardiac Arrest

Cardiac arrest occurs when the heart stops contracting and no blood is pumped through the blood vessels. Without a supply of blood, the cells of the body will die because they cannot get any oxygen or nutrients and they cannot eliminate waste products. As the cells die, organ damage occurs. Some organs are more sensitive to low oxygen levels than others. Brain damage begins within 4 to 6 minutes after the patient has gone into cardiac arrest. Within 8 to 10 minutes, the damage to the brain may become irreversible. Cardiac arrest may have many different causes, including the following:

- Heart and blood vessel diseases such as heart attack and stroke
- Respiratory arrest, if untreated
- Medical emergencies such as epilepsy, diabetes, allergic reactions, electric shock, and poisoning
- Drug overdose
- Drowning
- Suffocation
- Trauma and shock caused by massive blood loss

A patient who has experienced cardiac arrest is unresponsive, is not breathing or is only gasping, and does not have a detectable pulse. Regardless of the cause of cardiac arrest, the initial treatment is the same: provide CPR.

Words of Wisdom

Certain physiologic and lifestyle factors can increase the chance that a person will experience a heart attack. These factors include high blood pressure, uncontrolled diabetes, obesity, high blood cholesterol or lipids, and high stress. These factors can affect your patients, but they can also affect you. Developing and maintaining a healthy lifestyle will be beneficial in reducing your chance of experiencing a heart attack.

Components of CPR

The technique of CPR requires three types of skills: *A* (airway) skills, *B* (breathing) skills, and *C* (circulation) skills. From the airway and breathing skills discussed previously, you learned how to check patients to determine whether the airway is open and to correct a blocked airway by using the head tilt–chin lift or jaw-thrust maneuver. You learned how to check patients to determine whether they are breathing. You also learned to correct the absence of breathing by performing rescue breathing.

To perform CPR, you combine the *A* (airway) and *B* (breathing) skills with *C* (circulation) skills in a CAB sequence. You begin by checking for the patient's pulse. With practice, you will be able to check for a pulse at the same time you are

YOU are the EMR — CASE 1

You have just finished the morning report. You and your partner are in the middle of checking your equipment when you are dispatched for a report of a sick woman. As you arrive at the residence, you are met by the patient's husband. He informs you that his wife has been reporting indigestion since 0430 hours. She is sitting on the living room couch and has taken several antacids without relief. As you begin to question the woman, she suddenly stops breathing and her head falls forward. She does not respond to your questions, to shouting, or to gentle shaking of her shoulder.

1. On the basis of the patient's unresponsiveness, what should you do now for the patient?
2. What are the chances for a successful resuscitation on this call?
3. What role does your AED play in this call?

checking for signs of breathing. To reduce the time it takes to begin treating the patient, the pulse check should not last more than 10 seconds (but no less than 5 seconds). If the patient has no pulse, you must restore the patient's circulation by starting chest compressions. Airway and breathing techniques will then be used to push oxygen into the patient's lungs. Chest compressions move the oxygenated blood throughout the body. By compressing the patient's sternum (breastbone), you change the pressure in the patient's chest and force enough blood through the system to sustain life for a short time.

CPR by itself cannot sustain life indefinitely. However, once it is recognized that the patient is pulseless and is not breathing or only gasping, start CPR as soon as possible to give the patient the best chance for survival. By performing all three parts of the CPR sequence, you can keep the patient alive until an AED is available and more advanced medical care can be delivered. In many cases, the patient will need defibrillation and medication to be successfully resuscitated from cardiac arrest.

Street Smarts

Patients who are experiencing cardiac events, as well as their family members and friends, will usually be fearful and anxious about the episode. It is important for you to demonstrate a caring attitude and to acknowledge those feelings. Although your primary goal is to ensure that the patient receives appropriate and timely care, you should understand that compassion is an important part of your care for patients experiencing a cardiac event.

The Cardiac Chain of Survival

In most cases of cardiac arrest, CPR alone is not enough to save lives, but it is the first treatment in the out-of-hospital chain of survival presented by the American Heart Association (AHA). The cardiac chain of survival includes the following six links (**FIGURE 8-4**):

1. Recognition of cardiac arrest and activation of the emergency response system
2. Immediate CPR with emphasis on high-quality chest compressions
3. Rapid defibrillation
4. Advanced resuscitation by emergency medical services (EMS) and other health care clinicians
5. Post–cardiac arrest care
6. Recovery and survivorship

As an emergency medical responder (EMR), you can help the patient by providing early CPR with an emphasis on high-quality chest compressions and by making sure the EMS system has been activated. Some EMRs are trained in the use of AEDs. By keeping these links of the chain strong, you will help keep the patient alive until early advanced life support (ALS) care can be administered by paramedics and hospital personnel. Just as an actual chain is only as strong as its weakest link, the chain of survival is only as good as its weakest link. Your actions in performing early CPR are vital to giving patients in cardiac arrest their best chance for survival.

After cardiac arrest, survivors can have physical, cognitive, and emotional challenges and may need ongoing therapies and interventions. The AHA includes recovery and survivorship as the final link of the cardiac chain of survival to highlight the importance of caring for patients and their loved ones beyond the initial medical response. This step includes additional treatment, observation, rehabilitation, and psychological support.

Words of Wisdom

Patients with chest pain are often in denial as to the reason for their chest pain. Many people will try to deny that their pain could be caused by a cardiac event. They may tell you that they are experiencing indigestion or that they have a cold. This denial often results in long delays before the patient decides to call 9-1-1. Treat patients with chest pain as if their pain could be caused by a significant heart problem.

When to Start CPR

CPR should be started on all patients who are not breathing (or are only gasping) and pulseless, unless they are obviously dead or they have a do-not-resuscitate (DNR) order that is valid in your jurisdiction. (DNR orders are discussed more fully later in this chapter.) Few reliable criteria exist to determine death immediately.

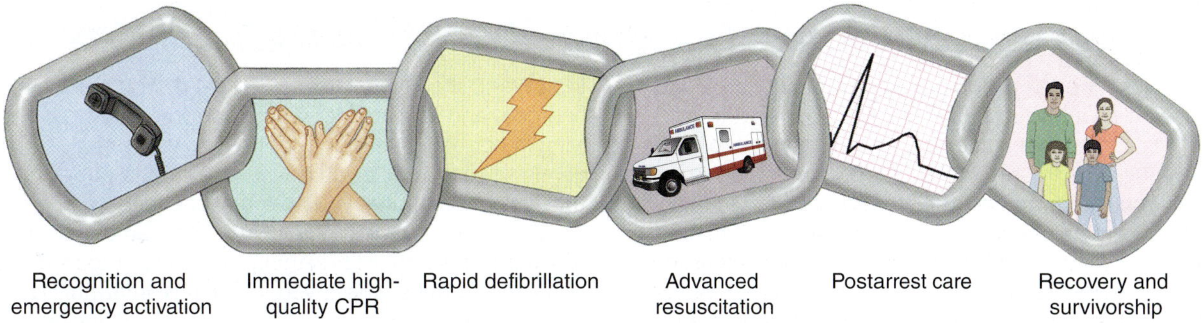

FIGURE 8-4 The six links of the cardiac chain of survival.

© Jones & Bartlett Learning. Courtesy of MIEMSS.

The following criteria are definitive signs of death and indicate that CPR should not be started:

1. **Decapitation.** Decapitation occurs when the head is separated from the rest of the body. When this occurs, there is obviously no chance of saving the patient.
2. **Rigor mortis.** This is the temporary stiffening of muscles that occurs several hours after death. Rigor mortis indicates the patient has been dead for a prolonged time and cannot be resuscitated.
3. **Evidence of tissue decomposition.** Tissue decomposition or actual flesh decay occurs only after a person has been dead for an extended time. It can occur sooner with hotter temperatures and depends on the initial condition of the patient.
4. **Dependent lividity.** Dependent lividity is the red or purple color that appears on the parts of the patient's body that are closest to the ground. It is caused by blood seeping into the tissues in the dependent, or lower, part of the person's body. Dependent lividity occurs after a person has been dead for several hours.

If any of the preceding signs of death are present in a pulseless, nonbreathing person, do not begin CPR. If none of these signs are present, you should activate the EMS system and then begin CPR. It is far better to start CPR on a person who is later declared dead by a physician than to withhold CPR from a patient whose life might have been saved.

When to Stop CPR

You should discontinue CPR only when:

1. Effective spontaneous circulation and ventilation are restored or the patient begins to move.
2. Resuscitation efforts are transferred to another person with an equal or higher level of training who continues CPR.
3. A physician orders you to stop.
4. The patient is transferred to properly trained EMS personnel.
5. Reliable criteria for death (as previously listed) are recognized.
6. You are too exhausted to continue resuscitation, environmental hazards endanger your safety, or continued resuscitation would place the lives of others at risk.

Cardiac Compression

Chest Compressions on an Adult

An adult patient in cardiac arrest is unresponsive, has no carotid pulse, and is not breathing or only gasping. If you suspect that the patient has experienced cardiac arrest, check the carotid pulse and observe breathing adequacy. To check the carotid pulse, place your index and middle finger on the larynx (Adam's apple); you may also include your ring finger. Slide your fingers into the groove between the larynx and the muscles at the side of the neck (see Figure 8-2A). Keep your fingers there for at least 5 seconds but no more than 10 seconds to be sure the pulse is absent and not just slow. At the same time, look for signs of chest movement and feel for air exchange.

If there is no carotid pulse in an unresponsive, nonbreathing patient, you must begin chest compressions. For chest compressions to be effective, the patient must be lying on a firm, horizontal surface. If the patient is on a soft surface, such as a bed, it is impossible to compress the chest. Immediately place all patients needing CPR on a firm, level surface.

Safety

Take standard precautions when performing CPR.

To position yourself so that you can perform chest compressions effectively, stand or kneel beside the patient's chest and face the patient. Place the heel of one hand in the center of the patient's chest, on the lower half of the sternum. Place the heel of your other hand on top of the hand that is on the chest and interlock your fingers (**SKILL DRILL 8-1**).

Treatment

Do not let your fingers touch the chest wall; your fingers could dig into the patient, causing injury. Interlocking your fingers will help to avoid this.

YOU are the EMR **CASE 2**

You have just finished your morning equipment check and are thinking about a cup of coffee when your alert tones break the calm of your station. You are dispatched to 2739 Bliss Avenue, Apartment 208, for a report of an unresponsive woman. You recognize the address, which is located in a retirement community for senior citizens. After a 7-minute response, you and your partner arrive at the address and are met by an excited woman. She tells you that she arrived a few minutes earlier to clean Mrs. Ward's apartment and let herself in with her key. When she was unable to awaken Mrs. Ward, she immediately called 9-1-1. You hurry into the bedroom and see an older woman dressed in nightclothes lying in her bed. She is unresponsive to your voice and to gentle shaking. While you check for a carotid pulse and look for signs of breathing, you note that she feels very cool to your touch. Neither you nor your partner can detect any signs of a pulse, gasping, or breathing. As you start to move her arm away from her chest, you realize it is amazingly stiff.

1. What are the next steps you should take?

SKILL DRILL 8-1

Performing Adult Chest Compressions

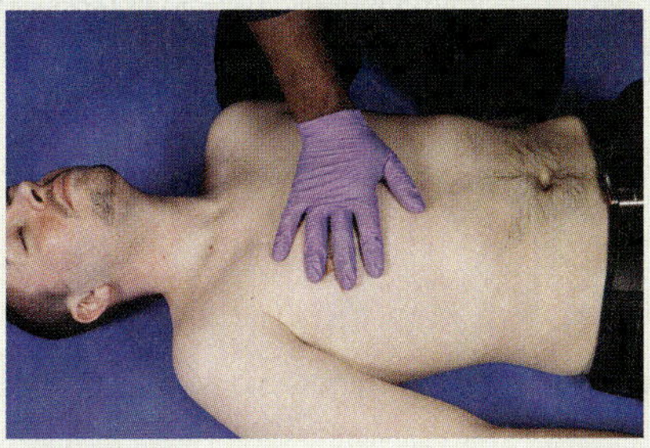

STEP 1 Locate the top and bottom of the sternum. Place the heel of your hand in the center of the chest, on the lower half of the sternum.

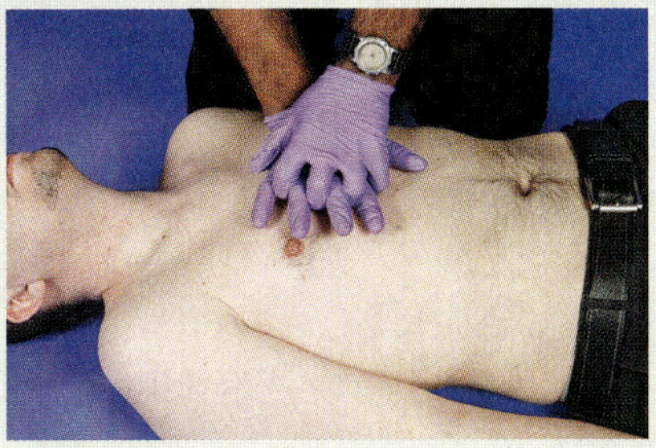

STEP 2 Place your other hand on top of your first hand and interlock your fingers. It is important to locate and maintain the proper hand position while applying chest compressions. If your hands are too high, the force you apply will not produce adequate chest compressions. If your hands are too low, the force you apply may damage the liver. If your hands slip sideways off the sternum and onto the ribs, the compressions will not be effective and you may damage the ribs and lungs.

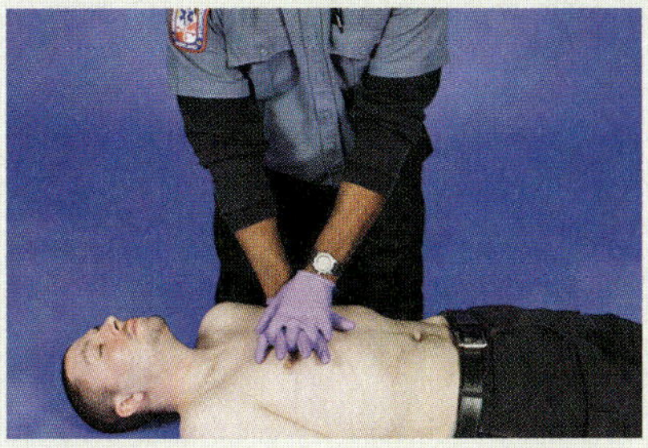

STEP 3 After you have both hands in the proper position, compress the chest of an adult at least 2 inches (5 cm) straight down. For compressions to be effective, stay close to the patient's side and lean forward so that your arms are directly over the patient. Keep your back straight and your elbows stiff so you can apply the force of your whole body to each compression, not just your arm muscles. Between compressions, make sure you completely release pressure on the chest to allow maximum filling of the patient's heart. Never lean on the chest during compressions. Compressions must be rhythmic and continuous.
Each compression cycle consists of one downward push followed by a rest so that the heart can refill with blood. Push hard and push fast. Compressions should be at the rate of 100 to 120 compressions per minute in all patients: adults, children, and infants. After every 30 chest compressions, give two rescue breaths (1 second per breath). Practice on a manikin until you can compress the chest smoothly and rhythmically.

© Jones & Bartlett Learning. Courtesy of MIEMSS.

Words of Wisdom

Hands-Only CPR

In 2012 the AHA adopted the approach of hands-only CPR (also called compression-only CPR). This successful campaign has helped save many lives. Hands-only CPR is a guideline created for the layperson who has not been trained in a comprehensive CPR course and who might hesitate to assist another person in cardiac arrest due to fear of performing mouth-to-mouth resuscitation. Two simple tasks are associated with hands-only CPR: (1) call 9-1-1, and (2) push hard and fast. As an EMR you should be aware of hands-only CPR, because when you arrive on scene you may encounter bystanders who have initiated this simplified version of CPR.

Chest Compressions on an Infant

An **infant** (a child younger than 1 year) who has experienced cardiac arrest will be unresponsive, not breathing or only gasping, and pulseless. To check for cardiac arrest, begin by checking responsiveness. If the infant is unresponsive, check the brachial pulse and look, listen, and feel for signs of breathing. If a pulse is absent and there are no signs of breathing, begin CPR starting with chest compressions.

To check an infant's circulation, feel for the brachial pulse on the inside of the upper arm (**FIGURE 8-5**). Use two fingers of one hand to feel for the pulse and use your other hand to maintain the head tilt. If the infant has no pulse and is not

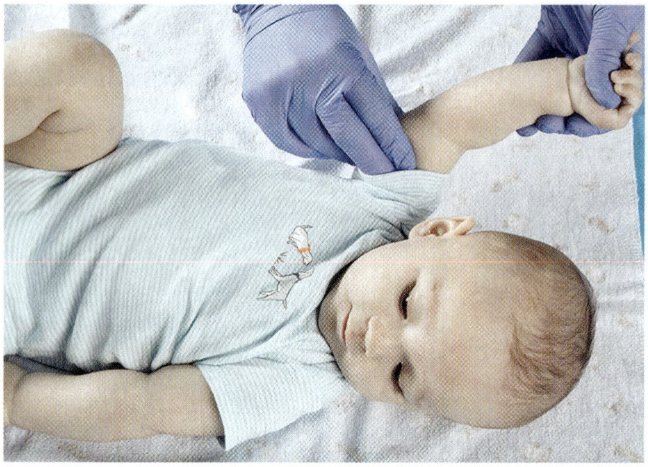

FIGURE 8-5 Check the brachial pulse on the inside of the infant's arm.
© Jones & Bartlett Learning

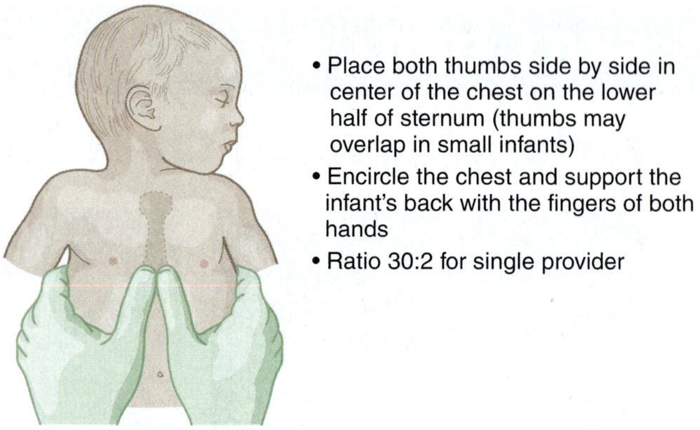

FIGURE 8-6 Performing infant chest compressions.
© Jones and Bartlett Learning

breathing or only gasping, begin CPR starting with chest compressions. When you perform chest compressions, place the infant on a solid surface such as a table or cradle the infant in your arm, as shown in **FIGURE 8-6**. You do not need to use much force to achieve adequate compressions on infants because they are so small and their chests are so flexible. Use the two-thumbs/encircling-hands technique to deliver chest compressions just below the nipple line on the lower half of the sternum, making sure to avoid the xiphoid process. Compress the sternum at least one-third the depth of the chest (approximately 1.5 inches [4 cm]). Compress the sternum at a rate of 100 to 120 times per minute. If you are the only rescuer, give two rescue breaths (1 second per breath) after every 30 chest compressions. If two rescuers are present, give two rescue breaths after every 15 chest compressions.

Special Populations

Circulatory Failure in Children

The most common cause of circulatory failure in children is respiratory failure. Uncorrected respiratory failure in children can lead to circulatory failure, and uncorrected circulatory failure can lead to cardiac arrest. Therefore, it is important for you to correct respiratory failure before it progresses to circulatory failure. Because this is not always possible, you should learn the signs of circulatory failure and its treatment. An increased heart rate, pallor or cyanosis, and changes in mental status indicate circulatory failure. If the child or infant's heart rate is more than 60 beats/min, your treatment should consist of completing the patient assessment sequence, supporting ventilations, administering oxygen if available, and observing vital signs for any changes. If the heart rate of a child or infant is less than 60 beats/min and there are signs of poor circulation, such as cyanosis, you should begin chest compressions and rescue breathing.

Chest Compressions on a Child

The signs of cardiac arrest in a **child** (from age 1 year to the onset of puberty [age 12 to 14 years]) are the same as those for an adult. Determine if the child is responsive. If the child is unresponsive, simultaneously check for a heartbeat at the carotid artery and for breathing. Check the carotid pulse in the same manner used for an adult. If there is no pulse and no breathing (or only gasping), the patient is in cardiac arrest and you need to begin chest compressions.

To perform chest compressions on a small child, place the heel of one hand in the center of the chest, on the lower half of the sternum. In larger children, perform chest compressions with two hands, as with the adult. Compress the sternum at least one-third the depth of the chest (approximately 2 inches [5 cm]). Compress the chest at a rate of at 100 to 120 times per minute. If you are the only rescuer present, give two rescue breaths after every 30 chest compressions. If two rescuers are present, give two rescue breaths after every 15 compressions.

Adult CPR

One-Rescuer Adult CPR

You learned previously how to open the airway and perform rescue breathing. Now that you have learned how to check for circulation and do chest compressions, you are ready to put all your skills together to perform CPR. If you are the only trained person at the scene, you must perform **one-rescuer CPR**. Follow the steps in **SKILL DRILL 8-2**.

Words of Wisdom

If you do not have a partner with you to help perform CPR, do not wait for another rescuer to arrive. Call 9-1-1 to activate EMS and then begin one-rescuer CPR immediately!

When performing one-rescuer CPR—whether the patient is an adult, child, or infant—deliver chest compressions and rescue breathing at a ratio of 30 compressions to two breaths. Immediately give two rescue breaths after each set of 30 chest compressions. Because you must interrupt chest compressions to ventilate, you should perform each series of 30 chest compressions in approximately 18 seconds (a rate of 100 to 120 compressions per minute).

SKILL DRILL 8-2

Performing One-Rescuer Adult CPR

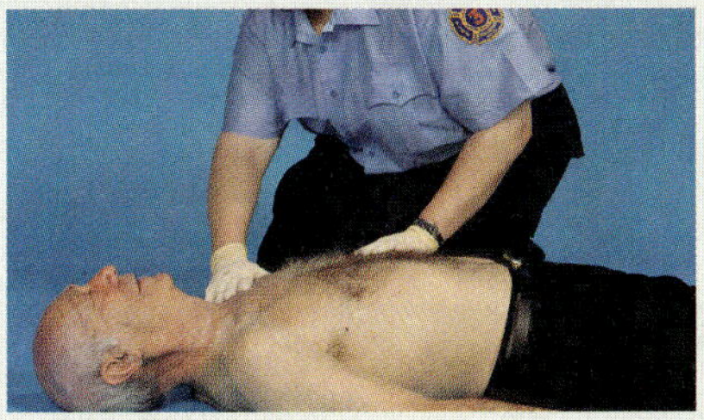

STEP 1 Determine responsiveness. Ask the patient, "Are you okay?" Gently shake the patient's shoulder. If you do not get a response, call for additional help, activate the EMS system, and send someone to get an AED if one is available.

Position the patient. The patient should be flat on their back on a firm, horizontal surface. Position yourself so that your knees are alongside the patient's chest.

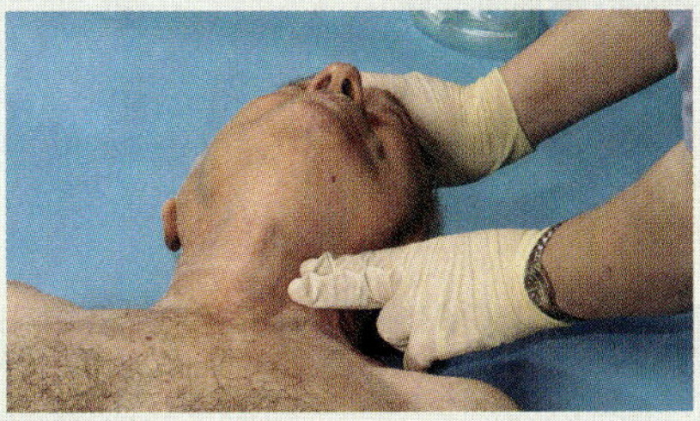

STEP 2 Assess circulation by checking for the presence of a carotid pulse and simultaneously observe breathing adequacy. This check should take no more than 10 seconds.

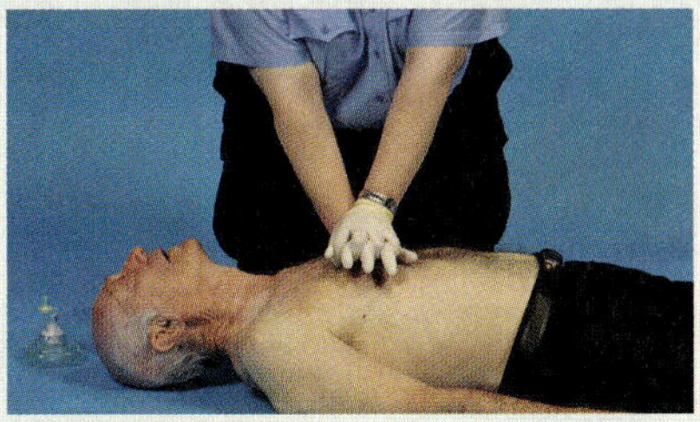

STEP 3 If the patient has no pulse and is not breathing or only gasping, begin chest compressions. Place the heel of one hand in the center of the chest, on the lower half of the sternum. Place your other hand on top of the first. Interlock your fingers and pull upward so that the only thing touching the patient's chest is the heel of your hand.

Lean forward so your shoulders are directly over your hands and the patient's sternum. Keep your arms straight and compress the sternum at least 2 inches (5 cm), using the weight of your body. Relax between compressions, allowing the chest to fully recoil. Give 30 compressions at a rate of 100 to 120 compressions per minute, and count each one out loud as follows: "One and two and three and . . ." Each set of 30 compressions should take between 15 and 18 seconds to complete.

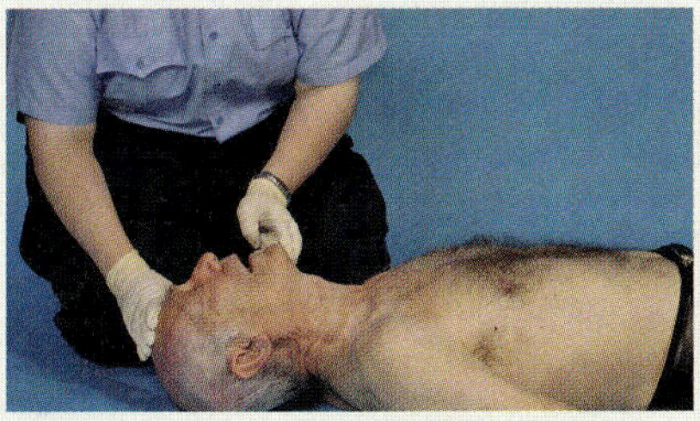

STEP 4 After 30 chest compressions, open the airway using a head tilt–chin lift maneuver or, if you suspect a head or spinal injury, a jaw-thrust maneuver.

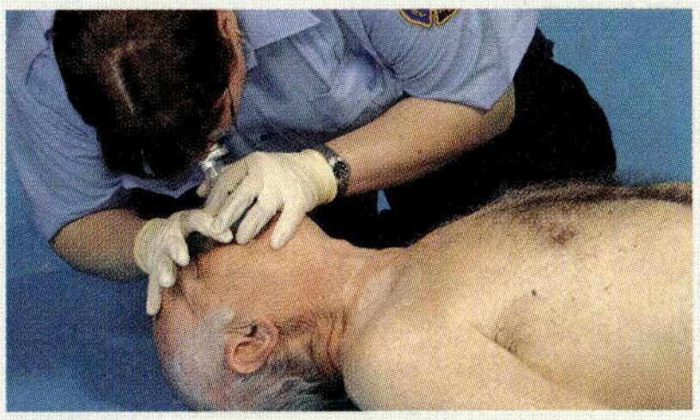

STEP 5 Give two rescue breaths (1 second each). Ensure that each breath produces visible chest rise. Continue cycles of 30 compressions and two rescue breaths until an AED arrives, patient care is assumed by other clinicians, or the patient starts to move.

© Jones & Bartlett Learning. Courtesy of MIEMSS.

A skill performance sheet titled One-Rescuer Adult CPR is shown in **FIGURE 8-7** for your review and practice.

Although one-rescuer CPR can keep the patient alive, two-rescuer CPR is preferable because it is less exhausting for the rescuers. Whenever possible, CPR for an adult should be performed by two rescuers.

Two-Rescuer Adult CPR

In many cases, a second, trained person will be on the scene to help you perform CPR. Two-rescuer CPR is more effective than one-rescuer CPR. One rescuer delivers chest compressions while the other performs rescue breathing. Chest compressions and ventilations can be given more regularly and without interruption. However, to avoid rescuer fatigue, which may result in less effective chest compressions, the two rescuers should switch roles after every five cycles of CPR (approximately every 2 minutes). Two rescuers should be able to switch roles quickly, interrupting CPR for 5 seconds or less. In any circumstance, CPR should not be interrupted for longer than 10 seconds.

In **two-rescuer CPR**, one rescuer delivers ventilations (mouth-to-mouth rescue breathing, bag-mask device, or mouth-to-mask breathing) and the other gives chest compressions. If possible, position yourselves on opposite sides of the patient: one rescuer near the head and the other near the chest. When working with multiple responders on a cardiac arrest victim, the responders must approach patient care as a team. It is crucial that team members communicate who will switch and who will perform the next task. Often, the patient's family or friends are watching what is happening; assigning a team member to explain what is occurring and what the team is doing to treat the patient has proven to be a benefit to the patient's loved ones in the healing process if there is not a successful outcome. The sequence of steps is the same as for one-rescuer CPR, but the tasks are divided (**SKILL DRILL 8-3**).

Words of Wisdom

When you have a patient who is in cardiac arrest, always be prepared for vomiting. It is a frequent event, and your preparation for it can be lifesaving.

Compressions and ventilations should remain rhythmic and uninterrupted. By counting out loud, rescuer 2 can continue to deliver compressions at the rate of 100 to 120 compressions per minute, briefly pausing as rescuer 1 delivers two rescue breaths. Once you and your partner establish a smooth pattern of CPR, you should limit interruptions in CPR to 10 seconds or less, such as when reassessing or moving the patient. A skill performance sheet titled Two-Rescuer Adult CPR is shown in **FIGURE 8-8** for your review and practice.

One-Rescuer Adult CPR	
Steps	**Adequately Performed**
1. Determine responsiveness by shouting and gently shaking the patient. If unresponsive and not breathing, activate the EMS system.	
2. Check for signs of circulation and breathing at the same time by checking the carotid pulse and watching for chest rise (within 10 seconds).	
3. If the patient has no pulse and is not breathing or only gasping, give cycles of 30 chest compressions at a rate of 100 to 120 compressions per minute.	
4. Open the airway using the head tilt–chin lift maneuver. (If trauma is present or you suspect a head or spinal injury, use the jaw-thrust maneuver.)	
5. Give two slow breaths (1 second per breath). If the chest does not rise, reposition the head and try to ventilate again. Watch for chest rise; allow for exhalation between breaths.	
6. Continue cycles of 30 chest compressions and two breaths until additional personnel arrive, an AED arrives, or the patient starts to move.	

FIGURE 8-7 Skill performance sheet: One-Rescuer Adult CPR.
© Jones & Bartlett Learning

SKILL DRILL 8-3

Performing Two-Rescuer Adult CPR

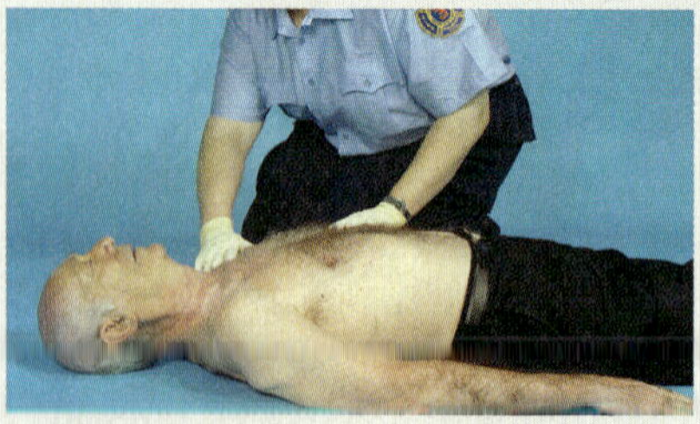

STEP 1 Rescuer 1 determines responsiveness. Rescuer 2 moves to the patient's side to be ready to deliver chest compressions. Rescuer 1 activates the EMS system.

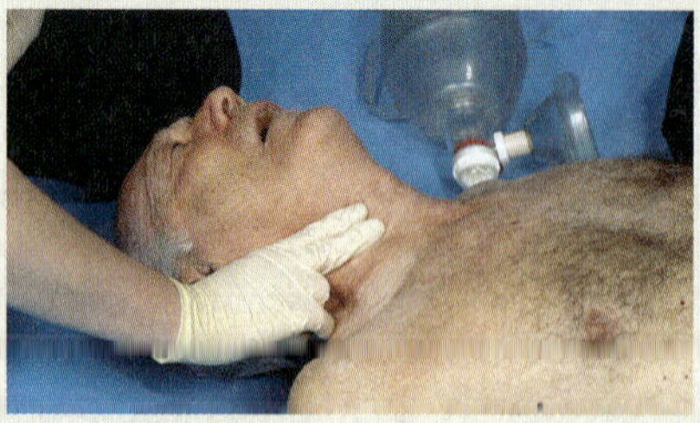

STEP 2 If the patient is unresponsive, rescuer 1 assesses circulation by checking for the presence of a carotid pulse and simultaneously observes breathing adequacy by watching for chest rise. This check should take no more than 10 seconds. If the patient has no pulse and is not breathing or only gasping, continue to step 3.

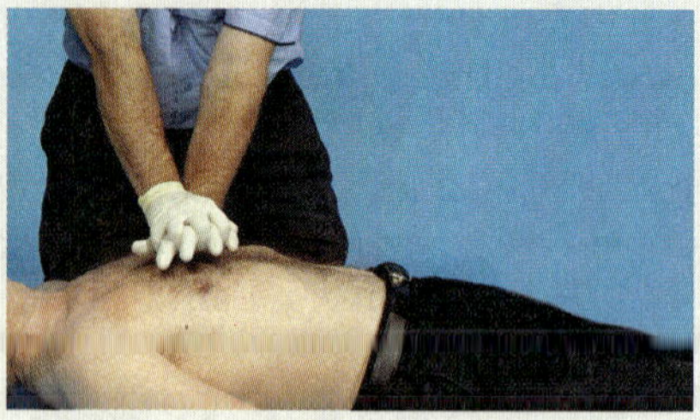

STEP 3 The rescuers begin CPR, starting with chest compressions. Rescuer 2 performs 30 chest compressions at a rate of 100 to 120 compressions per minute.

SKILL DRILL 8-3 *(continued)*

Performing Two-Rescuer Adult CPR

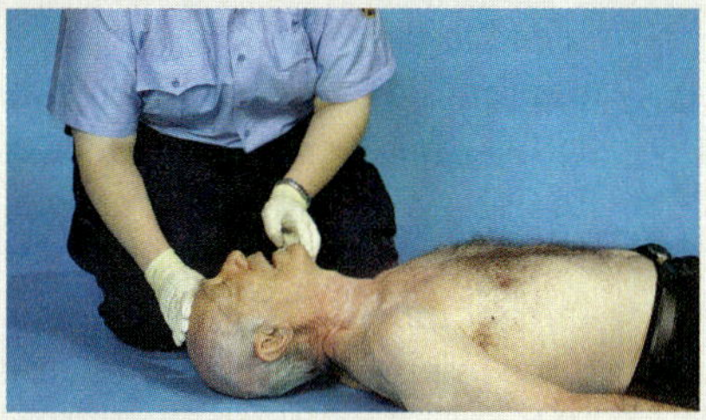

STEP 4 Rescuer 1 opens the airway with a head tilt–chin lift maneuver or, in the case of trauma or a suspected head or spinal injury, a jaw-thrust maneuver.

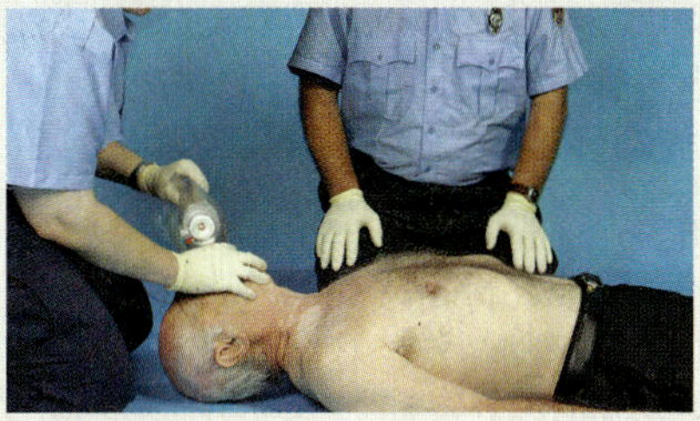

STEP 5 Rescuer 1 gives two ventilations of 1 second each and observes for visible chest rise.

The rescuers continue CPR for five cycles of 30 compressions and two ventilations (approximately 2 minutes). After 2 minutes of CPR, the rescuers switch positions. The switch time should take no longer than 5 seconds. Cycles of 30 chest compressions and two ventilations continue until an AED arrives, ALS personnel take over, or the patient starts to move.

© Jones & Bartlett Learning. Courtesy of MIEMSS.

Two-Rescuer Adult CPR	
Steps	**Adequately Performed**
1. Rescuer 1 checks for responsiveness by shouting and gently shaking the patient's shoulder.	
2. If the patient is unresponsive, rescuer 1 simultaneously checks the carotid pulse and looks for signs of no breathing or only gasping (within 10 seconds). Activate the EMS system.	
3. If the patient has no pulse and is not breathing or only gasping, rescuer 1 instructs rescuer 2 to begin compressions.	
4. Rescuer 2 begins chest compressions at the rate of 100 to 120 compressions per minute.	
5. After 30 compressions, rescuer 1 opens the airway and gives two rescue breaths.	
6. The rescuers continue for five cycles of CPR.	
7. After five cycles of CPR are completed, the rescuers switch positions. Rescuer 1 begins compressions and rescuer 2 takes over rescue breathing.	
8. As soon as an AED is available it is placed in operation.	
9. Continue cycles of CPR until the patient moves or other rescuers arrive to take over the care of the patient.	

FIGURE 8-8 Skill performance sheet: Two-Rescuer Adult CPR.

© Jones & Bartlett Learning

Switching Positions During CPR

If you and your partner must continue to perform two-rescuer CPR for any length of time, the rescuer performing chest compressions will become tired. Once a rescuer gets tired, the effectiveness of chest compressions decreases. Therefore, rescuers should switch positions after every five cycles of CPR (approximately every 2 minutes). This will improve the quality of chest compressions and give the patient the best chance for survival.

A switch allows the person giving compressions (rescuer 2) to rest their arms. Switching positions should be accomplished as smoothly and quickly (5 seconds or less) as possible to minimize the break in rate and regularity of compressions and ventilations. There are many orderly ways to switch positions. Learn the method practiced in your EMS system. One method is as follows:

1. Rescuer 2 says the following out loud (instead of counting): "We—will—switch—this—time." One word is spoken as each compression is done. These words replace the counting sequence for the first five compressions.
2. After 25 more chest compressions (a total of 30 compressions), rescuer 1 completes two ventilations and moves to the chest to perform compressions.
3. Rescuer 2 moves to the head of the patient to maintain the airway and ventilation.
4. Rescuer 1 then begins chest compressions.

Practice switching positions until you can do it smoothly and quickly. Switching positions is much easier if the rescuers work on opposite sides of the patient.

Street Smarts

Smartphones can be used in a voice-activated manner and allow rescuers to call 9-1-1 while using their hands to assess the patient. For example, people whose phones use the iOS system can simply call out, "Siri! Call 9-1-1." They can then speak with the dispatcher while performing chest compressions or maintaining an open airway.

Infant CPR

One-Rescuer Infant CPR

The principles of CPR are the same for adults and infants. In actual practice, however, you must use slightly different techniques for an infant. Follow these steps for one-rescuer infant CPR:

1. Position the infant faceup on a firm, flat surface.
2. Determine the infant's level of responsiveness. An unresponsive infant is limp. Gently shake or tap the infant to determine the level of responsiveness. If unresponsive, call for additional help and activate the EMS system.
3. If the infant is unresponsive, simultaneously assess circulation by checking the brachial pulse and observe breathing adequacy. The brachial pulse is on the inside of the arm. You can feel it by placing your index and middle fingers on the inside of the infant's arm, halfway between the shoulder and the elbow. Check for at least 5 seconds but no more than 10 seconds. Assess for breathing by looking at the infant's chest and abdomen.
4. If the infant has no pulse or a pulse of less than 60 beats/min with signs of poor circulation and is not breathing or only gasping, begin chest compressions. An infant's heart is located relatively higher in the chest than an adult's heart. Imagine a horizontal line drawn between the infant's nipples. Use the two-thumbs/encircling-hands technique for chest compressions (**FIGURE 8-9**). This technique is done by placing both thumbs side by side over the lower half of the infant's sternum and encircling the infant's chest with your hands.
5. With your thumbs in the correct location, compress the chest 30 times with the pads of your fingertips/thumbs. Compress the chest at least one-third the depth of the chest (approximately 1.5 inches [4 cm]) at a rate of 100 to 120 compressions per minute.
6. Open the infant's airway. This step is best done by the head tilt–chin lift maneuver. Gently tilt the infant's head to a neutral or slight sniffing position. Tilting it too far can obstruct the airway.
7. Give two breaths, each lasting 1 second. To breathe for an infant, place your mouth over the infant's mouth and nose. Because an infant has very small lungs, you should give only very small puffs of air, just enough

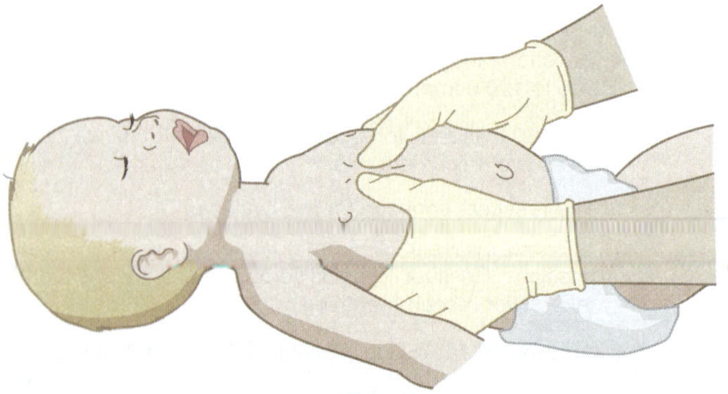

FIGURE 8-9 To perform chest compressions on an infant, use the two-thumbs/encircling-hands technique.
© Jones & Bartlett Learning

One-Rescuer Infant CPR	
Steps	**Adequately Performed**
1. Determine responsiveness by shouting and gently shaking the infant.	
2. If unresponsive, simultaneously check the brachial pulse and look for movement of the chest and stomach for signs or breathing. Call for help if anyone else is around or if you have a mobile phone.	
3. If there is no pulse or the pulse is less than 60 beats per minute with signs of poor circulation and no signs of breathing, begin chest compressions. Give 30 chest compressions by using two thumbs in the middle of the chest just below the nipple line. Maintain a rate of 100 to 120 compressions per minute. Compress the chest 1.5 inches (4 cm).	
4. Use the head tilt–chin lift maneuver to open the airway to a neutral or slight sniffing position. (If trauma is present, use the jaw-thrust maneuver.)	
5. Give two slow breaths (1 second per breath). If the chest does not rise, reposition the head and try to ventilate again. Watch for chest rise; allow for exhalation between breaths.	
6. Continue cycles of 30 chest compressions and two rescue breaths until the infant moves or until other EMS providers arrive to take over the care of the patient. If you are by yourself with no communications device, perform 2 minutes of CPR before leaving the victim to activate the EMS system.	

FIGURE 8-10 Skill performance sheet: One-Rescuer Infant CPR.
© Jones & Bartlett Learning

to make the chest rise. Do not use large or forceful breaths.

8. Continue compressions and ventilations. If you are alone, give 30 compressions and two breaths. Continue to give 30 compressions followed by two rescue breaths until other clinicians arrive to take over care or the infant begins to move.

Words of Wisdom

Due to the size of an infant's head, you may need to place a folded towel or other padding underneath the shoulders to maintain an open airway. Otherwise, the large occipital region (the back of the head) will force the head forward and close off the airway.

A skill performance sheet titled One-Rescuer Infant CPR is shown in **FIGURE 8-10** for your review and practice.

Two-Rescuer Infant CPR

If you are performing two-rescuer infant CPR, one clinician provides compressions as the other manages ventilations (**FIGURE 8-11**). This technique is done by placing both thumbs side by side over the lower half of the infant's sternum and encircling the infant's chest with your hands. Compress the sternum at a rate of 100 to 120 compressions per minute. When you are performing two-rescuer infant CPR, perform a compression-to-ventilation ratio of 15 to 2. Rescuers should switch roles after 10 cycles of CPR (approximately 2 minutes) when using a compression-to-ventilation ratio of 15:2.

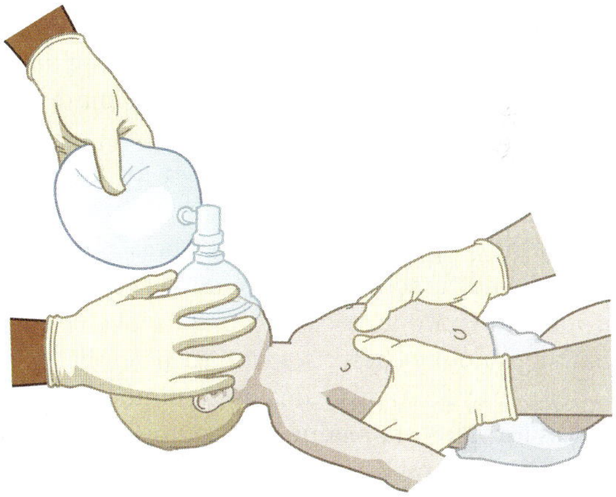

FIGURE 8-11 When performing two-rescuer infant CPR, one clinician uses the two-thumb/encircling-hands technique for chest compressions as the other clinician manages ventilations.
© Jones & Bartlett Learning

Child CPR

One-Rescuer and Two-Rescuer Child CPR

The steps for child CPR are essentially the same as for an adult; however, some steps may require modification for a child. These variations are as follows:

- Use less force to compress the child's chest.
- In small children, use only one hand to depress the sternum at least one-third the depth of the chest

(approximately 2 inches [5 cm]). Use two hands in larger children.
- Use less force to ventilate the child. Ventilate only until the child's chest rises.

Follow these steps to administer CPR to a child:

1. Assess the child's level of responsiveness. Tap and gently shake the shoulder and shout, "Are you okay?" If a second rescuer is available, have this person activate the EMS system and get an AED if available.
2. Place the child faceup on a firm, flat surface.
3. Assess circulation by checking for a carotid pulse and simultaneously observe breathing adequacy. Locate the larynx with your index and middle fingers. Slide your fingers into the groove between the larynx and the muscles at the side of the neck to feel for the carotid pulse. Check for at least 5 seconds but no more than 10 seconds.
4. If the child has no pulse or the pulse is less than 60 beats/min with signs of poor circulation and the child is not breathing or only gasping, begin chest compressions.
5. Begin a cycle of 30 chest compressions. Compress the chest at least one-third the diameter of the chest (approximately 2 inches [5 cm] in most children) at a rate of 100 to 120 compressions per minute (**FIGURE 8-12**). Count the compressions out loud: "One and two and three and . . ." In between compressions, allow the chest to fully recoil.
6. After 30 compressions, open the airway. Use the head tilt–chin lift maneuver or, if the child is injured, the jaw-thrust maneuver.
7. Give two rescue breaths. Blow slowly for 1 second, using just enough force to make the chest visibly rise. Allow the lungs to deflate between breaths.
8. Coordinate chest compressions and ventilations in a 30:2 ratio for one rescuer or 15:2 for two rescuers, making sure the chest rises with each ventilation.
9. After five cycles (approximately 2 minutes) of CPR, assess for signs of breathing or a pulse. If the child has no pulse and you have an AED, apply it now.

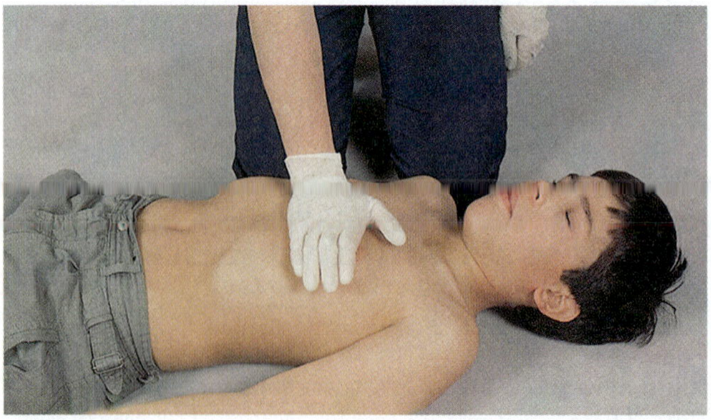

FIGURE 8-12 When performing chest compressions on a child, place the heel of your hand in the center of the chest, in between the nipples.
© Jones & Bartlett Learning. Courtesy of MIEMSS.

10. If you are alone with no communications device, perform 2 minutes of CPR before leaving the patient to activate the EMS system.
11. Continue until other EMS clinicians arrive to take over the care of the patient or the patient starts to move.

A skill performance sheet titled One-Rescuer Child CPR is shown in **FIGURE 8-13** for your review and practice. In large children, remember that you may need to use two hands to achieve an adequate depth of compression. When you are performing two-rescuer CPR on a child, administer 15 compressions followed by two rescue breaths. Switch compressors every five cycles (2 minutes).

Signs of Effective CPR

It is important to know the signs of effective CPR so you can assess your efforts to resuscitate the patient. The signs of effective CPR are as follows:

1. The patient's skin color improves (returns to its baseline color).
2. The chest visibly rises during ventilations.
3. Compressions and ventilations are delivered at the appropriate rate and depth.

If some of these signs are not present, evaluate and alter your technique to try to achieve these signs.

Note that CPR-assistive devices are sometimes used in the prehospital setting but may not be appropriate for pediatric patients. Examples include impedance threshold devices, mechanical chest compression devices, and load-distributing band devices. All of these devices assist with chest recoil and compression, with the goal of improving venous return and outflow. Although not all of these devices may be available to you as an EMR, it is important to know which patients they are appropriate for and how to use the devices employed by your local EMS system.

Complications of CPR

A discussion of CPR is not complete without mentioning its complications, but you can minimize these complications by using proper technique.

Broken Ribs

If your hands slip to the side of the sternum during chest compressions or if your fingers rest on the ribs, you may break a patient's ribs while delivering a compression. To prevent this complication, use proper hand positioning and do not let your fingers come in contact with the ribs. If you hear a cracking sound while performing CPR, check and correct your hand position but continue CPR. Sometimes you may break bones or cartilage even when using proper CPR technique. This risk is higher for geriatric patients, whose bones may be more fragile.

One-Rescuer Child CPR	
Steps	**Adequately Performed**
1. Determine responsiveness by shaking the child. If a second rescuer is available, have this person activate the EMS system.	
2. Check for signs of circulation by checking the carotid pulse and simultaneously checking for no breathing and only gasping.	
3. If the child has no pulse or the pulse is less than 60 beats per minute with signs of poor circulation and is not breathing or only gasping, give cycles of 30 chest compressions at a rate of 100 to 120 compressions per minute.	
4. Open the airway using the head tilt–chin lift maneuver. (If trauma is present or you suspect a head or spinal injury, use the jaw-thrust maneuver.)	
5. Give two effective breaths (1 second per breath). If the airway is obstructed, reposition the head and try to ventilate again. Watch for chest rise; allow for exhalation between breaths.	
6. Continue cycles of 30 chest compressions and two ventilations until additional personnel arrive or the patient starts to move. If you are alone with no communications device, perform 2 minutes of CPR before leaving the patient to activate the EMS system.	

FIGURE 8-13 Skill performance sheet: One-Rescuer Child CPR.

© Jones & Bartlett Learning

Gastric Distention

Bloating of the stomach is called **gastric distention**. It is caused when too much air is blown too fast and too forcefully into the stomach. A partially obstructed airway, which allows some of the air you breathe into the patient's airway to go into the stomach rather than into the lungs, can also cause gastric distention.

Gastric distention causes the abdomen to increase in size. A distended abdomen pushes on the diaphragm and prevents the lungs from inflating fully. Gastric distention also often causes regurgitation. If regurgitation occurs, quickly turn the patient to the side, wipe out the mouth with your gloved fingers, and then return the patient to a supine position.

You can prevent gastric distention by making sure you have opened the airway completely. Do not blow excessive amounts of air into the patient (deliver each breath over a period of 1 second). Be especially careful if you are a large person with a large lung capacity and the patient is smaller than you.

Regurgitation

Regurgitation (passive vomiting) is a common occurrence during CPR, so you must be prepared to manage this complication. You can minimize the risk of regurgitation by minimizing the amount of air that enters the patient's stomach. Regurgitation commonly occurs if the patient has experienced cardiac arrest. When cardiac arrest occurs, the muscle that keeps food in the stomach relaxes. If there is any food in the stomach, it backs up, causing the patient to vomit.

If the patient regurgitates as you are performing CPR, immediately turn the patient onto their side to allow the vomitus to drain from the mouth. Clear the patient's mouth of remaining vomitus, first with your fingers and then with a clean cloth (if one is handy). Use suction if it is available.

The patient may experience frequent episodes of regurgitation, so you must be prepared to take these actions repeatedly. EMS units carry a mechanical suction machine that can clear the patient's mouth. However, you cannot wait until the mechanical suction machine arrives before beginning or resuming CPR. You must manage the regurgitation as it occurs so that CPR is not delayed.

Do your best to clear any vomitus from the patient's airway. If the airway is not cleared, two complications may arise:

1. The patient may breathe in (aspirate) the vomitus into the lungs.
2. You may force vomitus into the lungs with the next artificial ventilation.

It takes a strong stomach and the realization that you are trying to save the patient's life to continue with resuscitation after the patient has regurgitated, but you must continue. Remove the vomitus from the patient's mouth with a towel, the patient's shirt, your gloved fingers, or a manual suction unit if available. As soon as you have cleared away the vomitus, continue rescue breathing.

Hyperventilation

Hyperventilation (ventilating too fast or with too much force) may cause increased pressure inside the patient's chest cavity. This increased pressure decreases the effectiveness of chest compressions and results in the heart and brain receiving less oxygen. As you incorporate breathing skills into your CPR training, you will need to be mindful of this risk. See Chapter 7, *Airway Management*, for further discussion of breathing skills.

Creating Sufficient Space for CPR

As an EMR, you will frequently find yourself alone with a patient in cardiac arrest. One of the first steps you must take is to create or find a space where you can perform CPR. Ask yourself, "Is there enough room in this location to perform effective CPR?" To perform CPR effectively, you need 3 to 4 feet (approximately 1 m) of space on all sides of the patient. This will provide you with enough space so that rescuers can change places, ALS procedures can be implemented, and an ambulance stretcher can be brought in. If there is not enough space around the patient, you have two options:

1. Quickly rearrange the furniture in the room or arrange objects at the scene to make space.
2. Quickly drag the patient into an area that has more space—for instance, out of the bathroom and into the living room, but not into a hallway (**FIGURE 8-14**).

Space is essential to a smooth rescue operation for a cardiac arrest patient. It takes a minimal amount of time to either clear a space around the patient or move the patient into a larger area.

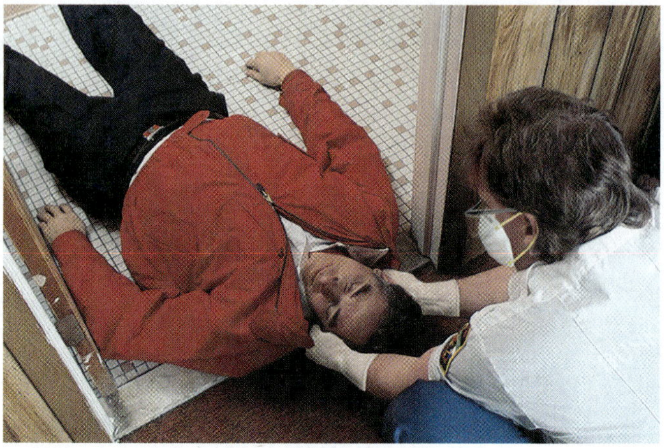

FIGURE 8-14 Create sufficient space for CPR.
© American Academy of Orthopaedic Surgeons

Early Defibrillation by EMRs

According to the AHA, more than 350,000 people experience out-of-hospital cardiac arrest each year. As noted earlier, more than 70% of all out-of-hospital cardiac arrest patients have an irregular heart electrical rhythm called **ventricular fibrillation**. This condition, often referred to as V-fib, is the rapid, disorganized, and ineffective vibration of the heart. An electric shock applied to the heart will defibrillate it and reorganize the vibrations into effective heartbeats. A patient in cardiac arrest stands the greatest chance for survival when early defibrillation is available.

As an EMR, you are often the first emergency health care clinician to reach a patient who has collapsed in cardiac arrest. When you perform effective CPR, you are helping to keep the patient's brain and heart supplied with oxygen until a defibrillator and ALS clinicians arrive at the scene.

To get defibrillators to cardiac arrest patients more quickly, increasing numbers of EMS systems are equipping EMRs with an **automated external defibrillator (AED)**

Words of Wisdom

AEDs are available in many public and private buildings, including schools, office buildings, athletic facilities, churches, and retail settings. Look for them as you move around your community. You should know where they are located in the event you encounter a patient who needs one while you are on duty, or even off duty without your equipment.

YOU are the EMR — CASE 3

On your way back from getting fuel, you are suddenly dispatched for the report of an unknown emergency. As you arrive at the address, you are led to a basement workshop in a suburban home. A 12-year-old girl tells you that her father went down into his woodworking shop to work on a project. The girl tells you that she was upstairs doing homework when she heard her father yell for help. She ran downstairs and found him slumped over his band saw. As you approach the scene, you notice your patient seems to be grasping the power switch in one hand.

1. What should you do first?
2. What steps should you take to assess this patient?
3. Do you think an AED is important in this situation?

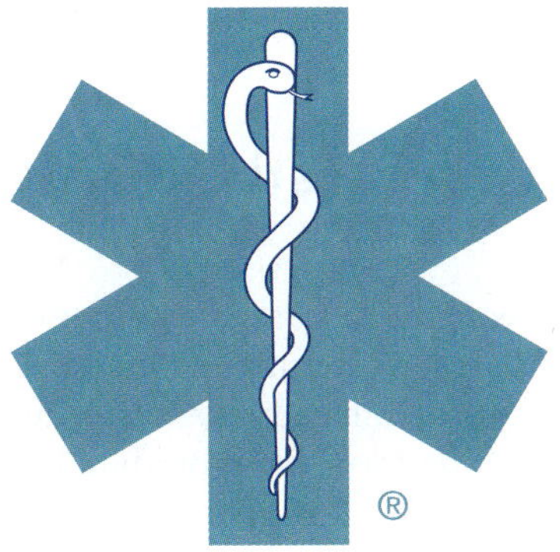

Voices OF Experience

Paul, my friend of 10 years, was 70 years old and very physically fit. One day, while mowing the lawn, he began experiencing shortness of breath. He went inside to rest and felt better. Later that day, he had the same problem when he walked up the stairs. Paul called his doctor and made an appointment to be seen in his office the next week.

The following day, while eating breakfast, he began to complain of chest pain. Paul's wife, Donna, called 9-1-1 and help was on the way, but before they arrived, Paul's wife says, "He turned green and that was it."

> **"When emergency medical responders arrived, they found Paul unconscious and unresponsive."**

When emergency medical responders arrived, they found Paul unconscious and unresponsive. With the ambulance still on the way, they immediately began to administer professional rescuer CPR. A pulse check was done and they opened his airway, but Paul had no pulse and was not breathing. The team initiated compressions and an AED was attached. It prompted: "Shock advised, stand clear of patient." A shock was delivered. Paul had been in cardiac arrest for 4 minutes and 30 seconds.

Two weeks after Paul's incident, I sat at a local restaurant listening to this story. As Paul's wife spoke, it sent chills up my spine. Paul was in cardiac arrest for over 4 minutes. Yet, due to rapid implementation of the cardiac chain of survival and the actions of the EMRs, my friend sat beside his wife with tears in his eyes that day thanking me for teaching others the lifesaving skills that had saved his life.

As you study the material in this textbook, consider the following: Will you someday be the Paul whose life is saved by someone, or will you be a lifesaver yourself and save someone's Paul?

Charles Dixon
President, American Heritage Training
Training Officer, American Heritage Ambulance
Ladson, South Carolina

Adapted from the personal Medical Identification Symbol of the American Medical Association.

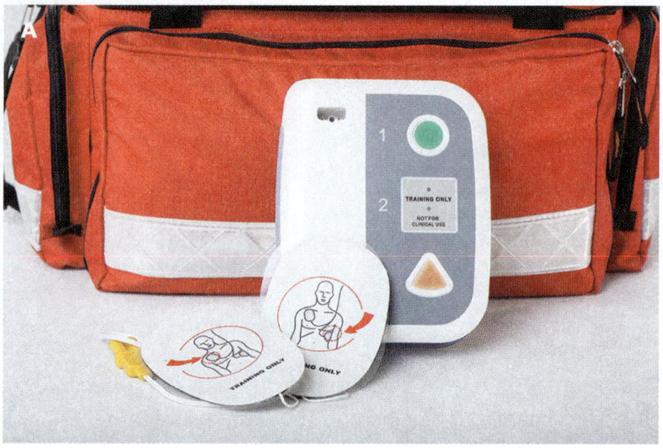

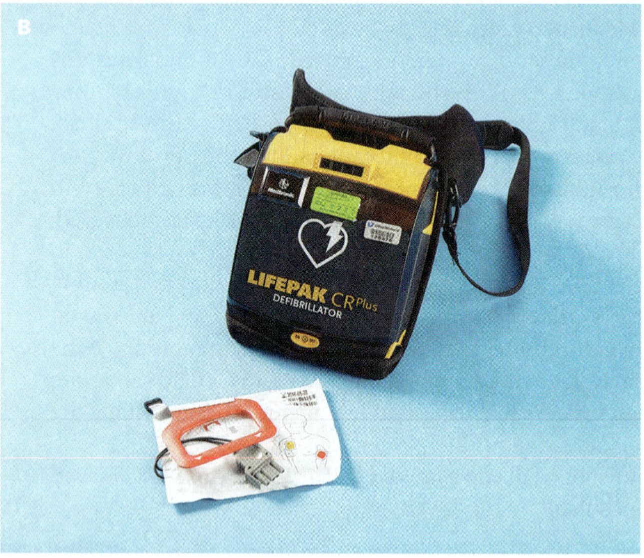

FIGURE 8-15 Automated external defibrillators can vary in their design, features, and operation.
A: © Photographee.eu/Shutterstock; **B:** © Jones & Bartlett Learning

(**FIGURE 8-15**). These machines accurately identify ventricular fibrillation (and ventricular tachycardia) and advise you to deliver a shock if needed. Such equipment allows you to combine effective CPR with early defibrillation to restore an organized heartbeat in a patient.

Performing Automated External Defibrillation

AEDs vary in design and operation, so learn how to use your specific AED. You must have the training required by your medical director to practice automated external defibrillation. Practice until you can perform the procedure quickly and safely. Because the recommended guidelines for using the AED change, always follow the most current CPR and Emergency Cardiac Care (ECC) guidelines.

Safety

Never apply an AED to a patient who has a pulse. AEDs are designed to recognize two rhythms: ventricular fibrillation and ventricular tachycardia. A patient in ventricular tachycardia may or may not have a pulse. Because the AED cannot detect the presence of a pulse, you could shock a patient who has a pulse and cause them to go into cardiac arrest.

Special Populations

AED Use With Pediatric Patients

You can safely use AEDs in pediatric patients using the pediatric-size pads and a dose-attenuating system (energy reducer). However, if these items are unavailable, use an adult AED. During CPR, the AED should be applied to infants or children after the first five cycles of CPR have been completed. Cardiac arrest in children is usually the result of respiratory failure; therefore, oxygenation and ventilation are vitally important. After the first five cycles of CPR, use the AED to deliver shocks in the same manner as with an adult patient.

If the child is between 1 month and 1 year of age (an infant), a manual defibrillator is preferred to an AED; however, manual defibrillation is a paramedic-level skill. Therefore, call for paramedic backup immediately if you suspect an infant may be in cardiac arrest. If paramedic backup with a manual defibrillator is not available, an AED equipped with a pediatric dose attenuator is preferred. If neither is available, an AED without a pediatric dose attenuator may be used. Follow the manufacturer's instructions for use of the AED for pediatric patients.

The steps for using an AED are listed in **SKILL DRILL 8-4**.

YOU are the EMR — CASE 4

You are en route to the station when you are dispatched for a man reporting shortness of breath and jaw pain. On arrival at the scene, you find a 60-year-old man leaning over in a chair; he is diaphoretic and breathing rapidly, and he reports severe pain in his jaw. As you begin your primary assessment, he clutches his chest and falls forward. After positioning the patient on the ground, your partner applies the AED while you begin the steps of CPR. You stop CPR to allow the AED to analyze the patient's rhythm. The AED indicates that no shock is advised and to continue CPR.

1. Why should you stop providing CPR while the AED is analyzing the patient's rhythm?
2. Which heart rhythms are considered to be shockable rhythms?

SKILL DRILL 8-4

Performing Automated External Defibrillation

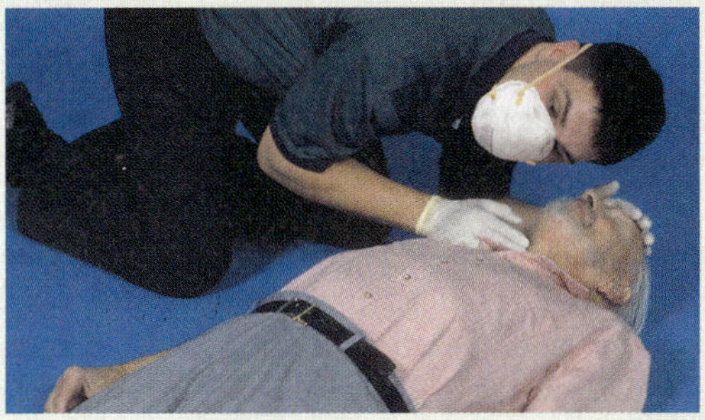

STEP 1 On reaching the patient, determine whether CPR has been initiated and whether the patient is responsive and has a pulse.

- *If the patient is responsive or has a pulse, do not apply the AED.*
- *If CPR is in progress*, verify that the patient is unresponsive and has no pulse. Continue chest compressions and ventilations at a ratio of 30 compressions to two ventilations until an AED is available and ready to shock the patient, as described in the following steps.
- *If no CPR is being performed*, check for responsiveness, pulse, and breathing. If the patient is unresponsive, has no pulse, and is not breathing, begin chest compressions. Continue chest compressions and ventilations at a ratio of 30 compressions to two ventilations until an AED is available and ready to shock the patient, as described in the following steps.

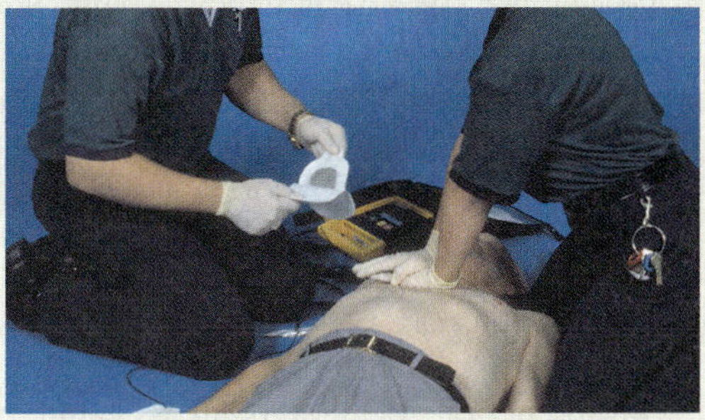

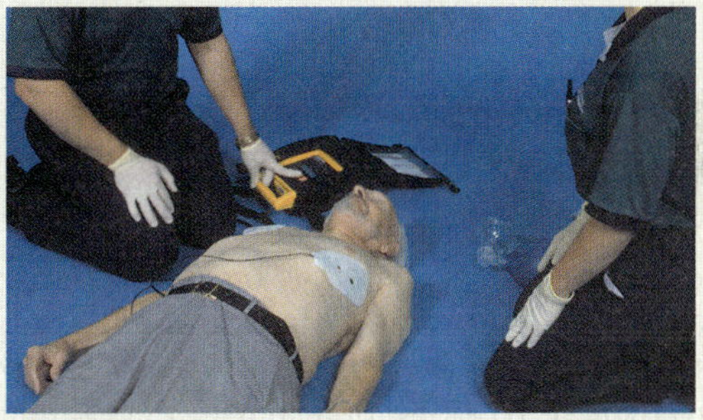

STEP 2 As soon as an AED is available, turn on the AED and follow the prompts. Remove clothing from the patient's chest area. Apply the pads to the chest: one just to the right of the breastbone (sternum) just below the collarbone (clavicle), the other on the left lower chest area with the top of the pad 2 to 3 inches (5 to 8 cm) below the armpit. Be sure the patient cables are attached to the pads and to the AED.

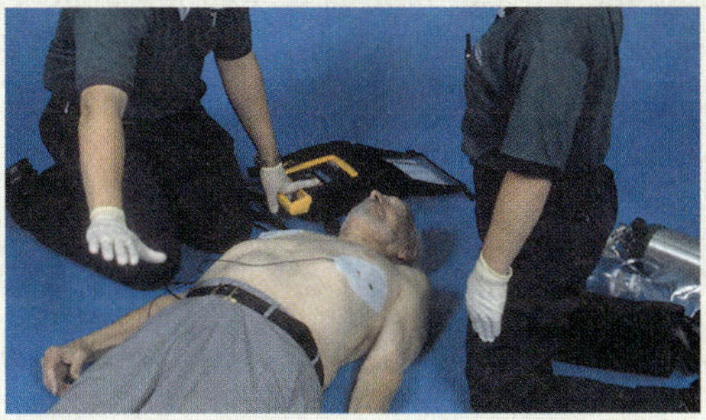

STEP 3 Stop CPR. State aloud, "Clear the patient," and be sure that no one is touching the patient. Push the Analyze button and wait for the AED to determine if a shockable rhythm is present. Listen for the voice prompt.

If the AED determines no shock is advised, perform five cycles (approximately 2 minutes) of CPR beginning with chest compressions. Then reassess the patient's pulse and reanalyze the cardiac rhythm.

If a shock is advised, reconfirm that no one is touching the patient and push the Shock button. After the shock is delivered, immediately resume CPR, beginning with chest compressions.

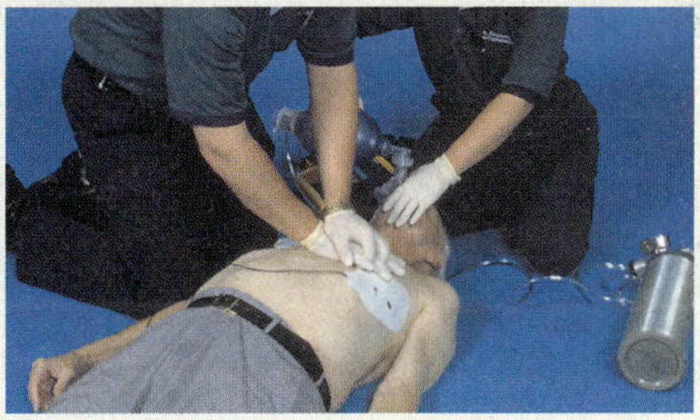

STEP 4 After five cycles (approximately 2 minutes) of CPR, reanalyze the patient's cardiac rhythm. Do not interrupt chest compressions for more than 10 seconds.

Repeat the cycle of 2 minutes of CPR, one shock (if indicated), and 2 minutes of CPR. Arrange for advanced care and transport. Contact medical control as needed.

© Jones & Bartlett Learning. Courtesy of MIEMSS.

Treatment

When preparing to defibrillate a patient, be alert for the following situations:

- If the patient is wet, dry the patient before initiating defibrillation. This will ensure that the defibrillation pads stick to the patient's chest and that the full shock is delivered safely. If the patient is lying in water, drag the person out of it and quickly dry the chest prior to applying the pads.
- If the patient has excessive chest hair and a razor is available, quickly shave the area where the pads will be placed.
- If the patient has a pacemaker, reposition one of the defibrillation pads so that it is not placed directly over the pacemaker.
- If the patient has a transdermal medication patch on the chest, remove the patch and wipe the skin before defibrillating the patient.

CPR Training

As an EMR, you should successfully complete a CPR course through a recognized agency such as the Emergency Care and Safety Institute, the AHA, or the American Red Cross. You should also regularly update your skills by successfully completing a recognized recertification course. You cannot achieve proficiency in CPR unless you have adequate practice on adult, child, and infant manikins. Manikin feedback devices help ensure that the trainee has the proper understanding of the depth and consistency in compressions needed for CPR to be effective. Your department should schedule periodic reviews of CPR theory and practice for all EMRs.

Legal Implications of CPR

Advance directives, living wills, and durable powers of attorney for health care are legal documents that indicate the patient's wishes regarding specified medical procedures. You may sometimes wonder whether you should start CPR on a person who has an advance directive or a living will. If you are familiar with the advance directive documents that are legally binding in your state and your agency has authorized you to evaluate and interpret these documents, you should withhold CPR in any case where the patient's documents express this wish. Because you are not always in a position to determine whether the advance directive or living will is valid, whenever you are not certain of the validity of the document or if any question is raised as to the degree to which the document represents the will of the patient, CPR should be started unless signs of obvious death are present (such as rigor mortis, tissue decay, or decapitation) or a resuscitation attempt would put you in harm's way. If a patient has an advance directive or living will, the physician at the hospital can also determine whether you should stop CPR. Follow your department's protocols regarding advance directives, living wills, and DNR orders.

Do not hesitate to begin CPR on a pulseless, nonbreathing patient. Without your help, the patient will certainly die. Make sure you perform a careful assessment of the patient before beginning CPR.

Another potential legal pitfall is abandonment, which is the discontinuation of CPR without the order of a licensed physician or without turning the patient over to someone who is at least as qualified as you are. If you avoid these pitfalls, you need not be overly concerned about the legal implications of performing CPR. Your most important protection against a possible lawsuit is to become thoroughly skilled in the theory and practice of CPR.

YOU are the EMR SUMMARY

You are the EMR: CASE 1

1. On the basis of the patient's unresponsiveness, what should you do now for the patient?

Because your patient does not respond to verbal stimuli or to gentle shaking of her shoulder, you need to simultaneously check for signs of circulation and breathing by checking the carotid pulse and watching for chest rise and movement. If the patient has no pulse and is not breathing or only gasping, move the patient from the couch to the floor and begin CPR. Perform cycles of 30 compressions and two breaths. Use the AED as soon as it is available. Make sure additional help has been dispatched. Give compressions at a rate of 100 to 120 compressions per minute at a depth of at least 2 inches (5 cm). Allow full chest recoil between compressions and minimize interruptions when switching between compressions and ventilations.

2. What are the chances for a successful resuscitation on this call?

A witnessed cardiac arrest has a higher probability for a successful resuscitation than an unwitnessed cardiac arrest. The sooner you are able to start CPR and apply the AED to the patient, the greater the chance for a successful outcome. However, note that only about one in four people who experience a witnessed cardiac arrest will regain a pulse with resuscitation efforts.

3. What role does your AED play in this call?

Having an AED available greatly increases the possibility that you can successfully resuscitate this patient. If you have an AED available, apply it as soon as possible. Allow the AED to analyze the cardiac rhythm. If a shock is indicated, shock the patient. During the resuscitation, avoid interruptions in chest compressions as much as possible. During a witnessed cardiac arrest, immediate defibrillation will sometimes result in spontaneous return to a normal heart rhythm.

YOU are the EMR SUMMARY

You are the EMR: CASE 2

1. What are the next steps you should take?

You have an unresponsive, pulseless, and nonbreathing patient. You do not have any way of determining when the patient went into cardiac arrest. The patient is cool and has rigid muscles. If you were to look under her clothing at her back, you would likely find dependent lividity. All are signs of a patient who has been dead for some time and cannot be resuscitated. When reliable signs of death are present, as in this case, do not start CPR. Know your local protocols regarding when to start and stop CPR and who you need to notify in cases of obvious death. In such situations, realize that you may still have other patients who need your understanding: the friends and family members who are grieving the loss of their loved one.

You are the EMR: CASE 3

1. What should you do first?

Your first step is to ensure the scene is safe. In this case, it appears there might be an electrical problem associated with the band saw. Before you assess the patient, ensure that the power to the saw has been disconnected. This step may involve pulling the plug from an outlet or disconnecting the main power switch. Do not come into direct contact or otherwise touch the patient until you have made sure the scene is safe. If you become a patient yourself, you cannot provide any further emergency care.

2. What steps should you take to assess this patient?

Begin by determining responsiveness. If the patient is responsive, ask him what happened, determine what signs and symptoms he has, and assess his breathing and circulation. If he is unresponsive, quickly assess his carotid pulse and breathing simultaneously. If the patient has no pulse and is not breathing or only gasping, begin chest compressions followed by rescue breathing. Make sure additional help has been dispatched.

3. Do you think an AED is important in this situation?

If the patient is in cardiac arrest from contact with an electrical source, he may be in ventricular fibrillation. In this case, an AED may be able to convert his heart rhythm to a normal pattern and increase his chance for survival. Begin CPR with cycles of 30 compressions and two breaths. Use the AED as soon as it is available.

You are the EMR: CASE 4

1. Why should you stop providing CPR while the AED is analyzing the patient's rhythm?

It is important to clear the patient while the AED is analyzing the heart rhythm. Touching the patient while the AED is analyzing the heart rhythm may affect the accuracy of the rhythm being analyzed. It is also important to clear the patient before delivering a shock because the person who is touching the patient may also get shocked.

2. Which heart rhythms are considered to be shockable rhythms?

The AED will automatically analyze the heart rhythm of a pulseless patient. If the patient's heart rhythm is ventricular fibrillation or ventricular tachycardia, the AED will indicate that a shock is advised. The AED will not advise delivering a shock and instruct you to continue CPR if the patient is not in ventricular fibrillation or ventricular tachycardia.

Prep Kit

Ready for Review

- The circulatory system transports oxygenated blood from the lungs to the rest of the body. Each beat of the heart produces a pulse, which can be felt at various sites on the body, such as the inside of the wrist (radial), the neck (carotid), the inside of the upper arm (brachial), and the groin (femoral).
- Cardiac arrest occurs when the heart stops contracting and no blood is pumped through the blood vessels. Brain damage begins within 4 to 6 minutes after the patient has experienced cardiac arrest. Within 8 to 10 minutes, the damage to the brain may become irreversible.
- The chain of survival includes six links that are essential to successful emergency cardiac care: (1) recognition of cardiac arrest and activation of the emergency response system; (2) immediate high-quality CPR; (3) rapid defibrillation; (4) advanced resuscitation by EMS and other health care clinicians; (5) post–cardiac arrest care; and (6) recovery and survivorship.
- When you arrive at an emergency scene, first assess the area for potential safety hazards. If the scene is unsafe,

Prep Kit

make it as safe as possible for yourself and the patient. As you approach the patient, look for possible causes of illness or injury. Next, determine responsiveness. If the patient is unresponsive, simultaneously check for signs of circulation and breathing by checking the pulse and watching for chest rise. If the patient has no pulse and is not breathing or only gasping, begin CPR with chest compressions, followed by rescue breathing.

- Basic life support for adults and children follows the same general steps: check responsiveness, circulation, airway, and breathing. Intervene at any point if the patient's airway is obstructed, the patient is not breathing or only gasping, or the patient has no pulse.
- To open the airway, use the head tilt–chin lift maneuver or, if you suspect a head or spinal injury, the jaw-thrust maneuver.
- Rescue breathing should be performed at a rate of one breath every 6 seconds (10 breaths/min) for adults and one breath every 2 to 3 seconds (20 to 30 breaths/min) for children and infants.
- Chest compressions should be performed at a rate of 100 to 120 compressions per minute for adults and children. Perform 30 compressions and two breaths for adults and for one-rescuer CPR. Perform 15 compressions and two breaths for two-rescuer child and infant CPR.
- BLS for infants is similar to that provided for adults and children. The techniques may vary somewhat, but the same general steps apply: check responsiveness and simultaneously check circulation and breathing adequacy. Intervene at any point if the infant's airway is obstructed, the infant is not breathing or only gasping, or the infant has no pulse.
- Open an infant's airway by using the head tilt–chin lift maneuver if you do not suspect a spinal injury. Be careful not to hyperextend the neck, which could obstruct the airway.
- If the infant has no pulse, begin CPR. Use the two-thumbs technique to compress the chest 30 times, at a rate of 100 to 120 compressions per minute, to a depth equal to at least one-third the depth of the chest. After 30 compressions, give two breaths. If two rescuers are present, one clinician compresses as the other ventilates, providing 15 compressions to two breaths.
- The single most important cardiac arrest survival factor is early defibrillation. The indications for using an AED are that the patient is unresponsive, pulseless, and not breathing or only gasping. After determining that a patient is in cardiac arrest, begin immediate CPR and apply the AED as soon as possible.
- Once you turn on the AED and attach it to the patient's bare chest, the AED will analyze the heart rhythm and advise whether a shock is indicated. If a shock is advised, ensure that no one is touching the patient, deliver the shock, and immediately perform CPR for 2 minutes before reanalyzing the patient's rhythm. If no shock is advised, perform CPR for 2 minutes and then reanalyze the patient's rhythm. Continue CPR and rhythm analysis until ALS personnel arrive.

Vital Vocabulary

automated external defibrillator (AED) A portable, battery-powered device that recognizes ventricular fibrillation (and ventricular tachycardia) and advises when a countershock is indicated. The device delivers an electric shock to patients with ventricular fibrillation.

brachial pulse The pulse located on the arm between the elbow and shoulder; used for checking the pulse in infants.

cardiac arrest Cessation of breathing and a heartbeat.

carotid pulse The pulse that can be felt on each side of the neck where the carotid artery is close to the skin.

chest compressions A means of applying artificial circulation by applying rhythmic pressure and relaxation on the lower half of the sternum.

child A person between the age of 1 year and the onset of puberty (age 12 to 14 years).

circulatory system The heart and blood vessels, which together are responsible for the continuous flow of blood throughout the body.

femoral pulse The pulse taken at the groin.

gastric distention Inflation of the stomach caused when excessive pressures are used during artificial ventilation and air is directed into the stomach rather than the lungs.

Prep Kit

infant A person younger than 1 year.

one-rescuer CPR Cardiopulmonary resuscitation performed by one rescuer.

plasma The clear, yellowish fluid of the blood that carries blood cells, transports nutrients, and removes cellular waste materials.

platelets Microscopic disk-shaped elements in the blood that are essential to the formation of a blood clot, the mechanism that stops bleeding.

pulse The wave of pressure created by the heart as it contracts and forces blood out into the major arteries.

radial pulse The pulse located on the inside of the wrist on the thumb side.

two-rescuer CPR Cardiopulmonary resuscitation performed by two rescuers.

ventilation The movement of air into and out of the lungs.

ventricular fibrillation An uncoordinated muscular quivering of the heart; the most common abnormal rhythm causing cardiac arrest; often referred to as V-fib.

References

CPR facts and stats. American Heart Association website. https://cpr.heart.org/en/resources/cpr-facts-and-stats. Accessed November 19, 2024.

Ludhwani D, Goyal A, Jagtap M. Ventricular fibrillation. *StatPearls*. National Library of Medicine website. https://www.ncbi.nlm.nih.gov/books/NBK537120/#. Updated August 8, 2023. Accessed November 19, 2024.

Mastenbrook J, Redinger KE, Vos D, Dickson C. Retrospective comparison of prehospital sustained return of spontaneous circulation (ROSC) rates within a single basic life support jurisdiction using manual vs Lund University Cardiac Assist System (LUCAS-2) mechanical cardiopulmonary resuscitation. *Cureus*. 2022;14(6):e26131. doi:10.7759/cureus.26131

Out-of-hospital chain of survival. American Heart Association website. https://cpr.heart.org/en/resources/cpr-facts-and-stats/out-of-hospital-chain-of-survival. Accessed November 19, 2024.

What is CPR? American Heart Association website. https://cpr.heart.org/en/resources/what-is-cpr. Accessed November 19, 2024.

Assessment IN ACTION

At 1147 hours on a Sunday, you are dispatched to the First Community Church for a report of a 72-year-old man with severe chest pain. On arrival, you find an older man lying on the floor. His skin appears to be blue in color. He is unresponsive to your questions and does not respond when you shake his shoulder. Bystanders tell you that when they first noticed the man, he was clutching his chest. Several minutes after they called 9-1-1, he collapsed and fell to the floor.

1. What is your first step in providing emergency care for this patient?
   - A. Check for a pulse.
   - B. Check for breathing.
   - C. Perform chest compressions.
   - D. Establish unresponsiveness.
2. Which of the following signs would indicate that CPR is needed?
   - A. Shallow breathing
   - B. Dilated pupils
   - C. Absence of a pulse and breathing
   - D. Shortness of breath
3. Knowing when to start CPR is important. Which of the following criteria is NOT a reliable sign of death?
   - A. Evidence of tissue decomposition
   - B. Rigor mortis
   - C. Decapitation
   - D. Dilated pupils
4. What is the appropriate depth of chest compressions for an adult patient?
   - A. 0.25 inch (6 mm) to 0.5 inch (1 cm)
   - B. 0.5 inch (1 cm) to 1 inch (3 cm)
   - C. At least 2 inches (5 cm)
   - D. One-half the depth of the chest
5. When CPR is performed on this patient, what is the correct ratio of chest compressions to rescue breaths?
   - A. 5:1
   - B. 15:2
   - C. 30:2
   - D. 50:2
6. What is the rate at which you should compress the chest during adult CPR?
   - A. At least 100 times per minute
   - B. Exactly 100 times per minute
   - C. 100 to 120 times per minute
   - D. More than 110 times per minute
7. Which of the following is considered an acceptable reason to stop providing CPR?
   - A. You are too physically exhausted to continue.
   - B. Your partner orders you to stop.
   - C. You cannot feel a pulse.
   - D. You determine CPR is not working.
8. Why is it important to ensure your hands are off the chest between compressions?
9. At what point in this scenario should the AED be applied to the patient?
10. Why is it important to minimize interruptions of chest compressions when switching positions during two-rescuer CPR?

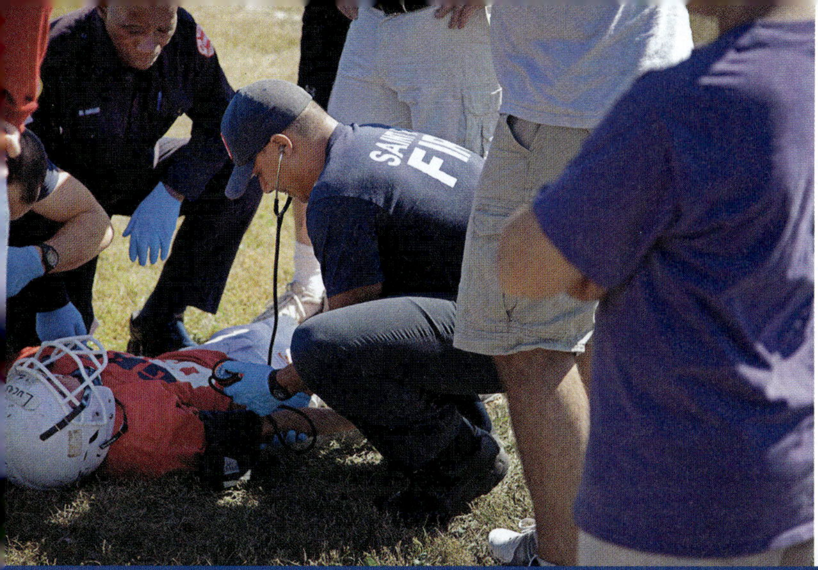

SECTION **3**

Patient Assessment

9 Patient Assessment

© Steve Skjold/Alamy Stock Photo

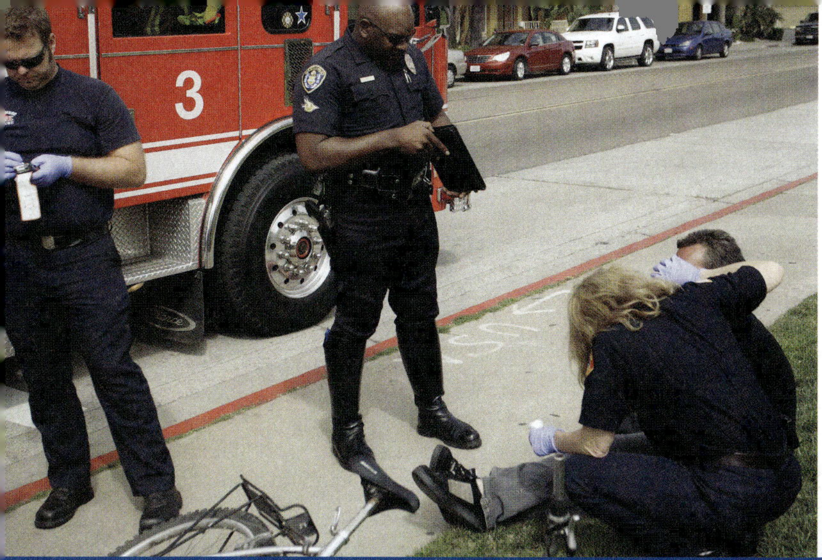

CHAPTER 9

Patient Assessment

National EMS Education Standard Competencies

Assessment

Use scene information and patient assessment findings to identify and manage immediate life threats and injuries within the scope and practice of the emergency medical responder (EMR).

Scene Assessment

- Scene safety/situational awareness (pp 179–180)
- Scene management (pp 180–182)
- Impact of the environment on patient care (pp 180–183)
- Addressing hazards (p 181)
- Violence (pp 178–183)
- Need for additional or specialized resources (p 183)
- Standard precautions (p 183)
- Multiple-patient situations (pp 182–183)

Primary Assessment

- Primary assessment for all patient situations (pp 184–187)
- Begin interventions needed to preserve life (pp 185–187)

History Taking

- Determining the chief complaint (pp 188–189)
- Mechanism of injury/nature of illness (p 189)
- Associated signs and symptoms (pp 188–190)

Secondary Assessment

- Assessment of vital signs (pp 196–202)
- Assessment of pain (pp 196–202)
- Performing a rapid full-body scan (pp 196–202)

Reassessment

- How and when to reassess patients (pp 203–204)

© Kevin Link/Science Source

Knowledge Objectives

1. Discuss the importance of each of the following five steps in the patient assessment sequence:
   - Step 1. Scene assessment (pp 180–183)
   - Step 2. Primary assessment (pp 184–187)
   - Step 3. History taking (pp 188–190)
   - Step 4. Secondary assessment (pp 199–202)
   - Step 5. Reassessment (pp 203–204)
2. Discuss the components of a scene assessment. (pp 180–183)
3. Explain why it is important to get an idea of the number of patients at an emergency scene as soon as possible. (pp 182–183)
4. List and describe the importance of the following steps of the primary assessment:
   - Forming a general impression of the patient (p 184)
   - Determining the patient's level of responsiveness (p 185)
   - Performing a rapid exam to identify life threats, including:
     - Assessing the patient's airway (p 186)
     - Assessing the patient's breathing (p 186)
     - Assessing the patient's circulation (pp 186–187)
   - Updating responding EMS units (p 187)
5. Describe the differences in checking airway, breathing, and circulation when the patient is an adult, a child, or an infant. (pp 186–187)
6. Explain the purpose for obtaining a patient's medical history. (pp 188–190)
7. Discuss the SAMPLE approach to obtaining a patient's medical history. (p 189)
8. Explain the difference between a sign and a symptom. (p 191)
9. Describe the sequence used to perform a secondary assessment of the entire body. (pp 192–196)

10. List the areas of the body that should be examined during the secondary assessment. (pp 192–196)
11. Explain the significance of the following signs: respiration, circulation, blood pressure, skin condition, pupil size and reactivity, and level of consciousness. (pp 196–202)
12. Describe how to implement the pediatric assessment triangle. (p 201)
13. List the information that should be obtained during reassessment. (pp 203–205)
14. List the information about the patient's condition that should be addressed in your handoff report. (p 204)

Skills Objectives

1. Demonstrate the following five steps of the patient assessment sequence:
   - Step 1. Scene assessment (pp 180–183)
   - Step 2. Primary assessment (pp 184–185)
   - Step 3. Obtaining the patient's medical history using the SAMPLE format (pp 188–190)
   - Step 4. Performing a secondary assessment, including:
     - Performing a secondary assessment of the entire body (pp 191–202; Skill Drill 9-1)
     - Identifying and measuring a patient's vital signs (pp 196–201)
   - Step 5. Performing an ongoing reassessment (pp 203–204)

Introduction

As an emergency medical responder (EMR), you will often be the first trained emergency medical services (EMS) clinician at the incident scene. Your initial actions, including your assessment of the scene and the patient, will help ensure a safe and effective response for everyone involved.

It is important that you are able to perform a systematic patient assessment to determine whether your patient has a medical condition or has sustained injuries from trauma. The patient assessment sequence consists of the following five steps:

Step 1. Perform a scene assessment.
Step 2. Perform a primary assessment.
Step 3. Obtain the patient's medical history.
Step 4. Perform a secondary assessment.
Step 5. Perform a reassessment.

By performing these five steps, you can systematically gather the information you need. After you have learned these steps, you will discover that you can modify the order in which you perform them to gather needed information about a patient who is experiencing a medical problem as opposed to a patient who has sustained trauma (a wound or injury).

The skills and knowledge presented in this chapter follow an **assessment-based care** model. With assessment-based care, the treatment rendered is based on the patient's signs and symptoms. Assessment-based care requires you to conduct a careful and thorough evaluation of the patient so that you can provide appropriate care. If a given condition has already been diagnosed by a physician and is known to the patient, you will sometimes have an idea of the patient's diagnosis. Other times, you will have to respond to the signs and symptoms you find during the assessment process.

Careful and thorough study of the skills and knowledge related to patient assessment will go a long way in helping you perform as a valuable member of the EMS team in your community.

Patient Assessment Sequence

The patient assessment sequence is designed to provide you with a framework so you can safely approach an emergency scene, determine the need for additional resources, examine the patient to determine whether injuries or illnesses are present, obtain the patient's medical history, and report the results of your assessment to other EMS clinicians.

YOU are the EMR — CASE 1

You are dispatched to a rural section of highway for the report of a crash involving a single vehicle. As you arrive on the scene, you observe that the vehicle left the road and collided with a tree, resulting in moderate damage to the front end of the vehicle. As you are preparing to get out of your vehicle, you note an older person slumped over the steering wheel.

1. Why is it so important to follow the five steps in the patient assessment sequence as you evaluate this scene and this patient?
2. Why is it important to complete all of the steps of the patient assessment before you determine what is wrong with this patient?

Patient Assessment

Scene Assessment

Ensure scene safety
Determine mechanism of injury/nature of illness
Determine number of patients
Consider additional resources
Take standard precautions

↓

Primary Assessment

Form a general impression
Assess level of responsiveness
Assess ABCs
Update responding EMS units

↓

History Taking

Investigate the chief complaint (SAMPLE history)

↓

Secondary Assessment

Systematically assess the patient
Assess vital signs

↓

Reassessment

Repeat the primary assessment
Reassess vital signs
Reassess the chief complaint
Recheck the effectiveness of any treatment and ensure all bleeding is controlled.
Identify and treat changes in the patient's condition
Reassess patient
- Unstable patients every 5 minutes
- Stable patients every 15 minutes

Patient Assessment

Scene Assessment

- Ensure scene safety
- Determine mechanism of injury/nature of illness
- Determine number of patients
- Consider additional resources
- Take standard precautions

↓

Primary Assessment

↓

History Taking

↓

Secondary Assessment

↓

Reassessment

Scene Assessment

The **scene assessment** is best defined as a general overview of the incident and its surroundings. On the basis of this information, you can determine the safety of the scene, the type of incident, any mechanism of injury, and the need for additional resources.

> **Safety**
>
> Even though scene assessment occurs toward the beginning of the response, its underlying principles apply throughout the entire call. These principles are embodied by the concept of situational awareness. **Situational awareness** involves paying attention to the conditions and people around you at all times and anticipating the risks that those conditions or people may pose.

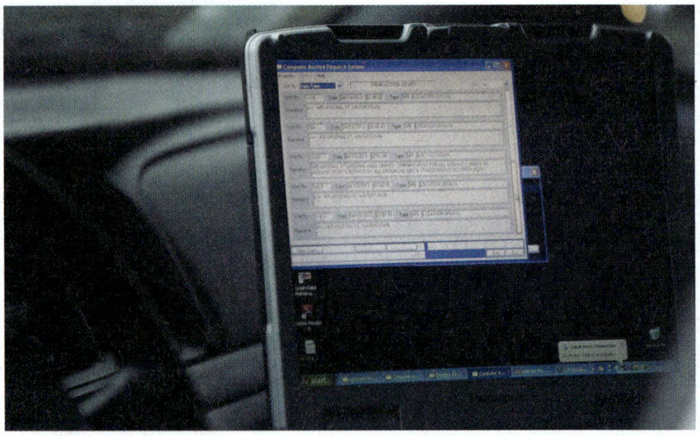

FIGURE 9-1 Begin your scene assessment by reviewing dispatch information.

© Julio Cortez/AP Photo

Review Dispatch Information

When dispatched to an emergency, your scene assessment actually begins before you arrive at the scene. When you are alerted for an emergency call, you can anticipate possible conditions by reviewing and understanding the information received from the dispatcher. Your dispatcher should have obtained the following information: the location of the incident, the main problem or type of incident, the number of people involved, and any safety issues at the scene. As you receive the dispatcher's information, you should begin to assess it (**FIGURE 9-1**).

In addition to the information obtained from the dispatcher, other factors can affect your actions. Consider, for example, factors such as the time of day, the day of the week, and weather conditions. A call from a school during school hours may require a different response than a call during the weekend. Finally, think about the resources that may be needed, and mentally prepare for other situations you may find when you arrive on the scene.

If you come across an emergency, notify the emergency medical dispatch center by using your two-way radio. If you do not have a two-way radio, use a cellular phone or send someone to call for help. Relay the following information: the location of the incident, the main problem or type of incident, the number of people involved, and any safety issues at the scene.

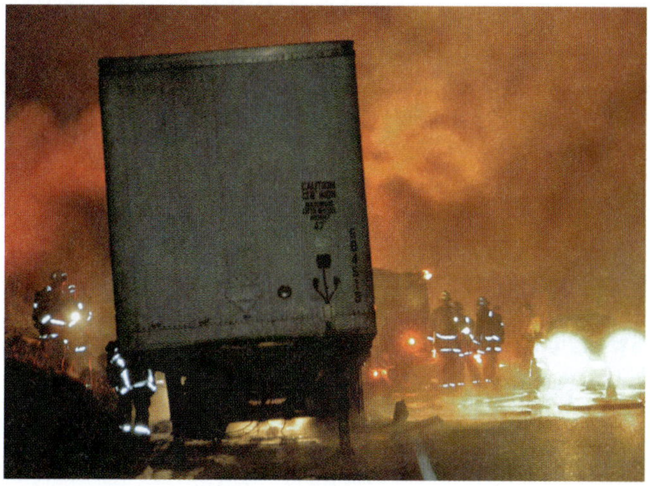

FIGURE 9-2 Perform a scene assessment.
© Keith D. Cullom/www.fire-image.com

Ensure Scene Safety

When you arrive at the scene, remember to park your vehicle so it helps to secure the scene and minimize traffic blockage. Do not park where it will impede the responding ambulance and/or fire truck. Be especially alert for traffic hazards as you exit your vehicle. As you approach the scene, scan the area to determine the extent of the incident, the possible number of people injured, and the presence of possible hazards (**FIGURE 9-2**). It is also important to scan the scene to ensure that you are not putting yourself in danger.

Hazards can be visible or invisible. Visible hazards include downed electrical wires, traffic, spilled gasoline, unstable buildings, a crime scene, weather, and crowds. Unstable surfaces such as slopes, ice, and water also pose potential hazards. Invisible hazards include electricity, biologic hazards, hazardous materials, and poisonous fumes. Downed electrical wires or broken poles may indicate an electrical hazard. Never assume a downed electrical wire is safe. Confined spaces such as farm silos, industrial tanks, and below-ground pits often contain poisonous gases or lack enough oxygen to support life. Hazardous materials placards on vehicles may indicate the presence of a chemical hazard.

As you take note of the hazards, consider your ability to manage them and decide whether to call for assistance. This assistance may include the fire department, additional EMS units, law enforcement officers, heavy-rescue equipment, hazardous materials teams, electric or gas company personnel, or other specialized resources. If a hazardous condition exists, make every effort to ensure that bystanders, rescuers, and patients are not exposed to it unnecessarily. If possible, see to it that any hazardous conditions are corrected or minimized as soon as possible. Noting such conditions early keeps them from becoming part of the problem later. Sometimes the first action needed at an incident scene is to prevent it from becoming worse. For example, it may be necessary to control traffic to prevent further crashes before it is safe to begin caring for injured patients.

Some emergency scenes will not be safe for you to enter. These scenes will require personnel with special training and equipment. If a scene is unsafe, keep people away until specially trained teams arrive. It is also important to identify potential exit routes from the scene in the event a hazard becomes life threatening to you or your patients and to wear appropriate personal protective equipment (PPE).

YOU are the EMR — CASE 2

It is a cold day in February when you are dispatched to a two-story house for a report of a sick child. As you and your partner enter the front door, you detect a slight odor. The boy's mother appears to be approximately 35 years old. She tells you that her 9-year-old son has been feeling sick. He has a headache and has been sleeping a lot. She tells you she was going to take the child to see a physician, but she also began experiencing a headache and has been feeling increasingly sick. She thinks she needs to see a physician also. She also tells you that she has been feeling light-headed in the last few minutes.

1. What are the first actions that you should take?
2. What additional resources do you need?

Safety

Never enter an enclosed space unless you have received proper training and are equipped with self-contained breathing apparatus (SCBA).

Determine the Mechanism of Injury or Nature of Illness

Patients generally can be divided into two main categories: those who have a sudden illness and those who sustain trauma. **Trauma** is the term used for any injury to a patient. The injury may be major or minor. Some incidents that cause trauma include falls, motor vehicle crashes, and sports-related injuries. The cause of the trauma is referred to as the mechanism of injury (MOI). In contrast, the cause of a sudden illness is referred to as the nature of the illness (NOI). Examples of sudden illnesses include heart attacks, strokes, asthma, and gallbladder conditions. If you can determine the MOI or NOI, you can sometimes predict what care the patient will require.

As you approach the scene, look for clues that may indicate how the incident happened (**FIGURE 9-3**). For example, a ladder lying on the ground next to a spilled bucket of paint most likely indicates that the patient fell from the ladder and may have sustained bone fractures or head or spinal injury. If the incident is a vehicle crash, knowing what type of crash occurred makes it possible to anticipate the types of injuries that may be present. For example, a rollover crash may result in different injuries than a vehicle that has collided head-on with a tree. It is also possible to anticipate injuries by examining the extent of damage to a vehicle. If the windshield is broken, look for head and spine injuries; if the steering wheel is bent, check for a chest injury. See Chapter 15, *Injuries to Muscles and Bones*, for more information on MOIs that result in musculoskeletal injuries.

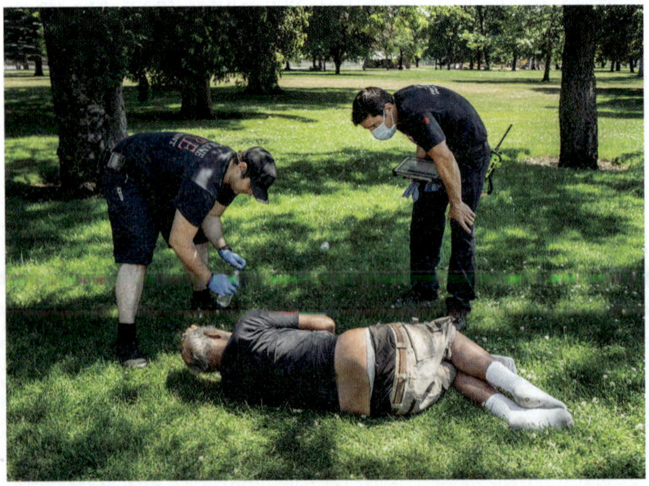

FIGURE 9-3 Determine the mechanism of injury, or MOI.
© Colin Mulvany/The Spokesman-Review/AP Photo

Although it is often helpful to consider whether the patient's problem is caused by trauma or sudden illness, avoid jumping to conclusions. Some patients need to be treated for both trauma and sudden illness.

Street Smarts

Always lift deployed airbags to note any damage to the structures underneath. Remember some cars have multiple airbags that may be located in different places to protect the knees, the head, or the torso. Multiple airbags may deploy in a crash.

Ask the patient (if alert), family members, or bystanders for additional information about the MOI or the NOI. This may provide you with important trauma or medical information that you can use to assist the patient. You can use the same type of overview that gives you information at the scene of an incident to help provide you with information about a patient's condition. Do not, however, rule out any injury without conducting a secondary assessment of the entire body of the patient. The mechanism of the accident may provide clues, but it cannot be used to determine what injuries are present in a particular patient. Using the previous example, the house painter may have fallen from the ladder because he had a heart attack.

Words of Wisdom

The five-step patient assessment sequence gives the information about the patient in a logical order. It allows you to assess the most critical factors first. Although you may have to vary the order of the steps somewhat for certain patients, you should generally try to follow this order. When caring for a trauma patient, modify the sequence slightly. Perform the scene size-up and the primary assessment just like you do for a medical patient. However, when examining a trauma patient, perform the secondary assessment before taking the patient's history. By performing the secondary assessment of the entire body before the history, you gain information about the patient's injuries. In trauma situations, this is often more important than obtaining the history.

Determine the Number of Patients

Check to see if there is more than one patient. Then determine the total number of patients who need emergency care. Call for additional assistance when there are multiple patients. It may be necessary to sort patients into groups according to the severity of their injuries to determine which patients should be treated and transported first. The topic of triage, or patient sorting, is covered more thoroughly in Chapter 19, *Incident Management*.

Consider Additional Resources

Many kinds of resources may be needed at the scene of an emergency. These resources include additional EMS units for treatment and transport; law enforcement personnel for traffic control or crowd control; fire department units for spilled fuel, fire, or extrication; utility company personnel for damaged utility lines; and wrecker operators for vehicle removal. As you prepare to make your initial report to the dispatcher, you may find it easier to report on the need for additional resources at the same time you report on the number of patients. Remember that your dispatcher cannot see the emergency scene. The only information the dispatcher has is the information you see and then report.

Words of Wisdom

Many of the same technologic advances that have enabled telemedicine have been adopted by 9-1-1 call centers. Many centers now use software that allows callers to share the video and camera features from their smartphones. These images can then be shared with emergency responders. For example, a person calling to report an unresponsive person in a public park could share video of the person's location, which could then be shared with responders via their vehicle's mobile data terminal, thus allowing the crew to more quickly locate the patient. This software incorporates other technology, such as artificial intelligence, to further improve the dispatcher's ability to immediately assist callers, triage calls (if the call center is experiencing a high call volume), gather information for responders, translate languages, and provide further services that are useful for quality management, such as taking accurate transcriptions, analyzing dispatcher performance, and identifying geographic patterns in calls.

Take Standard Precautions

Before arriving at the scene, prepare yourself by anticipating the types of standard precautions for infectious diseases that may be required. You should always have gloves readily available and use them. Consider whether the use of additional protection, such as eye protection, gowns, or masks, may be necessary. Try to anticipate your needs for equipment to ensure that you and your patients are well protected from exposure to infectious diseases. Regardless of the standard precautions you take, wash your hands thoroughly after contact with a patient or contaminated materials. See Chapter 2, *Workforce Safety and Wellness*, for more information on standard precautions.

Words of Wisdom

If you determine that additional resources are required, call for further assistance before beginning to treat the patient or patients. It will take time for more help to arrive, so the sooner you request aid, the better. In addition, you may be unable to call for help if you are already involved in patient care, such as controlling bleeding, which can be detrimental to the patient's chance for recovery.

YOU are the EMR — CASE 3

You are riding third for station 403 as part of your required clinical rotation hours. Your team is dispatched to a vehicle versus pedestrian collision in the parking lot of the local supermarket. On arrival, your team ensures that the scene is safe. The paramedic in charge requests that you hold the patient's head to manually stabilize the patient's spine.

1. Identify scene safety issues that you should consider when you arrive at the scene of a vehicle crash.
2. Why do you think manual stabilization of the spine is necessary for the patient in this incident?

Patient Assessment

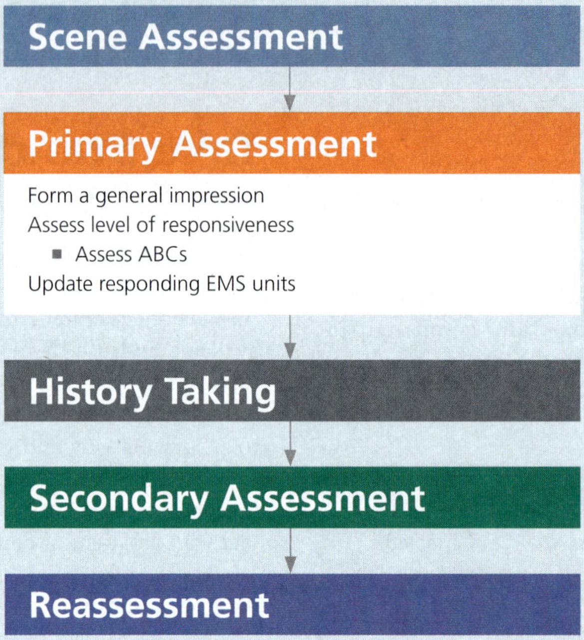

Primary Assessment

The second part of the patient assessment sequence is the **primary assessment**. This is sometimes called the primary patient assessment or the initial patient assessment. The purpose of the primary assessment is to identify and treat life threats. Life threats are defined as problems with the patient's airway, breathing, and circulation (the ABCs). It is important to quickly identify any life-threatening conditions and take immediate actions to correct these conditions. Notice that the primary assessment consists of evaluating the same functions that you evaluate when you are beginning to perform cardiopulmonary resuscitation (CPR).

The first step of the primary assessment is to form a general impression of the patient. You can do this as you approach the patient. The second step of the primary assessment is to determine the patient's level of responsiveness. The third step of the primary assessment consists of three parts: checking and correcting life-threatening problems connected to the ABCs. The fourth and final step of the primary assessment is to update responding EMS units about the patient's condition.

Form a General Impression

The general impression consists of those things you notice about the patient as you approach. If possible, always approach from in front of the patient so that the patient does not startle and turn their head. Note the sex, size or weight, and the approximate age of the patient. Look for clues that help determine whether the patient has experienced trauma or illness. If you are unsure if the patient has sustained an injury, err on the side of caution and treat the patient as a trauma patient. The patient's position or the sounds they are making may also help indicate to you the nature of the emergency. Talk to the patient to gain insight into the patient's level of consciousness. A quick look at the patient's face will often give you an idea of whether they are experiencing pain. Although your first impression is valuable, keep an open mind and do not let it block out later information that may lead you in another direction (tunnel vision).

Assess the Level of Responsiveness

The first part of determining the patient's level of responsiveness is to introduce yourself. Many patients will be alert and able to interact with you. As you approach the patient, tell the patient your name and the agency you are with (**FIGURE 9-4**). For example, say: "I'm Jesse Phillips from the sheriff's department, and I'm here to help you." This simple introduction helps establish:

- Your reason for being at the scene
- The fact that you will be helping the patient
- The patient's level of consciousness

The introduction is your first contact with the patient. You should be able to put the patient at ease by conveying that you are a trained person ready to help. Next, ask the patient's name and then use it when talking with the patient, family, or friends. The patient's response helps you determine their level of responsiveness. Avoid telling the patient that everything will be all right.

> **Safety**
>
> Remember, performing a patient assessment may bring you in contact with the patient's blood, other body fluids, and waste products. Wear approved gloves and PPE and take other standard precautions to prevent exposure to infected body fluids. Follow the latest standards from the Centers for Disease Control and Prevention and Occupational Safety and Health Administration.

Even if the patient appears to be unresponsive, introduce yourself and talk with the patient as you conduct the rest of the patient assessment. Many patients who appear to be unresponsive can hear your voice and need the reassurance it carries. Do not say anything you do not want the patient to hear!

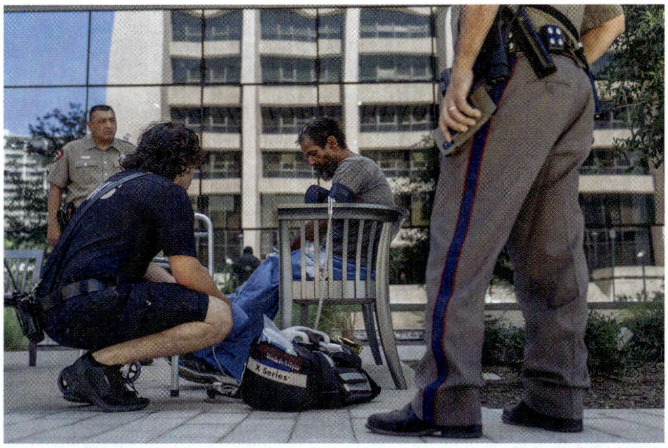

FIGURE 9-4 As you approach the patient, introduce yourself. If a patient appears unresponsive, gently touch or shake the patient's shoulder to get a response.

© Brandon Bell/Getty Images News/Getty Images

If a patient appears to be unresponsive, speak to the patient in a tone of voice that is loud enough for the patient to hear. If the patient does not respond to the sound of your voice, gently touch the patient or shake the patient's shoulder to see if you can generate a response from the patient.

The patient's level of consciousness can range from fully alert to unresponsive. Describe the patient's level of consciousness using the **AVPU scale**:

A **Alert.** An alert patient is able to answer the following questions accurately and appropriately: What is your name? Where are you? What is today's date? A patient who can answer these questions is said to be "alert and oriented."

V **Verbal.** A patient is said to be "responsive to verbal stimuli" if the patient opens their eyes and reacts only to loud sounds.

P **Pain.** A patient who is responsive to pain will not respond to a verbal stimulus but will move or cry out in response to pain. Response to pain is tested by pinching the patient's earlobe or pinching the patient's skin over the collarbone. A patient who withdraws from the painful stimulus is said to be "responsive to painful stimuli."

U **Unresponsive.** An unresponsive patient will not respond to either a verbal or a painful stimulus. This patient's condition is described as "unresponsive."

If the patient has sustained any type of major trauma, provide manual stabilization of the patient's neck as soon as possible. This step will prevent any further injury to the neck and spinal column.

> **Special Populations**
>
> **Assessing Responsiveness of Infants and Children**
>
> Infants and children may not have the verbal skills to answer the questions used to assess responsiveness in adults. Therefore, you should assess how the children and infants interact with their environment and with their parents or caregivers and understand appropriate responses for various ages.

Rapidly Assess the ABCs to Identify Life Threats

When assessing the ABCs, the first step is to check the airway and correct any serious problems, such as a blocked airway. The second step is to check for breathing and correct any serious breathing problems, such as a lack of breathing or open chest injuries that interfere with adequate breathing. The third step is to check the status of circulation and correct any life-threatening circulation problems, such as applying pressure to external bleeding. With practice, you will learn to check the patient's circulation and breathing at the same time.

Note that the ABC sequence is modified if you suspect cardiac arrest in an unresponsive person or if you are aware of life-threatening external bleeding. These conditions may be obvious on arrival or may be communicated to you en route by dispatch. When a patient is in cardiac arrest, you must first check for circulation followed by airway and breathing (CAB). This sequence minimizes the time to the beginning of chest compressions. When the patient is experiencing life-threatening external bleeding, you must first control the bleeding (such as by applying a tourniquet); in this case, the sequence becomes XABC, where the *X* stands for life-threatening eXternal bleeding (also referred to as eXsanguination).

Assess the Airway

If the patient is alert and able to answer questions without difficulty, then the airway is open. If the patient is unresponsive to verbal stimuli, then assistance may be needed to maintain an open airway. If the patient is unresponsive, open the airway by using the head tilt–chin lift maneuver for patients with medical problems and use the jaw-thrust maneuver (without tilting the patient's head) for patients who have sustained trauma. After the airway is open, inspect it for foreign bodies or secretions. Clear the airway as needed, using finger sweeps (if the obstruction is visible) or suction. You may need to insert an airway adjunct to keep the airway open. See Chapter 7, *Airway Management*, for information about airway adjuncts.

Assess Breathing

If the patient is alert, assess the rate and quality of the patient's breathing by looking at the chest. Does the chest rise and fall with each breath, or does the patient appear to be short of breath? If the patient is unresponsive, check for breathing by placing the side of your face next to the patient's nose and mouth while looking at the chest. You should be able to hear the sounds of breathing, see the chest rise and fall, and even feel the movement of air on your cheek (**FIGURE 9-5**). If the patient is having difficulty breathing or if you hear unusual breath sounds, check for an object in the patient's mouth, such as food, vomitus, dentures, gum, chewing tobacco, or broken teeth, and remove it.

If you cannot detect any movement of the chest and no sounds of air are coming from the nose and mouth, breathing is absent. Take immediate steps to check the patient's carotid pulse to assess whether there is any circulation. This step is described in the next section. If a carotid pulse is present but the patient is not breathing or is only gasping, perform rescue breathing. If you suspect trauma, protect the cervical spine by keeping the patient's head in a neutral position and using the jaw-thrust maneuver to open the airway. Maintain manual cervical stabilization until definitive spinal motion restriction has been established. These procedures are covered in Chapter 7, *Airway Management*.

Assess Circulation

Next, check the patient's circulation (heartbeat). If the patient is unresponsive, check the carotid pulse (**FIGURE 9-6**). Place your index and middle fingers together and touch the larynx (Adam's apple) in the patient's neck. (The pulse can also be checked using three fingers.) Then slide your fingers off the larynx toward the patient's ear until you feel a slight notch. Practice this maneuver until you are able to find a carotid pulse within 5 seconds of touching the patient's larynx. If you cannot feel the carotid pulse with your fingers in 10 seconds, begin CPR. CPR is covered in Chapter 8, *Professional Rescuer CPR*.

If the patient is alert, assess the radial pulse rather than the carotid pulse (**FIGURE 9-7**). Place your index and middle fingers on the patient's wrist at the thumb side. Practice taking the radial pulse often to develop this skill.

Next, quickly check the patient for any severe external bleeding. If you discover severe bleeding, you must take immediate action to control it by applying direct pressure over the wound or by applying a tourniquet. These procedures are covered in Chapter 14, *Bleeding, Shock, and Soft-Tissue Injuries*.

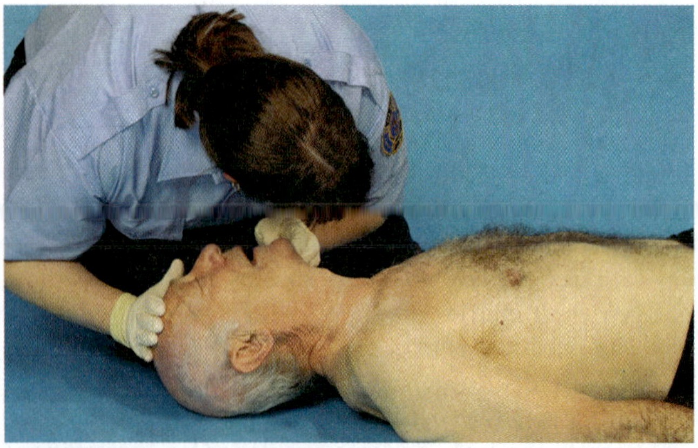

FIGURE 9-5 Check the patient's breathing.

© Jones & Bartlett Learning. Courtesy of MIEMSS.

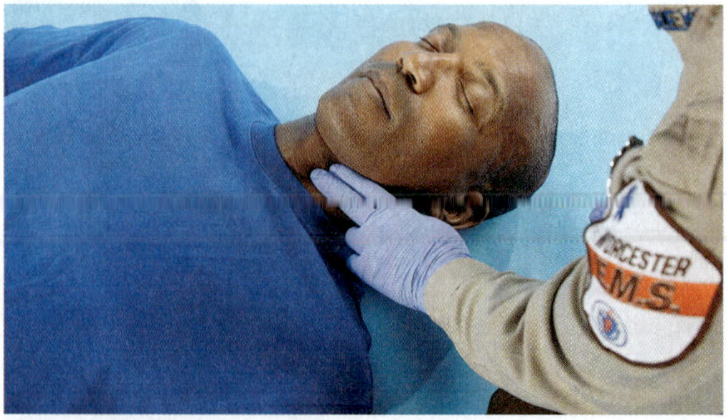

FIGURE 9-6 Check an unresponsive patient's circulation by checking the carotid pulse.

© Jones & Bartlett Learning

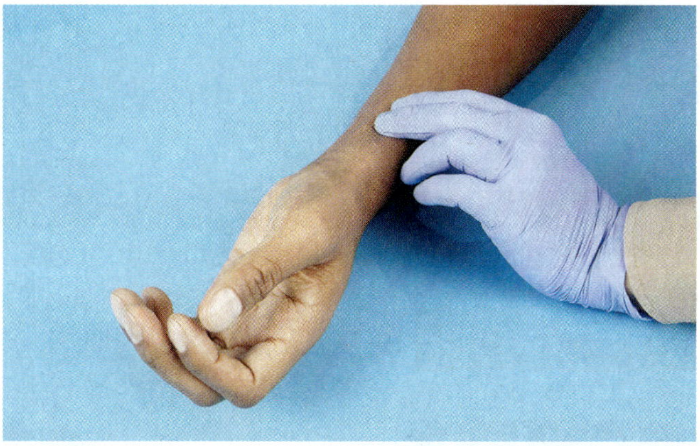

FIGURE 9-7 Take the radial pulse if the patient is alert.
© Jones & Bartlett Learning

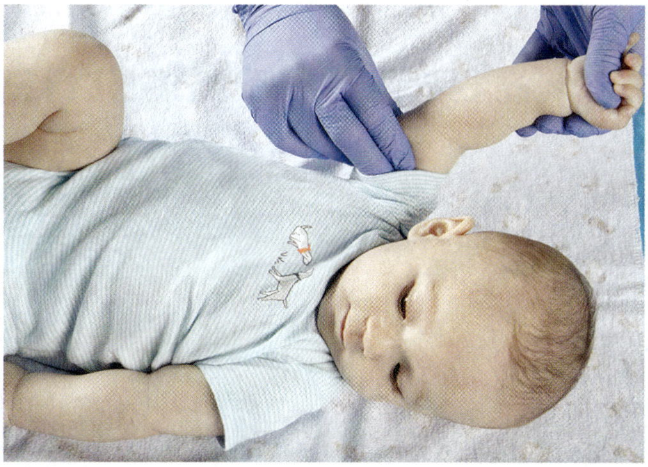

FIGURE 9-8 Take the brachial pulse if the patient is an infant.
© Jones & Bartlett Learning

Special Populations

Assessing Circulation in an Infant

To assess circulation in an infant, check the brachial pulse, located on the inside of the upper arm. You can feel the brachial pulse by placing your index and middle fingers on the inside of the infant's arm halfway between the shoulder and the elbow (**FIGURE 9-8**). Check for 5 to 10 seconds.

Quickly assess the patient's skin color and temperature. This assessment will help you determine whether the patient is experiencing internal bleeding and shock. It is important to check the color of the patient's skin when you arrive at the scene so that you can monitor the patient's skin for color changes as time goes on.

Assessment of skin color should take into account the patient's baseline skin color. Remember that changes to skin color will depending on the individual's baseline skin color and therefore will present differently from one person to another. For patients with deeply pigmented skin, color changes may be more apparent in the fingernail beds, in the whites of the eyes (conjunctiva), on the palm of the hand, or inside the mouth.

Skin color is described as follows:

- **Normal.** *Normal* refers to the patient's baseline skin color. Remember, it is a relative term and varies for each person. Often, someone on scene who knows the patient can tell you whether the patient's skin color looks "normal" or not.
- **Pale.** White or light skin coloration indicates decreased circulation to that part of the body or to all of the body. This could be caused by blood loss, poor blood flow, or low body temperature. Brown skin will appear yellow-brown, and very dark or black skin will appear ash gray. In these patients, pallor may be easier to detect by examining the mucous membranes, which may appear ash gray.
- **Flushed.** Red skin coloration indicates excess circulation to that part of the body. In patients with dark skin, it may present as skin that is darker than the person's baseline color.
- **Blue.** Blue skin coloration, called **cyanosis**, indicates lack of oxygen and possible airway problems. In patients with dark skin, it may be seen on the palms, soles, or conjunctiva; also, the nail beds, lips, and tongue will be gray or white.
- **Yellow.** Yellow skin coloration, called jaundice, indicates liver problems. In patients with dark skin, this finding may be easier to detect in the oral mucosa, especially the hard palate.

Update Responding EMS Units

In some EMS systems, you will be expected to update responding EMS units about the condition of your patient. This report should include the age and sex of the patient, the chief complaint, the level of responsiveness, and the status of the ABCs. This update helps other responders know what to expect when they arrive at the scene.

Because many conditions present an immediate threat to life, you should try to perform all four steps of the primary assessment quickly as you make contact with the patient.

Patient Assessment

Scene Assessment

Primary Assessment

History Taking

Investigate the chief complaint (SAMPLE history)

Secondary Assessment

Reassessment

History Taking

Investigate the Chief Complaint

As you perform the primary assessment, you will often form an impression of the patient's **chief complaint**. It is important to acknowledge the patient's primary problem or chief complaint and provide reassurance (**FIGURE 9-9**). An alert patient will often report a problem that is producing great pain or direct you to an injury that has obvious bleeding. However, keep in mind that this injury may not be the most serious problem the patient has sustained. Do not allow an alert patient's comments to distract you from completing the patient assessment sequence. Acknowledge the patient's chief complaint by saying something like, "Yes, I can see that your arm appears to be broken, but let me finish checking you completely in case there are any other injuries. I will then treat your injured arm." In an unresponsive patient, the primary "complaint" is unresponsiveness.

The purpose of obtaining a history is to gather a systematic account of the patient's current condition, past medical conditions, and events leading up to the present situation (**FIGURE 9-10**). It is important to question patients who are

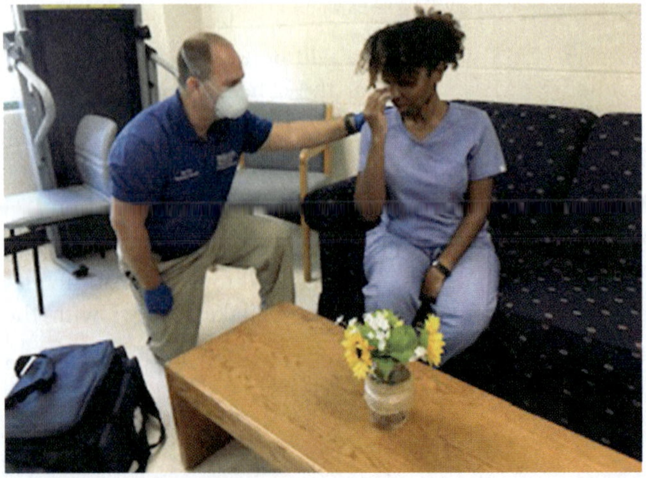

FIGURE 9-9 Acknowledge the patient's chief complaint.
Courtesy of Rhonda Hunt.

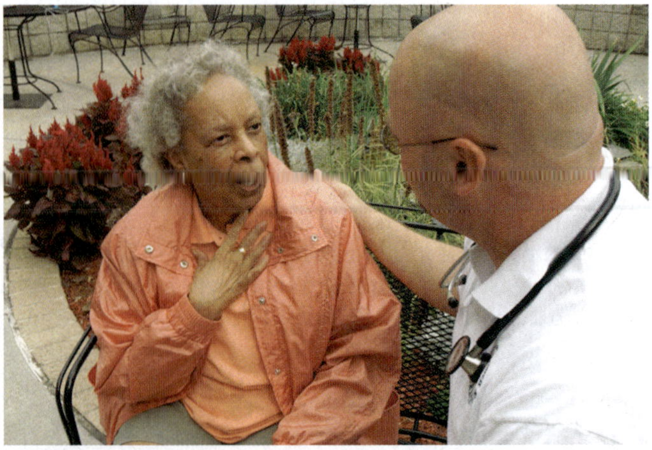

FIGURE 9-10 Obtain the patient's SAMPLE history.
© Jones & Bartlett Learning. Courtesy of MIEMSS.

alert and oriented in a clear and systematic manner to gain as much information as possible. Obtaining a history of the current illness or injury is an important part of the patient assessment sequence for all patients, and it will help tie together your findings from the primary assessment.

Words of Wisdom

Never let gathering a history interfere with your care of a critical patient. Patient care comes first!

Obtain SAMPLE History

To obtain a patient history in a consistent and thorough manner, remember the acronym SAMPLE, which stands for Signs and symptoms, Allergies, Medications, Pertinent past medical history, Last oral intake, Events leading up to the illness or injury. By using this easy-to-remember acronym, you can gain the information you need about past medical history as well as the events leading to the current episode of illness or injury.

The **SAMPLE history** provides a framework of pertinent questions. Remember to ask the patient one question at a time. Give the patient time to answer before you ask the next question. Listen carefully and maintain eye contact to let the patient know you are listening to the response. Designate one EMS clinician to ask questions to avoid confusing the patient.

TABLE 9-1 summarizes the SAMPLE acronym.

If the patient is not alert and oriented or is otherwise unable to answer your questions (for example, a young child

TABLE 9-1 SAMPLE Medical History

S	Signs and symptoms of the injury or illness. These should be the reasons that caused the patient to call for emergency medical services. Patients should describe signs and symptoms in their own words. Key considerations: • What signs and symptoms occurred at the beginning of the event? • What signs and symptoms is the patient experiencing now? • Is the patient experiencing any pain? If so, ask the patient to describe it.
A	Allergies. Patients may be allergic to medications, food, or airborne particles. Key considerations: • Does the patient have any known allergies? • How does the patient react to known allergens? • If the patient reports having no allergies, communicate this to other EMS personnel.
M	Medications. The patient may be taking prescribed medications, over-the-counter medications, herbal supplements, or illicit drugs. Key considerations: • What is the purpose of the patient's prescription medications? • What other drugs or supplements is the patient taking, and why? • Does the patient have a list of these medications that you can obtain and give to other EMS responders?
P	Pertinent past medical history. Try to keep this part of the history relevant to the current condition. A cardiac bypass operation may indicate cardiovascular disease; however, an appendectomy 10 years ago is probably not relevant to the current condition. Key considerations: • Is the patient currently under the care of a physician? • Does the patient have any existing medical conditions, such as diabetes or a heart condition? • Has the patient had a serious illness or injury or a recent hospitalization?
L	Last oral intake and last menstrual cycle. Key considerations: • When was the last time the patient had anything to eat or drink, and what did they eat or drink? • If the patient is experiencing abdominal pain, what (and how much) did the patient have to eat and drink in the past few hours? • If the patient is female, when was the last menstrual cycle? One or more missed cycles for a patient who is usually regular may point to the source of the problem.
E	Events associated with or leading up to this illness or injury. Knowing these events will help you put together the pieces of the medical history puzzle. Let patients describe these events in their own words. Key considerations: • What was the patient doing when the symptoms of this event started or when the injury occurred? • Did the patient notice anything unusual in the hours prior to the start of the illness or when the injury happened?

© Jones & Bartlett Learning

or a patient with dementia), a family member, friend, or co-worker may be able to answer your questions. Look for important information on a medical identification necklace, bracelet, or card, or an app on their phone. The information you gain will help determine what steps you need to take to treat the patient. Next, communicate this information to other EMS personnel to help them in their assessment and treatment of the patient.

Words of Wisdom

Pay particular attention to patients who tell you their pain feels just like the kidney stone episode they experienced last year or their pain feels just like the heart attack they had 2 years ago. Patients who have experienced a certain kind of pain before are often correct in identifying that pain if it recurs.

YOU are the EMR — CASE 4

You are working as an EMR for an outdoor summer camp. You receive a radio call that one of the campers is feeling sick and weak approximately one-half mile (less than 1 km) from the camp. You and your partner respond to the scene. You note the scene is safe. An 11-year-old girl is sitting on a log. The camp counselor tells you that they were returning from a 3-mile (5-km) hike around the lake when one of the campers, Mattie, started to lag behind the group. The counselor encouraged her to sit down on the log. Mattie states that she feels weak. You note that her pulse is slightly rapid and weak and that she is sweating.

1. What is Mattie's chief complaint?
2. Why is the SAMPLE history important when caring for a patient who has a vague chief complaint?

Patient Assessment

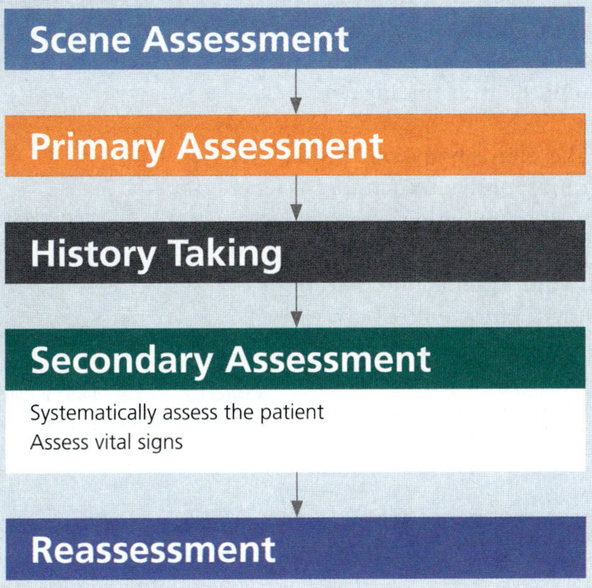

Secondary Assessment

After you have completed the primary assessment and stabilized any life-threatening conditions, perform a **secondary assessment** (the physical examination) of the patient from head to toe to assess for any other conditions. Vital signs are noted as part of the secondary assessment. They may be obtained before the physical examination is completed or after the examination is done. They can also be obtained by a second person while other parts of the patient assessment are being completed.

Information about signs and symptoms and vital signs is presented in this section because you need to understand how to measure some of these vital signs to provide a complete secondary assessment. The physical examination you conduct during the secondary assessment helps you to locate and begin initial management of the signs and symptoms of illness or injury. After you complete the secondary assessment, review any positive signs and symptoms of injury or illness. This review will give you a better picture of the patient's overall condition.

Signs and Symptoms

In a careful and systematic patient assessment, you need to understand the difference between a **sign** and a **symptom**. Simply put, a sign is something about the patient you can see, feel, or measure for yourself. A symptom is something the patient tells you about their condition, such as, "My back hurts" or "I think I am going to vomit." It is not visible or measurable. You need to be able to assess any signs and report them systematically when you transfer care. You also need to be able to understand and report the symptoms that the patient reports.

Systematically Assess the Patient

As you perform the secondary assessment, look and feel for the following signs of injury: deformities, open injuries, tenderness, and swelling. Use the mnemonic DOTS to remember these signs:

D Deformities
O Open injuries
T Tenderness
S Swelling

Alternatively, some EMS clinicians find it helpful to use the mnemonic DCAP-BTLS when performing a full body examination to help them remember the patient's injuries:

D Deformities
C Contusions (bruises)
A Abrasions
P Punctures or Penetrations
B Burns
T Tenderness
L Lacerations
S Swelling

Secondary Assessment of the Entire Body

Conduct a thorough, hands-on, secondary assessment of the entire body in a logical, head-to-toe, systematic manner. It is important to conduct the examination the same way each time to be sure you inspect all areas of the body for injuries. Use a clear, concise format to communicate your findings to other medical personnel.

The secondary assessment of the entire body can be done whether the patient is alert or unresponsive. Watch the reactions of an alert patient during your examination. If you detect signs of discomfort, you may want to ask what the patient is feeling as you proceed with your examination. Remember that your secondary assessment of the entire body is the main focus of this part of the patient assessment. It is permissible to question the patient during your assessment, but do not let the questions distract you from completing a thorough assessment.

> **Treatment**
>
> Continue talking to the patient throughout the entire patient assessment. Tell the patient what you are doing and why, even if they are not alert.

If the patient is unresponsive, it is vital that you assess the ABCs during the primary assessment. After you have addressed any problems with the patient's airway, breathing, and pulse, begin a secondary assessment of the entire body. Assessing an unresponsive patient is difficult because the patient cannot cooperate or tell you where something hurts, although your assessment often will elicit grimaces or moans.

> **Words of Wisdom**
>
> As your hands move down the patient's scalp and onto the neck, check for the presence of an emergency medical identification neck chain. Look for medical identification (MedicAlert) emblems as an indication of the patient's medical history. The internationally recognized symbol shown in **FIGURE 9-11** is found on necklaces, arm bracelets, ankle bracelets, watches, rings, and wallet cards and is carried by people who have a medical condition that warrants special attention if they become ill or injured. These items serve as a patient directive that allows EMS personnel to access the patient's stored medical information by calling the MedicAlert Foundation. Each MedicAlert member has a unique, secure patient identifier engraved at the bottom of the emblem. By wearing this emblem, the patient has consented to the release of information to attending medical personnel. The stored patient history can include conditions, allergies, medications and dosages, and implanted devices. Note that some of these bracelets, or other forms of identification, include QR codes or USB flash drives that provide the stored information. If you find such a warning on a patient, it is your responsibility to give this information to the next person in the EMS system.

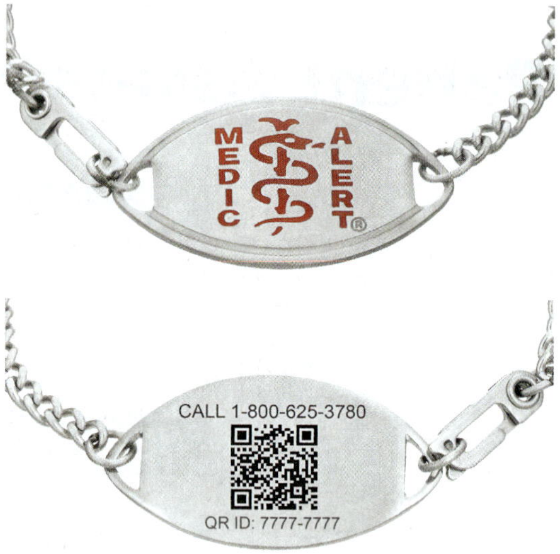

FIGURE 9-11 Medical identification is found on wrist and ankle bracelets, necklaces, watches, rings, and wallet cards.
Used with permission from MedicAlert Foundation.

Assume all unresponsive, injured patients have spinal injuries. Manually stabilize the head and spine to minimize movement during the patient examination. It is essential to stabilize all injured, unresponsive patients on a **backboard** or another effective spinal stabilization device before transporting them.

> **Treatment**
>
> Be careful not to move the neck or head during your assessment if there is any possibility of spinal injury!

Follow the steps in **SKILL DRILL 9-1** to perform a secondary assessment of the entire body.

When you reach the final step of the secondary assessment, assessment of the extremities, note that the considerations and procedures differ between the upper and lower extremities. Each **upper extremity** consists of the **arm**, the forearm, the wrist, and the hand. The arm extends from the shoulder to the elbow; the forearm extends from the elbow to the wrist. Examine one upper extremity at a time as follows:

1. Observe the extremity. Start by looking at its position. Is it in a normal or an abnormal position? Does it look broken (deformed) to you? Compare it to the opposite extremity.
2. Examine for tenderness. Encircle the upper extremity with your hands. Work from the shoulder downward to the hand. Firmly squeeze the limb to locate any possible fractures.
3. Check for movement. Take the patient's hand in yours and ask the patient to squeeze your hand. Squeezing is usually painful for a patient who has a fracture or other injury. If an alert patient cannot squeeze your hand, assume the extremity is seriously injured or paralyzed.

SKILL DRILL 9-1

Performing a Secondary Assessment

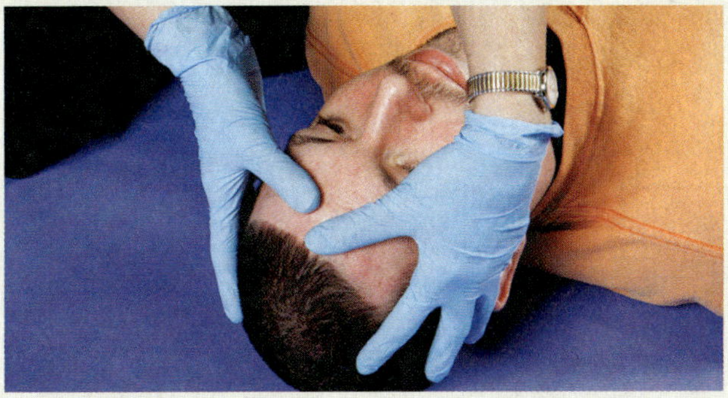

STEP 1 Assess the head. Use both hands to thoroughly examine all areas of the scalp. Do not move the patient's head! This precaution is especially important if the patient is unresponsive or has sustained a spinal injury. Injuries to the head tend to bleed excessively. Be sure to find the actual wound; do not be fooled by areas of matted, bloody hair. If necessary, remove the patient's eyeglasses and put them in a safe place. Be considerate of the patient. If the patient is wearing a wig, it may be necessary to remove the hairpiece to complete the head examination. Be sure to check the entire head for bumps, areas of tenderness, and bleeding.

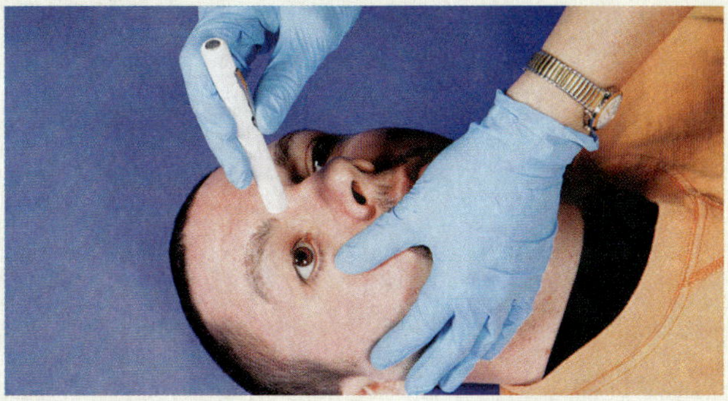

STEP 2 Assess the eyes. Cover one of the patient's eyes for 5 seconds. Then quickly open the eyelid and watch the pupil, the dark part at the center of the eye. The normal reaction of the pupil is to constrict (get smaller) within approximately 1 second. If you are examining a patient's eyes at night or in the dark, use a flashlight to assess the pupillary reaction to light. A pupil that fails to react to light or pupils that are unequal in size may be important diagnostic signs; report this information to personnel at the next level of medical care.

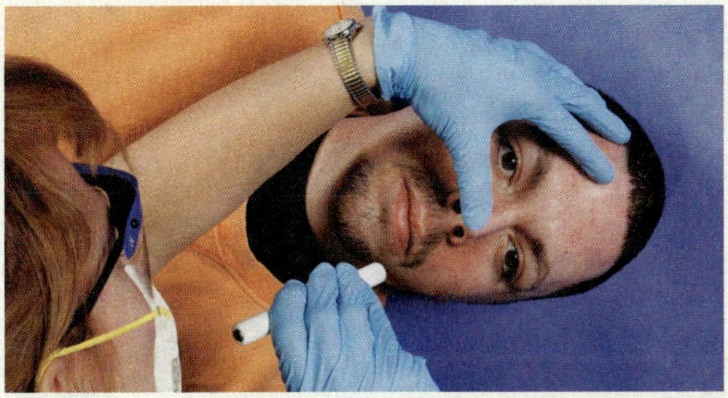

STEP 3 Assess the nose. Assess the nose for tenderness or deformity, which may indicate a broken nose. Check to see if there is any blood or fluid coming from the nose.

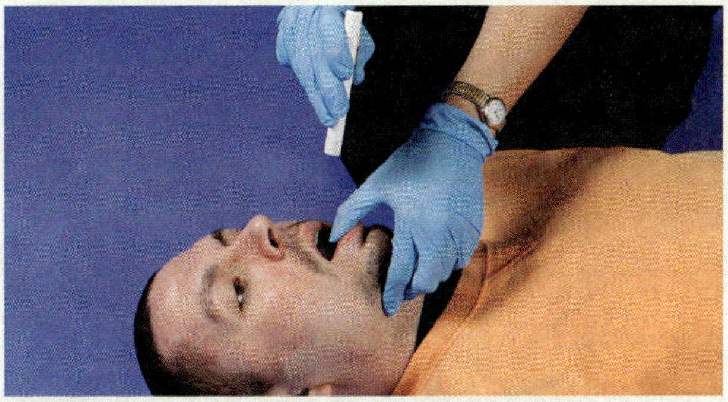

STEP 4 Assess the mouth. Your first assessment of the mouth should have taken place when you checked to see whether the patient was breathing. Now recheck the mouth for foreign objects or fluid. Be sure to carefully clear away any material that obstructs the patient's airway. Use finger sweeps if the obstruction is visible or a suction machine if it is available. In addition, be ready to manage any vomiting. It is important to prevent **aspiration** (inhalation) of vomitus into the lungs.

(continues)

SKILL DRILL 9-1 *(continued)*

Performing a Secondary Assessment

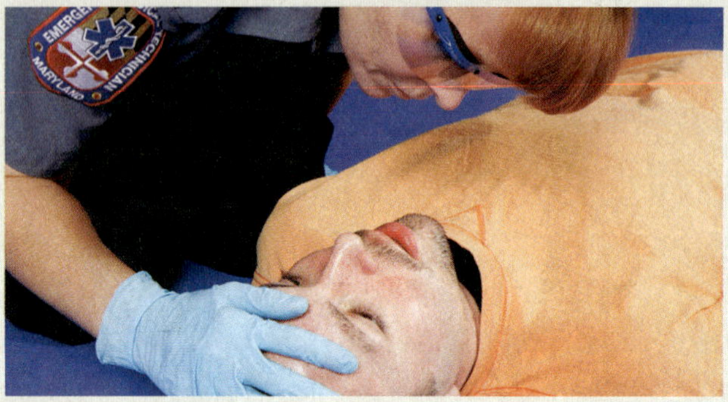

STEP 5 **Check for unusual breath odors.** Use your sense of smell to aid in the assessment. A patient who has diabetes may have a fruity breath odor. Do not allow the presence of alcohol on the patient's breath to change the way you treat the patient. In fact, if you detect the smell of alcohol, you should conduct an especially careful physical examination, particularly if the patient appears to be severely injured. Remember to place any unresponsive patient who has not sustained trauma in the recovery position. This position helps keep the patient's airway open and prevents aspiration of vomitus into the airway or lungs.

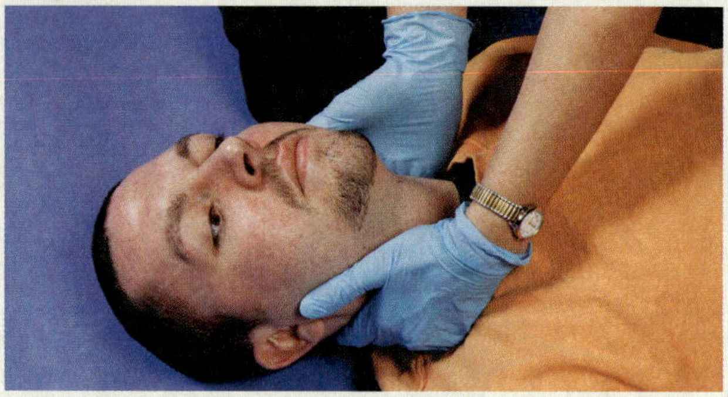

STEP 6 **Assess the neck and face.** Assess the neck carefully using both hands, one on each side of the patient's neck. Be sure to touch the vertebrae (the bony protrusions at the back of the neck) to see whether gentle pressure produces pain. Check the neck veins. Swollen (distended) neck veins may indicate heart conditions or major trauma to the chest. Examine the neck for a stoma (opening), which indicates that the patient is a neck breather. A neck breather is a person who has undergone a surgical procedure in which the airway above the stoma has been removed. The stoma may be the patient's only means of breathing, and the patient may not be able to speak normally. The stoma is often concealed behind an article of clothing or a bib.

While you are performing the hands-on assessment of the head and neck, note the color of the facial skin, its temperature, and whether it is moist or dry (**TABLE 9-2**). After you have completed the head examination, note any bumps, bruises, cuts, or other abnormalities.

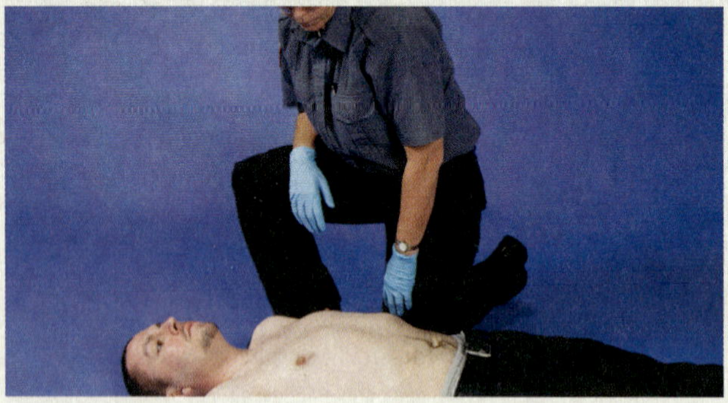

STEP 7 **Assess the work of breathing.** If the patient is alert, ask them to take a deep breath and tell you whether they feel any pain on **inhalation** or **exhalation**. Note whether the patient breathes with difficulty.

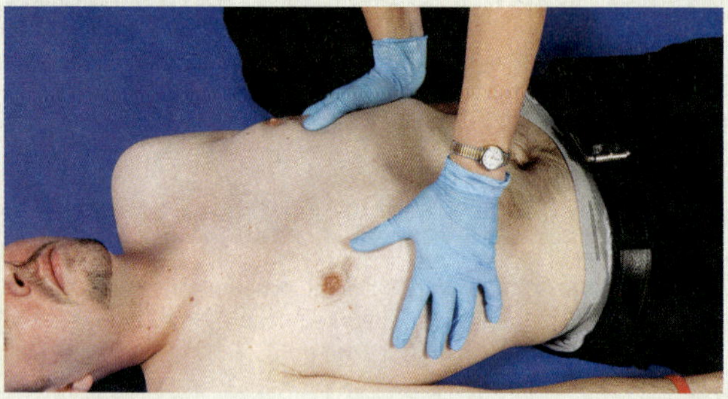

STEP 8 **Assess the chest for injury.** Look and listen for signs of difficult breathing such as coughing, wheezing, or frothy sputum in the mouth. It is important to look at both sides of the chest completely, noting any injuries, bleeding, or sections of the chest that move abnormally, unequally, or painfully. Unequal motion of one side or section of the chest may be a sign of a serious condition, called a **flail chest**, which can result from multiple rib **fractures**. Be sure to run your hands over all parts of the chest. Like the head and neck examinations, try to move the patient as little as possible while you assess the chest.

Apply firm but gentle pressure to the collarbone (**clavicle**) to check for fractures. Check the chest for fractured ribs by placing your hands on the chest and pushing down gently but firmly. Then put your hands on each side of the chest and push inward, gently squeezing the chest.

SKILL DRILL 9-1 *(continued)*

Performing a Secondary Assessment

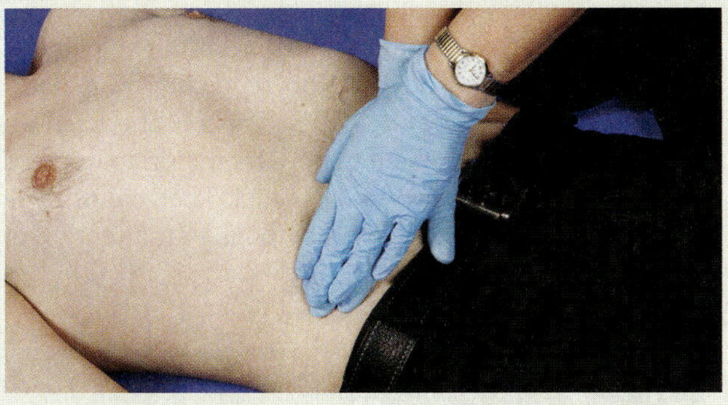

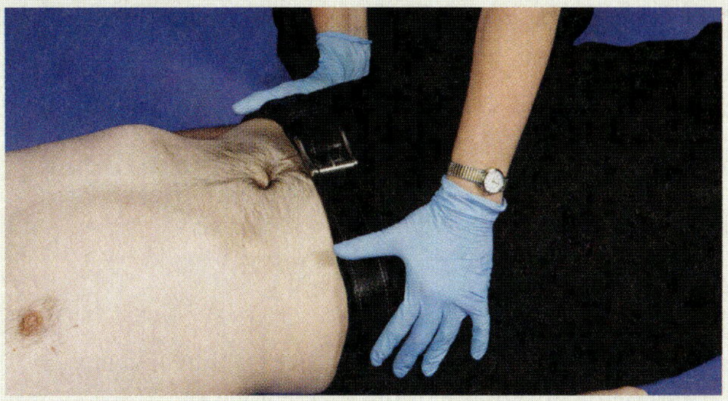

STEP 9 **Assess the abdomen.** Continue your assessment downward to the **abdomen** (stomach and groin). Look for any signs of external bleeding, penetrating injuries, or protruding parts, such as intestines. Ask the patient to relax the stomach muscles and observe whether the stomach remains rigid. Rigidity is often a sign of abdominal injury. Swelling is also a sign of abdominal injury.

Note whether the clothing has been soiled with urine or feces. This finding may be an important diagnostic sign for certain illnesses or injuries, such as stroke. Make sure you check the genital area for external injuries. Although both the patient and you may be socially uncomfortable during this examination, it must be done if there is any suspicion of injury.

STEP 10 **Assess the pelvis.** Next, check for fractures of the pelvis. First check for signs of obvious bruising, bleeding, or swelling. If no pain is reported by the patient, then gently press on the pelvic bones. If the patient reports pain or tenderness or if you note any movement, a severe injury may be present in this region.

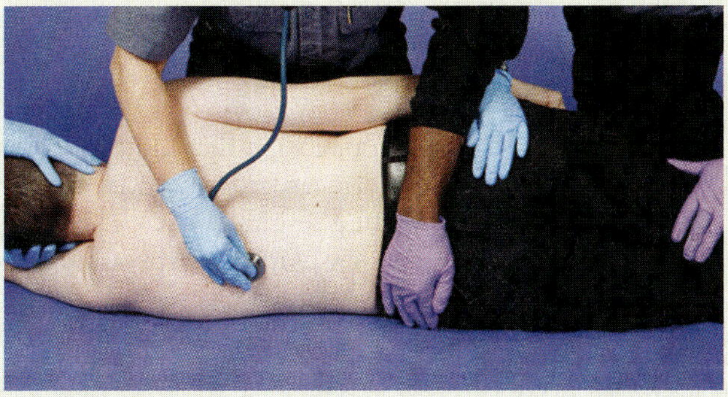

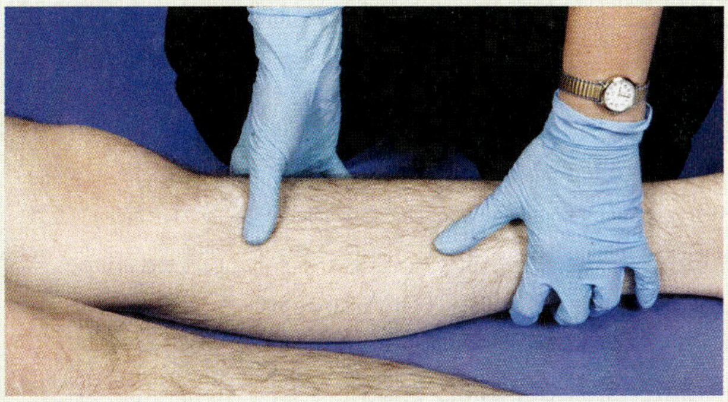

STEP 11 **Assess the back.** The patient's back should be checked one side of the back at a time. Move the patient as a unit, taking care to support the head and spine to keep them in proper alignment. As you check each side of the back, be sure that your hand goes all the way to the midline of the patient's body so you can feel the spinal column. Check half the back from one side, then switch sides and check the other side in the same manner. This ensures that no part of the back is missed during the examination. Also, look for any bleeding from the rectum. If the patient is lying on their side or stomach, it will be much easier to examine the patient's back. If the patient must be rolled onto a backboard, you can examine the patient's back while the patient is on their side. Do not wait for a backboard if doing so will delay your examination of the patient.

Remember that for patients with potential back or neck trauma, you will need to continue to stabilize the head and neck to prevent movement as you examine the back. You must have a second person available to provide cervical spine control before rolling the patient onto their side.

STEP 12 **Assess the extremities.** Do a systematic assessment of each extremity to determine whether there are any injuries. This examination consists of the following five steps:

1. Observe the extremity to determine whether there is any visible injury and compare it to the opposite extremity. Look for bleeding and deformity.
2. Examine for tenderness in each extremity by encircling it with both hands and gently, but firmly, squeezing each part of the limb. Watch the patient's face and listen to determine if the patient shows any signs of pain.
3. If no injury is found, ask the patient to move the extremity. Check for normal movement. Determine whether there is any pain when the patient moves the extremity.
4. Check for sensation by touching the bare skin of each extremity. See if the patient can feel your touch.
5. Assess the circulatory status of each extremity by checking for the presence of a distal pulse in that extremity and by checking for capillary refill (discussed later in this chapter).

© Jones & Bartlett Learning. Courtesy of MIEMSS.

TABLE 9-2 Skin Color[a]

Color	Term	Indicates
Red	Flushed	Fever or sunburn
White or light in color	Pale	Shock
Blue	Cyanotic	Airway obstruction
Yellow	Jaundiced	Liver disease

[a] Depending on the patient's baseline skin tone, from light to very dark, the degree to which you will be able to see these skin color changes, or the actual colors observed, will vary.

© Jones & Bartlett Learning

4. Check for sensation. Ask the patient if they feel any tingling or numbness in the extremity. Sensations such as tingling or numbness may be a sign of a spinal injury. Check for sensation by touching the palm of the patient's hand. See if the patient can feel your touch.
5. Assess the circulatory status. Check the patient's radial pulse. Absence of a radial pulse indicates blood vessel damage. Check the fingers for capillary refill. Check the color, temperature, and moisture of the hand.

Treatment

Do not ask the patient to move an extremity if you find any deformity or tenderness during your examination.

Each **lower extremity** consists of the thigh, the **leg**, the ankle, and the foot. The thigh extends from the hip to the knee. The leg extends from the knee to the ankle. Examine one lower extremity at a time, as follows:

1. Observe the extremity. Look at the position and shape of the lower extremity. Is it deformed? Is the foot rotated inward or outward? Compare it to the opposite extremity.
2. Examine for tenderness. Encircle the lower extremity with your hands, as you did with the upper extremities. Move from the groin to the foot. Be sure to make contact with all surfaces of the limb. Use firm but gentle pressure to identify tender (injured) areas.
3. Check for movement. Ask the patient to move the limb only if you have found no signs of injury in the first two steps. If there is a significant injury, movement most likely will be painful. If an alert patient cannot move the foot or toes, the limb is seriously injured or paralyzed.
4. Check for sensation. Ask the patient whether they can feel your touch as you examine the extremity. Tingling or numbness in a limb is a sign of spinal injury.
5. Assess circulatory status. Check the posterior tibial pulse, located just behind the ankle bone on the medial (inner) side of the ankle. Absence of this pulse indicates blood vessel damage, which is sometimes caused by fractures. Check the toes for capillary refill. Check the skin color, temperature, and moisture of the extremity.

Focused Exam of a Specific Area of the Body

A focused exam is generally performed on patients who have sustained nonsignificant MOIs or on responsive medical patients complaining of injury or illness to a specific area of the body. This type of examination is based on the chief complaint. For example, in a person reporting head pain, you should carefully and systematically assess the head and/or neurologic system. A person with a laceration to the arm may need to have only that arm evaluated. The goal of the exam of a specific area of the body is to focus your attention on the immediate problem.

Words of Wisdom

While you are examining patients, it is important to preserve patient privacy and to maintain body temperature. Patients who are in public places need to be covered with a sheet or blanket to maintain their privacy. It is often necessary to cover patients to preserve their body temperature. Ill or injured patients will often be cold even when it does not feel cold to you.

Assess Vital Signs

The patient's **vital signs** consist of respiration, pulse, blood pressure, skin condition, temperature, and oxygen saturation (if the means to measure it are available).

Respiration

The **respiratory rate** is a vital sign that indicates how fast the patient is breathing. It is measured as breaths per minute. In a normal adult, the resting respiratory rate is between 12 and 20 breaths/min. One cycle of inhaling (breathing in) and exhaling (breathing out) is counted as one breath (respiration). Count the patient's breaths for 1 minute to determine the respiratory rate.

Respirations may be rapid and shallow (characteristic of shock) or slow (characteristic of a stroke or drug overdose). Respirations may also be described as deep, wheezing, gasping, panting, snoring, noisy, or labored. If the patient is not breathing, respiration is described as absent, a condition that would have been addressed during the primary assessment.

When you are checking the rate or noting the quality of respirations, make sure that your face or hand is close enough to the patient's face to feel the exhaled air on your skin. Also watch for the rise and fall of the chest. When counting respirations in an alert patient, try not to let the patient know that you are counting. If the patient knows you are counting respirations, you may not get an accurate count.

To calculate the respiratory rate of a child, count respirations for 30 seconds and multiply by two. Counting for less than 30 seconds can cause inaccurate results because children often have irregular breathing patterns.

As you examine children, look to see how much work they are doing to breathe. This work of breathing will help to determine whether they are in respiratory distress. Look for abnormal breath sounds such as noisy breathing, snoring, crowing, grunting, or wheezing. Look to determine whether they are holding themselves in an abnormal position. Are they supporting themselves with their arms while leaning forward (known as the tripod position) or do they refuse to lie down? Check for retractions of the neck or chest. Look for flaring of the nostrils. These signs and symptoms of breathing difficulty are the same as the ones you use to assess breathing difficulty as part of the pediatric assessment triangle, discussed later in the chapter. The presence of any of these signs indicates that the child is having some difficulty breathing and may be experiencing respiratory distress.

When the demands on a child's respiratory system change, the child is able to compensate quickly by increasing the breathing rate and breathing efforts. However, these compensatory mechanisms will function for only a short time, because the child will become exhausted. When this happens, the child may begin to show signs of severe respiratory distress and rapidly progress into respiratory failure if left untreated. Therefore, it is important for you to perform a thorough patient assessment and monitor the child's vital signs at least every 5 minutes when caring for seriously ill or injured pediatric patients.

Words of Wisdom

From birth to approximately 6 months of age, children are "nose breathers." They are not yet able to breathe through their mouths. They show signs of distress very quickly when their noses are filled with mucus.

Street Smarts

When assessing the respirations of an adult patient who is alert, place your hand on the wrist where you would feel for a pulse. The patient will breathe normally if they think you are counting the pulse instead of respirations.

Pulse

The second vital sign is the **pulse**, which indicates the speed and force of the heartbeat. A pulse can be felt anywhere on the body where an artery passes over a hard structure such as a bone. Although there are many such places on the body, the four most common pulse points used by the EMR are the radial (wrist), the carotid (neck), the brachial (arm), and the posterior tibial (ankle).

The most commonly assessed pulse is the **radial pulse**, located on the thumb side of the wrist where the radial artery passes over one of the forearm bones, the radius (see Figure 9-7). The **carotid pulse** is assessed over a **carotid artery**, located on either side of the patient's neck, just under the jawbone (see Figure 9-6). The **brachial pulse** is assessed on the inside of the arm, halfway between the shoulder and the elbow (see Figure 9-8). The **posterior tibial pulse** is located on the inner aspect of the ankle, just behind the ankle bone (**FIGURE 9-12**).

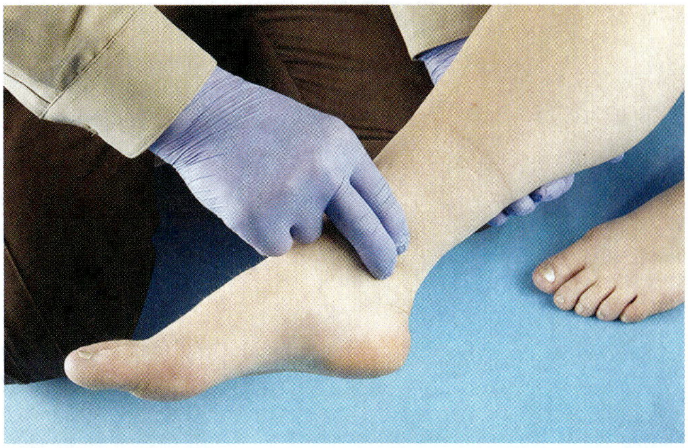

FIGURE 9-12 Assessing the posterior tibial pulse.
© Jones & Bartlett Learning

In general, take the radial pulse of an alert patient and the carotid pulse of an unresponsive patient. When examining an infant, use the brachial pulse. The posterior tibial pulse is used to assess the circulatory status of a leg. When checking a patient's pulse, determine three things: rate, rhythm, and character. To determine the pulse rate (heartbeats per minute), find the patient's pulse with your fingers, count the beats for 30 seconds, and multiply by two. Do not allow your thumb to touch the patient because it has a pulse of its own. In a normal adult, the resting pulse rate is approximately 60 to 100 beats/min, although in a physically fit person (such as a jogger) the resting rate may be lower (approximately 40 to 60 beats/min). In children, the pulse rate is normally faster (approximately 70 to 150 beats/min). A very slow pulse (fewer than 40 beats/min) can be the result of a serious illness, whereas a very fast pulse (more than 120 beats/min) can indicate that the patient is in shock. A person who is simply anxious or worried could have a fast pulse rate (more than 110 beats/min).

You should also be able to determine the rhythm and describe the character of the pulse. Note whether the pulse is regular or irregular. A particularly strong pulse is often referred to as a **bounding pulse**. This is similar to the heart rate that follows physical exertion such as running or lifting heavy objects. The beats are very strong and well defined. A pulse that is so weak that it is barely palpable is often called a **thready pulse** and is typically fast. The pulse is present, but the beats are not easily detected. A thready pulse is a more dangerous sign than a bounding pulse. A bounding pulse can be dangerous if the patient has high blood pressure and is at risk for a stroke. A more detailed explanation of where each pulse point is located was presented in the section on primary assessment.

Capillary Refill

Capillary refill is the ability of the circulatory system to return blood to the capillary vessels after the blood has been squeezed out. The capillary refill test is done on the patient's fingernails or toenails. To perform this test, squeeze the patient's nail bed firmly between your thumb and forefinger (**FIGURE 9-13**). The patient's nail bed will look pale. Release

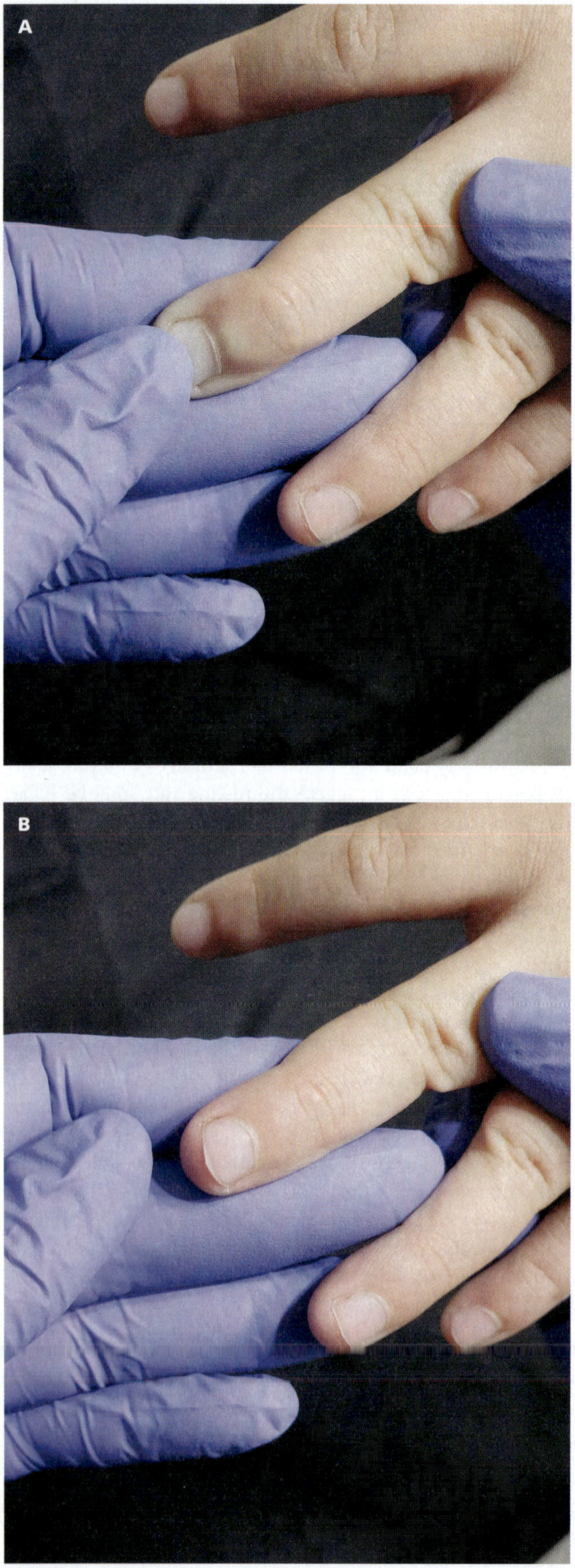

FIGURE 9-13 Checking capillary refill time. **A.** Squeeze the nail bed between your thumb and forefinger. **B.** Release the pressure.
© Heidi Jones

the pressure. Count 2 seconds by saying "capillary refill." The patient's nail bed should become pink. This indicates a normal capillary refill time.

If the patient has lost a significant amount of blood and is in shock, or if the blood vessels supplying that limb have been damaged, the capillary refill will be delayed or entirely absent. Capillary refill will be delayed in a cold environment and should not be used as the sole means for assessing the circulatory status of an extremity. Check with your medical director to determine whether you should use the capillary refill test.

Blood Pressure

Blood pressure is another way to measure the condition of a patient's circulatory system. High blood pressure may indicate that the patient is susceptible to a stroke. Low blood pressure generally indicates one of several possible types of shock.

The blood pressure measurement consists of a reading of two numbers (for example, 120 over 80, or 120/80). These numbers represent the pressures found in the arteries as the heart contracts and relaxes. The numbers are determined by the pressure exerted in millimeters of mercury (mm Hg), as shown on the dial. The higher number (120 mm Hg in the example of 120 over 80) is called the **systolic pressure**. The systolic pressure is the force exerted on the walls of the arteries as the heart contracts (pumps). The lower number (80 mm Hg in the example of 120 over 80) is known as the **diastolic pressure**. The diastolic pressure represents the arterial pressure during the relaxation phase of the heart.

Normal Blood Pressure

Blood pressure ranges may vary greatly. Excitement or stress may raise a person's blood pressure. **Hypertension** (high blood pressure) exists when the blood pressure remains greater than 130/90 mm Hg after repeated examinations over several weeks. Hypertension is a serious medical condition that requires treatment by a physician.

Hypotension (low blood pressure) exists when the systolic pressure (the higher number) is 90 mm Hg or lower. A patient with this condition is usually in serious trouble. Immediately start treatment of shock if the patient is also experiencing other signs of shock (for example, cold, clammy, pale skin or dizziness) or if repeat measurements of blood pressure are decreasing.

Checking Blood Pressure by Palpation

To take a patient's blood pressure by **palpation** (by feeling it), apply the blood pressure cuff to the uninjured (or less injured) arm. Wrap the cuff around the upper arm. The bottom of the cuff should be 1 to 2 inches (3 to 5 cm) above the crease of the elbow. The arrow should point to the brachial artery, which is located on the medial side of the arm at the crease of the elbow (**FIGURE 9-14**).

Blood pressure cuffs come in different sizes for adults, children, and infants. Be sure to use the appropriate size for your patient, such as a narrow cuff for a child and an

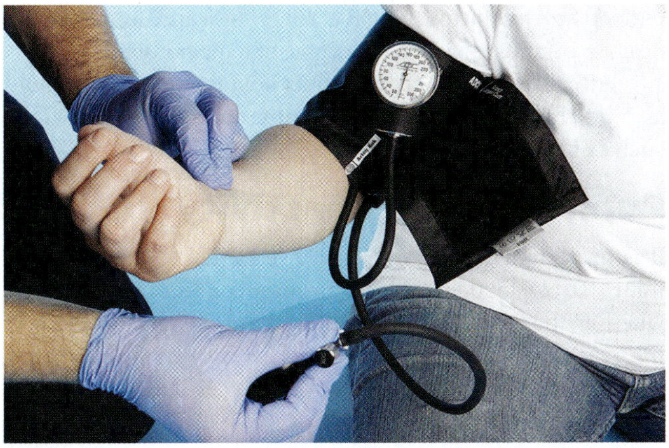

FIGURE 9-14 When using the palpation method, place your fingertips on the radial artery so you can feel the radial pulse.
© Jones & Bartlett Learning

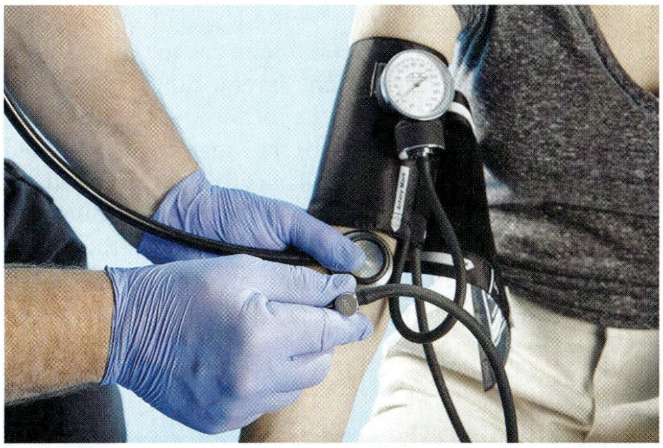

FIGURE 9-16 Taking blood pressure by auscultation.
© Jones & Bartlett Learning

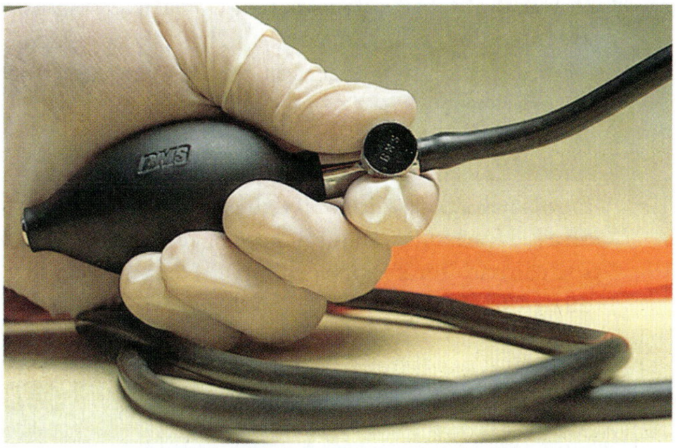

FIGURE 9-15 Slowly release pressure on the blood pressure cuff by turning the valve counterclockwise.
© American Academy of Orthopaedic Surgeons

extra-large cuff for an adult with obesity. Cuffs that are too small may give falsely high readings, and cuffs that are too large may give falsely low readings. Place the indicator dial in a position where you can easily see the movement of the indicator needle. Turn the control knob on the blood pressure inflator bulb clockwise to close the valve. Do not tighten it too much. With the fingers of your other hand, locate the radial pulse at the patient's wrist. Slowly pump up the blood pressure cuff until you can no longer feel the radial pulse. Continue to pump up the cuff for another 10 to 20 mm Hg beyond the disappearing point of the radial pulse. Slowly release the pressure in the cuff (at 2 to 4 mm per second), by turning the valve counterclockwise (**FIGURE 9-15**). Continue to feel for the radial pulse; when you first feel the pulse return, carefully note the position of the indicator needle on the dial. This number is the systolic pressure.

The palpation method of taking blood pressure does not give you a diastolic pressure. You will have only one number, the systolic pressure, instead of the two numbers. Report the results as "the blood pressure by palpation is 90" or "90/p."

Checking Blood Pressure by Auscultation

To take blood pressure by **auscultation** (by hearing it), you need both a blood pressure cuff and a stethoscope. Apply the blood pressure cuff in the same manner and position as in the palpation method. After you apply the cuff, locate the brachial artery pulse on the medial side of the arm at the crease of the elbow.

Put the earpieces of the stethoscope in your ears with the earpieces pointing forward. Place the diaphragm of the stethoscope over the site of the brachial pulse. Using your index and middle fingers, hold the diaphragm snugly against the patient's arm. Do not use your thumb! If you use your thumb, you may hear your own heartbeat in the stethoscope.

Listen as you inflate the blood pressure cuff. When you can no longer hear the sound of the brachial pulse, note the pressure on the dial. Continue to inflate the cuff for another 20 mm over the pressure at which the brachial pulse disappeared. Then slowly and smoothly release air from the cuff by opening the control valve at a rate of 2 to 4 mm per second. Carefully watch the indicator needle, listen for the pulse to return, and note the pressure reading when you first hear the pulse return. This is the systolic pressure. As the cuff pressure continues to fall (at 2 to 4 mm per second), listen for the moment when the pulse disappears. Note the number when you can no longer hear the pulse; this is the diastolic pressure.

Blood pressure measured by auscultation (**FIGURE 9-16**) is reported as systolic pressure over diastolic pressure (the larger number over the smaller number). Blood pressure readings from auscultation provide more accurate and detailed information about a patient and should be used when possible.

It takes practice to become skilled in taking blood pressures. Take every opportunity to practice on as many healthy, uninjured people as possible. Practice on children and older people as well as on your friends and coworkers. This will help prepare you to measure the blood pressure of a seriously ill or injured patient.

Many EMS systems use electronic blood pressure devices. These devices may be set to operate automatically or may require manual activation. Several different types of electronic devices are used in the prehospital setting. These may be small portable devices or they may be incorporated into the cardiac monitor defibrillators used by advanced life support (ALS) services. The operation of these devices varies from one machine to another. If your EMS system uses an electronic blood pressure device and you will be expected to use it, you need to receive training on that specific machine.

TABLE 9-3 presents a table of typical vital sign values based on age.

Skin Condition

Check the patient's skin for color, temperature, and moisture. Normal body temperature is approximately 98.6°F (37°C). Precise body temperature is obtained with a thermometer, but you can estimate a patient's body temperature by placing the back of your hand on the patient's forehead or abdomen under their clothing. The patient's skin temperature is judged, in relation to your skin temperature, as hot or cold.

Some illnesses can cause the skin to become excessively moist or excessively dry. Therefore, together with its relative temperature, the patient's skin might be described as hot and dry, hot and moist, cold and dry, or cold and moist. Normal skin conditions often are described as warm and dry.

Flushed skin, sweating, and restlessness often accompany high temperatures in children. You can often feel a high temperature just by touching the child's chest and head. A child's heart rate increases with each degree of temperature rise.

After determining the patient's vital signs, you should also be able to identify and measure other important signs such as pupil size and reactivity.

Pupil Size and Reactivity

It is important to examine each eye to detect signs of head injury, stroke, drug overdose, or other condition. Look to see whether the **pupils** (the circular openings in the middle of the eyes) are of equal size and whether they both react (constrict) when you shine a light into them (**FIGURE 9-17**). The following findings are abnormal:

- **Pupils of unequal size.** Unequal pupils can indicate a stroke or injury to the brain (**FIGURE 9-18**). A small percentage of people normally have unequal pupils, but in an unresponsive patient, unequal pupils are often a sign of serious illness or injury.
- **Pupils that remain constricted.** Constricted pupils are often present in a person who has taken opioids. They are also a sign of certain central nervous system diseases.
- **Pupils that remain dilated (enlarged).** Dilated pupils indicate a relaxed or unresponsive state. Pupils will dilate within 30 to 60 seconds of cardiac arrest. Head injuries and the use of certain drugs, such as barbiturates or sleeping pills, can also cause dilated pupils.

TABLE 9-3 Typical Vital Sign Values Based on Age

Age	Pulse Rate (Heart Rate) (beats/min)	Respirations (breaths/min)	Systolic Blood Pressure (mm Hg)
Infants (birth to age 1 year)	90–180	30–60	50–95
Children (ages 1 to 12 years)	70–150	18–40	80–110
Adults	60–100	12–20	90–140

© Jones & Bartlett Learning

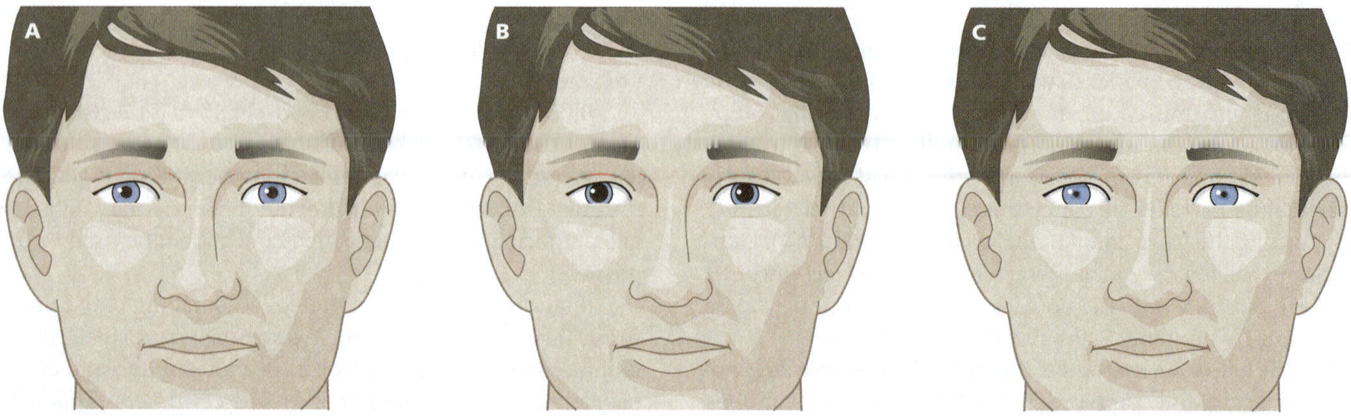

FIGURE 9-17 Normal pupils **(A)**, dilated pupils **(B)**, and constricted pupils **(C)**.

© Jones & Bartlett Learning

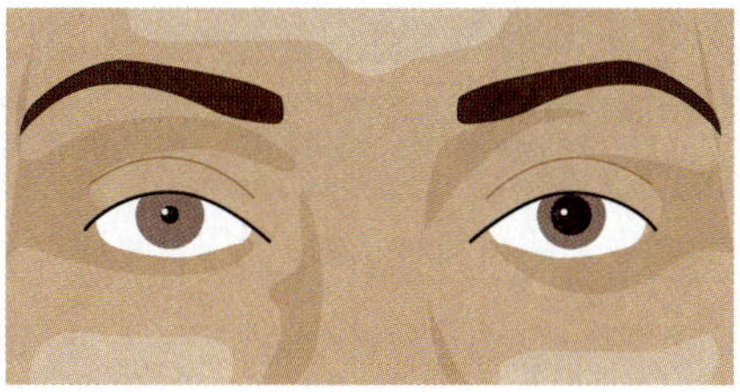

FIGURE 9-18 Unequal pupils may indicate a stroke or injury to the brain.
© Jones & Bartlett Learning

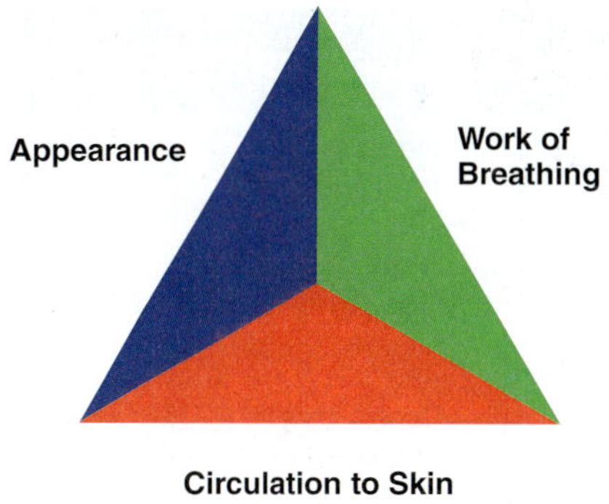

FIGURE 9-19 The three components of the pediatric assessment triangle include overall appearance, work of breathing, and circulation to the skin.
Used with permission of the American Academy of Pediatrics, *Pediatric Education for Prehospital Professionals*. © American Academy of Pediatrics, 2000.

Level of Responsiveness

You will usually assess the patient's level of responsiveness as part of your primary assessment. However, it is important to observe and note any changes that occur between the time of your arrival and the time you turn over the patient's care to personnel at the next level of the EMS system. Report any changes from one level of consciousness to another, using the AVPU scale.

Signs Review

Signs are indicators of illness or injury that you can observe in a patient. They help you determine what is wrong with the patient and the severity of the patient's condition. Vital signs include the patient's respirations (respiratory status), pulse, capillary refill, blood pressure (circulatory status), skin condition, and temperature. Other signs include pupil size and reactivity and level of responsiveness.

To assess a patient's respiratory status, determine the patient's breathing rate and determine whether breaths are rapid or slow, shallow or deep, noisy or quiet. In assessing a patient's circulatory status, determine the rate, rhythm, and character of the patient's pulse. You can also determine whether the patient's capillary refill is normal, slow, or absent. Determine the patient's blood pressure. Although you may not be able to determine the patient's exact temperature, you will be able to state whether the patient is hot or cold. Skin condition is measured by color and moisture and can be described as pale, flushed, cyanotic, jaundiced, normal or baseline, dry, or moist. To assess the patient's pupils, check to see whether the pupils are equal or unequal in size and whether they remain constricted or dilated. Use the AVPU scale to assess the patient's level of consciousness: awake and alert, responsive to verbal stimuli, responsive to pain, or unresponsive.

The Pediatric Assessment Triangle

It is important for you to be able to quickly determine when a child is seriously ill or injured. The **pediatric assessment triangle (PAT)** was developed to help you quickly form a general impression of a pediatric patient's condition as part of your primary assessment. It does not change the steps of the patient assessment sequence you have already learned.

The PAT uses your senses of sight and hearing to gain an accurate initial picture of the child's ABCs and level of responsiveness. This helpful tool allows you to quickly obtain valuable information without touching and agitating the child, and it helps set the priorities for further assessment and treatment. The three components of the PAT are (1) the child's overall appearance, (2) the work of breathing, and (3) circulation to the skin (**FIGURE 9-19**). Each of these three components is discussed in this section.

Appearance

The first element of the PAT is appearance. Does the child appear to be ill or injured? The child's general appearance is important when you are trying to determine the severity of the child's illness or injury. The general appearance is an indicator of how well the heart and lungs are working. Appearance is also a good indication of how well the central nervous system is working. As you assess a child, compare their appearance and actions with what you would expect from a healthy child of the same age.

Consider the following when assessing the child's appearance:

- Does the child have good muscle tone?
- Is the child crying or able to speak? Infants and young children normally cry in response to fear or pain; a child who is not crying may have a decreased level of consciousness, an upper airway infection, or swelling in the airway. If the child is crying, does the cry sound like a normal, healthy cry, or is it a subdued whimper?
- Does the child have a blank, unfocused stare, or does the child look at others? Carefully evaluate a child who is unresponsive or lackluster; lack of activity and interest can signal serious illness or injury.
- Is the child able to interact in a manner that is age appropriate?

If the child is alert, it is better to start your assessment from across the room than to disturb the child by removing them from the caregiver's arms. A child with good eye contact, good muscle tone, and good color would seem to be normal. A child who makes poor eye contact, whose skin is

TABLE 9-4 Characteristics of Appearance

Characteristic	Healthy Reaction	Unhealthy Reaction
Movement	Moving vigorously	Limp, listless, flaccid
Interaction	Reaches for a toy Reacts to a person or sound	Uninterested in playing or toys
Reassurance	Reassured by caregivers	Crying or agitated Unrelieved by gentle reassurance
Eye movement	Eyes follow movement of a person or toy	Glassy-eyed stare
Speech	Age-appropriate speech	Garbled or confused speech
Cry	Strong cry	Weak or high-pitched cry

© Jones & Bartlett Learning

pale compared with baseline, and who is listless should be of concern to you.

As you evaluate the initial appearance of a child, keep in mind that the child's appearance can change quickly. Therefore, you need to reassess the child's appearance regularly. **TABLE 9-4** lists the characteristics of appearance you should look for in a pediatric patient.

Work of Breathing

The second element of the PAT is the work of breathing. In children, assessing the work of breathing is a more accurate indicator of a child's condition than merely determining the rate of respirations. You can determine the child's work of breathing by measuring four factors: (1) abnormal breath sounds, (2) abnormal positioning, (3) retractions of the neck or chest, and (4) flaring of the nostrils (**TABLE 9-5**). You can perform this assessment from across the room without touching the child.

TABLE 9-5 Characteristics of Work of Breathing

Characteristic	Features to Look For
Abnormal breath sounds	Noisy breathing, snoring, crowing, grunting, or wheezing
Abnormal positioning	Leaning forward while using the arms for support, refusal to lie down
Retractions	Retractions above the collarbone or between the ribs or depression of the sternum
Flaring	Flaring of the nostrils during inhalation

© Jones & Bartlett Learning

Circulation to the Skin

The third element of the PAT is circulation to the skin. The three characteristics for determining circulation to the skin are pallor, mottling, and cyanosis. The presentation and indications of pallor and cyanosis are the same in children as they are for adults, as described previously. **Mottling** refers to a patchy skin discoloration that is caused by too little or too much circulation to the skin.

You can establish the status of the circulation to the skin without touching the child. Assessment of skin changes can be more challenging in children with dark skin tone or pigmentation. Evaluation of lips or mucous membranes, such as the inside of the mouth, may be a helpful alternative in these cases.

Patient Assessment

Scene Assessment

↓

Primary Assessment

↓

History Taking

↓

Secondary Assessment

↓

Reassessment

Repeat the primary assessment
Reassess vital signs
Reassess the chief complaint
Recheck the effectiveness of any treatment and ensure all bleeding is controlled
Identify and treat changes in the patient's condition
Reassess patient
- Unstable patients every 5 minutes
- Stable patients every 15 minutes

Reassessment

The first four steps of the patient assessment sequence help you determine the patient's initial condition. If other EMS personnel arrive to take over the care of the patient at any point, all you need to do is provide them with a report of your findings in the form of a handoff report. However, if you need to continue to care for the patient, it is necessary to regularly repeat some parts of the patient assessment. This is the process of reassessment.

Repeat the Primary Assessment

The first step is to repeat the primary assessment. Recheck the patient's level of responsiveness and recheck the patient's ABCs. Continue to maintain an open airway and to monitor breathing and the pulse for rate and quality.

Reassess Vital Signs

The second step is to reassess the patient's vital signs. Observe the patient's skin color and temperature. Reassess the patient's blood pressure.

Reassess the Chief Complaint

The third step is to reassess the chief complaint to see if there is any change.

Recheck the Effectiveness of the Treatment

Check to see if the interventions you took were effective. When there is a change, determine whether you need to alter your care of the patient.

Identify and Treat Changes in the Patient's Condition

The next step is to identify and treat changes you have noticed in the patient's condition.

Reassess the Patient

Patients who appear stable can become unstable quickly. Therefore, it is essential that you reassess all patients carefully for changes in status. Reassess all stable patients every 15 minutes. If the patient is unstable, repeat the reassessment every 5 minutes.

The Handoff Report

It is important that you describe your findings concisely and accurately to the EMS personnel who take over the care of your patients in a handoff report (**FIGURE 9-20**).

The easiest way to report your patient assessment results is to use the same systematic approach you followed during the patient assessment:

1. Provide the age and sex of the patient.
2. Describe the history of the incident.
3. Describe the patient's primary problem or chief complaint.
4. Describe the patient's level of responsiveness.
5. Describe how you found the patient.
6. Report the status of the vital signs: ABCs (including severe bleeding).
7. Describe the results of the secondary patient assessment.
8. Report any pertinent medical conditions using the SAMPLE format.
9. Report the interventions you provided and how the patient responded to them.

Working in a systematic manner will help ensure that you do not overlook any significant symptoms, signs, or injuries and will help to make the handoff report complete and accurate. For example, a handoff report on a 23-year-old man injured in a motor vehicle crash might include the following information:

1. The patient is a 23-year-old male.
2. He was involved in a two-vehicle, head-on collision.
3. He is reporting stomach pain and has a 2-inch (5-cm) cut on his forehead.
4. He is alert and oriented.
5. His pulse rate is 78 beats/min and strong. His blood pressure is 128/82 mm Hg. His respirations are 16 breaths/min and are regular and deep.
6. Examination revealed a 2-inch (5-cm) cut on his forehead, marks on his stomach, and moderate pain midway between his right knee and ankle.
7. He has no known medical conditions or allergies.
8. The patient is on his back, covered with a blanket to preserve his body heat. We have bandaged his laceration and stabilized his leg with an inflatable splint.

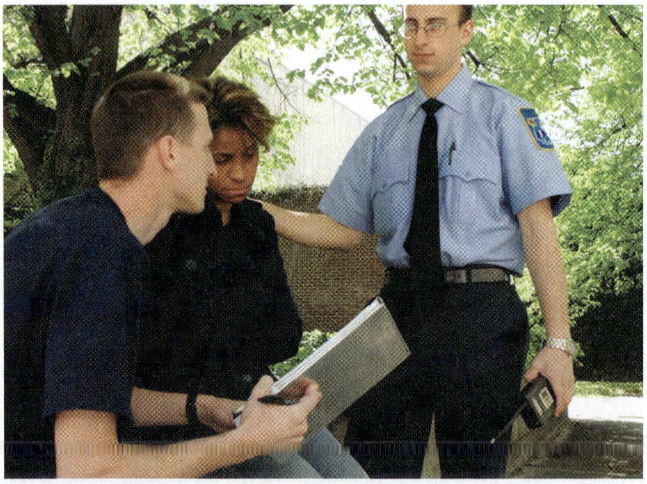

FIGURE 9-20 Communicate your findings in a handoff report.
© Jones & Bartlett Learning

Remember that the purpose of the patient assessment sequence is to:

- Assist in finding the patient's injuries so you can treat them.
- Obtain information about the patient's condition, which you provide to the EMS personnel at the next level of medical care.

With practice, you can complete the entire patient assessment sequence in approximately 2 minutes. This is not a complete medical examination, but it allows you to perform a systematic patient assessment to determine what injuries or illnesses the patient may have. Remember that there are times when you may need to perform some of the steps of the patient assessment sequence in a slightly different order. Each step is numbered only to help you keep track of where you are in the patient assessment sequence.

Examine every patient involved in an incident before you begin major treatment of any single patient. The exceptions to this rule are patients with airway, breathing, and circulatory problems (severe bleeding or shock). These emergencies must be treated as you encounter them during patient assessment. Except for these life-threatening conditions, do not begin treatment until you have examined all patients to determine the extent and severity of injuries and to make sure you treat injuries in the order of severity.

A Word About Medical and Trauma Patients

Although it is often helpful to consider whether the patient's problem is caused by trauma or sudden illness, avoid jumping to conclusions. Some patients need to be treated for both traumatic injury and a sudden medical illness. For example, a person who has a heart attack while driving a vehicle needs to be treated for the heart attack and for any trauma sustained in the motor vehicle crash. The most important factor to remember is to follow a system of patient assessment that will gather all the information needed.

Voices OF Experience

The call came in a little before noon for ALS backup at the nearby motocross racetrack. A BLS unit, staffed by an EMT and an EMR, was on standby for the event. According to dispatch information, they had already helped the patient to the medical tent and initiated treatment.

We arrived at the medical tent 5 minutes later and found the patient, a 26-year-old woman, sitting on the edge of the cot as the EMT obtained vital signs and the EMR administered oxygen with a nonrebreathing mask. The crew gave us an update: The patient had laid down her motorcycle while attempting a turn and had slid on her left side for about 5 feet before going end over end into the protected side wall of the racetrack. She was wearing full racing equipment, including head gear and other protective items, and had not been struck by any other bikes. When they reached her, she was already on her feet and was breathing adequately but had signs of injury and seemed disoriented. She agreed to let them help her to the medical tent for evaluation. She reported pain in her right hip, and the crew observed damage to her helmet and other protective equipment. She consented to transport to the hospital for further evaluation, but the EMR was growing concerned. Aside from the patient's inability to remember the crash, her breathing was becoming labored and her lips and nail beds were cyanotic. The EMR suggested to her partner that they request ALS support on scene. He initially felt she was being overly cautious, but after she explained her concern, that the patient's cyanosis may indicate a respiratory condition, he agreed to request an ALS unit.

"The EMR suggested to her partner that they request ALS support on scene."

My partner and I, who were both paramedics, began our initial assessment on arrival. Our neurologic assessment suggested minor impairment. Due to the mechanism of injury and the patient's signs and symptoms, we initiated cervical-spine precautions, but the patient said she was not comfortable being restrained. The EMR reminded us that the patient was able to walk after the accident; she also told us that the patient's breathing difficulty had increased while lying down, so they had allowed her to sit up. As such, we discontinued cervical-spine precautions.

In addition to confirming the patient's cyanosis, I noted a delayed capillary refill time. She reported pain in her right side and said it was becoming harder to take a deep breath. I assessed her right side and noticed a crackling sound on touch. I was concerned she might have a tension pneumothorax, but I didn't want to get too aggressive just yet. Once we had secured her to the stretcher and placed her in the ambulance, she reported increased breathing difficulty. I listened again to her right side and detected subcutaneous popping and decreased breath sounds. She was definitely experiencing a tension pneumothorax. With our ambulance still on scene, I performed a decompression with my partner assisting. As we did so, the EMR and EMT set up our cardiac monitor and monitored vital signs. Once the decompression relieved the pressure, the patient's condition returned to stable. As we prepared to depart, the EMR, with her EMT partner's guidance, helped spike an IV bag.

During transport, we continued assessment and provided further care. She was delivered without further incident.

This call reminded me how important the initial clinician's assessment is. The EMR had paid attention in class and recognized the signs of a breathing condition that could deteriorate rapidly. She understood that an advanced intervention may be required in the length of time that it would take the BLS ambulance to reach the hospital. Had she not employed her training and asserted her knowledge, the patient may not have survived her crash.

Jamie Rossborough, NRP, CCP-C, FP-C
South Davis Community Hospital / Western Peaks Specialty Hospital
Bountiful, Utah

Adapted from the personal Medical Identification Symbol of the American Medical Association.

YOU are the EMR SUMMARY

You are the EMR: CASE 1

1. Why is it so important to follow the five steps in the patient assessment sequence as you evaluate this scene and this patient?

The five steps in the patient assessment sequence are designed to protect you, the patient, and the bystanders. The steps help you focus on the most important factors—responsiveness, airway, breathing, circulation, and shock—before evaluating additional factors. This sequence helps you to determine the need for additional resources so you can call for them as soon as possible. It assists you in performing a systematic examination of the patient so you do not miss signs and symptoms of illness and injury. Finally, it provides a framework for you to report your findings to other health care clinicians. By following the patient assessment sequence, you have a framework to provide appropriate care to your patients. It helps you perform these tasks in a systematic manner so you do not forget any parts of this important fact-gathering sequence.

2. Why is it important to complete all of the steps of the patient assessment before you determine what is wrong with this patient?

Often the injuries and symptoms that are most visible initially are not the most serious conditions. Complete the patient examination and the patient history before determining a course of action unless the patient has a problem with the ABCs. Conditions are usually best treated if you acknowledge them as discovered, but perform the complete patient examination before attempting to determine the order in which you should treat various injuries or conditions. Remember that a patient who is injured may also have medical conditions, and a patient with medical conditions may also be injured. Keep an open mind. Do not get tunnel vision when assessing a patient.

You are the EMR: CASE 2

1. What are the first actions that you should take?

Your first responsibility at any scene is to ensure that the scene is safe. At different incident scenes, this may require different types of actions. In this situation you have two patients who have the same symptoms along with the suspicion of an odor in the house. Also, this situation is occurring in the middle of the winter when the house is closed tightly and the heating unit is in operation. All these factors should lead you to suspect that there may be a high level of a poisonous gas such as carbon monoxide. If you suspect that the environment may contain a poisonous gas, you need to make sure that you do not become a patient yourself, and you need to protect the occupants of the building from further potential harm. This process may involve removing them from the house and placing them in your vehicle or in a nearby house. These actions may be necessary to ensure scene safety for you and for the building occupants before you are able to determine the NOI. In some situations, it may be necessary to request personnel with self-contained breathing apparatus to remove patients from a building.

2. What additional resources do you need?

Additional resources are needed to determine if there is carbon monoxide or another poisonous gas in the house, to assess the patients for poisoning, and to provide proper treatment and transport for these patients. Most fire departments are equipped with meters to assess the levels of carbon monoxide in the house. Many ALS clinicians carry equipment to evaluate the level of carbon monoxide in a patient's blood. In addition, you need to ensure that there are adequate transport units to care for and transport these patients to an appropriate medical facility for treatment. Your most important role at this scene is to carefully evaluate the information available to you and develop a plan. It is important to remove the patients from a potentially hazardous environment and to call for additional resources to evaluate the situation and to provide care and transport for these patients.

You are the EMR: CASE 3

1. Identify scene safety issues that you should consider when you arrive at the scene of a vehicle crash.

Vehicle crashes involve many safety hazards that should be considered as you begin providing patient care. Some of the considerations include: Is the scene safe so that additional crashes do not occur? Are the vehicles stable? Is there a fuel leak or threat of fire? Is there a chance that another vehicle could become involved? In this case, where a vehicle traveling at a low speed hit a pedestrian, your primary concern should be for the safety of the pedestrian. Make sure the scene is protected with your vehicle or by diverting traffic. Ensure that the vehicle that struck the pedestrian is stabilized and will not move. Place the vehicle in park, apply the parking brake, and shut off the engine. Chock the wheels if you have a wheel chock. In an incident such as this, there is little chance of a fuel leak. Be certain that your vehicle or some other object is blocking traffic in a way that is likely to prevent you or your patient from being struck by another vehicle. Once these steps have been taken, take standard precautions for infectious diseases and begin the other steps in the patient assessment sequence.

YOU are the EMR — SUMMARY

2. Why do you think manual stabilization of the spine is necessary for the patient in this incident?

After completing a primary assessment and forming a general impression of the patient, the paramedic had determined that spinal precautions are necessary. The MOI, a motor vehicle hitting a pedestrian, makes it likely that a spinal injury is present. Stabilization of the spine should be initiated on patients who have sustained trauma. Follow your local protocols.

You are the EMR: CASE 4

1. What is Mattie's chief complaint?

The patient's chief complaint in this scenario is weakness. At this point in your patient assessment, you do not know what is causing this weakness, but you know that you need to complete all five steps of the patient assessment process to get as much information as possible. Focusing on the patient's chief complaint helps you to listen carefully to the patient to gain additional information and to be alert as you examine the patient.

2. Why is the SAMPLE history important when caring for a patient who has a vague chief complaint?

The SAMPLE history is a means to systematically obtain information about the patient's current illness or injury and to learn more about their past medical history. In this case, you learn the following about this patient: Mattie started to feel weak about 20 minutes earlier. She is not allergic to any foods or medications. She takes insulin twice a day for her diabetes. She has had diabetes for 4 years but does not have any other illnesses or medical conditions. Because she woke up late that morning, she only had a glass of milk and one piece of toast for breakfast 3 hours earlier. She took her regular insulin shot this morning before breakfast. By completing a SAMPLE history on this patient, you are able to gather a lot of additional information that helps you to determine what the patient's problem is and then you are able to determine what steps you can take in this situation to care for this patient. In this case, you may be able to give the patient some food or juice that contains sugar to help alleviate her weakness.

Prep Kit

Ready for Review

- A complete patient assessment consists of five steps: (1) perform a scene assessment, (2) perform a primary assessment, (3) obtain a patient's medical history, (4) perform a secondary assessment, and (5) provide reassessment.
- Patients can generally be divided into two main categories: medical and trauma. When examining medical patients, follow the preceding five-step patient assessment sequence. When examining trauma patients, perform the secondary assessment before obtaining the patient's medical history.
- The scene assessment is a general overview of the incident and its surroundings. On the basis of this information, you can make decisions about the safety of the scene, the type of incident, the MOI or NOI, the number of patients, and the need for additional resources.
- During the primary assessment, determine and correct any life-threatening conditions. The steps of the primary assessment are as follows: form a general impression of the patient, assess responsiveness, and perform a rapid exam to identify life threats that consists of checking and correcting problems with the patient's ABCs. Finally, update responding EMS units.
- The purpose of obtaining a medical history is to gather a systematic account of the patient's past medical conditions, illnesses, and injuries to determine the signs and symptoms of the current condition. The SAMPLE history provides a framework to ask needed questions of the patient.
- The secondary assessment of the patient consists of a secondary assessment of the entire body used to assess non–life-threatening conditions. It is done only after completing the primary assessment and stabilizing any life-threatening conditions. This assessment helps you locate and begin management of the signs and symptoms of illness or injury. After completing the secondary assessment of the entire body, assess the patient's vital signs.
- The pediatric assessment triangle (PAT) is designed to give you a quick general impression of a child using only your senses of sight and hearing. The three components of the PAT are overall appearance, work of breathing, and circulation to the skin.

Prep Kit

- Carefully evaluate the child who is unresponsive or lackluster; the lack of activity and interest signal serious illness or injury.
- It is essential that you reassess all patients carefully to evaluate them for any changes in their status. If the patient is stable, repeat the vital signs every 15 minutes. If the patient is unstable, repeat the vital signs every 5 minutes. If the patient's condition changes, repeat the primary assessment and identify any changes in the patient's condition.
- Provide a concise and accurate handoff report to EMS personnel.

Vital Vocabulary

abdomen The body cavity between the thorax and the pelvis that contains the major organs of digestion and excretion.

arm The upper portion of the upper extremity; from the shoulder to the elbow.

aspiration Breathing in foreign matter such as food, drink, or vomitus into the airway or lungs.

assessment-based care A system of patient evaluation in which the chief complaint of the patient and other signs and symptoms are gathered. The care given is based on this information rather than on a formal diagnosis.

auscultation Listening to sounds with a stethoscope.

AVPU scale A scale to measure a patient's level of consciousness. The letters stand for Alert, Verbal, Pain, and Unresponsive.

backboard A straight board used for splinting, extricating, and transporting patients with suspected spinal injuries.

bounding pulse A very strong pulse (similar to the pulse that follows physical exertion such as running or lifting heavy objects).

brachial pulse The pulse located on the arm between the elbow and shoulder; used for checking the pulse in infants.

capillary refill The ability of the circulatory system to restore blood to the capillary blood vessels after it has been squeezed out by the examiner.

carotid artery The principal arteries of the neck; they supply blood to the face, head, and brain.

carotid pulse A pulse that can be felt on each side of the neck where the carotid artery is close to the skin.

chief complaint The patient's response to questions such as "What happened?" or "What's wrong?"

clavicle The collarbone.

cyanosis Blue discoloration of the skin or mucous membranes resulting from poor oxygenation of the circulating blood.

diastolic pressure The measurement of pressure exerted against the walls of the arteries while the left ventricle of the heart is at rest.

exhalation The act of breathing out.

flail chest A chest injury in which three or more ribs are broken in two or more places, resulting in the injured part of the chest moving in the opposite direction from the rest of the chest.

fractures Breaks in a bone.

hypertension High blood pressure.

hypotension Low blood pressure.

inhalation The act of breathing in.

leg The lower portion of the lower extremity; from the knee to the foot.

lower extremity The body part consisting of the thigh, leg, ankle, and foot.

mottling Patchy skin discoloration caused by too little or too much circulation.

palpation Examination by touch.

pediatric assessment triangle (PAT) An assessment tool that measures the severity of a child's illness or injury by evaluating the child's appearance, work of breathing, and circulation to the skin.

posterior tibial pulse The pulse that can be felt on the inner aspect of the ankle, just behind the ankle bone.

primary assessment The first actions taken to form an impression of the patient's condition; to determine the patient's responsiveness and introduce yourself to the patient; to check the patient's airway, breathing, and circulation; and to acknowledge the patient's chief complaint. Sometimes called the initial patient assessment.

pulse The wave of pressure that is created by the heart when it contracts as a result of forcing the blood out and into the major arteries.

pupils The circular openings in the middle of the eye.

radial pulse The pulse located on the inside of the wrist on the thumb side.

Prep Kit

respiratory rate The speed at which a person is breathing (measured in breaths per minute).

SAMPLE history A patient's medical history. The letters stand for Signs and Symptoms, Allergies, Medications, Pertinent past medical history, Last oral intake, Events associated with or leading up to the illness or injury.

scene assessment A step within the patient assessment process that includes a visual survey, or an overview of the incident and its surroundings, and a quick assessment of the scene and the surroundings to provide information about scene safety and the mechanism of injury or nature of illness before you enter and begin patient care.

secondary assessment The step in the patient assessment sequence in which you carefully examine the patient from head to toe and measure vital signs.

sign A condition that you observe in a patient, such as bleeding or the temperature of a patient's skin.

situational awareness Knowledge and understanding of one's surroundings and the ability to recognize potential risks to the safety of the patient or EMS team.

symptom A condition the patient tells you, such as "I feel dizzy."

systolic pressure The measurement of blood pressure exerted against the walls of the arteries during contraction of the heart.

thready pulse A barely palpable pulse.

trauma In the context of emergency response, a physical wound or injury; in other contexts, trauma may also refer to events producing psychological distress.

upper extremity The body part consisting of the arm, forearm, wrist, and hand.

vital signs Measurements or critical parameters used to assess the patient's immediate health condition, including pulse, capillary refill, skin condition, temperature, respirations, and blood pressure.

References

American Heart Association (AHA). *Pediatric Advanced Life Support Provider Manual.* Dallas, TX: AHA; 2020.

Improving 9-1-1 operations with artificial intelligence. National Telecommunications and Information Administration website. https://www.ntia.gov/category/next-generation-911/improving-911-operations-with-artificial-intelligence. Published August 2, 2024. Accessed December 4, 2024.

National Association of Emergency Medical Technicians. *PHTLS: Prehospital Trauma Life Support.* 10th ed. Burlington, MA: Jones & Bartlett Learning; 2024.

National Association of State EMS Officials. *National Model EMS Clinical Guidelines: Version 3.0.* https://nasemso.org/wp-content/uploads/National-Model-EMS-Clinical-Guidelines_2022.pdf. Updated March 2022. Accessed December 4, 2024.

National Highway Traffic Safety Administration. *National Emergency Medical Services Education Standards.* https://www.ems.gov/assets/EMS_Education-Standards_2021_FNL.pdf. EMS.gov website. Published January 2021. Accessed December 4, 2024.

Pusey-Reid E, Quinn L, Samost ME, Reidy PA. Skin assessment in patients with dark skin tone. *Am J Nurs.* 2023;123(3):36–43.

Assessment IN ACTION

You are dispatched to a convenience store for the report of a person who has fallen. On arrival, you find a 69-year-old man lying on the ground. He reports pain in the area of his left hip.

1. In what order should you perform the five steps of the patient assessment process on this patient?

1. Secondary assessment
2. Primary assessment
3. History taking
4. Scene assessment
5. Reassessment

A. 4, 2, 3, 1, 5
B. 3, 1, 4, 2, 5
C. 4, 2, 1, 3, 5
D. 1, 3, 2, 5, 4

2. Which of the following steps should you perform first during the scene assessment?

A. Take standard precautions.
B. Ensure scene safety.
C. Determine the need for additional resources and assistance.
D. Determine the mechanism of injury/nature of illness.

3. Place the following parts of the primary assessment in the order in which you should perform them.

1. Assess the patient's airway.
2. Assess the level of responsiveness.
3. Assess the patient's circulation.
4. Update the responding EMS units.
5. Form a general impression of the patient.
6. Assess the patient's breathing.

A. 5, 2, 1, 6, 3, 4
D. 6, 5, 3, 4, 1, 2
C. 3, 2, 1, 5, 6, 4
D. 2, 6, 3, 4, 5, 1

4. Which of the following measurements will give you the most information about this patient's condition?

A. Taking blood pressure by palpation
B. Taking blood pressure by auscultation

5. Your initial blood pressure reading on a patient who has been involved in a motor vehicle crash is 146/86 mm Hg. You reassess his blood pressure every 5 minutes and get the following readings: 142/82 mm Hg, 134/76 mm Hg, 126/68 mm Hg, and 106/54 mm Hg. What do these results tell you about this patient's condition?

A. The patient's condition seems to be stable.
B. The patient appears to be exhibiting signs of increasing shock.
C. The patient is becoming more relaxed.
D. The patient is probably not seriously injured.

6. How often do you need to monitor the vital signs of a patient in stable condition?

A. Every 3 to 5 minutes
B. Every 5 minutes
C. Every 15 minutes
D. Only when you see a change in the patient's condition

7. How often do you need to reassess a patient in unstable condition?

A. Every 3 to 5 minutes
B. Every 5 minutes
C. Every 15 minutes
D. Only when you see a change in the patient's condition

8. Pale skin indicates which of the following conditions?

A. Increased circulation to that part of the body
B. Poisoning
C. A normal condition
D. Decreased circulation to that part of the body

9. The SAMPLE mnemonic is part of which step in the patient assessment sequence?

A. Primary assessment
B. History taking
C. Secondary assessment
D. Reassessment

10. Why is it important to obtain a medical history for a patient who has sustained trauma?

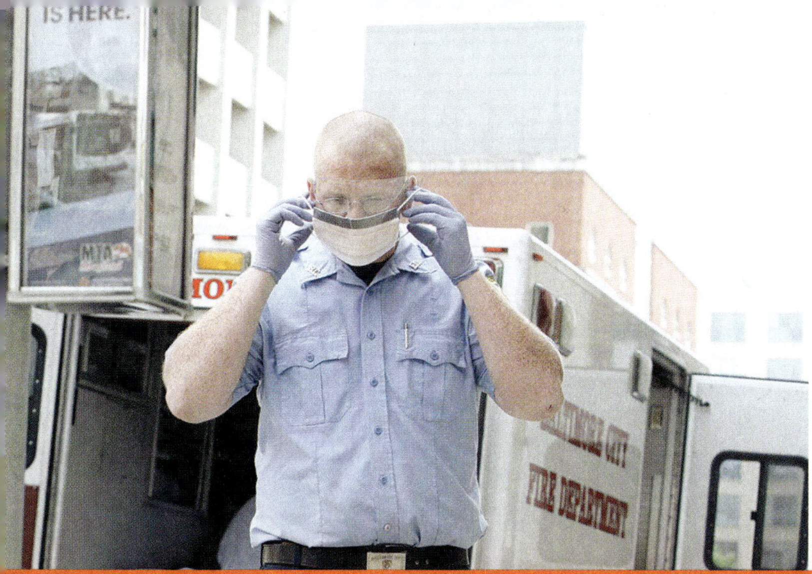

SECTION 4

Medical

10 Medical Emergencies

11 Poisoning and Substance Use

12 Behavioral Emergencies

13 Environmental Emergencies

© Jones & Bartlett Learning. Courtesy of MIEMSS.

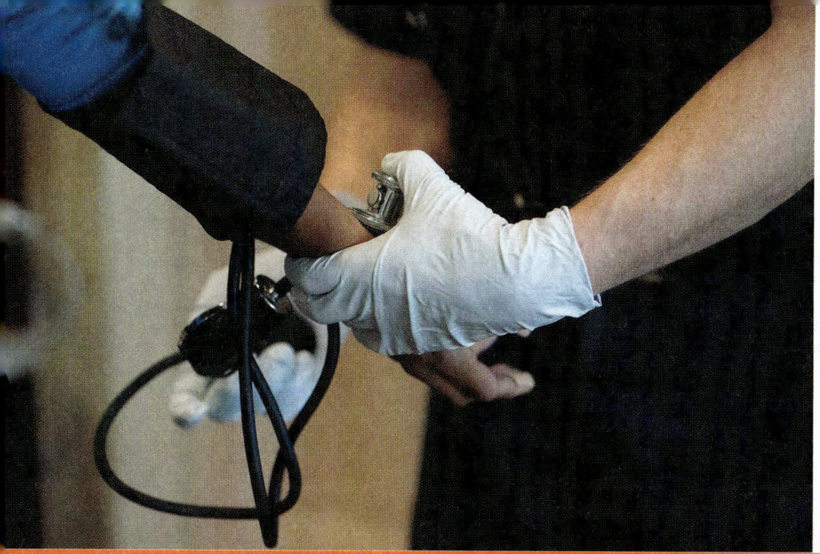

CHAPTER 10

Medical Emergencies

National EMS Education Standard Competencies

Medicine

Recognizes and manages life threats based on assessment findings of a patient with a medical emergency while awaiting additional emergency response.

Medical Overview

- Assessment and management of a medical complaint (pp 215–218)

Neurology

- Decreased level of responsiveness (p 216)
- Seizure (pp 216–217)
- Stroke (pp 224–225)

Abdominal and Gastrointestinal Disorders

- Anatomy, presentations, and management of shock associated with gastrointestinal bleeding (pp 228–229)

Endocrine Disorders

- Awareness that diabetic emergencies cause altered mental status (pp 226–228)

Cardiovascular

- Chest pain (pp 218–220)

Respiratory

- Respiratory distress/failure/arrest (Chapter 7, *Airway Management*)
- Upper airway obstruction (Chapter 7, *Airway Management*)
- Lower airway disease: asthma, bronchiolitis, pneumonia, chronic obstructive pulmonary disease (pp 222–225)

Genitourinary/Renal

- Blood pressure assessment in hemodialysis patients (p 230)

© ALEX EDELMAN/AFP/Getty Images

Pharmacology

- Uses knowledge of the medications that the EMR may administer in an emergency (pp 231–233)

Principles of Pharmacology

- Medication safety (p 232)
- Kinds of medications used during an emergency (pp 231–233)

Medication Administration

- Use of a medication cross-check procedure (pp 231–233)
- Use of an auto-injector (Chapter 11, *Poisoning and Substance Use*)
- Use of a unit-dose, premeasured intranasal device (Chapter 11, *Poisoning and Substance Use*)
- Use of tools/resources to facilitate safe administration of weight-based dosing (pp 231–233)

Acute Medications

- Names (pp 231–234)
- Effects (pp 231–234)
- Indications (pp 231–234)
- Contraindications (pp 231–234)
- Side effects (pp 231–234)
- Routes of administration (pp 231–234)
- Dosages (pp 231–234)

Knowledge Objectives

1. Describe the general approach to a medical patient. (pp 215–218)
2. Explain the causes, signs, symptoms, and treatment of a patient with altered mental status. (pp 215–216)
3. Explain the causes, signs, symptoms, and treatment of a patient with seizures. (pp 216–217)
4. Describe how to place an unresponsive patient in the recovery position. (pp 216–217)
5. Describe the causes, signs, symptoms, and initial treatment of a patient with angina pectoris. (pp 218–219)

6. Describe how to assist a patient with administering nitroglycerin pills or spray. (p 218)
7. Describe the major causes, signs, symptoms, and initial treatment of a patient with a heart attack. (pp 219–220)
8. Describe the cause, signs, symptoms, and initial treatment of a patient with heart failure. (pp 221–222)
9. Describe the causes, signs, symptoms, and initial treatment of a patient with dyspnea. (p 222)
10. Describe the causes, signs, symptoms, and initial treatment of a patient experiencing an asthma attack. (pp 222–223)
11. Describe the causes, signs, symptoms, and initial treatment of a patient experiencing croup. (p 223)
12. Describe the causes, signs, symptoms, and initial treatment of a patient experiencing epiglottitis. (pp 223–224)
13. Describe the causes, signs, symptoms, and initial treatment of a patient experiencing chronic obstructive pulmonary disease or acute respiratory distress syndrome. (pp 224–225)
14. Describe the major cause, signs, symptoms, and initial treatment of a patient with a stroke. (pp 224–225)
15. Explain the use of the Cincinnati Prehospital Stroke Scale as a stroke assessment tool. (p 225)
16. Describe the signs, symptoms, and initial treatment of hypoglycemia. (p 226)
17. Describe the signs, symptoms, and initial treatment of hyperglycemia. (pp 226–228)
18. Describe the causes, signs, symptoms, and initial treatment of an abdominal condition. (pp 228–230)
19. Explain how to measure blood pressure in a dialysis patient. (p 230)
20. Discuss potential complications for dialysis patients. (p 230)
21. Describe the responsibilities of emergency medical responders (EMRs) when treating patients with infectious diseases. (p 230)
22. Describe the responsibilities of EMRs when treating patients during disease outbreaks, including epidemics and pandemics. (pp 230–231)
23. Discuss situations that may require you to assist higher-level emergency medical services clinicians, including emergencies involving advanced medical equipment or medication administration. (pp 231–234)

Skills Objectives

1. Demonstrate a patient assessment for a medical patient. (pp 214–215)
2. Demonstrate placing an unresponsive patient in the recovery position. (p 216)
3. Demonstrate how to protect a patient who is seizing from sustaining further harm. (pp 216–217)
4. Demonstrate how to assist a patient with administering nitroglycerin pills or spray. (p 218)
5. Demonstrate how to support a patient experiencing a heart attack. (p 219)
6. Demonstrate care of a patient with heart failure. (pp 220–222)
7. Demonstrate the steps to treat a patient with dyspnea. (p 222)
8. Demonstrate the use of the Cincinnati Prehospital Stroke Scale as a stroke assessment tool. (p 225)
9. Demonstrate treatment of a patient with hypoglycemia. (p 226)
10. Demonstrate treatment of a patient with hyperglycemia. (pp 226–228)
11. Demonstrate treatment of a patient with abdominal pain. (pp 228–230)
12. Demonstrate how to measure blood pressure in a dialysis patient. (p 230)

Introduction

This chapter discusses medical conditions as either general medical complaints or specific medical conditions. General medical complaints may result from a wide variety of medical conditions. You will need to be able to use your understanding of the patient's signs and symptoms to initiate treatment of these patients. Some specific medical conditions you will encounter include angina pectoris, heart attack, heart failure, dyspnea, asthma, croup, epiglottitis, stroke, hypoglycemia, hyperglycemia, and abdominal pain. Recognizing and having familiarity with these conditions can greatly enhance the treatment you provide to these patients.

This chapter will also discuss principles you must understand when responding to a medical emergency. Some of these emergencies will involve infectious disease. Some may involve advanced medical equipment or medication considerations. You must know how to help within your capacity as an emergency medical responder (EMR).

Medical emergencies can test the knowledge and skills of even the most experienced emergency medical services (EMS) clinicians. As an EMR, your familiarity with these conditions will prepare you to provide reassuring and sometimes lifesaving care.

Patient Assessment in Medical Emergencies

Your approach to a patient who has a general medical complaint should follow the systematic patient assessment sequence (**FIGURE 10-1**). Review your dispatch information to help you decide on possibilities for the patient's condition. Carefully assess the scene to determine safety issues for you and your patient. As you perform the primary assessment, first try to form an impression of the patient's condition. Then determine the patient's level of responsiveness; introduce yourself; check the patient's airway,

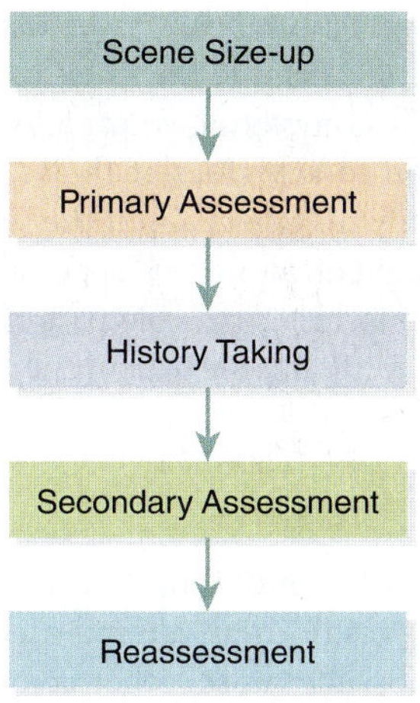

FIGURE 10-1 Patient assessment sequence.
© Jones & Bartlett Learning

breathing, and circulation (ABCs); and acknowledge the patient's chief complaint.

Usually, it is best to obtain a medical history on a patient experiencing a medical condition before you perform the secondary patient assessment. The medical history should be complete and include all factors that may relate to the patient's current illness.

The SAMPLE history format will help you secure the information you need:

S Signs and symptoms
A Allergies
M Medications
P Pertinent past medical history
L Last oral intake and Last menstrual cycle
E Events leading up to the illness or injury

Although the secondary assessment focuses on the areas related to the patient's current illness, patients may not always be aware of all the aspects of their condition. It is better to perform a complete physical examination and find all the conditions than to perform a partial examination and miss an underlying condition. Obtain the patient's vital signs. Be sure to monitor your patient through ongoing reassessment if the arrival of additional EMS personnel is delayed.

As you perform the patient assessment, remember to reassure the patient. Any call for emergency medical care is a frightening experience for the patient. Stress aggravates many medical conditions. Reducing the patient's stress will go a long way toward making the patient more comfortable.

Medications

As part of your assessment, it is important to determine what types of medication a patient takes, including any over-the-counter drugs or supplements. The patient is often a good source of information about their medications and condition. For example, the patient may be able to tell you, "The white pill is for my high blood pressure, and the green pill is a blood thinner."

While you are not expected to have a textbook knowledge of every medication you may encounter, having familiarity with the effects of common medications can help you understand the patient's presenting signs and symptoms. Many medications have negative side effects, such as dizziness, when taken in excess. Many patients with heart conditions take blood thinners (anticoagulants) to prevent blood clots, which make them more likely to bleed from even minor cuts. Knowing such details can help you determine the appropriate care for the patient.

Keep in mind that not all medications are taken by mouth. Some patients receive medication, such as nitroglycerin, through skin patches. Some patients use inhalers or auto-injectors. Be sure to ask about all forms of medication, not just pills.

Also keep in mind that older adults can have a variety of chronic conditions and may be taking multiple medications every day. They may see several physicians for different conditions. If the various physicians do not communicate effectively, there is a chance that some medications may interfere with the action of other medications. Older adults may not take their medications as instructed, accidentally taking the wrong dosage of a particular medication or missing doses altogether.

Finally, consider whether the patient is reporting not just what they *are* taking but also what they are *supposed* to be taking. For example, a patient may not be taking a prescribed medication because they cannot afford it. This patient may report not being on any medications, but the key detail for you to understand is that the patient has a diagnosis that is not being appropriately treated.

If the patient is being transported to a medical facility, gather all prescription medications and bring them to the hospital with the patient.

General Medical Complaints

General medical complaints may have different causes, but they result in similar signs and symptoms. By becoming skilled at recognizing the signs and symptoms of various general medical complaints and learning about general treatment guidelines, you will be able to provide immediate care for your patients even if you cannot determine the exact cause of the conditions. This initial treatment can stabilize the patient and allow other EMS and hospital clinicians to diagnose and further treat the condition.

Altered Mental Status

Altered mental status is a decrease in the patient's level of responsiveness. This change may range from a decrease in the level of understanding to unresponsiveness. Any patient who is unresponsive has experienced a severe change in mental status.

When you are assessing altered mental status, remember the AVPU scale:

- **A Awake and alert.** An alert patient will answer simple questions accurately and appropriately.
- **V Responsive to Verbal stimuli.** A patient who is responsive to verbal stimuli will react to loud voices.
- **P Responsive to Pain.** A patient who is responsive to a painful stimulus will react to the pain by moving or crying out.
- **U Unresponsive.** An unresponsive patient will not respond to either verbal or painful stimuli.

When assessing the patient's mental status, consider two factors: the patient's initial level of consciousness and any change in that level of consciousness. A patient who is initially alert but later responds only to verbal stimuli has experienced a decreased level of consciousness.

Many different conditions may cause an altered level of consciousness, including:

- Head injury
- Shock
- Decreased level of oxygen to the brain
- Stroke
- Slow heart rate
- High fever
- Infection (sepsis)
- Poisoning, including drugs and alcohol
- Low level of blood glucose (diabetic emergencies)
- Insulin reaction
- Psychiatric condition
- Drug use

Some of the specific conditions that cause altered mental status are explained in the second part of this chapter. Even if you cannot determine what is causing the patient's altered level of consciousness, you can help by treating the symptoms of the condition.

Sometimes you will be able to determine the cause of the altered mental status and take steps to correct the condition. For example, if the patient reports having diabetes and is experiencing insulin shock, you can administer glucose to increase the patient's blood glucose level. However, in many situations, you will not be able to determine the cause of the altered mental status and will have to treat the patient's symptoms. Initial treatment consists of maintaining the patient's ABCs and normal body temperature and keeping the patient from additional harm. Carefully note the patient's initial vital signs. Recheck vital signs regularly to monitor any changes. If the patient is unresponsive and has not sustained trauma, place the patient in the recovery position or use an airway adjunct to help maintain an open airway. Be prepared to provide suctioning if there is a chance that the patient may vomit or if secretions are accumulating in the airway.

Altered Mental Status in Pediatric Patients

Altered mental status in children can be caused by a variety of conditions, including low blood glucose level, poisoning, postseizure state, infection, head trauma, and decreased oxygen levels. To help determine the cause of the child's altered mental status, while completing your patient assessment, pay particular attention to any clues at the scene. Question any bystanders or family members about the situation and try to get as much of the medical history as possible.

Emotional support may be a big part of your role at these scenes. If needed, try to calm the patient and the patient's family.

Altered Mental Status in Geriatric Patients

Many of the medical conditions that commonly occur in older patients can result in an altered mental status. While dementia is one possible cause, other common causes of altered mental status in older patients are lack of adequate oxygen to the brain, low blood glucose level, and hypothermia. Never assume that an altered mental status or confusion is a patient's baseline unless you have definite confirmation that this is true. Confusion in older patients is often the result of acute illness that can be corrected with appropriate and timely medical care.

Seizures

A **seizure** can result from a high fever or from disorders such as **epilepsy**. This section discusses **generalized seizures**, in which the entire body stiffens and shakes severely, as these are the types of seizures most likely to require emergency response. Other forms of seizures exist but may not involve the patient's full body or awareness (referred to as focal seizures), and are therefore unlikely to result in an emergency call. Although seizures can be frightening to family members, bystanders, and rescuers, they are not usually dangerous.

Seizures are caused by sudden episodes of uncontrolled electrical impulses in the brain. Instead of discharging electrical impulses in a controlled manner, the brain cells keep firing impulses. During generalized seizures, a person becomes unresponsive, the eyes roll back, the teeth become clenched, and the person may experience loss of bladder and bowel control. These seizures usually last 1 to 2 minutes, although prolonged seizures may continue for more than 2 minutes. Patients are usually unresponsive during generalized seizures and do not remember them afterward.

Although most seizures are not life threatening, they are a serious medical emergency. If seizures last more than 5 minutes, they can be a life-threatening emergency. Often, you will not able to determine the cause of the patient's seizure. The patient's family may be able to tell you whether a physician has diagnosed the patient as having a seizure disorder.

Usually, the seizure will be over by the time you arrive at the scene. If it has not ended, focus your treatment on protecting the patient from injury. Do not restrain the patient's movements. If you attempt to restrain the patient, you may cause further injury. If a patient experiences a seizure while on a hard surface, control the arms by grasping them at the wrists. Allow the patient's arms to move but prevent the elbows from hitting the hard surface. To prevent the patient's head from hitting a hard surface, quickly slide the toes of your shoes under the patient's head, replacing with a pillow or cushion as soon as possible. Move the patient only if they are in a dangerous location, such as in a busy street or close to something hard, hot, or sharp.

Words of Wisdom

There are many different types of seizures, and many factors that can cause them, including:

- Epilepsy
- Trauma
- Head injury
- Stroke
- Shock
- Decreased level of oxygen to the brain
- High fever (As mentioned, some patients, typically infants and young children, may experience febrile seizures.)
- Infection
- Poisoning
- Overdose of drugs or alcohol
- Brain tumor or infection
- Diabetic emergencies (low blood glucose level)
- Complication of pregnancy
- Unknown causes

During a seizure, the patient generally does not breathe and the skin may show signs of decreased perfusion by turning pale or cyanotic. You cannot do anything about the patient's airway during the seizure, but once the seizure has stopped, it is essential that you ensure an open airway. Usually the best method to accomplish this is the head tilt–chin lift maneuver. Observe the seizure activity and report your observations and assessment findings to other EMS clinicians. This information may be important in determining the cause of the seizure.

Words of Wisdom

Remember that findings related to skin color, such as pallor and cyanosis, are relative to the patient's baseline skin color. For patients with deeply pigmented skin, color changes may be more apparent in the fingernail beds, in the whites of the eyes, on the palm of the hand, or inside the mouth.

If your patient is a child, reassure the parents, who may be frightened by the seizure. If they become too emotional as you are trying to care for the patient during the seizure, ask them to leave the room.

After you have opened the airway, place the patient in the recovery position to help keep the airway open and to allow any secretions (saliva or blood from a bitten tongue) to drain from the mouth. Patients who have experienced a seizure may have excess oral secretions. Review Chapter 7, *Airway Management*, for a detailed discussion of clearing and maintaining an open airway.

Most patients start to breathe soon after the seizure ends. If the patient does not resume adequate breathing after a seizure or if the seizure is prolonged, begin rescue breathing. Supplemental oxygen should be administered as soon as it is available.

Treatment

Treatment for a seizure patient is as follows:

- Stay calm. You cannot stop a seizure once it has started.
- Do not restrain the patient.
- Note the duration of the seizure.
- Protect the patient from contact with hard, sharp, or hot objects. If possible, place the person on a soft surface (sofa, bed, or rug) to protect them from injury during the seizure.
- Loosen ties or anything else around the neck that may obstruct breathing.
- Do not force anything between the patient's teeth.
- Do not be concerned if the patient stops breathing temporarily during the seizure.
- After the seizure, turn the patient onto their side and make sure breathing is not obstructed.
- Provide supplemental oxygen after the seizure if it is available and you are trained to use it.
- If the patient does not begin breathing after a seizure, begin rescue breathing.
- Arrange for prompt transport to an appropriate medical facility.
- Continue to monitor the patient's vital signs and support the ABCs if necessary.
- Cool the patient if the patient has a high fever.

YOU are the EMR — CASE 1

You are returning from a call and as you slow down for a traffic light ahead, you notice a small crowd of people on the sidewalk. When they see you, several people excitedly wave you down. You quickly pull your vehicle to the side and exit your vehicle. A patient is lying on the sidewalk. One of the bystanders tells you that the man was walking down the street and suddenly paused and then slumped to the ground. While you approach the patient, his legs and arms begin to vigorously contract in a seizure that seems to involve his whole body.

1. What can you do to prevent this patient from hurting himself during the seizure?
2. What actions should you take to provide care for this patient immediately after the seizure stops?
3. What additional care does this patient need during the first few hours after the seizure stops?

Following a seizure, the patient will experience a state of confusion that may last for 30 to 45 minutes. The patient may also become anxious, hostile, or belligerent. Continue to monitor the patient's breathing. At this point, the patient needs privacy. Because the person may be embarrassed about what happened or where it happened (perhaps in a public place such as a restaurant or shopping mall), move the patient to a more comfortable, private place if other EMS personnel have not arrived. Do not leave the patient, even if the patient insists that they are now awake and alert. Encourage any patient who experiences a seizure to go to a medical facility for examination and treatment.

Safety

Do not attempt to put anything in the mouth of a patient who is actively seizing. A person having a seizure cannot swallow their tongue, but the object can become a choking hazard or break teeth.

Treatment

Although you may be inclined to quickly categorize patients as medical patients or as trauma patients, many of the patients you encounter may have both a medical condition and a traumatic injury. For example, the altered level of consciousness experienced by a patient with diabetes who has severe hypoglycemia may contribute to a motor vehicle crash. As you study this chapter, try to imagine how you can use your knowledge to treat patients with a single condition or a variety of conditions. Remember to carefully assess each patient and treat the conditions that you identify.

Specific Medical Conditions

While knowing how to assess and treat general medical complaints will prepare you to manage a great many situations, some calls require more specialized knowledge. Sometimes the patient or the patient's family will tell you that the patient has a certain medical condition. Other times, your careful assessment of the patient will reveal information that leads you to suspect a particular condition. The added knowledge you gain from the second part of this chapter will help you assess, treat, and communicate more effectively with these patients. Specific medical conditions discussed include heart conditions, respiratory conditions, stroke, diabetic conditions, and abdominal pain.

With increasing age comes an increase in the incidence of many different medical conditions. The two types of medical conditions that cause the greatest number of deaths are cardiovascular diseases and respiratory diseases. As people get older, they are generally less able to fight off diseases. Their immune systems become less effective. They are unable to cough as effectively and may have increased difficulty clearing secretions, thus increasing the need for suctioning. Pay particular attention to these aging-related conditions when assessing a geriatric patient.

Heart Conditions

The heart must receive a constant supply of oxygen or it will die. The heart receives its oxygen through a complex system of coronary (heart) arteries. As long as these arteries continue to supply the heart with an adequate amount of oxygen, the heart can continue to function properly.

As a person ages, the body's ability to speed up the rate of heart contractions decreases. At the same time, the blood vessels become stiffer and narrowed, a disease process called **atherosclerosis**. Atherosclerosis causes layers of fat to coat the inner walls of the arteries. Progressive atherosclerosis can cause angina pectoris, heart attack, and even **cardiac arrest**.

Angina Pectoris

As atherosclerosis progresses in the coronary arteries, it can reduce the blood (oxygen) supply to the heart enough to cause pain or pressure in the chest. This pain is known as **angina pectoris**, or more simply, angina. The heart needs more oxygen than the narrowed coronary arteries can deliver.

When a patient has chest pain, first ask the person to describe the pain. Patients often describe angina as pressure or heavy discomfort. The patient may say something like, "It feels like an elephant is sitting on my chest." Angina attacks are usually brought on by exertion, emotion, or eating. The patient may feel crushing pain in the chest. The pain may radiate to either or both arms, the neck, jaw, or any combination of these sites. The patient is often short of breath and sweating, is extremely frightened, and feels a sense of doom. The patient may experience nausea and vomiting.

Ask whether the patient is already being treated for a diagnosed heart condition. If the answer is "yes," ask if the patient has a pill or spray to take for chest pain. Patients who have experienced previous episodes of angina usually have medication that they can place or spray under the tongue to relieve the pain. The most common medication of this type is **nitroglycerin**, and the patient may have already taken a dose by the time you arrive at the scene (**FIGURE 10-2**).

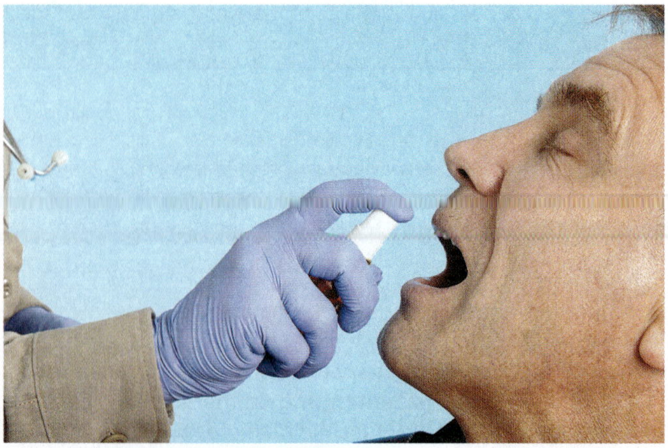

FIGURE 10-2 Nitroglycerin pills, ointment, patch, and spray (shown here) relieve chest pain.

© Jones & Bartlett Learning

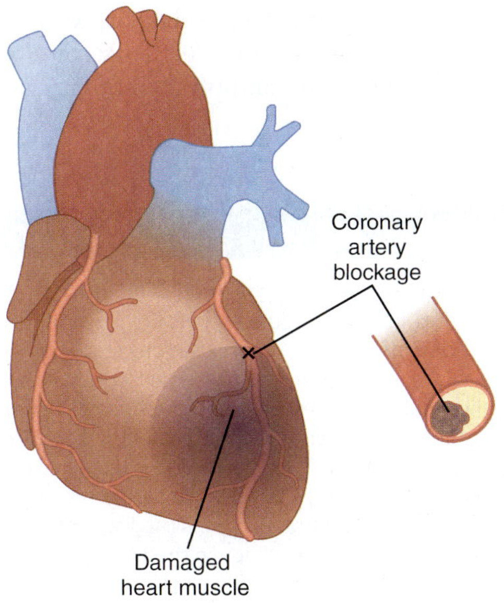

FIGURE 10-3 A blocked coronary artery results in a heart attack.
© Jones & Bartlett Learning

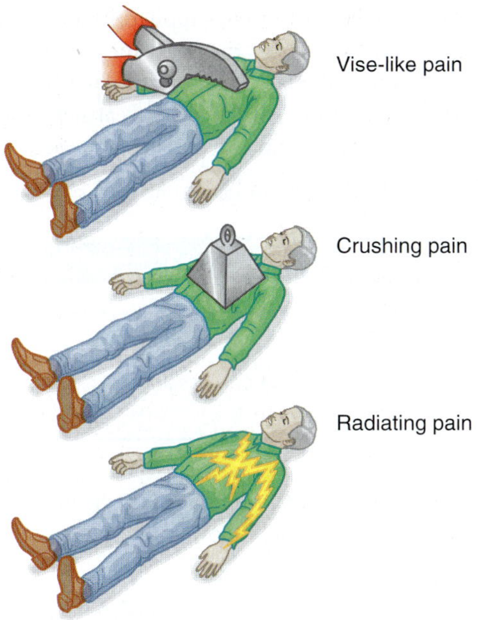

FIGURE 10-4 Descriptions of pain caused by heart attack.
© Jones & Bartlett Learning

In some states and locations, EMRs are authorized to help patients self-administer medication that has been prescribed for them by a physician. If the patient has nitroglycerin but has not taken it during the past 5 minutes, help place one of the tiny pills under the patient's tongue or help the patient administer the aerosol spray if you are authorized to do so. Follow your local protocols regarding the administration of nitroglycerin. Nitroglycerin usually relieves angina pain within 5 minutes. If the pain has not diminished after 5 minutes, help the patient take a second dose. If the pain still has not lessened 5 minutes after the second dose, assume the patient is having a heart attack. Before you assist with the administration of nitroglycerin, you need to receive training and have permission from your medical director.

Heart Attack

A heart attack (myocardial infarction) results when one or more of the coronary arteries is completely blocked. The two primary causes of coronary artery blockage are severe atherosclerosis and a blood clot from somewhere else in the circulatory system that breaks free and lodges in the artery. If one of the coronary arteries becomes blocked, the part of the heart muscle served by that artery is deprived of oxygen and dies (**FIGURE 10-3**).

Blockage of a coronary artery causes the patient to experience immediate and severe pain. The pain of angina pectoris and a heart attack may be similar at first. Most heart attack patients describe the pain as crushing. The pain may radiate from the chest to the left arm, or to the jaw, or to the back (**FIGURE 10-4**). Remember, however, that not all heart attacks present with this pain; nor is all chest pain caused by heart conditions. Pneumonia and muscle strains to the chest wall can also cause chest pain. It is better for the patient to treat the pain as if it is a heart attack than to undertreat the symptoms. The patient is usually short of breath, weak, sweating, and nauseated, and may vomit.

Nitroglycerin pills or spray help to reduce the workload on the heart, increase the supply of blood to the heart, and relieve the pain of a heart attack by dilating blood vessels. Because nitroglycerin can reduce blood pressure, it should not be given to a patient with a systolic blood pressure of less than 100 mm Hg, and the patient should be seated or lying down when it is administered. Aspirin (or acetylsalicylic acid) is also recommended for patients exhibiting signs and symptoms of a heart attack. Giving one adult aspirin (325 mg) or two to four low-dose aspirins (81 mg each) may help to reduce the chance of death from a heart attack. Instruct the patient to chew the aspirin and then swallow it. Be sure the patient is not allergic to aspirin and has not had any recent internal bleeding such as a stomach ulcer.

Treatment

As an EMR, you may administer aspirin and should understand its medication properties.

Aspirin

Effects. Blocks the formation of blood clots, helps to reduce deaths from heart attacks

Indications. Any person with symptoms of pressure, heavy weight, squeezing, or crushing that seems to be related to possible heart attack

Contraindications. Patients who are hypersensitive or allergic to aspirin

Side effects. None

Routes of administration. Oral (chewing is preferable)

Dosages. 160-mg to 325-mg tablet (taken as two low-dose tablets or one full-dose tablet)

Medication properties are discussed later in this chapter.

If the area of heart muscle supplied by the blocked artery is either critical or large, the heart may stop completely. Complete cessation of heart is called cardiac arrest. Cardiopulmonary resuscitation (CPR) is the treatment for cardiac arrest. Most patients do not experience immediate cardiac arrest with a heart attack.

Signs and Symptoms

The signs and symptoms of cardiac arrest are as follows:

- Unresponsiveness
- Absence of respirations or only gasping
- Absence of a carotid pulse

To support the patient and reduce the probability of cardiac arrest, you can take the following actions:

- Summon additional help.
- Talk to the patient to relieve their anxiety.
- Reassure the patient that you are there to help. The person is afraid that death is close, and fear can create tension and make the pain worse.
- Do not allow the person to walk! You and other bystanders must move the patient if necessary.
- Place the patient in the position they find most comfortable. This is usually a semi-reclining or sitting position.
- If your local protocols permit, help the patient take one adult aspirin (325 mg) or two to four low-dose aspirins (81 mg each). Instruct the patient to chew and then swallow the aspirin tablets.
- If oxygen is available and you are trained to use it, administer it to the patient. Supplemental oxygen increases the amount of oxygen the blood can carry. The increase in oxygen reduces pain and anxiety. It also eases the minds of the patient's family and friends to see that you are doing something to relieve the patient's physical distress.
- Be prepared to perform CPR, if necessary.
- If an automated external defibrillator (AED) is available, have it brought to the patient and make sure it is ready for use, if needed.

As an EMR, you may not have extensive equipment available to help a patient experiencing a heart attack; therefore, your primary role is to provide emotional support and arrange for prompt transport to an appropriate medical facility. Because the patient's emotional state can affect their physical condition, emotional support is valuable.

Words of Wisdom

Research has shown that the administration of one adult aspirin (325 mg) or two to four low-dose aspirins (81 mg each) may decrease the risk of death from a heart attack by reducing the size of the blood clot in the heart. The American Heart Association recommends that patients experiencing chest pain take aspirin as soon as possible. The patient should chew and then swallow the aspirin tablets. Check to be sure the patient is not allergic to aspirin and has not had any recent internal bleeding such as a stomach ulcer. Check with your supervisor or medical director to see if your department recommends aspirin administration in patients with chest pain.

Treatment

Not everyone having a heart attack has severe chest pain. Older people, women, and people with diabetes are more likely to have "silent" heart attacks. People experiencing silent heart attacks may report vague feelings of discomfort and not feel the classic chest pain associated with heart attacks. Do not discount vague complaints in these patients. The only way to rule out a heart attack is to undergo a thorough examination by a physician.

Special Populations

Recognizing Signs and Symptoms in Geriatric Patients

When caring for geriatric patients, it is important to understand that the signs and symptoms of medical conditions may be different from the classic signs and symptoms you would expect in a younger patient. Remember, older patients often have a decreased awareness or sensation to the pain of a medical or trauma condition. Older patients are more likely to have a silent heart attack, where they do not experience acute pain; hence, they may not realize they are experiencing a heart attack. Maintain a high degree of suspicion when assessing older adults. It is better to err on the side of overtreating than undertreating. Arrange for transport to the hospital.

YOU are the EMR — CASE 2

You are at a local diner where you have just placed your order for dinner when dispatch informs you there is an incident just around the corner. A 58-year-old woman is complaining of not feeling right, but she cannot give any specific reason other than an odd sensation in her chest.

1. You ask if she has pain in her chest and she says no. Does that mean she is not having a heart attack?
2. The woman is nervous and repeatedly asks if she is going to die. What should you do?
3. Should you administer oxygen if you are trained to use it?

Treatment

Within the past 20 years, clot-busting drugs and nonsurgical treatments, such as percutaneous coronary intervention (PCI), have been important advances in treating patients experiencing a heart attack. Clot-busting drugs and PCI can often open the blocked coronary vessels and prevent the need for costly and painful surgery. These treatments are most effective when administered as soon after the onset of the symptoms of a heart attack as possible. Your prompt response and attentive care of a patient experiencing a heart attack may be the first step in returning that patient to a comfortable, healthy, and productive life.

Words of Wisdom

Many EMS units are equipped with electrocardiography (ECG) machines that can produce a computer-generated assessment of the patient's heart rhythm. This assessment helps qualified EMS clinicians determine whether the patient is experiencing a heart attack and ensures they have correctly evaluated the patient's signs and symptoms, enabling them to begin the proper treatment before the patient is transported to the hospital.

Heart Failure

Heart failure is not directly caused by narrow or blocked coronary arteries, but by failure of the heart to pump adequately. The heart has two sides. The right side receives deoxygenated blood from the body and sends it to the lungs; the left side receives newly oxygenated blood from the lungs and pumps it to the body. If one side of the heart becomes weak and cannot pump as well as the other side, the circulatory system becomes unbalanced, resulting in circulatory congestion. In heart failure, the failure is in the heart muscle, but the congestion is in the blood vessels. **FIGURE 10-5** shows what happens if heart failure occurs on the left side of the heart, which sends blood to the body. Because the left side cannot send blood to the body as efficiently as the right side can send blood to the lungs, more blood goes to the lungs than to the body. This results in congestion (overload) in the blood vessels of the lungs.

The major symptom of heart failure is difficulty breathing, not chest pain. If you are assisting a patient who has respiratory difficulty but no airway obstruction or signs of injury, look for the signs and symptoms of heart failure. As blood pressure builds in the vessels of the lungs, fluid is forced into the lung tissue, causing it to swell. The patient may make a gurgling sound when breathing and start spitting up a white or pink froth or foamy fluid. At this point, the patient is "drowning" in their own body fluids. The patient is very anxious but is usually in little or no pain (unless they are experiencing a heart attack coupled with heart failure).

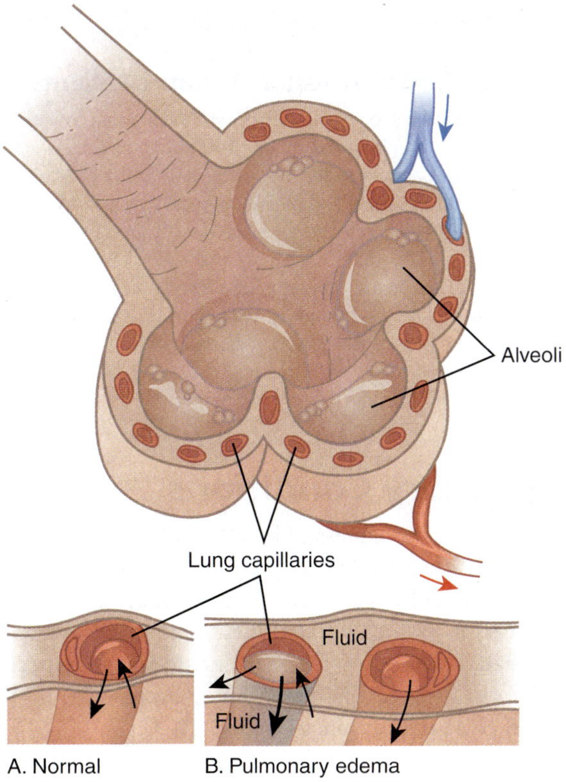

FIGURE 10-5 **A.** Normal exchange of oxygen and carbon dioxide between a capillary and an alveolus. **B.** Pulmonary edema: heart failure causes fluid to leak from the capillary and build up in the alveolus, impeding exchange of oxygen and carbon dioxide.
© Jones & Bartlett Learning

Signs and Symptoms

Signs and symptoms of heart failure include the following:

- Shortness of breath
- Rapid, shallow breathing
- Moist or gurgling respirations
- Profuse sweating
- Enlarged neck veins
- Swollen ankles
- Anxiety

As soon as you determine that your patient is experiencing heart failure, take these simple, lifesaving actions:

1. Place the patient in a sitting position, preferably on a bed or chair. Having the legs hang down over the edge of the bed or chair helps drain some of the fluid back into the lower parts of the body and may improve breathing.
2. Administer oxygen (if it is available and you are trained to give it) in large quantities and at a high flow rate.
3. Summon additional help.
4. Arrange for prompt transport to an appropriate medical facility.

The most important action you can perform is to place the patient in a sitting position with the legs down. This position helps relieve heart failure symptoms until more highly trained EMS personnel arrive.

Special Populations

Causes of Cardiac Arrest in Pediatric Patients

While adults usually experience cardiopulmonary arrest as a result of a heart attack, children may go into respiratory arrest followed by cardiac arrest because of the lack of oxygen to the heart. It is important for you to open and maintain the airway and to ventilate adequately any child with a respiratory condition. Some of the specific causes of cardiopulmonary arrest in children include suffocation caused by the aspiration of a foreign body, infections of the airway such as croup and acute epiglottitis, sudden infant death syndrome, accidental poisonings, and injuries involving the head and neck.

Respiratory Conditions

Dyspnea means shortness of breath or difficulty breathing. Although healthy people may experience shortness of breath during intense physical exertion or at high altitudes, this situation usually does not represent a medical emergency. Heart-related causes of dyspnea include angina pectoris, heart attack, and heart failure. Many pulmonary (lung) diseases can also cause dyspnea (**TABLE 10-1**).

As an EMR, you will not always be able to determine what is causing a patient to be short of breath. Do not spend too much time trying to determine the specific cause. Focus on treating the symptoms of dyspnea.

General treatment for patients with dyspnea consists of the following steps:

1. Check the patient's airway to ensure that it is not obstructed.
2. Check the rate and depth of the patient's breathing. If the rate is less than 8 breaths per minute or more than 40 breaths per minute, be prepared to assist with mouth-to-mask, mouth-to-barrier device, or bag-mask rescue breathing.
3. Place the patient in a comfortable position. An alert patient is usually most comfortable when sitting.
4. Provide reassurance.
5. Loosen any tight clothing.
6. Administer oxygen if it is available and you are trained to do so.

Special Populations

Respiratory Conditions in Pediatric Patients

A respiratory condition in an infant or child can range from a minor cold to complete blockage of the airway. Because infants breathe primarily through their noses, even a minor cold can cause breathing difficulties. The excessive mucus in the nose resulting from a cold makes it more difficult for an infant to breathe than for an older child, who can breathe through both the nose and mouth. Although colds cause most common respiratory conditions in children, you should also be able to recognize and treat the three more serious conditions: asthma, croup, and epiglottitis.

Asthma

Asthma is an acute spasm (narrowing) of the smaller air passages (bronchioles) associated with excess mucus production and swelling of the lining of the respiratory passages. A type of allergic reaction can cause an asthma attack. Severe emotional stress, exercise, or a respiratory infection can also cause an asthma attack. Asthma is a common condition, affecting people of all ages. In the United States, almost 25 million people have asthma.

TABLE 10-1 Examples of Pulmonary Conditions That May Cause Dyspnea

Condition	Description
Acute respiratory distress syndrome (ARDS)	ARDS is caused by severe lung injury that produces swelling and fluid buildup in the alveoli, possibly leading to respiratory failure.
Asthma	Asthma is caused by a clamping down or spasm of the smaller air passages.
Bronchiolitis	Bronchiolitis is caused by inflammation of the smaller airways (bronchioles) in the lungs.
Bronchitis	Bronchitis is caused by an inflammation of the larger airways (bronchi) in the lungs.
Chronic obstructive pulmonary disease (COPD)	COPD is a slow process in which the airways, alveoli, and pulmonary blood vessels are destroyed.
Emphysema	Emphysema is caused by damage to the small air sacs (alveoli) in the lungs. This damage decreases the amount of working lung capacity, resulting in shortness of breath. Emphysema results in COPD; thus, the conditions are closely associated and patients may refer to them interchangeably. As an EMR, it is important to understand that both COPD and emphysema are ongoing pulmonary diseases caused by damage to the lungs.
Pneumonia	Pneumonia is caused by an infection in the lungs.

© Jones & Bartlett Learning

Patients experiencing an asthma attack have great difficulty exhaling through partially obstructed air passages. The situation can be compared with trying to exhale through a narrow straw. You will often hear a wheezing sound, even without a stethoscope, during exhalation. The patient can inhale air without difficulty but must labor to exhale the air. The effort to exhale is both frightening and tiring for the patient, particularly if the patient is a child who does not understand what is happening. In this case, your primary treatment consists of calming and reassuring both the parents and the child. Tell them everything possible is being done and encourage them to relax.

If there is a limited amount of air moving through the small air passages, wheezing may be absent. Fatigued patients may be so short of breath that they are unable to talk. It is important that you follow the preceding steps for treating dyspnea. In addition to these steps, you can instruct the patient to perform pursed-lip breathing (**FIGURE 10-6**). Many patients with asthma are already being treated for the condition by a physician and will have taken medications before your arrival. If a child has asthma medication but it has not been administered, help the patient or caregiver administer the medication. Arrange for prompt transport to the emergency department.

Treatment

Patients who are short of breath or receiving oxygen should have their breathing and pulse monitored at least every 5 minutes. Underlying illness or trauma may cause certain patients to stop breathing and require you to begin rescue breathing.

Treatment by paramedics or in the hospital includes medications that help to relax the constricted air passages. If the patient has medication that has been prescribed by a physician, make sure the patient has taken it as prescribed.

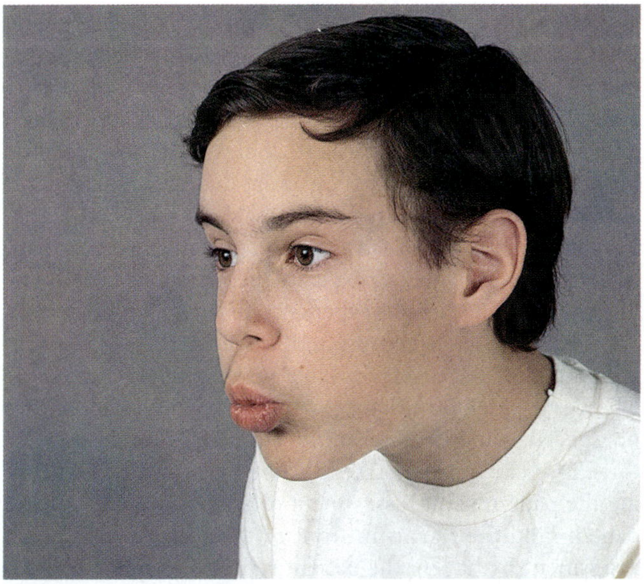

FIGURE 10-6 Pursed-lip breathing may help relieve an asthma attack.

© American Academy of Orthopaedic Surgeons

If advanced life support (ALS) is not available, arrange for prompt transport to an appropriate medical facility.

Croup

Croup is an infection of the upper airway that occurs mainly in children who are between 6 months and 6 years old. The lower throat swells and compresses (narrows) the airway, resulting in a characteristic hoarse, whooping noise during inhalation and a seal-like, barking cough.

Croup occurs often in colder climates (during fall and winter) and is frequently accompanied by a cold. The child usually has a moderate fever and a croupy noise that has developed over time. When you encounter noisy breathing, do not assume that croup is the cause. Look to see if the child is choking on a toy, food, or foreign object lodged in the airway.

The worst episodes of croup usually occur in the middle of the night. A lack of fright or anxiety in the child and the willingness to lie down are important signs for you to note because they can help you recognize the condition as croup rather than epiglottitis. Epiglottitis is a more serious condition that is discussed in the next section. Although the child may not feel frightened by the signs and symptoms of croup, parents will likely be distressed. As in many childhood emergencies, you must respond to the emotional needs and concerns of the parents as well as the medical needs of the child.

Signs and Symptoms

Signs and symptoms of croup include the following:

- Noisy, whooping inhalations
- Seal-like, barking cough
- History of a recent or current cold
- Lack of fright or anxiety
- Willingness to lie down

If the EMS unit is delayed, ask the parents to turn on the hot water in the shower and close the bathroom door. After the bathroom steams up, ask a parent to take the child into the warm bathroom. Continue to closely monitor the child's respiratory status while the child is with you and the parent in the bathroom. The moist, warm air relaxes the vocal cords and lessens the croupy noise. This effectively treats the child and reassures the parents. Arrange for transport to an appropriate medical facility.

Epiglottitis

Epiglottitis is a severe inflammation of the epiglottis, the small flap that covers the trachea during swallowing. In this condition, the flap is so inflamed and swollen that air movement into the trachea is completely blocked. Epiglottitis usually occurs in children between ages 3 to 6 years. Because of the widespread vaccination of infants against the bacteria that causes epiglottitis (*Haemophilus influenzae* type b), the incidence of this disease is much less common now than in the past. This condition also occurs in adult patients who have not received the vaccination for *H influenzae* type b.

Safety

Do not examine a child's throat if you suspect epiglottitis! An examination can cause more swelling of the epiglottis, resulting in a complete airway blockage.

While you conduct your initial examination, you may think the child has croup. However, because epiglottitis poses an immediate threat to life, you must be able to recognize the differences between croup and epiglottitis and know the signs and symptoms of epiglottitis; this is a very serious respiratory emergency. There is little that you can provide in the way of treatment except to make the child comfortable with as little handling as possible, keep everyone calm, administer oxygen (if you have it available and have been trained to use it), and arrange for prompt transport to an appropriate medical facility. You may consider letting a parent hold the child during transport if the emotional attitudes of the child and parent are appropriate.

Signs and Symptoms

The signs and symptoms of epiglottitis include the following:

- The child is usually sitting upright (does not want to lie down).
- The child cannot swallow.
- The child is not coughing.
- The child is drooling.
- The child is anxious and frightened (knows that something is seriously wrong).
- The child's chin is thrust forward.

Treatment

The child with epiglottitis must receive medical attention to ensure an open airway.

Special Populations

Respiratory Conditions in Geriatric Patients

Respiratory diseases are a major cause of sickness and death in older adults. As a person ages, the alveoli lose elasticity. This condition makes it harder to inhale oxygen and to exhale carbon dioxide. Older adults usually have a reduced lung capacity, which means they do not exchange as much air with each breath as they did when they were younger. Also, the muscles associated with respiration become weaker with age. This condition makes it harder to cough, increasing susceptibility to a variety of respiratory infections.

Chronic Obstructive Pulmonary Disease and Acute Respiratory Distress Syndrome

Patients with COPD may live with this condition for many years. They call for EMS assistance when a change to their baseline functioning, such as a cold or other respiratory infection, causes them to experience shortness of breath.

ARDS can strike a patient quickly. Pneumonia is a common infectious disease. Because many older patients have a weakened immune system, they are especially susceptible to pneumonia. Pneumonia frequently kills older people. Minor symptoms can become a major illness in a short time. A physician should examine any older patient who has congestion and a possible fever.

As usual, your role in caring for patients with a possible respiratory condition, including COPD or ARDS, is to carefully examine them, secure an accurate medical history (past and present), treat their presenting symptoms, and arrange for transport to an appropriate medical facility when indicated.

Stroke

Stroke is a leading cause of death and long-term disability in the United States. Each year, approximately 795,000 adults in the United States experience strokes. Most strokes (87%) are caused by a blood clot that lodges in an artery of the brain. The clot blocks the blood supply to a part of the brain. Without treatment, that part of the brain will be damaged or die. Think of a stroke as a "brain attack," similar to a heart attack.

Words of Wisdom

Being aware of the key risk factors for stroke is helpful in recognizing one:

- High blood pressure is the most important risk factor for stroke.
- Approximately 62% of patients hospitalized for stroke are older than 65 years; however, strokes can occur at any age.
- The risk of strokes in current smokers is almost double that of nonsmokers.

The signs and symptoms of a stroke vary depending on what portion of the brain is affected. They can be similar to the signs and symptoms of a head injury, hypoglycemia, or seizures. When you are caring for a patient who has experienced a stroke, the person may be alert, confused, or unresponsive. Responsive patients may not be aware that they have signs of a stroke. Some stroke patients are unable to speak; others are unable to move one side of their body. The patient may have a headache and may describe it as "the worst headache of my life." Some stroke patients experience seizures.

The Cincinnati Prehospital Stroke Scale is an easy-to-administer and accurate tool that you can use to determine whether a patient may have experienced a stroke. It requires no special equipment to administer. This test consists of three assessments: assessment of the facial muscles by having the patient smile, assessment of arm drift by having the patient hold their arms in front of themselves, and speech assessment by having the patient repeat a simple phrase. If the patient is not able to complete one or more of these tasks, suspect a stroke. **TABLE 10-2** describes the specific steps for administering the Cincinnati Prehospital Stroke Scale.

TABLE 10-2 The Cincinnati Prehospital Stroke Scale

The Cincinnati Prehospital Stroke Scale is a tool you can use to tell if there is a high probability that a patient has experienced a stroke. This scale requires you to quickly assess three things: facial droop, arm drift, and abnormal speech.

Facial droop	**Have patient show teeth or smile.**
Normal	Both sides of the face move equally.
Abnormal	One side of the face does not move as well as the other side.
Arm drift	**Patient closes eyes and holds both arms straight out for 10 seconds.**
Normal	Both arms move the same or both arms do not move.
Abnormal	One arm does not move or one arm drifts down compared with the other.
Speech	**Have patient say, "You can't teach an old dog new tricks."**
Normal	Patient uses correct words with no slurring.
Abnormal	Patient slurs words, uses the wrong words, or is unable to speak.

© Jones & Bartlett Learning. Courtesy of MIEMSS.

Signs and Symptoms

The signs and symptoms of stroke include the following:

- Headache
- Numbness or paralysis on one side of the body
- Dizziness
- Confusion
- Drooling
- Inability to speak
- Difficulty seeing
- Unequal pupil size
- Unresponsiveness
- Seizures
- Respiratory arrest
- Incontinence

Your first priority is to maintain an open airway. Administer oxygen (if it is available and you are trained to use it) using a nasal cannula. If the patient is having a seizure, try to prevent further injury from occurring. Be prepared to administer rescue breathing if the patient stops breathing. Place an unresponsive patient in the recovery position to help maintain an open airway. This is especially important because some stroke patients are unable to swallow. Give emotional support by talking to and touching the patient. Be especially careful if you must move a patient because some patients may not be able to feel one side of their body.

Some stroke patients can be treated with special drugs to dissolve the blood clot in their brain. These clot-busting drugs must be administered in the hospital within the first few hours after the stroke. For this reason, it is important for you to determine the time the stroke began by questioning the patient, family, or bystanders. If the patient has signs or symptoms of a stroke, it is important for you to arrange for *prompt transport* of the patient to a medical facility that is equipped to treat stroke patients. Some facilities are equipped to acutely remove blood clots that have formed that are causing strokes to occur. These interventions can be successful in certain situations for a longer period after the onset of stroke symptoms.

Treatment

Many communities have hospitals that have been designated as stroke centers, and some larger areas actually have mobile stroke units. These hospitals have specifically trained physicians and equipment and are capable not only of administering clot-busting drugs but also of performing surgical procedures to remove or break up blood clots in the vessels of the brain. These procedures are most effective when performed as soon as possible after the onset on the symptoms of a stroke. Therefore, it is important that EMS systems have protocols in place to ensure that suspected stroke patients are promptly transported to stroke centers that can provide a high level of care to stroke patients.

Street Smarts

Patients experiencing a stroke may be able to hear what you are saying even if they cannot speak or appear to be unresponsive. Be careful not to say anything that would increase the patient's anxiety.

YOU are the EMR — CASE 3

Your alert tones go off at 0517 hours. You are dispatched to a residence approximately 4 miles (6 km) from your location for the report of a sick person. While you are responding, your dispatcher informs you that the patient is a 71-year-old woman. Her husband reports that she is having trouble speaking and cannot move her right side.

1. What are your priorities for assessing this patient?
2. What tool do you have to help you with this assessment?
3. Why is it important for this patient to be transported without delay?

Diabetes

Diabetes is caused by the body's inability to process and use glucose (sugar) that is carried by the bloodstream to the body's cells. Glucose is an essential nutrient. The body's cells need both oxygen and glucose to survive. The body produces a hormone (chemical) called insulin that enables glucose carried by the blood to enter individual cells, which use it as fuel.

If the body does not produce enough insulin, the cells become "starved" for glucose. This condition is called diabetes. Many people with diabetes must take supplemental insulin injections to maintain normal blood sugar levels. Oral medicine, rather than insulin that must be injected, is sometimes used to treat mild diabetes.

Diabetes is a serious medical condition. Therefore, all patients with diabetes who are sick must be evaluated and treated in an appropriate medical facility. Two specific medical conditions can occur in patients in the course of managing their diabetes: hypoglycemia and hyperglycemia. Consider both of these conditions as medical emergencies.

Hypoglycemic Emergencies

Hypoglycemia, or low blood sugar, occurs if the body has enough insulin but not enough blood glucose. An older term for hypoglycemia is insulin shock. A person with diabetes may take insulin in the morning and then alter their usual routine by not eating or by exercising vigorously. In either case, the level of blood glucose drops and the patient experiences hypoglycemia.

The signs and symptoms of hypoglycemia (insulin shock) are similar to those of other types of shock. Suspect low blood sugar if your patient has a history of diabetes or is wearing medical emergency information, such as a medical alert necklace or bracelet.

Hypoglycemia is a serious medical emergency that can occur quickly, often within a few minutes. With low levels of blood sugar, a person with diabetes may become unresponsive. If hypoglycemia is not diagnosed and corrected by the rapid administration of glucose in some form, the patient may die or experience permanent brain injury.

A person experiencing hypoglycemia may appear to be drunk or confused. It is important not to jump to conclusions and misinterpret hypoglycemia as intoxication. If you suspect that a patient is experiencing hypoglycemia, try to get answers to the following questions:

- Do you have diabetes?
- Did you take your insulin today?
- Have you eaten today?

If the patient has diabetes and has taken insulin that day, but has not yet eaten, suspect that the patient is experiencing hypoglycemia. If the patient is able to swallow, attempt to get the patient to eat or drink something sweet. For example, you could use a drink that has a high sugar concentration such as a cola or orange juice. Honey is another possibility. Do not give a diet beverage to these patients. Diet beverages do not contain sugar.

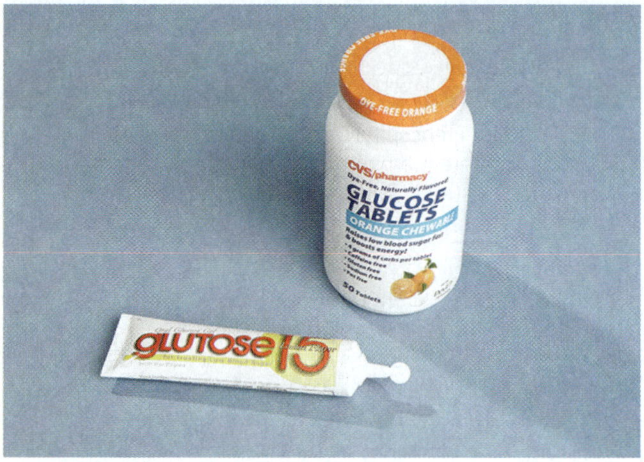

FIGURE 10-7 Instant glucose provides high concentrations of sugar.
© Jones & Bartlett Learning

Signs and Symptoms

Signs and symptoms of hypoglycemia include the following:

- Pale, moist, cool skin
- Rapid, weak pulse
- Dizziness or headache
- Confusion or unresponsiveness
- Sweating
- Hunger
- Rapid onset of symptoms (within minutes)

If the patient is unresponsive, do not try to administer anything by mouth because the patient may choke and aspirate the fluid into the lungs. Summon help immediately. Open the patient's airway, and assist breathing and circulation, if necessary. The patient must have glucose administered intravenously as soon as possible. A paramedic or a physician can do this.

Some EMRs carry glucose tablets or a tube of oral glucose gel. The preferred route for oral glucose administration is for the patient to swallow oral glucose tablets. If the patient is not able to safely swallow these, some people place a tablet or glucose gel inside the cheek. Make sure the patient is able to sit upright so there is no chance of aspiration. Some glucose will be absorbed through the inside of the patient's cheek (**FIGURE 10-7**). Glucose can be administered orally to patients who are able to swallow. Even though the patient's body may absorb only a small amount of glucose, it may be enough to keep the patient alert until they receive further medical treatment.

Words of Wisdom

Progression into hypoglycemia is rapid and may be fatal; progression into hyperglycemia usually takes several days.

Hyperglycemic Emergency

Hyperglycemia occurs when the body has too much blood glucose and not enough insulin. For example, a person with diabetes may not take insulin for several days, resulting in

Voices OF Experience

Some people end up attracting the same type of call throughout their shift or even series of shifts. That was me when I first started in EMS; I was almost guaranteed a seizure call.

Prior to my involvement with EMS, I had never witnessed a seizure. The terms *generalized seizure*, *status epilepticus*, and *postictal* were foreign.

We were dispatched to a community center for a man having a seizure. Seizures can have a variety of causes, but this patient was known to have epilepsy. When we arrived, people had cleared the area around him and he was still seizing. It was a little overwhelming to see someone writhing uncontrollably on the floor, and it took me a second to absorb what was happening. Then, the training kicked in. One of several concerns is the patient's airway, which is virtually impossible to assess while the patient is actively seizing. The patient's respiratory rate and tidal volume are compromised during a seizure. The patient may vomit during and after the seizure, presenting the possibility of aspiration. We had suction ready, along with a bag-mask device, high-flow oxygen, and an airway. The paramedic was prepared to start an IV line for both fluid and medication administration. Drugs like diazepam (Valium) are used to break or stop seriously prolonged seizure activity in a condition known as status epilepticus.

> **"It was a little overwhelming to see someone writhing on the floor uncontrollably, and it took me a second to absorb what was happening."**

As the muscular activity subsided, the patient lay still. His breathing was shallow but present. We opened his airway, verified there were not any secretions, put a nonrebreathing mask on him, providing high-flow oxygen, and placed him on his side in the recovery position. He began to show purposeful movement and mumble a little. Seizure patients in their postictal phase (after the seizure, when the body is recovering) often are not able to communicate for some time, so it is our responsibility as EMRs to look out for what they may need. The paramedic started the IV line and we prepared to load the patient onto the gurney for our 35-minute transport to the nearest hospital.

Some patients will have a medical bracelet indicating their condition; some scenes will have family or friends available to give us a medical history. Other times, we have to wait until the patient is able to provide us with information, but obtaining a SAMPLE history helps us to provide the best care possible. It is also important to keep in mind that, while someone who has been susceptible to seizures might be a little more comfortable in communicating with us after a seizure, someone who has experienced one for the first time could be scared, embarrassed, or confused, complicating the information-gathering process. Either way, be patient and understanding. The worst part is over. Give the patient a gentle, comforting ride to the hospital.

Carl M. Prather, EMSI
Santa Fe Community College
Santa Fe, New Mexico

Adapted from the personal Medical Identification Symbol of the American Medical Association.

TABLE 10-3 Comparing Hypoglycemia and Hyperglycemia

Hypoglycemia	Hyperglycemia
Pale, moist, cool skin	Warm, dry skin
Rapid, weak pulse	Rapid pulse
Normal breathing	Deep, rapid breathing
Dizziness or headache	—
Confusion or unresponsiveness	Confusion or unresponsiveness
Rapid onset of symptoms (minutes)	Slow onset of symptoms (days)

© Jones & Bartlett Learning. Courtesy of MIEMSS.

blood glucose levels that build to higher and higher levels, but there is no insulin to process it for use by the body's cells.

A patient experiencing a hyperglycemic emergency (sometimes referred to as diabetic coma) may be unresponsive. This patient may appear to have the flu (influenza) or a severe cold. As with hypoglycemia, misdiagnosis is common. It is not always easy to tell the difference between hypoglycemia and hyperglycemia (**TABLE 10-3**).

Treatment

During your initial examination of every patient, look for an emergency medical alert device (such as a necklace or bracelet) to find out whether the patient has a preexisting medical condition such as diabetes.

If the patient is alert and you cannot get definite answers to your questions to determine whether the patient is experiencing hypoglycemia or hyperglycemia, you can do no harm by administering a liquid substance that contains sugar. In a patient who is experiencing low blood sugar, the sugar may improve the patient's condition. If the patient is experiencing a hyperglycemic emergency, the sugar will not raise blood glucose levels enough to do any further harm to the patient. In general, give alert patients with diabetes sugar by mouth and arrange for prompt transport to an appropriate medical facility.

Signs and Symptoms

Signs and symptoms of hyperglycemia include the following:

- History of diabetes
- Warm, dry skin
- Rapid pulse
- Deep, rapid breathing
- Fruity or acetone odor on the patient's breath
- Weakness, nausea, and vomiting
- Increased hunger, thirst, and urination
- Slow onset of symptoms (days)

If the patient with diabetes is unresponsive, arrange for prompt transport to an appropriate medical facility. Every patient with diabetes who is experiencing illness should be transported to an appropriate medical facility for further treatment and examination.

Abdominal Pain

The abdomen is separated from the chest by the diaphragm. It is a crossroads for several body systems, including the circulatory, skeletal, nervous, digestive, and genitourinary systems. For example, the aorta carries blood from the heart through the abdomen to the lower parts of the body. Conversely, a large vein, the inferior vena cava, carries blood back to the heart. The spine, with its large trunks of nerves, runs through this area. Parts of the rib cage surround the abdominal cavity. Most of the digestive system, including the stomach, small intestine, large intestine, liver, gallbladder, and pancreas, are in the abdomen. The kidneys and ureters are located in the abdominal area, as are parts of the male and female reproductive systems.

The abdomen has both hollow and solid structures. Hollow structures, such as the small intestine, are tubes through which digestive contents pass. Solid structures, such as the pancreas, spleen, and liver, produce or process various substances used by the body. The structures in the abdomen are usually identified by quadrant, according to their location (**FIGURE 10-8**). As an EMR, you do not have to learn the names, types, and locations of all the abdominal structures, but it is helpful for you to have a basic understanding of abdominal anatomy.

The abdomen occupies a large part of the body, and abdominal pain is a common complaint. Because of the number of body systems and organs located in the abdomen, even

YOU are the EMR — **CASE 4**

You are dispatched to the Chippewa City Park for a report of a sick woman. After a 6-minute response, you arrive at the park and a concerned bystander directs you to a park bench. You find a 25- to 30-year-old woman slumped on the park bench. She is dressed in a jogging outfit. You introduce yourself and attempt to determine her primary complaint. The woman responds to verbal stimuli, but she seems confused when you ask her questions. You note that she is sweaty and has a weak pulse at a rate of 88 beats per minute.

1. What types of medical conditions or situations can cause confusion?
2. What steps can you take to determine the cause of the patient's confusion?
3. If you determine that this woman has diabetes, what steps can you take to improve her condition?

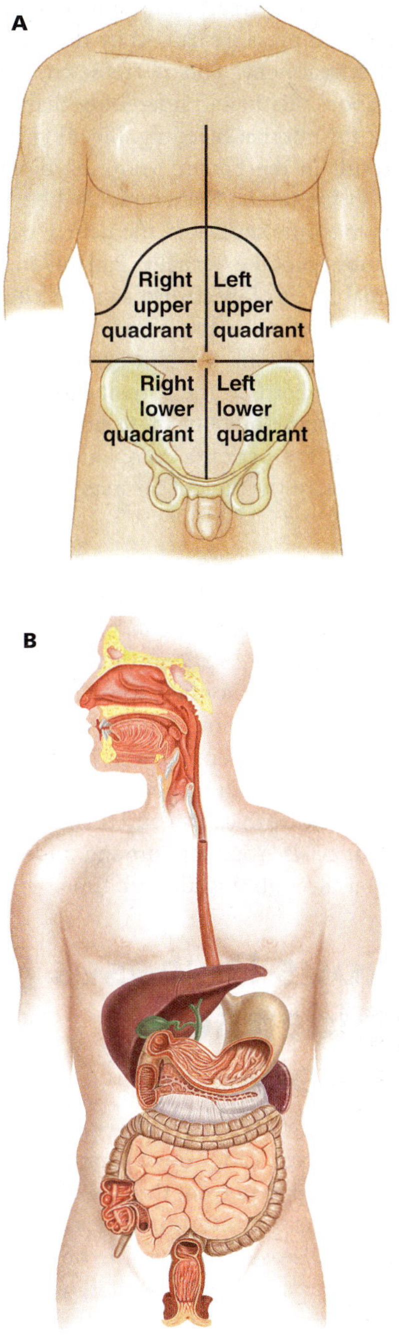

FIGURE 10-8 A. Locations on the abdomen are often designated according to four quadrants. **B.** Many organs lie in more than one quadrant.

A: © Jones & Bartlett Learning; B: © leonello calvetti/Shutterstock

physicians may have a difficult time identifying the cause of abdominal pain. As an EMR, you need to be able to recognize that a patient has an abdominal condition. You do not have to determine the cause of the abdominal pain.

One condition you may encounter is called an **acute abdomen**. Irritation of the abdominal wall causes an acute abdomen. This irritation may be the result of infection or due to the presence of blood or leakage from the gastrointestinal tract in the abdominal cavity as a result of disease or trauma. A patient with an acute abdomen may have referred pain in other parts of the body such as the shoulder. The abdomen may feel as hard as a board. These patients may have nausea and vomiting, fever, and diarrhea, as well as pain.

Some patients with abdominal pain will vomit blood because they are bleeding from the esophagus or the stomach. Bleeding from the lower part of the gastrointestinal tract may produce bloody stools that contain bright red blood, or the stools may be black and tarry. Treat these patients for shock. Arrange for prompt transport to an appropriate medical facility.

If a patient has abdominal pain, monitor vital signs, treat symptoms of shock, keep the patient comfortable, and arrange for transport to an appropriate medical facility. It is important for a physician to examine these patients.

One of the most serious causes of abdominal pain in children is appendicitis. Although it can occur at any age, appendicitis is often seen in people who are between 10 and 25 years. A cramping pain usually starts in the belly button area of the abdomen. Within a few hours, the pain moves to the right lower quadrant of the abdomen, becoming steady and more severe. Usually the child is nauseated, has no appetite, and occasionally will vomit. Because appendicitis is only one of several potential causes of abdominal pain, do not try to make a diagnosis in the field. A good rule is to treat every child with a sore or tender abdomen as an emergency and arrange for transport to an appropriate medical facility for an appropriate diagnosis.

Special Populations

Recognizing Appendicitis in Geriatric Patients

In geriatric patients, the signs and symptoms of appendicitis are less apparent and can be easily overlooked. As a result, there is an increased chance of a ruptured appendix in geriatric patients.

Another cause of abdominal pain is an **abdominal aortic aneurysm (AAA)**. An abdominal aortic aneurysm occurs when one or more layers of the aorta become weak and separate from other layers of the aorta. Patients who have diabetes, high blood pressure, or atherosclerosis, as well as heavy smokers, are at high risk of experiencing an AAA. The weakening of the aorta causes a ballooning of the vessel, much like a weak spot on thin rubber tubing. If this weak spot or aneurysm ruptures, the patient will rapidly lose large quantities of blood into the abdomen. This massive internal blood loss will cause profound shock.

Patients with an AAA may report pain in the abdomen. Some patients describe this pain as a tearing sensation. They may have pain referred to the shoulder. If an AAA ruptures, the patient will experience severe pain and profound shock from the blood spilling into the abdomen.

Signs and Symptoms

Signs and symptoms of an acute abdomen include the following:

- Nausea and vomiting
- Loss of appetite
- Pain in the abdomen
- Rigid abdomen
- Distention
- Shock

Place any patient who experiences these signs and symptoms in a comfortable position. This is often a side-lying position with the legs drawn up. Treat the patient for shock. Handle these patients gently and arrange for prompt transport to an appropriate medical facility. The sooner these patients receive medical care, the better their chance of survival will be.

Special Populations

Vomiting and Diarrhea in Pediatric Patients

Children are very susceptible to vomiting and diarrhea, which are often caused by gastrointestinal infections. Prolonged vomiting and diarrhea may produce severe dehydration. The dehydrated child is lethargic and has very dry skin, which can be especially noticeable around the mouth and nose. Hospitalization may be required to replace fluids through the veins. If you suspect that a child may be dehydrated, arrange for transport to an appropriate medical facility.

Kidney Dialysis

People with certain types of kidney disease are unable to filter waste products from their bloodstream. Many patients with chronic kidney disease must undergo a treatment called hemodialysis, usually three times per week. During hemodialysis, the patient's blood passes through a machine that filters out the waste products and returns the cleansed blood to the patient (**FIGURE 10-9**). Most hemodialysis patients undergo a medical procedure to create a fistula or shunt in their arm or leg. The fistula is a surgically created connection between an artery and a vein. The fistula is used to connect the patient to the hemodialysis machine. A fistula looks like a raised bump on the patient's arm or leg. If you are caring for a person who is on dialysis, find out if they have a fistula. If a fistula is in place, be sure to take the patient's blood pressure in the arm without the fistula to prevent damaging it.

Patients who are receiving dialysis treatment may experience medical emergencies related to the treatment. During or shortly after dialysis treatment, patients may experience a decrease in blood pressure caused by the changes in their body from the treatment. This decrease in blood pressure can produce shock. Patients undergoing dialysis treatment are also at risk for internal bleeding. Bleeding from stomach ulcers may result in the patient vomiting blood or having bloody stools. If the tubing that connects the patient's shunt to the dialysis machine separates, the patient can lose a substantial amount of blood externally. Patients may also experience abnormal levels of electrolytes in their blood that can cause cardiac dysrhythmias that sometimes result in cardiac arrest. For these conditions, treat the symptoms presented by the patient. Remember that the patient can most likely supply you with information about these situations. If not, seek information from the patient's companions and caregivers because they are with the patient for many hours each week.

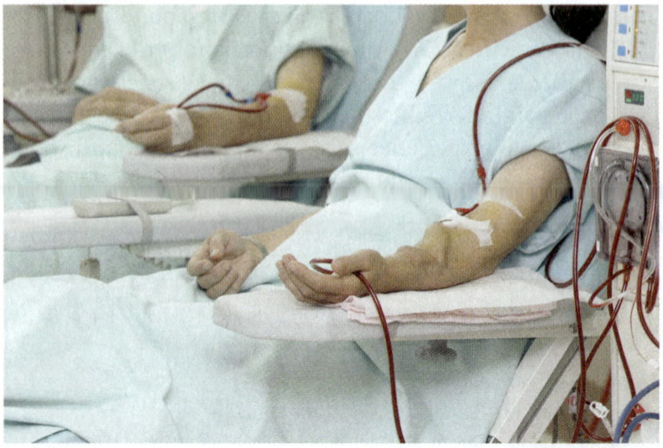

FIGURE 10-9 Patients receiving hemodialysis at a community-based dialysis clinic.

© Picsfive/Shutterstock

Cancer

Cancer is a frequent cause of disability and death in older patients, although it can affect patients of any age. Cancer can strike any part of the body. Patients do not call EMS because they have cancer. They call for help when complications from the cancer result in acute pain, shortness of breath, shock, or some other medical condition. These patients require prehospital support and then transport to a medical facility for stabilization. Patients with cancer and their families are experiencing a major crisis. Your support and understanding will help them to get through this difficult time.

Infectious Diseases and Epidemics

Infectious Diseases

As an EMR, you must understand a few principles about infectious diseases so you can protect yourself, provide proper patient care, and help to prevent the spread of infectious diseases to other people. An infectious disease is an illness that is transmitted by disease-carrying microorganisms (pathogens), such as bacteria, viruses, parasites, or fungi.

Infectious diseases can be spread from one person to another by direct contact, indirect contact, or contact with blood. Methicillin-resistant *Staphylococcus aureus* (MRSA) is an example of an infectious disease that is spread by direct contact between the patient's skin and contaminated clothing or towels.

Coughing, sneezing, and spitting produce droplets or aerosols, small particles of fluids, which are propelled into the air. Contaminated droplets or aerosols can produce an indirect transmission of infectious diseases. Examples of infectious diseases transmitted by indirect contact include influenza, coronavirus disease 2019 (COVID-19), and tuberculosis.

Some infectious diseases are transmitted by coming in contact with blood from an infected patient. Examples of diseases that are spread by contact with blood or other body fluids are HIV, hepatitis B, and hepatitis C. These infectious

Special Populations

High Fever in Pediatric Patients

Fevers occur quite commonly in children and can be caused by many different infections, especially ear and gastrointestinal infections. Because the temperature-regulating mechanism in young children has not fully developed, a very high temperature (104°F to 106°F [40°C to 41°C]) can occur quickly even with a relatively minor infection. Most children can tolerate temperatures as high as 104°F (40°C), but a high fever may require that the child be hospitalized so that the underlying cause can be identified and treated.

Your first step in treating a child with a high fever is to uncover the child so that body heat can escape. Layers of clothing or blankets retain body heat and can increase the patient's body temperature high enough to cause convulsions. Between 2% and 5% of children between 3 months and 6 years of age will experience seizures brought on by high fevers, called febrile seizures. These seizures usually last approximately 20 seconds.

Remember that in attempting to reduce a high fever, you are treating only the symptom and not the source. A physician must see the child as soon as possible to determine the cause of the fever.

If you encounter a child with a temperature higher than 104°F (40°C), take these steps to treat the fever symptoms:

1. Make certain the child is not wrapped in too much clothing or too many blankets.
2. Attempt to reduce the high temperature by undressing the child.
3. Fan the child to provide cooling. However, never cool a patient to the point of shivering.
4. Protect the child during any seizure (do not restrain the child's motion), and make certain that normal breathing resumes after each seizure.

agents are called bloodborne pathogens. You need to follow standard precautions to prevent the spread of infectious diseases to yourself and to others.

Epidemics and Pandemics

An **epidemic** is an infectious disease or condition that affects many people at the same time in the same geographic area. If an epidemic spreads to many different parts of the world at the same time, it is called a **pandemic**. Pandemics, global outbreaks of a disease, can occur when a novel strain of a virus emerges and is able to infect people easily and spread from person to person in an efficient and sustained manner. Transmission from one person to another is enhanced when people have no natural immunity to a new virus and no vaccine is available against the new disease. This sequence of conditions occurred in 2020 and resulted in the COVID-19 pandemic.

The specific steps needed to protect patients and caregivers from contracting or spreading a virus may not be known during the beginning of an epidemic or pandemic. However, as more information is learned about a new disease, valuable guidance and protocols will be made available through reputable organizations such as the Centers for Disease Control and Prevention, the Occupational Safety and Health Administration (OSHA), and public health officials. This information will be made available to you through your medical director and department supervisors. Avoid obtaining information from sources that lack scientifically based information. During an epidemic or pandemic, it is important that you follow established protocols to prevent spread of the disease organisms to yourself and to others. You have an important part in preventing the spread of a disease during an epidemic.

Although epidemics and pandemics may seem like rare events, it is important to remember that they do occur with some regularity. **TABLE 10-4** outlines epidemics and pandemics that have occurred since 2000.

Pharmacology

Pharmacology is the study of the effects of drugs on people and animals. Drugs are defined as chemical substances, including medications, that affect living organisms. As an EMR, you may need to administer certain emergency medications. It is important that you understand how these medications

TABLE 10-4 Epidemics and Pandemics That Have Occurred Since 2000

Epidemic/Pandemic Name	Disease	Date	Location and Number of Cases
SARS pandemic	Severe acute respiratory syndrome (SARS)	2002–2004	China, Hong Kong, Taiwan, Canada, Singapore; 8,096 reported cases, 774 deaths
Mweka Ebola epidemic	Ebola	2007	Democratic Republic of the Congo; 264 reported cases, 187 deaths
Swine flu pandemic	Pandemic H1N1/09 virus	2009–2010	Worldwide; 0.7–1.4 billion estimated cases, 151,700–575,400 deaths
MERS pandemic	Middle East respiratory syndrome (MERS)	2012–2020	Worldwide; 2,613 confirmed cases, 943 deaths
COVID-19 coronavirus pandemic	COVID-19/novel coronavirus	2019–2023	Worldwide; 704 million estimated cases, more than 7 million deaths

© Jones & Bartlett Learning

function, when they should or should not be used, and how to safely administer them.

Medication Safety Principles

To ensure safe administration of medications, EMS systems use a medication cross-check procedure. A **medication cross-check** is a team-based communication method to verify that the proper medication is being given by the correct route of administration to the correct patient. It requires two people to implement. There are many different medication cross-check systems. You should learn the steps to the specific cross-check used in your EMS system if you are expected to assist in this process. If you are by yourself, you will need to double-check each step when administering emergency medications.

One widely used method to prevent errors in medication administration is to review the rights of medication administration, which include the following:

- Right patient
- Right medication and indication
- Right dose
- Right route of administration
- Right time
- Right documentation

Using a medication cross-check with attention to these rights has been proven to reduce the risk of medication errors.

Routes of Administration

Medications can be administered in several different ways, including the following:

- Orally, such as by helping the patient swallow a pill with water
- Nasally, by spraying the medication inside the nostril
- By inhalation, such as by applying a mask to the patient's face so they can breathe the medication in through the mouth and nose
- By injection, by using a needle to place the medicine under the skin, into a muscle, or into a vein

A medication taken orally will usually be absorbed more slowly than one that is inhaled, injected, or administered nasally.

Medication Properties

You must understand the basic properties of any medication you are authorized to administer. Drugs are typically described by the following properties:

- **Name.** Medications are referred to by their generic name or their trade name.
- **Effects.** Medications produce desired outcomes. They can also produce undesired outcomes, referred to as adverse effects or side effects.
- **Indications.** There is always a reason or condition for which a particular medication is given.
- **Contraindications.** There are situations in which a medication should not be given, even if it usually is indicated for that person's condition.
- **Routes of administration.** As discussed, medications can enter the body through various routes.
- **Dosage.** The amount of the medication that is given often depends on the patient's weight or age. It also depends on the desired effect the medication.

Special Populations

Weight-Based Dosing in Children

The dosages of medications that paramedics give to children are based on the child's weight. It is not possible to weigh a child in an emergency setting. However, because a child's weight is related to their height, it is possible to determine proper dosing of a medication based on the child's height. Several reference tools are commonly used by paramedics to determine the proper medication dosage. If the advanced-level EMS clinicians in your community use one of these reference tools and you will be expected to assist them, you should receive training in this dosing system.

Words of Wisdom

In addition to the four drugs that EMRs may administer, patients may be prescribed many other medications that they take regularly to treat chronic conditions. As such, these medications are sometimes referred to as chronic medications. EMRs are not expected to have knowledge of these chronic medications.

Special Populations

End-of-Life Issues

Caring for geriatric patients or those with a terminal condition can be emotionally challenging. A **hospice** is a health care program that brings together a variety of caregivers to provide physical, emotional, spiritual, social, and economic care for patients who have terminal illnesses and who are expected to die within the next 6 months. Hospice care is provided in the patient's home or in a special facility.

The hospice's interdisciplinary programs are designed to provide pain relief and other supportive care when there is no hope that the patient can recover from the illness. One of the goals of a hospice is to provide pain relief without the use of needles or intravenous lines. Pain relief is provided through oral medications, medication patches, and medicine placed in the mouth between the gum and the cheek. Many hospice patients have some type of cancer.

When the hospice care is working well, EMS clinicians are usually not called. However, if the patient experiences unexpected conditions such as shortness of breath, EMS may be requested by a family member or by a caregiver. In the event that you are called to care for someone who is in hospice care, it is helpful for you to know the purpose of the hospice and the types of care being provided. Patients who are under hospice care may have advance directives requesting that they not be resuscitated. If there is any question about whether you should begin treatment, begin treatment and let the physician at the hospital make any further decisions. See Chapter 4, *Medical, Legal, and Ethical Issues*, for further discussion of legal considerations relating to end-of-life care.

EMR-Administered Medications

There are four medications you may be authorized to administer as an EMR: oxygen, aspirin, epinephrine, and naloxone. Oxygen is used for patients who are having difficulty breathing. It is administered by inhalation. Aspirin is used for patients who exhibit signs of a possible heart attack. It is administered orally. Epinephrine is used for patients who are experiencing an acute allergic reaction. It is administered intramuscularly by using an auto-injector or nasally with a premeasured unit-dose device. Naloxone is used to reverse the effects of an overdose of an opioid drug. It is administered intranasally with a premeasured unit-dose device.

A description of each of these four medications is included in the chapter of this text where that medication's use is most relevant.

Patients With Advanced Medical Needs

Modern medical science has made great advances in treating patients with chronic conditions. In the past, most patients with serious chronic medical conditions were treated in hospitals or rehabilitation facilities; many died shortly after their conditions were diagnosed. Today, many patients are treated at home by nurses, home health aides, or family members. The life expectancy of people with chronic conditions has greatly increased. Patients with chronic conditions may be of any age. Most patients with chronic conditions are older. However, remember that young children with complex chronic conditions are often treated at home as well.

As an EMR, you may be called to assist with these patients for a variety of reasons, ranging from trauma or illness to mechanical failures or transport needs. A minor illness for a healthy person can be life threatening for a patient with a chronic condition. Some patients fall and sustain musculoskeletal trauma, whereas others simply need help getting back into bed. Medical equipment may stop working because the power or backup batteries failed. Patients may need transport to a hospital for assessment and treatment.

When you receive such a call, remember your role as an EMR is to assess the emergency and to use your training to take the appropriate steps in caring for the patient. Do not get overwhelmed or distracted by the complex equipment. You are not expected to understand how these complex medical devices work. The people caring for the patient are familiar with the equipment they use each day. Do not be afraid to ask them about the equipment and the condition of the patient. Do not hesitate to question the patient and the patient's caregivers about the issue. They can probably tell you what the issue is and how you can help. Keep in mind the principles of your training. These patients need an open airway and adequate breathing and circulation. In most situations, you need to help stabilize the patient for only a few minutes until more highly trained EMS personnel arrive to provide care.

Advanced Medical Devices

A variety of complex medical devices are used with patients who require long-term care. Devices that help patients breathe include ventilators that push oxygen into the patients' lungs, oxygen-enrichment devices, surgically inserted breathing tubes, and monitors that sound an alarm if a patient stops breathing. Patients with certain heart conditions may have pacemakers and automatic defibrillators inserted under their skin (**FIGURE 10-10**). Tubes inserted into a patient's arm, neck, or stomach may provide fluids or food. Catheters drain urine from the patient's bladder. To make matters even more complex, patients who require long-term care must often take a variety of medications.

Some cardiac patients you encounter may have a type of cardiac assist device that has been implanted to assist or correct a heart-related problem. The three most common devices you may encounter are a cardiac pacemaker, an implantable defibrillator, and a ventricular assist device (VAD).

A cardiac pacemaker is a small, battery-operated device. This device senses when the patient's heart is beating too

A

B

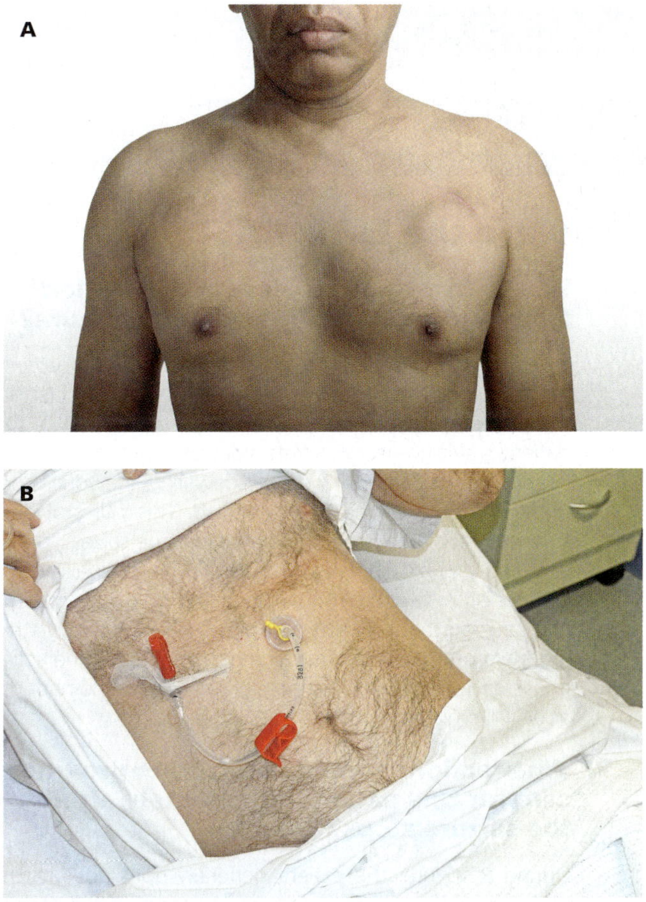

FIGURE 10-10 Complex medical devices may be used to treat patients who need chronic care. **A.** Patient with a surgically implanted pacemaker in the upper left chest. **B.** Patient with a feeding tube inserted into the stomach.

A: © NUTTANART KHAMLAKSANA/Shutterstock; B: © Douglas Cliff/Shutterstock

slowly or irregularly. It then sends an electrical impulse or signal to the heart that makes it beat at the correct rate. Pacemakers weigh as little as 1 ounce (28 g) and consist of two parts. A generator contains a battery and electrical circuitry to control the heartbeat, and wires connect the heart to the generator. The pacemaker is implanted under the skin, often just under the left collarbone. You can often feel or see a small lump in this location.

An implantable defibrillator is a device that detects any life-threatening or rapid heartbeat or dysrhythmia. If a life-threatening dysrhythmia occurs, the defibrillator quickly sends an electrical shock to the heart to stop the rhythm and allow the heart's pacemaker to resume a normal pattern. These defibrillators contain two main parts. The pulse generator is about the size of a large pocket watch and contains a battery and electrical circuits to read the electrical activity of the heart. The electrodes are the wires or leads that go through the veins to the heart and connect to the generator. Some defibrillators also contain a pacemaker in case the heart is beating too slowly. Defibrillators are also usually placed under the skin on the left side of the chest just below the collarbone.

VADs help the heart to pump blood from one of the ventricles to the rest of the body or to the other side of the heart. These devices are implanted in patients who have a weakened heart that is not capable of pumping enough blood. In most cases, VADs are connected to machinery outside the body. VADs consist of three parts. The first part is a pump that weighs up to 2 pounds (1 kg). It may be implanted inside the body or placed outside the body. The second part is an electronic controller that controls how the pump works. The third part is the battery, which is carried outside the patient's body. The battery is connected to the pump through a cable that goes into the patient's abdomen. Patients with a VAD may not have a detectable pulse because the pump produces a steady flow of blood instead of the pulsing from a natural heartbeat.

If patients with any of these devices are unresponsive, lack a pulse, and are not breathing, you should begin CPR as you would with any other patient. If you need to attach an AED to a patient with a pacemaker or a defibrillator, be careful to avoid placing a defibrillator pad over the lump where the pacemaker or defibrillator is located. Place the defibrillator pad below the device in such a manner that the electrical charge will still pass through the heart.

Patients who have these devices usually have identification in the form of a bracelet or card that indicates which type of device they have. Although you are not expected to completely understand how these devices work, it is important to inform other EMS personnel about the presence of these devices.

YOU are the EMR SUMMARY

You are the EMR: CASE 1

1. What can you do to prevent this patient from hurting himself during the seizure?

Focus care for a patient experiencing a seizure on protecting the patient from further harm. Move any objects that the patient may strike or hit out of his way. Because this patient is seizing on a concrete sidewalk, try to prevent his head from violently striking the sidewalk. Slide your shoes under the back of the patient's head. This will provide a softer surface for the back of his head as he seizes. To prevent injury to his elbows as they strike the sidewalk, grasp each wrist with one of your hands and hold his wrists up in a position that prevents his elbows from forcefully striking the ground without restraining them. During the active phase of a seizure, it is not possible to control the patient's airway. Do not attempt to restrain the patient.

2. What actions should you take to provide care for this patient immediately after the seizure stops?

During a seizure, the patient generally does not breathe and their skin tone may change. As soon as the seizure stops, take steps to ensure that the patient has an open airway. The best way to accomplish this is to use the head tilt–chin lift maneuver. After you have opened the airway, make sure the patient starts to breathe. When you are sure the patient is breathing adequately, place the patient in the recovery position. This position will help to keep the airway open and to allow any secretions (saliva or blood from a bitten tongue) to drain from the patient.

3. What additional care does this patient need during the first few hours after the seizure stops?

After you have ensured that the airway is open and the patient is breathing adequately, the patient needs additional care. Remember that following a seizure the patient will experience a state of confusion that may last 30 to 45 minutes. The patient may become anxious, hostile, or belligerent. Often this confusion will resolve with time and adequate respirations. Immediately after a seizure the patient needs privacy. It may help to move the patient to a more comfortable private place until EMS personnel arrive. Arrange for transport to an appropriate medical facility. Usually, you will not be able to determine the cause of a seizure. A physician needs to carefully evaluate the patient to determine the cause of the seizure. Once the physician determines the cause of the seizure, the patient can begin appropriate treatment. Remember that seizures can be caused by many different conditions, including stroke, epilepsy, head injury, shock, high fever, infection, poisoning, brain tumors, and low levels of blood sugar and of

YOU are the EMR SUMMARY

oxygen to the brain. Your role as an EMR is to ensure that the patient receives careful evaluation and further care at an appropriate health care facility.

You are the EMR: CASE 2

1. You ask if she has pain in her chest and she says no. Does that mean she is not having a heart attack?

Not every person having a heart attack has the classic symptom of chest pain. Older people, women, and people with diabetes can have what is referred to as a silent heart attack with symptoms that tend to be vague. Like this woman, people experiencing a silent heart attack may report discomfort that does not seem like the classic crushing chest pain associated with most heart attacks. As an EMR, do not discount vague symptoms. Assure the woman that the best treatment is a thorough evaluation by an emergency department physician.

2. The woman is nervous and repeatedly asks if she is going to die. What should you do?

Patients with heart issues are often frightened and feel a sense of doom. As always, as a trained EMR at the scene, you must remain calm. Your confidence will help reduce her stress. Reassure the woman that you are there to help. Establish a bond with the patient by talking with confidence, and hold her hand. Fear can create tension, resulting in additional pain or causing the condition to worsen. Your steps toward lowering her anxiety level may improve her condition. Make sure she is in a position of comfort and move her as little as possible.

3. Should you administer oxygen if you are trained to use it?

Yes, you should administer oxygen if allowed to do so. Supplemental oxygen boosts the amount of oxygen the blood can carry and can help reduce pain and anxiety. The simple action of administering oxygen can help ease the minds of family members by showing them that you are doing something to help their loved one. If providing oxygen, check the patient's breathing and pulse at least every 5 minutes and follow your local protocols for oxygen administration.

You are the EMR: CASE 3

1. What are your priorities for assessing this patient?

Obtaining information about the patient's condition before you arrive on the scene is always helpful. With this information, you can start thinking about what conditions might cause the signs and symptoms communicated to you. However, this information should not distract you from carefully completing the steps of the patient assessment sequence. For this situation, it is important for you to assess the scene for safety and then perform a primary assessment. Determine the patient's level of responsiveness, and then assess her airway, breathing, and circulation. Correct any problems, if necessary. For example, if secretions in the airway are creating breathing difficulty, it may be necessary to place her lying on her side. Once you have completed the primary assessment, continue by obtaining the patient's medical history and performing a secondary assessment. After completing these steps, perform an ongoing reassessment every 5 minutes.

2. What tool do you have to help you with this assessment?

The Cincinnati Prehospital Stroke Scale is a valuable tool for assessing a person who has signs or symptoms of a stroke. Assume that a patient who shows signs of facial droop, arm drift, or abnormal speech is experiencing a stroke. The results obtained from administering the Cincinnati Prehospital Stroke Scale also help the paramedics and physicians who will be treating the patient.

3. Why is it important for this patient to be transported without delay?

Some stroke patients can be treated with special drugs or procedures to dissolve or retrieve the blood clot in their brain. These interventions must occur soon after the stroke occurs. It is important that you try to determine when the patient's symptoms began and to arrange for prompt transport of this patient because she has signs and symptoms of a stroke. Your assessment and care will help ensure that this patient has the best chance of a full recovery.

You are the EMR: CASE 4

1. What types of medical conditions or situations can cause confusion?

There are many reasons a person may become confused. As an EMR, you will sometimes not be able to determine the cause of a patient's confusion. One way to approach a confused patient is to consider some of the conditions that might cause confusion. One category of conditions that may cause confusion is trauma. Patients who have experienced an open or closed head injury, recently or in the past, may be confused. Shock from internal or external blood loss or other causes can result in confusion. A second category of conditions that may result in confusion is medical conditions. Some heart conditions can result in a slow heart rate and in confusion. Heart attack and strokes can result in confusion. Patients with irregularities in blood sugar levels, including diabetes, become confused. People who just had a seizure are confused. A third category of conditions that can result in confusion is improper levels of medications and drugs. The intentional or unintentional overdose of prescribed medications or unprescribed drugs

YOU are the EMR SUMMARY

or alcohol can result in confusion. Taking too small an amount of certain medications can have the same effect. A fourth category of conditions that can cause confusion is mental illness. Medication may play a role in these patients' confusion, too. Finally, a broad consideration for patients experiencing confusion is oxygenation. Patients without sufficient oxygen will become confused. Insufficient levels of oxygen can occur for many reasons. This list is a review of some conditions that can cause confusion and is not comprehensive. Rather, it gives you an idea of how you can systematically approach patients with this symptom.

2. What steps can you take to determine the cause of the patient's confusion?

Always attempt to talk with the patient to gather as much information as possible. The SAMPLE history format provides a good framework to gather appropriate information. If the patient is not able to give you this information, consider other approaches. If there is a friend, relative, or caregiver with the patient, this person can often assist you with gathering this information. Bystanders who have witnessed the scene before you arrive can sometimes help. Carefully look for any medical alert devices on the patient's neck, wrist, and ankle. Check to see if the patient has any identification. Often the patient will have information related to a medical condition that might result in an altered level of consciousness. If you are not able to determine the cause of the patient's confusion, treat any symptoms you find. Finally, make sure the next level of EMS personnel takes over the patient's care or the patient is transported to an appropriate medical facility.

3. If you determine that this woman has diabetes, what steps can you take to improve her condition?

If you suspect the patient has diabetes, try to ask her specific yes/no questions. Do you have diabetes? Have you taken your insulin today? When did you last have anything to eat? Even though she is confused, she may be able to answer these questions. Next, if she is able to swallow, try to give her some sugar to increase her blood glucose level. If you have some instant glucose tablets or gel, follow the instructions for administering this. If this is not available, try to find some orange juice or a carbonated drink that has sugar in it. These drinks can sometimes raise the blood sugar level enough to help the patient. If nothing is available to give the woman, remember that the EMS transport crew will be able to give her glucose either orally or through a vein. Make sure to turn over this patient to EMTs for additional care.

Prep Kit

Ready for Review

- Your approach to a patient who has a general medical complaint should follow the systematic patient assessment sequence. Usually, it is best to collect a medical history on the patient experiencing a medical condition before you perform a physical examination. The SAMPLE history format will help you secure the information you need.
- General medical complaints may have different causes, but they may result in similar signs and symptoms. By becoming skilled at recognizing the signs and symptoms of various general medical complaints and learning about general treatment guidelines, you will be able to provide immediate care for patients even if you cannot determine the exact cause of the condition.
- Altered mental status is a sudden or gradual decrease in the patient's level of responsiveness. When you are assessing altered mental status in a patient, remember the AVPU scale. Complete the patient assessment sequence to ensure scene safety and proper assessment. Initial treatment should consist of maintaining the patient's ABCs and normal body temperature and keeping the patient safe from incurring any additional harm. If the patient is unresponsive and has not sustained trauma, place the patient in the recovery position or use an airway adjunct to help maintain an open airway.
- Seizures are caused by sudden episodes of uncontrolled electrical impulses in the brain. Usually, the seizure will be over by the time you arrive at the scene. If it has not ended, focus your treatment on protecting the patient from injury. Do not restrain the patient's movements. You cannot do anything about the patient's airway during the seizure, but once the seizure has stopped, it is essential that you ensure an open airway. After you have opened the airway, place the patient in the recovery position and arrange for transport to an appropriate medical facility.
- As an EMR, you should be familiar with the specific medical conditions that you are likely to encounter, including angina pectoris, heart attack, heart failure, dyspnea, asthma, stroke, hypoglycemia, hyperglycemia, and abdominal pain. Although a physician must

Prep Kit

diagnose and treat these conditions, you can greatly improve the patient's chances of survival by taking the simple actions described here until more highly trained EMS personnel arrive on the scene to assist you.

- Preventing the spread of infectious diseases and safely responding to patients who have been exposed to these diseases are important skills for the EMR. Recent epidemics and pandemics have demonstrated just how dangerous infectious diseases can be.
- Some situations may require you to assist higher-level EMS clinicians. You should understand your potential role at emergencies involving advanced medical equipment or medication administration.

Vital Vocabulary

abdominal aortic aneurysm (AAA) A condition in which the layers of the aorta in the abdomen weaken. This causes blood to leak between the layers of the artery, causing it to bulge and sometimes rupture.

acute abdomen The sudden onset of abdominal pain caused by disease or trauma that irritates the lining of the abdominal cavity and requires immediate medical or surgical treatment.

acute respiratory distress syndrome (ARDS) A condition in which severe lung injury produces swelling and fluid buildup in the alveoli, possibly leading to respiratory failure.

altered mental status A sudden or gradual decrease in the person's level of responsiveness; measured using the AVPU scale.

angina pectoris Chest pain with squeezing or tightness in the chest caused by an inadequate flow of blood to the heart muscle.

asthma A disease in which the airway becomes narrowed and inflamed, resulting in episodes of shortness of breath because of air being trapped in the small air sacs of the lungs.

atherosclerosis A disease characterized by thickening and destruction of the arterial walls and caused by fatty deposits within them; the arteries lose the ability to dilate and carry blood.

bronchiolitis Inflammation of the small airways (bronchioles) in the lungs.

bronchitis Inflammation of the airways (bronchi) in the lungs.

cardiac arrest Cessation of breathing and a heartbeat.

chronic obstructive pulmonary disease (COPD) A slow process of destruction of the airways, alveoli, and pulmonary blood vessels caused by chronic bronchial obstruction (emphysema).

croup Inflammation and narrowing of the air passages in young children, causing a barking cough, hoarseness, and a harsh, high-pitched breathing sound.

diabetes A disease in which the body is unable to use glucose normally because of a deficiency or total lack of insulin.

dyspnea Shortness of breath or difficulty breathing.

emphysema Damage to the small air sacs (alveoli) in the lungs, which decreases the amount of working lung capacity, resulting in shortness of breath.

epidemic An infectious disease or condition that affects many people at the same time in the same geographic area.

epiglottitis Severe inflammation and swelling of the epiglottis; a life-threatening situation.

epilepsy A disease manifested by seizures, caused by an abnormal focus of electrical activity in the brain.

generalized seizures Seizures characterized by contractions of all the body's muscle groups that may last for 1 to 2 minutes; formerly known as grand mal seizures.

hospice A health care program that brings together a variety of caregivers to provide physical, emotional, spiritual, social, and economic care for patients who have terminal illnesses and a short life expectancy.

hyperglycemia A condition of high blood sugar that occurs when the body has too much glucose and not enough insulin.

hypoglycemia A condition of low blood sugar that occurs in a person with diabetes who has taken too much insulin or has not eaten enough food.

medication cross-check A team-based communication method to verify that the proper medication is being given by the correct route of administration to the correct patient.

nitroglycerin A medication used to treat angina pectoris; increases blood flow and oxygen supply to alleviate the pain of angina pectoris.

pandemic An infectious disease or condition that affects many people at the same time in the many geographic areas of the world; a global disease outbreak.

Prep Kit

pharmacology The study of the effects of drugs and chemicals on people and animals.

pneumonia An infection that causes inflammation of the air sacs within the lungs.

seizure A neurologic episode that causes uncoordinated muscular activity, resulting from a surge of electrical activity in the brain.

stroke A brain attack caused by a blood clot or a broken blood vessel in the brain. Strokes can result in trouble speaking, inability to move parts of the body, confusion, or unresponsiveness.

References

Health conditions: lower your risk of stroke. My Health Finder website. https://health.gov/myhealthfinder/topics/health-conditions/heart-health/reduce-your-risk-stroke. Updated January 14, 2025. Accessed January 14, 2025.

Most recent national asthma data. Centers for Disease Control and Prevention website. https://www.cdc.gov/asthma/most_recent_national_asthma_data.htm. Reviewed May 10, 2023. Accessed January 14, 2025.

Primiani CT. Febrile seizures. Epilepsy Foundation website. https://www.epilepsy.com/what-is-epilepsy/seizure-types/febrile-seizures. Accessed January 14, 2025.

Stroke facts. Centers for Disease Control and Prevention website. https://www.cdc.gov/stroke/data-research/facts-stats/index.html. Published October 24, 2024. Accessed January 14, 2025.

Assessment IN ACTION

You are sent to a local high school in the middle of a championship basketball game for a man experiencing chest pain. When you arrive at the scene, you find a 72-year-old man sweating, leaning forward, and breathing rapidly.

1. You begin to take a SAMPLE history. What does the *P* stand for?

A. Pulse
B. Patient
C. Presumption
D. Pertinent past medical history

2. Obtaining a medical history will give you all of the following information, EXCEPT:

A. allergies.
B. medications.
C. signs and symptoms.
D. name of the illness.

3. If the patient is not able to answer your questions, how should you obtain a medical history?

A. Call the patient's physician.
B. Ask the basketball coach if he knows the man.
C. Ask the patient's son, who is standing nearby.
D. Contact medical control.

4. Complete cessation of a heartbeat is called:

A. cardiopulmonary resuscitation.
B. angina.
C. indigestion.
D. cardiac arrest.

5. During your assessment of the man, you note that he has shortness of breath, moist or gurgling respirations, and enlarged neck veins. These are signs and symptoms of:

A. asthma.
B. diabetes.
C. heart failure.
D. respiratory distress.

6. When you introduce yourself to the man, what are you looking for?

7. Why must the heart receive a constant supply of oxygen?

8. Which of the following is NOT a part of the Cincinnati Prehospital Stroke Scale?

A. Listening for abnormal speech
B. Assessing arm drift
C. Measuring the patient's blood pressure
D. Looking for facial droop

9. Which of the following is NOT helpful for a person with diabetes who has low blood sugar?

A. Instant glucose tablets
B. Diet cola
C. Orange juice
D. Oral glucose gel

10. Which of the following is NOT a sign or symptom of an acute abdomen?

A. Distention
B. Nausea and vomiting
C. Paralysis of one leg
D. Pain in the abdomen

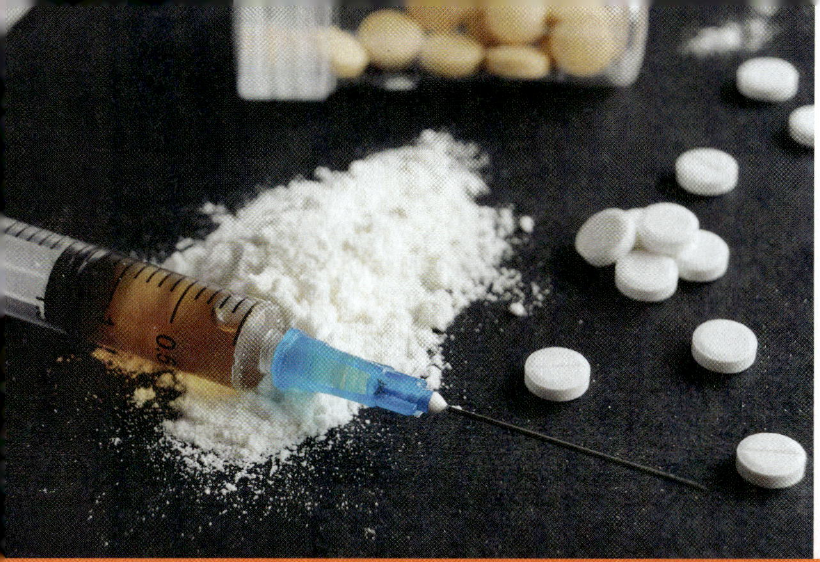

CHAPTER 11

Poisoning and Substance Use

National EMS Education Standard Competencies

Medicine

Recognizes and manages life threats based on assessment findings of a patient with a medical emergency while awaiting additional emergency response.

Toxicology

- Carbon monoxide poisoning (p 245)
- Nerve agent poisoning (pp 249–250)
- Opioid toxicity (pp 251–253)
- How and when to contact a poison control center (pp 246–250; p 254)

Immunology

- Anaphylactic reactions (pp 246–248; p 254)

Pharmacology

Uses knowledge of the medications that the EMR may administer in an emergency.

Medication Administration

- Use a medication cross-check procedure (Chapter 10, *Medical Emergencies*)
- Use an auto-injector (pp 249–253)
- Use a unit-dose, premeasured intranasal device (pp 251–254)
- Use of tools/resources to facilitate safe administration of weight-based dosing (Chapter 10, *Medical Emergencies*)

Knowledge Objectives

1. Define poison. (p 242)
2. Describe the signs and symptoms of ingested poisons. (p 243)
3. Explain how to treat a patient who has ingested a poison. (pp 243–244)
4. Describe the signs and symptoms of inhaled poisons. (pp 245–246)
5. Explain how to treat a patient who has inhaled a poison. (pp 245–246)
6. Describe the signs and symptoms of injected poisons. (p 248)
7. Explain how to treat a patient who has been injected with a poison. (pp 246–248)
8. Explain how to assist a patient with an auto-injector. (p 249)
9. Describe the signs and symptoms of absorbed poisons. (p 249)
10. Explain how to treat a patient who has absorbed a poison. (p 249)
11. Describe how to brush off a dry chemical from a patient and then flush with water. (p 249)
12. Describe how to use water to flush a patient who has come in contact with liquid poison. (p 249)
13. Describe the signs and symptom of exposure to a nerve agent. (p 249)
14. Describe the role of emergency medical responders (EMRs) in an incident involving exposure to a nerve agent. (p 249)
15. Explain how to administer a nerve agent auto-injector. (p 249)
16. Describe the signs and symptoms of a drug overdose caused by amphetamines, opioids, hallucinogens, and inhalants. (pp 250–254)
17. Explain the general treatment of a patient who has experienced a drug overdose. (p 254)
18. Explain how to administer intranasal naloxone for an opioid overdose. (pp 251–254)

Skills Objectives

1. Demonstrate treatment of a patient who has ingested a poison. (pp 243–244)
2. Demonstrate treatment of a patient who has inhaled a poison. (pp 245–246)

© New Africa/Shutterstock

3. Demonstrate treatment of a patient who has been injected with a poison. (pp 246–248)
4. Demonstrate how to assist a patient with an epinephrine auto-injector. (p 248)
5. Demonstrate treatment of a patient who has absorbed a poison. (p 249)
6. Demonstrate how to brush off a dry chemical from a patient and then flush with water. (p 249)
7. Demonstrate how to use water to flush a patient who has come in contact with a liquid poison. (p 249)
8. Demonstrate administration of nerve agent auto-injectors. (p 249)
9. Demonstrate treatment of a patient who has experienced a drug overdose. (p 254)
10. Demonstrate administration of intranasal naloxone for an opioid overdose. (pp 251–254)

Introduction

A **poison** is a substance that causes illness or death when eaten, drunk, inhaled, injected, or absorbed in relatively small quantities. This chapter covers the signs, symptoms, emergency care, and treatment of patients who have experienced an emergency relating to accidental or intentional poisoning, bites or stings, or alcohol or substance use. You can save a patient's life by quickly recognizing and promptly treating a serious poisoning.

Patient Assessment for Poisoning

As an emergency medical responder (EMR), you need to be a good detective when caring for patients who have come in contact with poisons. Poisoning can be classified according to the four primary routes by which it enters the body:

1. *Ingestion* occurs when a poison enters the body through the mouth and is absorbed by the digestive system.
2. *Inhalation* occurs when a poison enters the body through the mouth or nose and is absorbed by the mucous membranes lining the respiratory system.
3. *Injection* occurs when a poison enters the body through a small opening in the skin and spreads through the circulatory system. Injection can occur as a result of an insect sting, a snakebite, or use of a hypodermic needle.
4. *Absorption* occurs when a poison enters the body through intact skin and spreads through the circulatory system.

Even though poisons can be introduced into the body by different routes, some of the effects of the poison on the body may be similar. In general, when you assess and treat patients who have been poisoned, begin with a thorough assessment that follows the patient assessment sequence

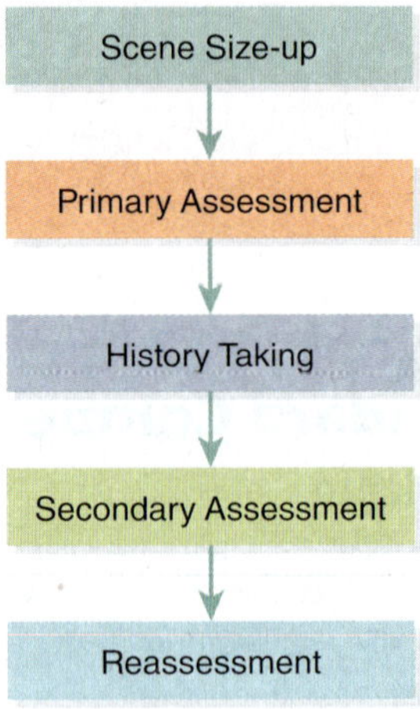

FIGURE 11-1 Patient assessment sequence.
© Jones & Bartlett Learning

(**FIGURE 11-1**). If you suspect poisoning, obtain a thorough history from the patient or from bystanders. A good history of the incident will help guide you in your patient assessment.

Be alert for any visual clues that may indicate the patient has been in contact with a poison. These findings include traces of the substance on the patient's face and mouth (ingested poisons), traces of the substance on the skin (absorbed poisons), needle pricks or sting marks (injected poisons), and respiratory distress (inhaled poisons).

Safety

Conduct a scene size-up (overview) to determine whether it is safe for you to enter. Be alert for odors. Look for containers close to the patient. Be suspicious of scenes where multiple patients are exhibiting similar symptoms. If you believe the scene is unsafe, stay a safe distance away and call for specialized assistance. To help identify potential hazardous substances and determine whether the scene is safe to enter, refer to the *Emergency Response Guidebook*, which is described in Chapter 19, *Incident Management*.

TABLE 11-1 General Signs and Symptoms of Poisoning

History	History of ingesting, inhaling, injecting, or absorbing a poison
Respiratory	Difficulty breathing or decreased respirations
Digestive	Nausea and vomiting Abdominal pain Diarrhea
Central nervous system	Unresponsiveness or altered mental status Dilation or constriction of the pupils Convulsions
Other	Excess salivation Sweating Cyanosis Empty containers at the scene

© Jones & Bartlett Learning

Much of the emergency care you provide will be based on the patient's signs and symptoms. A patient with a poisonous substance on the skin needs to have the substance removed, which may require special training or the assistance of a hazardous materials (hazmat) team. A patient who shows signs of respiratory distress needs to receive respiratory support. A patient who is exhibiting signs of digestive distress needs to receive support for that condition. Sometimes the patient's signs and symptoms will be less specific, and you will have to base your treatment on general signs and symptoms. The general signs and symptoms of poisoning are shown in **TABLE 11-1**.

Special Populations

Age Groups at Increased Risk of Drug Poisoning

The rate of deaths caused by drug poisoning varies widely across different age groups. In the past, the rate of deaths from accidental poisoning was higher in children between birth and age 12 years. The advent of child-resistant caps and other safety containers has significantly decreased poisoning deaths among children. Today, the rate of overdose deaths is highest in adults (**FIGURE 11-2**). According to the Centers for Disease Control and Prevention, there were 107,941 drug overdose deaths in the United States in 2022. In 1999, there were 6.1 drug overdose deaths per 100,000 people, and in 2022, there were 32.6 drug overdose deaths per 100,000 people. Thus, there has been a 5.3-fold increase in the rate of drug overdose deaths from 1999 to 2022. Drug overdoses, or drug poisonings, account for 96% of poisoning deaths, and more than three out of four of these deaths involve an opioid, such as fentanyl, heroin, oxycodone, morphine, or hydrocodone.

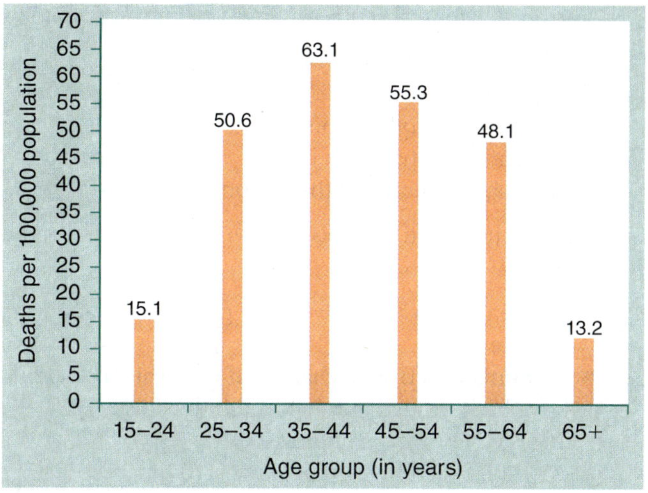

FIGURE 11-2 Drug poisoning death rates by age in the United States in 2022.

Adapted from Spencer MR, Garnett MF, Miniño AM. Drug overdose deaths in the United States, 2002–2022. Hyattsville, MD: National Center for Health Statistics; 2024: NCHS Data Brief No. 491.

Ingested Poisons

An ingested poison is taken by mouth. Often, you will find chemical burns, odors, or stains around the patient's mouth. The person may also be experiencing nausea, vomiting, abdominal pain, or diarrhea. Later symptoms may include abnormal or decreased respirations, unresponsiveness, or seizures.

Signs and Symptoms

Signs and symptoms of ingested poisons include the following:

- Unusual breath odors
- Discoloration or burning around the mouth
- Nausea and vomiting
- Abdominal pain
- Diarrhea
- Any of the other signs and symptoms of poisoning listed in Table 11-1

Treatment for Ingested Poisons

To treat a person who has ingested a poison, do the following:

- Try to identify what was swallowed, attempt to estimate the amount ingested, and send the bottle or container along with the patient to the emergency department (ED).
- Gather any spilled tablets and replace them in the bottle so they can be counted. The emergency physician may then be able to determine how many tablets the patient has taken.
- Call poison control (1-800-222-1222) and follow the instructions given.

The poison control center will need to know the following information:

- Age of the patient
- Identification of the poison
- Weight of the patient
- Estimated quantity of the poison taken

Actions indicated by poison control may include the following:

- Dilute the poison by giving the patient large amounts of water.
- Administer activated charcoal if it is available, if you have been trained to use it, and if the poison was ingested less than 1 hour ago.
- Monitor breathing and pulse closely. This step is crucial. You must be prepared to provide emergency care, including rescue breathing and cardiopulmonary resuscitation (CPR).
- Arrange for prompt transport to an appropriate medical facility.

Activated Charcoal

Administering activated charcoal is a method of treating ingested poisons (**FIGURE 11-3**). Activated charcoal is a finely ground powder that is mixed with water to make it easier to swallow. It works by binding to the poison, thereby preventing the poison from being absorbed in the patient's digestive tract.

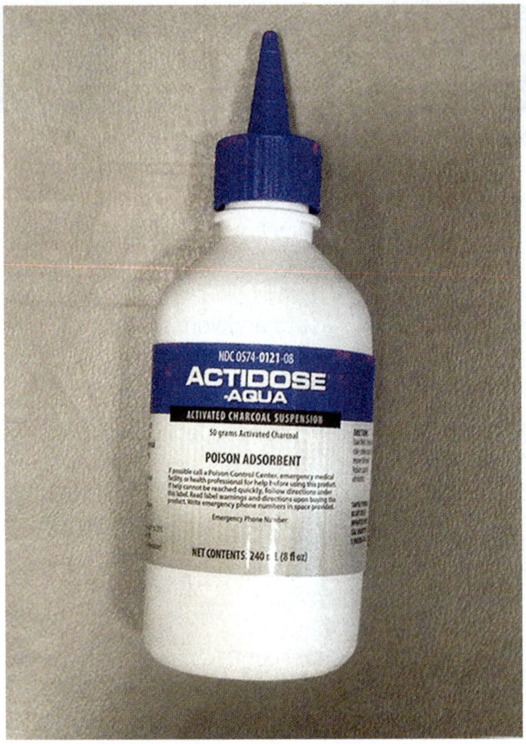

FIGURE 11-3 Activated charcoal.
© Chuck Stewart, MD, EMDM, MPH

Activated charcoal may be used by some emergency medical services (EMS) systems to treat poisonings if the nearest medical facility is a long distance away. However, give activated charcoal only if you are trained in its use and have approval from your medical director or your poison control center.

Do not give activated charcoal if the patient cannot swallow, is unresponsive, or has ingested an acid, a base, or a petroleum-based product. An **acid** is a chemical substance with a pH level of less than 7.0 that can cause severe burns; an example of an acid is battery acid. A **base**, also known as an alkali or caustic, is a chemical that has a pH level greater than 7.0; an example of a base is liquid drain cleaner. Petroleum-based products include gasoline and charcoal fire starter. The usual dose of activated charcoal for an adult patient is 25 to 50 g. The usual dose for a pediatric patient is one-half of an adult dose, or 12.5 to 25 g. Because the mixture looks like mud, you can serve the mixture in a covered cup and give the patient a straw. This step may make it easier for the patient to drink.

Treatment

Place an unresponsive patient in the recovery position to help keep the airway open and to facilitate the drainage of mucus and vomitus from the mouth and nose. Do not attempt to give liquids or induce vomiting in an unresponsive or partially responsive patient because of the risk of aspiration.

Special Populations

Laundry Detergent Pods and Children

Young children are curious and often like to sample the contents of brightly colored bottles or cans looking for something good to eat or drink. However, many common household items contain poisonous substances. The two most common types of poisonings in children are caused by ingestion and absorption.

Many people use laundry detergent pods because they are premeasured, easy to handle, and do not spill. The coating on the pod dissolves in the wash, releasing the liquid detergent into the washing machine. These multicolored pods present a poisoning hazard for children, who may mistake them for candy and bite into them. Serious side effects can occur quickly and include difficulty breathing, severe vomiting, burns to the esophagus, and possible unresponsiveness. In addition, the liquid detergent can cause burns to the skin and eyes.

If a child bites into a detergent pod, immediately remove it from the child's mouth. Wash the child's face and hands. Gently wipe out the child's mouth. Call poison control for assistance and arrange for transport to an appropriate medical facility.

Treatment

Two general treatments for poisoning by ingestion are as follows:

1. Dilution using water
2. Activated charcoal

Follow the directions from your local poison control center or medical director.

Inhaled Poisons

Poisoning by inhalation occurs if a **toxic** substance is breathed in and absorbed through the lungs. Some toxic substances such as carbon monoxide are poisonous but are not irritating to the respiratory tract. **Carbon monoxide** is an odorless, colorless, tasteless gas that cannot be detected by your normal senses. Other toxic gases such as chlorine gas and ammonia are irritating to the respiratory tract and will cause coughing and severe respiratory distress. These gases can be classified as irritants.

Carbon Monoxide

One of the most common causes of carbon monoxide poisoning is an improperly vented heating appliance, such as a furnace or space heater, or a water heater. Grills or generators used indoors can also cause carbon monoxide poisoning. Carbon monoxide is also present in smoke. People caught in building fires often experience carbon monoxide poisoning. When a person inhales even a relatively small quantity of carbon monoxide gas, severe poisoning can result because carbon monoxide combines with red blood cells approximately 200 times more readily than oxygen does. Therefore, a small quantity of carbon monoxide can "monopolize" the red blood cells and prevent them from transporting oxygen to all parts of the body.

The signs and symptoms of carbon monoxide poisoning include headache, nausea, disorientation, and unresponsiveness. Low levels of carbon monoxide poisoning often cause signs and symptoms that are very similar to influenza. If you find several patients together who are all reporting these symptoms (especially in winter), suspect carbon monoxide poisoning and remove everyone from the structure or vehicle. If the fire department is not already on scene, request their assistance, as fire departments carry carbon monoxide detectors.

Safety

Residential carbon monoxide detectors have been installed in many homes. These detectors are designed to sound an alarm before the residents of the house show signs and symptoms of carbon monoxide poisoning. Once the residential carbon monoxide detector is activated, specifically trained and equipped personnel must be summoned to investigate the source of the carbon monoxide and to verify that everyone is out of the building. Many newer detectors are combination alarms, which will activate in the presence of either smoke or carbon monoxide.

Signs and Symptoms

Signs and symptoms of carbon monoxide poisoning include the following:

- Headache
- Nausea
- Disorientation
- Unresponsiveness
- Multiple people with flulike symptoms in the same location

Signs and Symptoms

Signs and symptoms of inhaled poisons include the following:

- Respiratory distress
- Dizziness
- Cough
- Headache
- Hoarseness
- Confusion
- Chest pain
- Any other signs and symptoms of poisoning listed in Table 11-1

Irritants

Many gases irritate the respiratory tract. Two of the more frequently encountered gases are:

1. **Ammonia.** Inhalation of ammonia often occurs in agricultural settings where it is used as a fertilizer (**FIGURE 11-4**). Ammonia is also a chemical that is used to manufacture amphetamine. It has a strong, irritating odor and is highly toxic. Inhaling large amounts of ammonia gas deadens the sense of smell and severely irritates the lungs and upper respiratory tract, causing violent coughing. Ammonia can also severely burn the skin. Anyone who enters an environment containing ammonia must wear a proper encapsulating suit with a **self-contained breathing apparatus (SCBA)** (**FIGURE 11-5**). This apparatus contains a mask, regulator, and air supply and delivers air to rescuers when they enter contaminated areas.

YOU are the EMR — CASE 1

Just as you are finishing your dinner at the station, you are dispatched to a residence in a middle-class neighborhood for a report of an unresponsive patient experiencing an overdose. The dispatcher does not know the age of the patient.

1. If this patient is a young child, what types of overdose will you most likely encounter?
2. If this patient is a young adult, what types of overdose will you most likely encounter?
3. If this patient is an older adult, what types of overdose will you most likely encounter?

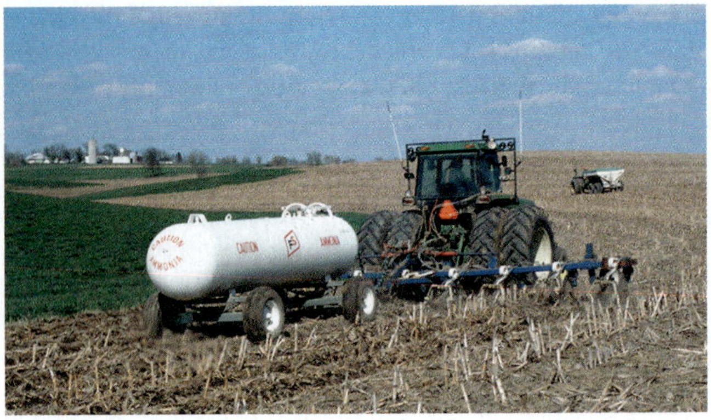

FIGURE 11-4 Fertilizer trucks on farms often carry ammonia.
Courtesy of Lynn Betts/NRCS.

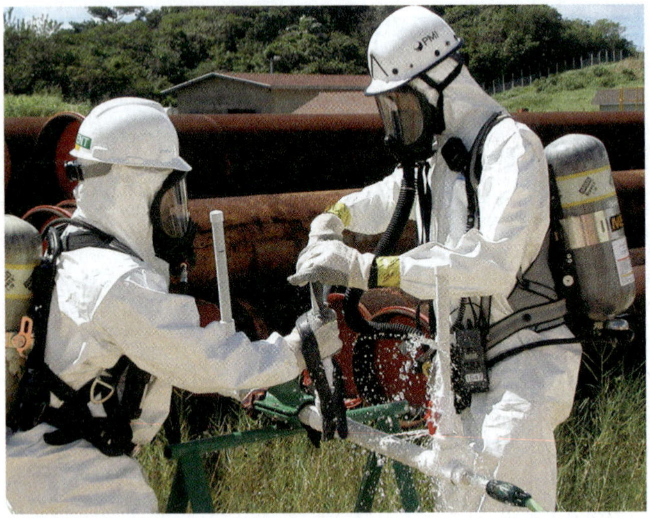

FIGURE 11-5 Encapsulated suit with self-contained breathing apparatus (SCBA).
© Jones & Bartlett Learning. Courtesy of MIEMSS.

2. **Chlorine.** Chlorine gas is commonly found in large quantities around swimming pools and water treatment plants. The odor of chlorine is familiar to anyone who has used chlorine bleach or been in a swimming pool or hot tub. Chlorine gas can severely irritate the lungs and the upper respiratory tract, causing violent coughing. Chlorine gas can also cause skin burns. Anyone who enters an environment containing chlorine gas must wear a proper encapsulating suit with an SCBA.

The presence of hazardous materials that are toxic (poisonous) and those that present a danger of fire or explosion should be indicated by the appropriate hazmat warning placard (**FIGURE 11-6**). Refer to Chapter 19, *Incident Management*, for more information about hazmat emergencies.

Treatment for Inhaled Poisons

The first step to take in treating a patient who has inhaled any poisonous gas is to remove the individual from the source of the gas while protecting yourself. If the patient is not breathing,

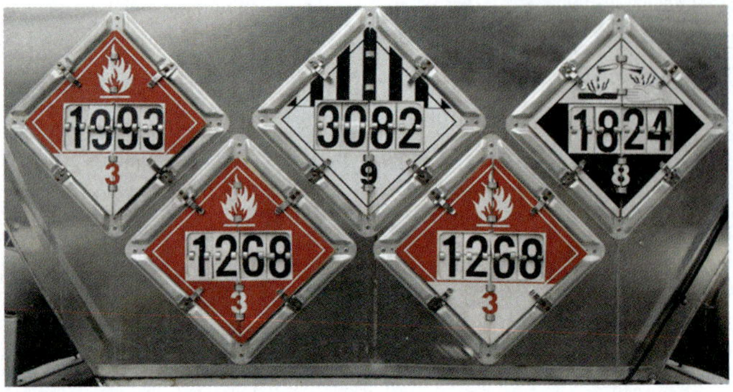

FIGURE 11-6 Placards used to identify the presence of hazardous materials.
© Mark Winfrey/Shutterstock

begin resuscitation with a bag-valve mask if available; if not available, perform mouth-to-mask breathing. If the patient is breathing, administer large quantities of oxygen (if available and if you are trained to do so). Promptly arrange transport for any patient who has inhaled a poisonous gas to an appropriate medical facility for further examination because the patient may have a dangerous reaction to the poison.

In some situations, your first response is to evacuate people. If you are called to the scene of a large poisonous gas leak (or other hazmat leak), you may have to evacuate large numbers of people to prevent further injuries. Once this has been done, begin to evaluate and treat the evacuees as necessary.

Safety

Do not venture into areas where poisonous gases may be present. Call an agency (such as the fire department) that is equipped with SCBA and other appropriate personal protective equipment. Be especially aware of the hidden dangers found in tanks, confined spaces, farm silos, sewers, and other below-ground structures. Every year, rescuers lose their lives by venturing into such areas to save a person who may already be dead. Often these calls are initially reported as a sick person or a person who has experienced a heart attack. Confined space rescue is discussed further in Chapter 18, *Vehicle Extrication and Special Rescue*.

Injected Poisons

The two major causes of poisoning by injection are (1) animal bites and stings and (2) toxic injection. This section covers animal bites and stings; toxic injection will be discussed later, as part of substance use. A person who has received a large amount of poison (for example, multiple bee stings) or who is especially sensitive to the poison (has an anaphylactic reaction) may become unresponsive and may go into cardiac arrest.

Treatment for Insect Bites and Stings

Encourage a person who has been bitten or stung by an insect to keep calm and still. This step will help slow the spread of the poison throughout the patient's body. Remove

Signs and Symptoms

Signs and symptoms of injected poisons from bites and stings include the following:

- Obvious injury site (bite or sting marks)
- Tenderness
- Swelling
- Red streaks radiating from the injection site
- Weakness
- Dizziness
- Localized pain
- Itching
- Any other signs and symptoms of poisoning listed in Table 11-1

the stinger by scraping a driver's license or other card over the area to dislodge it from the skin. Never squeeze the stinger or use tweezers because more poison may be injected into the patient. Wash the site with soap and water. Apply ice to reduce swelling, if available. Avoid scratching the sting because this may increase swelling, itching, and the risk of infection.

Some people experience an extreme allergic reaction to stings and bites and may go into anaphylactic shock. The signs and symptoms of **anaphylactic shock** include itching; **hives** (patches of swelling, redness, and intense itching on the skin); swelling; wheezing and severe respiratory distress; generalized weakness; unresponsiveness; rapid, weak pulse; and rapid, shallow breathing. The patient's blood pressure drops, and the patient may experience hypovolemic shock and go into cardiac arrest.

Your first step should be to maintain the patient's Airway, Breathing, and Circulation (ABCs). Administer oxygen if available and if you are trained to do so. Treating the patient for shock may help in some cases. Remove the allergen if possible. Monitor the patient's vital signs. If the patient's condition progresses to the point of respiratory or cardiac arrest, begin bag-mask breathing or CPR.

If a patient shows signs of anaphylactic shock, immediately arrange for rapid transport to a medical facility where the patient can receive treatment with specific medications. Advanced emergency medical technicians (AEMTs), paramedics, nurses, and physicians can give medications that may reverse the allergic reaction. Some patients who have severe allergies carry an epinephrine auto-injector so they can give themselves a shot of epinephrine. If the patient has a prescribed auto-injector, help the patient to use it. Instructions for using an EpiPen, a common type of epinephrine auto-injector, are as follows:

1. Remove the safety cap from the auto-injector. Use extreme caution to ensure your hands and fingers are not near the auto-injector needle once the safety cap has been removed. If possible, quickly clean the site with an alcohol pad, but do not delay administration of the drug. In extreme emergencies, it is possible to administer the auto-injector through the patient's clothing.
2. Place the tip of the auto-injector against the lateral (outer) part of the patient's thigh, halfway between the hip and the knee, at a 90° angle.
3. Push the injector firmly against the thigh until a click is heard. This sound indicates that the injector has activated and medication is being administered. Be sure to keep your thumb off either end of the injector. Maintain steady pressure to prevent kickback from the spring in the syringe and to prevent the needle from being pushed out of the injection site too soon. Hold the injector in place for 3 seconds, counting slowly ("one, two, three") to administer all of the medication (**FIGURE 11-7**).
4. Remove the injector from the patient's thigh and dispose of it in the proper container.
5. Massage the area for 10 seconds.
6. Reassess the patient's vital signs. If vital signs do not improve after 5 minutes, consider administering a second dose of the medication if available.

A device that administers epinephrine as a nasal spray (Neffy) has recently been approved to treat anaphylaxis. This device avoids the need for an injection and functions similarly to the naloxone nasal spray discussed later in this chapter.

You can administer epinephrine if you have been trained in its use and have permission from your local medical director. Be aware of and follow your local protocols.

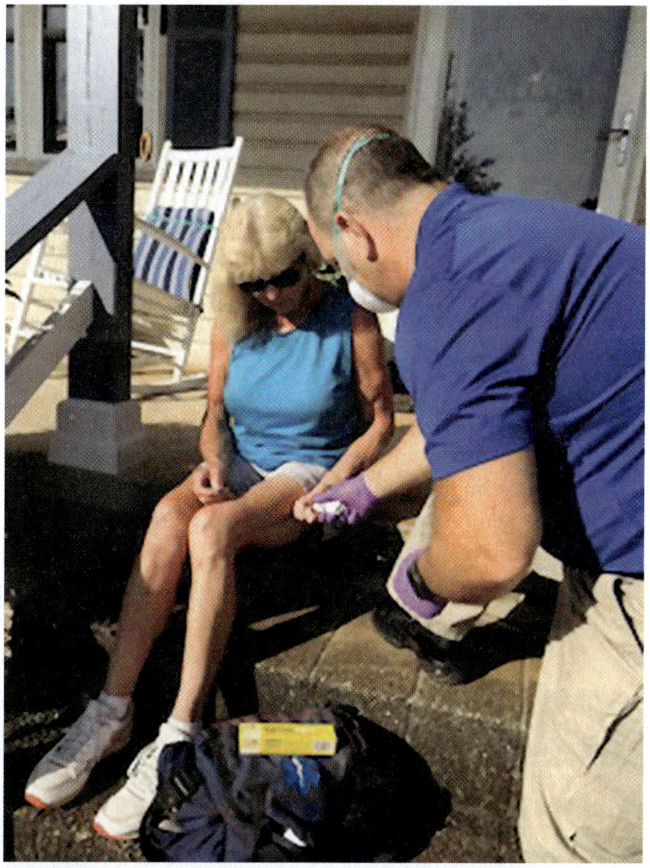

FIGURE 11-7 Depending on local protocols, EMRs may assist patients with the use of an auto-injector.
Courtesy of Rhonda Hunt.

Signs and Symptoms

Signs and symptoms of anaphylactic shock include the following:

- Itching all over the body
- Hives, swelling
- Generalized weakness
- Unresponsiveness
- Rapid, weak pulse
- Rapid, shallow breathing

Treatment

As an EMR, you may administer epinephrine and should understand its medication properties.

Epinephrine (EpiPen, EpiPen Jr, Neffy)

Effects. Reduces vasodilation, reduces wheezing and shortness of breath, reduces the formation of hives and itching
Indications. Allergic reaction to food; insect sting with difficulty breathing, wheezing, hives, or swelling of the face, lips, mouth, or tongue; fast heartbeat; weak pulse; dizziness; unresponsiveness
Contraindications. Known hypersensitivity to sympathomimetic amines, angle-closure glaucoma, nonanaphylactic shock
Side effects. Anxiety, restlessness, sweating, headache
Routes of administration. Intramuscular auto-injector, nasal spray
Dosages. Patients >66 pounds (30 kg): EpiPen 0.3 mg or 1 Neffy nasal spray; patients <66 pounds (30 kg): EpiPen Jr 0.15 mg

For more information about medication properties, see Chapter 10, *Medical Emergencies*.

Treatment of Snakebites

There are four kinds of venomous snakes native to the United States: rattlesnake, cottonmouth (water moccasin), copperhead, and coral snake. When a snake bites, it injects its venom into a person's skin and muscle with its fangs. This toxic venom can cause local injury to the skin and muscle and may even involve the entire extremity. Signs and symptoms may affect the entire body. A bite from a venomous snake is rarely fatal. The US Centers for Disease Control and Prevention estimates that 7,000 to 8,000 people per year are bitten by venemous snakes in the United States. Only about five people die from these bites each year. However, permanent injury can result if proper medical care is not obtained.

The field treatment of a poisonous snakebite is basically the same as the treatment of shock. Keep the patient calm and still; have the patient lie down and try to relax. This step can slow the spread of venom. Gently wash the bite area with soap and water. Use a pen to draw a circle around the perimeter of the redness or swelling. This will allow the doctor to see any changes. If the bite occurred on the arm or leg, snugly wrap an elastic bandage around the extremity from the shoulder (or hip) to just above the bite. This will slow the spread of the venom. Splint the affected extremity to decrease movement. Place the splinted extremity below the level of the patient's heart to decrease the absorption of the poison. Treat the patient carefully and arrange for prompt transport to the hospital or appropriate medical facility. The only effective treatment of venomous snakebites is the administration of **antivenin** in the hospital.

Signs and Symptoms

Signs and symptoms of snakebites include the following:

- Immediate pain at the bite site
- Swelling and tenderness around the bite site
- Fainting (from the emotional shock of the bite)
- Sweating
- Nausea and vomiting
- Shock

The bite of the coral snake delivers a slightly different venom that is neurotoxic and may cause these additional signs and symptoms:

- Respiratory difficulties
- Slurred speech
- Paralysis
- **Coma** (a state of unresponsiveness from which the patient cannot be roused)
- Seizures

Absorbed Poisons

Poisoning by absorption occurs when a poisonous substance enters the body through the skin. Insecticides and industrial chemicals are two common poisons absorbed through the skin. Common household products can also result in poisoning by absorption. For example, because aspirin is included as an ingredient in many common ointments, excess amounts can be absorbed and result in poisoning, especially in young children. A person who has absorbed a poison may have localized symptoms, such as skin irritation or burning,

YOU are the EMR — CASE 2

You and a partner are out on a lunch break when dispatch calls on the radio. You are sent to a local park where a woman has called because she has been stung by a bee. She told the call center it felt like her throat was closing.

1. On arrival at the scene, what should you check first?
2. What are some of the signs and symptoms of anaphylactic shock?
3. What should you ask the woman about her past medical history?

or may have systemic signs and symptoms, such as nausea, vomiting, dizziness, and shock.

Signs and Symptoms

Signs and symptoms of absorbed poisons include the following:

- Traces of powder or liquid on the skin
- Inflammation or redness of the skin
- Chemical burns
- Rash
- Burning
- Itching
- Nausea and vomiting
- Dizziness
- Shock
- Any other signs and symptoms of poisoning listed in Table 11-1

Treatment for Absorbed Poisons

Your first step in treating a patient who has absorbed a poisonous substance through the skin is to ensure that the patient is no longer in contact with the toxic substance. Protect yourself from exposure to the poison. Remove the patient's clothing if it is contaminated. Brush off—do not wash—any dry chemical from the patient. Contact with water may activate the dry chemical and result in a burning or caustic reaction.

After removing all the dry chemical, wash the patient completely for at least 20 minutes. Use any water source that is available: an industrial shower, a home shower, a garden hose, or even a fire engine's booster hose. Wash off any liquid poisons by flushing with water for at least 20 minutes.

If additional EMS personnel are delayed, contact the poison control center or your medical director for additional treatment information. Try to identify the poison and send any containers with the patient to the ED.

Monitor the patient for any changes in respiration and pulse. Be prepared to administer rescue breathing or CPR if needed. If the patient has vomited, save a sample in a clean container and send it with the patient to the hospital if you can perform this action without disrupting patient care. If the patient is experiencing shock, place them in a supine position and cover them to maintain body temperature. If the patient is having difficulty breathing, administer oxygen if it is available and you are trained to use it. Arrange transport to an appropriate medical facility for examination by a physician.

Management of chemical burns to the eyes is discussed in Chapter 14, *Bleeding, Shock, and Soft-Tissue Injuries*.

Treatment

Never pull clothing over a patient's head. Doing so could cause a dry chemical to become airborne, posing a respiratory problem for all involved, as well as possibly introducing it into the patient's mouth, nose, and eyes. Always cut clothing if there are no buttons or snaps.

Nerve Agents

Nerve agents represent a special type of poison that attacks the central nervous system. These agents can be absorbed through the skin, inhaled, or injected. Nerve agents are among the deadliest chemicals developed. Small quantities of these chemicals can kill large numbers of people by causing cardiac arrest within minutes of exposure. Four of the most commonly mentioned nerve agents are sarin (GB), soman (GD), tabun (GA), and V agent (VX). Nerve agents were discovered by scientists who were in search of a superior pesticide; however, nerve agents are much stronger organophosphates than those found in insecticides. Nerve agents, like insecticides, block an essential enzyme in the nervous system. The symptoms can be remembered using the mnemonic SLUDGEM:

S Salivation, sweating
L Lacrimation (excessive tearing of the eyes)
U Urination
D Defecation, drooling, diarrhea
G Gastrointestinal upset and cramps
E Emesis (vomiting)
M Muscle twitching, miosis (pinpoint pupils)

Additional symptoms include shortness of breath, slow heart rate, muscle weakness or paralysis, slurred speech, seizures, and loss of consciousness.

In the event you are called to the scene of an organophosphate or nerve agent poisoning, your primary responsibility is to keep yourself, other rescuers, and bystanders from becoming contaminated. Refer to the *Emergency Response Guidebook* for assistance identifying these scene threats. A well-trained hazmat team in special protective equipment (SCBA and encapsulating suits) is needed to remove patients from the contaminated area and decontaminate them before they are turned over to you for treatment.

Treatment of an exposed patient includes assessing and supporting the patient's ABCs. A nerve agent antidote called the DuoDote auto-injector can be administered to exposed patients or to yourself if you have become exposed. Use the DuoDote auto-injector only if you or the patient have signs and symptoms of organophosphate or nerve agent poisoning (SLUDGEM). You must have the approval of your medical director and have received proper training in its use. Organophosphate and nerve agents may require large quantities of medication.

The DuoDote auto-injector is a two-chamber device that administers two drugs: atropine and pralidoxime chloride. The instructions for using it are as follows:

1. Check that the DuoDote auto-injector has not expired.
2. Tear open the plastic pouch and remove the auto-injector.
3. Grasp the auto-injector in your dominant hand with the green tip pointing down. Remove the gray protective cap with your other hand.
4. Press the green end of the injector firmly against the lateral (outer) thigh, midway between the hip and knee, at a 90° angle.

5. Hold in place for 10 seconds to allow the medication to enter the muscle.
6. Dispose of the syringe in a medical sharps container, or place it back in its plastic pouch.
7. Reassess the patient's vital signs and symptoms.

Substance Misuse

Substance misuse is a widespread problem in the United States. According to the National Survey on Drug Use and Health, 16.5% of the US population (more than 46 million people) meet the criteria of having a substance use disorder; that is, they are dependent on alcohol or other drugs. Substance use results in an increased incidence of injuries and illness; therefore, many of your emergency calls will involve people who are under the influence of alcohol or other drugs. Even if the primary reason for the call is not substance use, it will still be a contributing factor in many calls.

Alcohol

Alcohol is the most commonly misused drug in the United States today. Alcohol intoxication may be seen in people of any age, including children, teenagers, and older adults. More than 178,000 people die from excessive drinking each year in the United States, making it a leading cause of preventable death. In 2022, alcohol intoxication played a role in approximately 32% of all traffic fatalities. As an EMR, many of the patients you encounter may be under the influence of alcohol.

When you have a patient who appears to be under the influence of alcohol, do not always assume that the symptoms (including the smell of alcohol on someone's breath) are caused by intoxication, because the symptoms of alcohol intoxication can be similar to those of other medical illnesses or severe injuries. If you are unsure about whether a patient who appears to be intoxicated has a serious injury or illness, be extra careful with your examination. For example, insulin shock and diabetic coma (hyperglycemia) may produce the same symptoms as alcohol intoxication. If you have the equipment and training, you may assess the patient's blood glucose level. Altered levels of blood sugar can present in a similar fashion as alcohol intoxication. In addition, keep in mind the possibility of head injury, traumatic shock, and drug reactions. Arrange for prompt transport to an appropriate medical facility, where a physician can make a complete assessment.

Alcohol is an addictive depressant drug. A person who is physically dependent on alcohol and then is suddenly deprived of it may experience withdrawal symptoms, such as convulsions or seizures. The most severe withdrawal symptoms are called **delirium tremens (DTs)**. The signs and symptoms of DTs include shaking, restlessness, confusion, hallucinations, gastrointestinal distress, chest pain, and fever. These signs and symptoms usually appear 3 to 4 days after the person stops drinking. Arrange for prompt transport of a person experiencing DTs to an appropriate medical facility. DTs are a serious medical emergency and can be fatal.

Words of Wisdom

Public safety personnel are not immune to substance use disorders. If you are having a problem with alcohol or other drugs, seek help through your employee assistance program or through a self-help program such as Alcoholics Anonymous.

Drugs

People of all ages use many different prescription and illegal street drugs (**FIGURE 11-8**). Drugs may be ingested, inhaled, injected, or absorbed into the body. As an EMR, you may not be able to identify the type of drug used, although this information will be helpful to medical clinicians. As you perform your scene size-up, look for clues that can indicate what type of drug was used and how it was administered. The most commonly encountered drugs fall into four categories: amphetamines, opioids (painkillers), hallucinogens, and inhalants.

Street Smarts

The types of drugs that cause adverse reactions and overdoses can change over time within a community. Stay informed about the drugs that are currently causing problems in your community.

In recent years, the misuse of prescription drugs has increased. Prescription drugs can have deadly effects when taken in large quantities and when mixed with other drugs. Many overdoses are the result of mixing alcohol with other drugs.

YOU are the EMR **CASE 3**

At 1337 hours, you are dispatched to a dairy farm approximately 7 miles (11 km) from your location for a report of an injured 32-year-old farmworker.

1. What factors should you consider as you are responding?
2. As you arrive, the farmer's wife meets you and tells you that her husband spilled a concentrated pesticide on himself while he was filling the tanks on his tractor-mounted sprayer. He has washed himself off and is sitting under a shade tree away from the tractor. How does this information change your plan?
3. What are the first steps you should take to assess and treat this patient?

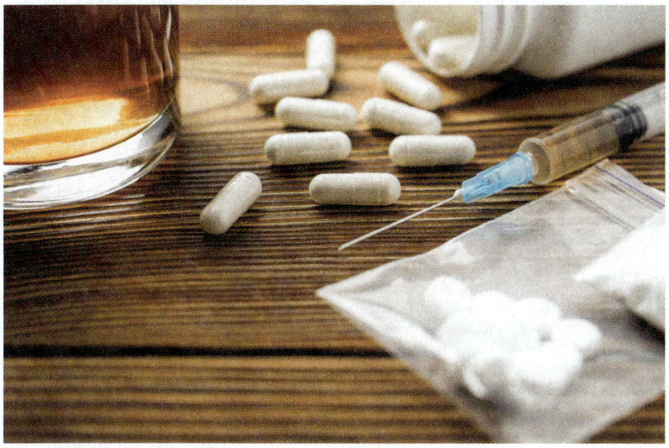

FIGURE 11-8 Examples of drugs that are commonly misused.
© Farion_O/Shutterstock

Amphetamines

Amphetamines are drugs that stimulate the **central nervous system (CNS)** (the brain and spinal cord). Drugs in this category are often called uppers, speed, ice, or crystal and include the drugs **cocaine** (coke, crack, rock) and methamphetamine (crack meth, ice, crystal meth). Patients under the influence of these mind-altering substances show signs of restlessness, irritability, and talkativeness. They may need to be kept from harming themselves and should be taken to a facility where they can be monitored until the effects of the drug wear off.

Synthetic stimulant-type drugs are commonly called **bath salts** (synthetic cathinones). Bath salts should not be confused with products such as Epsom salt (magnesium sulfate). These drugs copy the effects of naturally occurring mind-altering drugs and can be strong and dangerous. Often labeled as "not for human consumption," these drugs can be swallowed, snorted, smoked, or injected. Bath salts can produce effects that include paranoia, panic attacks, inappropriate sexual behavior, hallucinations, and agitated behavior.

Pain Relievers (Opioids and Heroin)

Opioids are a type of medication used to relieve pain by reducing the intensity of pain signals reaching the brain. Opioids also affect the areas of the brain that control emotion. This class of medications includes fentanyl (Duragesic), hydrocodone (Vicodin), oxycodone (OxyContin), morphine, and codeine. Opioids are named for the opium in poppy seeds, from which codeine and morphine are derived. When used appropriately and as prescribed, opioids are a valuable part of medical care. However, if these medications are misused (that is, taken without a prescription or used in excess quantities), dependency or overdose can occur.

Heroin is an illegal street drug that is powerful and addictive. Heroin is made from morphine.

An increasing number of drug overdoses are the result of taking a combination of drugs. One particularly deadly combination is heroin and fentanyl. Some drug dealers are using an illegal version of fentanyl, an analgesic (pain reliever) and anesthetic, to increase the potency of heroin that has been diluted. This combination of drugs acts quickly and is deadly even in very small quantities. According to the Drug Enforcement Administration, fentanyl produced in illicit labs is up to 100 times more powerful than morphine and 50 times more powerful than heroin. A dose of 2 mg is enough to kill the average person. Fentanyl may be snorted, smoked, taken orally as a pill, or spiked onto paper or patches.

Signs and Symptoms

Signs and symptoms of an opioid drug overdose include the following:

- Slow, difficult, shallow breathing, or no breathing
- Small or pinpoint pupils
- Weak pulse
- Clammy skin
- Low blood pressure
- Blue nail beds and lips (cyanosis), or possibly a gray or white appearance in individuals with dark skin
- Drowsiness
- Disorientation
- Delirium
- Coma

Words of Wisdom

Expect opioid intoxication if the patient presents with the classic triad of symptoms:

- Respiratory depression
- Pinpoint pupils
- Coma

Treating a Patient With an Opioid Overdose. An overdose of opioid drugs can result in respiratory depression or arrest. A person who has overdosed on opioids may be breathing shallowly or not at all. If the person is not breathing, begin resuscitation with a bag-valve mask if available; if not available, perform mouth-to-mask breathing. If cardiac arrest occurs, begin CPR immediately and arrange for prompt transport to an appropriate medical facility.

After initiating rescue breathing, administer naloxone (Narcan). Naloxone is an opioid antagonist that can rapidly reverse the effects of opioid drugs on the CNS. In the past, naloxone was administered exclusively by injection or through an intravenous (IV) line and the use of this drug was limited to ALS clinicians. Recently, however, naloxone has become available in a form that can be administered by spraying it into the patient's nostrils where it is absorbed by the mucous membranes. This method of administration is called intranasal administration (**FIGURE 11-9**).

To administer naloxone nasal spray, follow these instructions:

1. Determine that the person has experienced an opioid overdose.
2. Remove the naloxone nasal spray device from its package. Hold the device with your thumb on the

Voices OF Experience

In July of 1994, my advanced life support (ALS) unit was requested to evaluate two patients found unresponsive in a dirt alley in rural southern Georgia by the local police. We arrived to find two teenage males lying prone on the ground, not moving. Beside the patients were two paper bags and several cans of spray paint. My partner and I rolled the patients onto their backs and found both to be unresponsive with gasping respirations and slow carotid pulses. Their faces were speckled with gold spray paint. Faced with two critical patients, I immediately requested another ambulance for backup. We each took a patient and initiated airway management. While waiting for the second ambulance, two EMRs from the local fire department arrived on scene and quickly began to assist. One EMR went to the aid of my partner while the other assisted me. With no obstruction of the airway noted, I inserted an oral airway as the EMR prepared the bag-mask device and connected it to the oxygen cylinder. He initiated ventilations while I continued with my assessment, searching for injuries as well as any other signs of possible illicit substance use.

"En route, the EMR assisting me continued to ventilate our patient, freeing up my hands to provide additional care."

Unfortunately, calls like this one were becoming all too familiar to EMS systems in the mid-90s, before public awareness of the huffing problem had spread and laws were passed to regulate the sale of these dangerous products to minors. Even with today's precautions in place, EMS clinicians find themselves responding to these calls to resuscitate otherwise perfectly healthy young people who have chosen to poison themselves. Why would someone do this to themselves? Inhaling the vapors from the spray paint releases endorphins in the brain, producing an intoxication similar to that of alcohol. Unfortunately for these patients, not only do they get the desired sensation, they also experience extreme hypoxia as the chemicals in the paint take the place of oxygen in the blood. The metallic gold and silver spray paint colors are the most common ones used for huffing because they contain toluene. The toluene causes a euphoria that gives the recipient that much-craved high.

We had been on scene for 10 minutes when the second ambulance arrived. My partner's patient was already loaded into our unit awaiting the arrival of the second truck, and one EMR was assisting ventilations while my partner started IV lines. One EMT from the arriving unit climbed into the cab to drive them to the hospital. My patient was quickly lifted onto the stretcher from the second ambulance in preparation for transport.

Both patients were transported emergency status to the local hospital. En route, the EMR assisting me continued to ventilate our patient, freeing up my hands to provide additional care. The patient transported by the other EMS unit started seizing and went into cardiac arrest on the way to the hospital. He was pronounced dead approximately 45 minutes after arrival at the emergency center. My patient remained in respiratory arrest during transport. He eventually recovered after spending almost 2 weeks on a ventilator.

"Nobody trains to be backup" is a motto I teach each of my EMR students. You may very easily be the first on scene, requiring you to assess the patient and initiate care before an ALS unit arrives. Every skill you learn as an EMR is beneficial and may save someone's life. My crew was overwhelmed with two critical patients, and having the two knowledgeable EMRs to assist with patient care truly saved the day!

Matt Hunt, BS Ed, EMT-P
Paramedic Instructor
Albany State University
Albany, Georgia

Adapted from the personal Medical Identification Symbol of the American Medical Association.

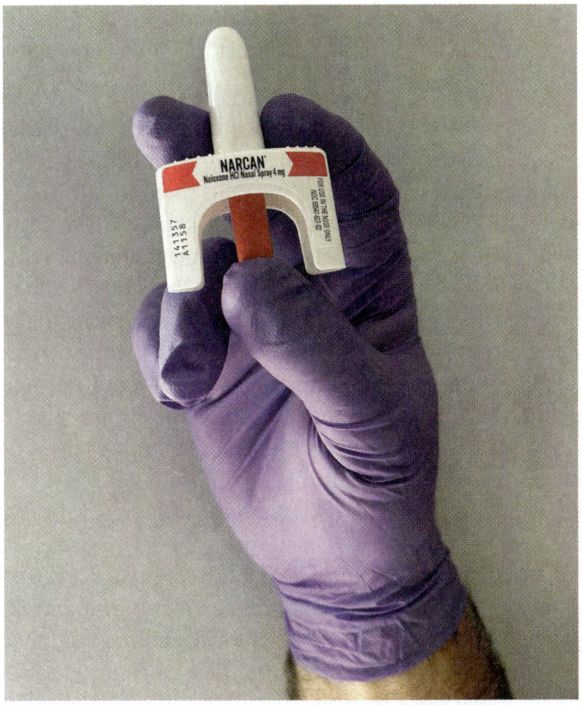

FIGURE 11-9 Depending on local protocols, some EMRs may administer naloxone intranasally to treat opioid overdose.
Courtesy of Rhonda Hunt.

bottom of the plunger and your first and middle fingers on either side of the nozzle.

3. Insert the nozzle into one nostril until your fingers rest against the bottom of the patient's nose.
4. Press the plunger firmly until the dose is fully discharged, then remove the device from the nostril.
5. Place the patient in the recovery position. Reassess the patient and document appropriately.
6. If the person does not become responsive or begin breathing normally within 2 to 3 minutes, you may administer another dose of naloxone.

Naloxone is also available in the form of an auto-injector. As an EMR, you can give this medication only if you are trained in its use and have approval from your medical director.

Hallucinogens

Hallucinogens include PCP (phencyclidine), LSD (lysergic acid diethylamide), peyote, mescaline, and some types of mushrooms. **Hallucinogens** are chemicals that cause people to see things that are not there. A patient who is hallucinating may become frightened and unable to distinguish between reality and fantasy. PCP also blocks the body's pain receptors. People taking PCP may feel no pain and may seriously injure themselves or others. Large doses of PCP can produce convulsions, coma, heart and lung failure, or stroke.

Your treatment for these patients is primarily supportive. Try to reduce auditory and visual stimulation. Avoid the use of bright lights and loud noises, including sirens. Because some of the patients who have taken these drugs are prone to violent behavior, approach each emergency scene with caution. Maintain safety for yourself, other rescuers, bystanders, and the patient. Arrange for transport to an appropriate medical facility for treatment.

Safety

Fentanyl and its analogs (drugs that are similar in structure or function) are powerful opioids that are 50 times more potent than heroin. There has been some concern that first responders and health care workers who are in close contact with people using these drugs could sustain effects from absorbing the drug while caring for a patient. Although fentanyl and related opioid drugs have rapid and potent effects when injected, absorbed through mucous membranes, or ingested, the risk of clinically significant exposure to emergency responders is extremely low, according the American College of Medical Toxicology and the American Academy of Clinical Toxicology. They state that incidental skin absorption is unlikely to cause opioid toxicity (symptoms of opioid overdose). Nonetheless, individuals who may come in contact with fentanyl should follow these recommendations:

- Take standard precautions.
- Wear nitrile gloves.
- Wash exposed skin surfaces with soap and water as soon as possible. (The use of alcohol-based hand sanitizers is not recommended because this may increase the absorption of these drugs.)
- Wash clothing that has been exposed to opioids.
- Consider the use of N95 masks if fine dust or particles are present.
- Consider the use of splash protection if you are in danger of a liquid containing this drug splashing into your eyes.

Treatment

As an EMR, you may administer naloxone and should understand its medication properties.

Naloxone (Narcan)

Effects. Reverses the effects of an opioid overdose, including respiratory depression, shock, and unresponsiveness

Indications. Emergency medical treatment of known or suspected opioid overdose when there is respiratory depression or unresponsiveness

Contraindications. None

Side effects. May produce rapid heartbeat, sweating, nausea and vomiting, restlessness, and trembling; in severe cases, possibly convulsions

Routes of administration. Premeasured intranasal device

Dosages. Initial dose: one nasal spray, which delivers 4 mg of Narcan; may be repeated if patient does not become responsive and resume normal breathing after 2 to 3 minutes

For more information about medication properties, see Chapter 10, *Medical Emergencies*.

Inhalants

Individuals, particularly teenagers, may intentionally inhale volatile chemicals (huffing) to achieve a high resembling that of alcohol. Many of these substances can be bought in hardware stores and include gasoline, paint thinners, cleaning compounds, lacquers, and a wide variety of substances used as aerosol propellants. Age requirements, similar to laws governing the sale of tobacco and alcohol, have been instituted to address this problem.

Huffing involves placing the chemical in a plastic bag and inhaling from the bag. The combination of a lack of oxygen and the effects of the poisonous substance can lead to unresponsiveness and death. Some types of inhalants cause drowsiness or unresponsiveness, and others cause seizures. Some of the chemicals can overstimulate the heart and produce sudden cardiac death from ventricular fibrillation.

Treat these patients carefully. Try to keep them calm and still. Support the ABCs. Give high-flow oxygen as soon as it is available and if you are trained to use it. Carefully monitor their vital signs and arrange for prompt transport to an appropriate medical facility.

Toxic Injection From Drugs

Drugs that are injected into the bloodstream can result in toxic injection. The patient's reaction depends on the quantity and type of drug injected. Because street drugs such as heroin and cocaine may be diluted ("cut") with sugar or other substances that should not be injected into the bloodstream, the patient may be unaware of exactly what has been injected. After a toxic injection, the patient may report weakness, dizziness, fever, or chills. This type of emergency requires you to support the patient, treat the symptoms, and provide transport to an appropriate medical facility. You should also check the injection site for redness, swelling, and increased skin temperature. The presence of any of these signs may indicate an infection that requires medical care.

Safety

People who use IV drugs have a high incidence of bloodborne diseases such as hepatitis B and acquired immunodeficiency syndrome (AIDS). Take standard precautions to reduce your chances of coming in contact with bloodborne pathogens.

General Treatment for a Drug Overdose

Once you have determined that a patient is experiencing a drug overdose, your care should consist of the following:

- Provide basic life support (clear the airway and perform mouth-to-mask breathing or CPR, as necessary).
- Keep the patient from hurting self and others.
- Provide reassurance and emotional support.
- Arrange for prompt transport to a medical facility for treatment.

The effects of some drugs can be counteracted only by other drugs administered by a paramedic or a physician.

If a patient is acting out, speak to them in a calm, reassuring tone of voice and try to keep the patient from harming anyone. If the patient reports seeing things that are not there, say, "I believe you are seeing those things, but I don't see them myself." This statement lets the patient know that you understand their experience, but that in reality, the perceived object is not present. Call immediately for law enforcement if the patient appears to be a danger to self or others.

For overdoses involving opioids or heroin that result in decreased or absent breathing, administer naloxone if you have been trained in its use and have the approval of your local medical director.

Patients who are experiencing adverse reactions from a drug overdose require specialized treatment. You and other EMS personnel should be aware of local facilities equipped to deal with such cases. Keep in mind that a person experiencing a drug overdose may also have other injuries or medical conditions that require medical treatment. Avoid classifying or judging the patient.

Safety

The 9-8-8 Suicide and Crisis Lifeline provides free and confidential support for people in distress, and prevention and crisis resources for anyone needing them. This three-digit code routes callers to help and is available 24/7.

Intentional Self-Poisoning

Intentional self-poisoning is attempted suicide and may involve ingested poisons (such as drugs) or inhaled poisons (such as carbon monoxide). Regardless of whether the poisoning was accidental or intentional, the medical treatment you provide is the same. A patient who has attempted suicide needs both medical and emotional support; however, the patient may not want your help and may be difficult to treat. Nevertheless, you and all other EMS personnel must make every effort to preserve life and offer reassurance to the patient.

YOU are the EMR **CASE 4**

On a rainy night, you are dispatched to a residence for a report of a sick man. As you are responding, your dispatcher informs you that the caller now reports the patient is unresponsive. As you arrive on the scene and enter the house, you discover a 26-year-old man who is lying on the couch in the living room. He is not responsive to verbal stimuli, and as you check his pulse, you determine that he is breathing at a rate of approximately 6 breaths per minute. Your partner checks the empty pill bottles on the coffee table and tells you the drugs are pain medication and sleeping pills.

1. What should be your first concern when approaching the patient?
2. Where should you look for clues in this situation?
3. As you begin to care for the patient, his friend tells your partner that the patient's wife left him about 5 days ago and the patient called his friend this morning sounding depressed. Does this comment have any significance?

YOU are the EMR **SUMMARY**

You are the EMR: CASE 1

1. If this patient is a young child, what types of overdose will you most likely encounter?

Young children tend to put objects in their mouths. Medications without child-resistant safety caps that are left within the reach of unsupervised children may result in accidental overdoses. Young children are most at risk for ingesting cosmetics and personal care products, household cleaning supplies, pain medications, and foreign bodies that are within their reach.

2. If this patient is a young adult, what types of overdose will you most likely encounter?

Overdoses in young adults are frequently the result of attempted suicide or the result of an accidental overdose of alcohol or recreational drugs. Alcohol is the most widely used drug in young adults. Most drug overdose deaths involve opioids. Since 1999, the rate of overdose deaths involving an opioid or heroin has nearly quadrupled.

3. If this patient is an older adult, what types of overdose will you most likely encounter?

Many geriatric patients take a wide variety of medications for a multitude of ailments. Taking large numbers of medications, coupled with confusion, often leads to unintentional double dosing, synergistic reactions between medications, or overdoses of prescribed medications. There is also the risk that an older patient may unintentionally take a medication that is prescribed for their spouse. The most common patterns of overdose change with the age of the patient. Recognizing these patterns may help you to gain a better picture of a given incident.

You are the EMR: CASE 2

1. On arrival at the scene, what should you check first?

The patient is concerned that her throat is closing, which suggests her airway could be at risk. Here, as in all cases, your first step (after scene safety) is to ensure that the patient has a patent (open) airway. Place the patient on high-flow oxygen if available and if you are trained to do so. Ask the woman if she has an auto-injector, EpiPen, or other medication that she can take. If you have been trained to administer an EpiPen and have permission to use it, you can administer it.

2. What are some of the signs and symptoms of anaphylactic shock?

The signs and symptoms are itching; hives; swelling; rapid, shallow breathing; wheezing and respiratory distress; weakness; and a rapid, weak pulse. The patient's blood pressure will decrease, which may result in hypovolemic shock and possible cardiac arrest.

3. What should you ask the woman about her past medical history?

Ask the patient if she knows if she is allergic to bee stings. Some people who have severe, life-threatening allergies carry an epinephrine auto-injector so they can give themselves an injection in those situations. If the woman has an auto-injector prescribed by a physician, you may help her use it. The injection is delivered through the clothes into the patient's outer thigh. Press the tip of the auto-injector firmly against the woman's leg, press the injector into the leg, and hold for several seconds. Rub the spot for a few moments after removing the injector. If the patient's condition does not improve, arrange for rapid transport to an appropriate medical facility.

You are the EMR: CASE 3

1. What factors should you consider as you are responding?

While you are responding to the scene, review the dispatch information. Considering the rural location and the possible difficulty finding the patient on a large farm, see if you can arrange with the dispatcher to have someone meet you to take you to the patient. Remember that calls to rural locations may require you to travel off the road to get to patients. Be sure that adequate resources have been dispatched. Consider the hazards you may encounter at a farm, including heavy machinery, motorized equipment, electrical hazards, animals, tall structures, confined spaces, chemicals, and hazardous materials such as pesticides, herbicides, and fertilizers.

2. As you arrive, the farmer's wife meets you and tells you that her husband spilled a concentrated pesticide on himself while he was filling the tanks on his tractor-mounted sprayer. He has washed himself off and is sitting under a shade tree away from the tractor. How does this information change your plan?

This information changes your focus from dealing with one sick patient to dealing with an incident that involves materials that are hazardous to both the patient and to responders. First, ensure scene safety for all people working at this scene. Make sure responders are not exposed to the pesticide, and remove the patient from the source of the pesticide. This type of call exceeds the limits of your training and requires additional resources. Inform the dispatcher that hazardous materials are involved and request a hazmat team to respond to your location.

3. What are the first steps you should take to assess and treat this patient?

The first step is to request a hazmat team. Determine how long it will take the team to arrive at your location. Because the farmer has washed off the pesticide and has removed

Assessment IN ACTION

Three days after a massive snowstorm, several parts of your response area are still without electricity. More than 30 inches (76 cm) of snow fell in the region. You and your partner are dispatched to a home in an area where the power has been out since the storm began. A family of four is reporting flulike symptoms. When you enter the home, you notice a kerosene heater in the middle of the room, which you know is a hazard for carbon monoxide poisoning.

1. Which of the following is NOT a sign or symptom of carbon monoxide poisoning?

A. Headache
B. Vomiting
C. Itching
D. Disorientation

2. Carbon monoxide enters a person's body by what route?

A. Ingestion
B. Inhalation
C. Absorption
D. Injection

3. Carbon monoxide attaches to the red blood cells, affecting the transportation of:

A. white blood cells.
B. carbon dioxide.
C. oxygen.
D. glucose.

4. Which of the following drugs is NOT an opioid?

A. Oxycodone
B. Heroin
C. Morphine
D. Amphetamine

5. Opioid overdose can cause all of the following symptoms EXCEPT:

A. pinpoint pupils.
B. an increase in the rate of respiration.
C. weak pulse.
D. low blood pressure.

6. What drug is administered to reverse an opioid overdose?

A. Epinephrine
B. Naloxone
C. Insulin
D. DuoDote

7. Which class of drugs includes the synthetic drugs commonly called bath salts?

A. Amphetamines
B. Opioids
C. Inhalants
D. Hallucinogens

8. A patient who is frightened and seeing things that are not there has most likely taken which type of drug?

A. Amphetamine
B. Opioid
C. Inhalant
D. Hallucinogen

9. If you find that a residential carbon monoxide detector is sounding an alarm, what should you do?

10. A patient who exhibits a weak pulse, shallow or absent breathing, delirium or coma, and blue lips is most likely experiencing which type of drug overdose?

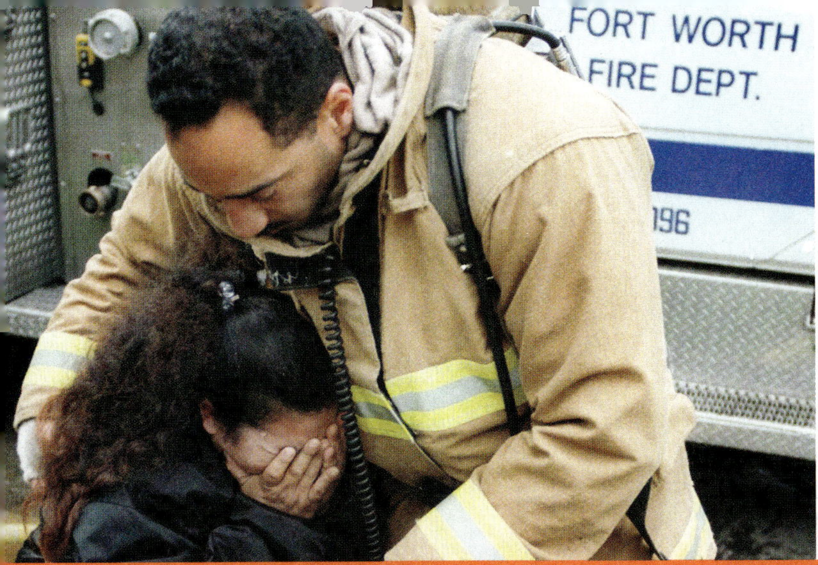

CHAPTER 12

Behavioral Emergencies

National EMS Education Standard Competencies

Medicine

Recognizes and manages life threats based on assessment findings of a patient with a medical emergency while awaiting additional emergency response.

Psychiatric or Behavioral Emergencies

- Recognition of behaviors that pose a risk to the EMR, patient, or others (p 260; pp 262–272)
- Recognition of suicide risk (pp 268–270)

Special Patient Populations

Recognizes and manages life threats based on simple assessment findings for a patient with special needs while awaiting additional emergency response.

Patients With Special Challenges

- Recognizing and reporting abuse and neglect (p 262; pp 265–268)

Knowledge Objectives

1. Identify the signs and symptoms of a patient experiencing a behavioral emergency. (pp 260–261)
2. List the five factors that may contribute to behavioral emergencies. (p 261)
3. List the phases of a situational crisis. (pp 261–262)
4. Explain the role of an emergency medical responder (EMR) in caring for a patient experiencing a behavioral emergency. (p 262)
5. List the steps for assessing a patient experiencing a behavioral emergency. (p 260)
6. Explain how to calm a patient experiencing a behavioral emergency. (pp 260–263)
7. Explain the following communication skills:
   - Restatement (p 263)
   - Redirection (p 263)
   - Empathy (pp 263–264)
8. Recognize the general signs and symptoms of an abused patient. (p 266)
9. Describe the signs and symptoms of elder abuse. (p 266)
10. Explain the steps you should take to care for a child who has signs of child abuse or sexual assault. (pp 265–266)
11. Describe the method for dealing with domestic violence situations. (p 264)
12. Describe the method for assessing potentially violent patients. (p 266)
13. Describe the safety precautions that should be taken when responding to a call involving a potentially violent patient. (pp 266–268)
14. Describe the EMR's role when responding to a call involving an armed or potentially violent patient. (p 266; p 268)
15. Explain the medical and legal considerations related to responding to behavioral emergencies. (p 268)
16. Describe the approaches to use when responding to calls involving the following:
    - Attempted suicide (pp 268–269)
    - Posttraumatic stress disorder (pp 269–270)
    - Sexual assault (pp 270–271)
    - Death and dying (p 271)
    - Dementia (p 272)
17. Explain the purpose of critical incident stress debriefing and peer support. (pp 273–274)

Skills Objectives

1. Demonstrate how to calm a patient experiencing a behavioral emergency. (p 261)
2. Demonstrate the following communication techniques:
   - Restatement (p 263)
   - Redirection (p 263)
   - Empathy (p 263)
3. Demonstrate management of the following crises:
   - Suicide attempt (pp 268–269)
   - Posttraumatic stress disorder (pp 269–270)
   - Sexual assault (p 270)
   - Death and dying (p 271)

© Glen E. Ellman

Introduction

Every emergency situation, whether it is an illness or an injury, has emotional and psychological effects for everyone involved—you, the patient, the patient's family and friends, and even bystanders. When you respond to the scene of a behavioral emergency, you will need to provide not just the necessary emergency medical care, but also the necessary psychological support to your patient.

This chapter explains the major factors that cause behavioral emergencies and describes the simple interventions that will allow you to safely care for patients and others on scene during these stressful experiences. As an emergency medical responder (EMR), your ability to recognize the nature of a person's crisis and effectively communicate with the individual will be the foundation for the initial assessment and care provided until further emergency medical support arrives.

This chapter also considers the potential effects of these calls on the EMR. While responders must know how to remain physically safe, they must also know how to avoid the legal and ethical perils unique to behavioral emergencies. Moreover, they must have the tools to maintain their emotional well-being during and after these high-stress encounters.

Patient Assessment in Behavioral Emergencies

When you are assessing a patient who appears to be experiencing a behavioral emergency, you should follow the steps of the patient assessment sequence. You should complete a scene assessment, being especially careful to ensure that the scene is safe for you and for the patient. If the patient is oriented and responsive, you can complete your primary assessment by observing the patient's responsiveness, airway, and breathing and measuring the pulse to determine the rate and strength of the heartbeat. Use the SAMPLE mnemonic (Signs and symptoms, Allergies, Medications, Pertinent past medical history, Last oral intake, Events leading up to the illness or injury) to aid you when obtaining the patient's past medical history. You may need to ask additional questions about the events leading up to the call for assistance. Do not neglect to ask about medical problems. Many of the calls you receive for situations that appear to be behavioral will have a medical cause or a medical component. It is important that you do not overlook this part of your examination.

The secondary assessment should rule out any obvious injuries and focus on signs of medical illnesses. Some patients experiencing a behavioral emergency may not be aware of injuries or illnesses that might contribute to their condition. An underlying medical illness or injury may be the cause of the behavioral emergency. Complete your secondary assessment by taking a set of vital signs. As you are performing your patient assessment, inform the patient what you are doing at each step of the way. Complete the last step of the patient assessment by reassessing the patient every 15 minutes for a stable patient and every 5 minutes for an unstable patient.

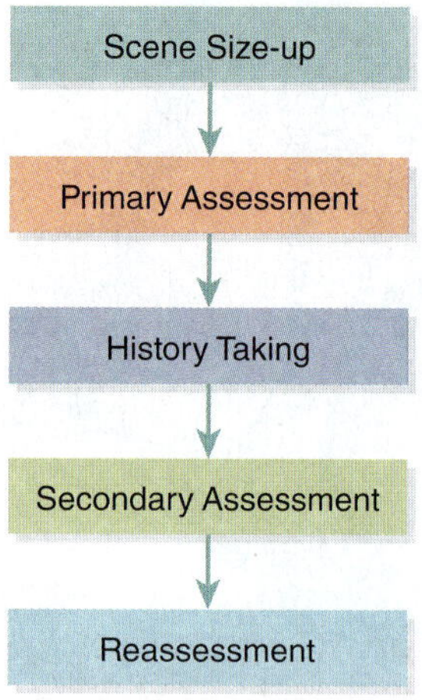

FIGURE 12-1 Patient assessment sequence.

© Jones & Bartlett Learning

> **Special Populations**
>
> **Assessing the Older Adult's Environment**
>
> As you are assessing an older patient's medical condition, try to also assess the patient's general well-being and environment. Consider the patient's ability to manage activities of daily living (ADLs) by observing the patient's hygiene and ability to walk, feed self, and take medications. Consider the condition of the patient's home. Is it reasonably clean? Is it kept at a suitable temperature? Are there fall hazards on the floor? Are hoarding conditions present? In general, does the patient seem to be able to meet the necessary functions of maintaining a healthy lifestyle? Does the patient have assistance from family members, home health aides, or meal delivery services?
>
> If you identify unsafe or unhealthy conditions on a medical call, sometimes the most important help you can provide an older patient will be to raise these concerns by making a referral to a social services agency. This may be done through your supervisor, a hospital, or a law enforcement agency. You need to know the process for contacting social services in your agency.

Some patients will not let you assess them. In this case, try to communicate to the patient that you are trying to help. However, in cases where you cannot complete the assessment, be sure to document your assessment findings and the reason for not completing all the steps. **FIGURE 12-1** lists the steps of the patient assessment sequence.

Behavioral Emergencies

As an EMR, you will encounter situations in which patients exhibit abnormal behavior. Sometimes this abnormal behavior is the primary reason that you have been called to the scene, and sometimes it is a secondary reaction to another situation such as an accident or illness. A **behavioral emergency** is a situation in which the patient exhibits abnormal behavior that is unacceptable or cannot be tolerated by the patient or by family, friends, or the community. Some behavioral emergencies will involve your patient, whereas others will involve the patient's family or friends.

Five main factors contribute to behavioral emergencies:

1. Medical conditions such as uncontrolled diabetes that cause low blood glucose, respiratory conditions that prevent the patient's brain from receiving enough oxygen, strokes, head injuries, high fevers, infections, and excessively low body temperature.
2. Physical trauma conditions such as head injuries and injuries that result in shock and an inadequate blood supply to the brain.
3. Psychiatric illnesses such as depression, panic disorders, or **psychotic behavior** (mental disturbance characterized by abnormal thought processes and/or the loss of contact with reality).
4. Mind-altering substances such as alcohol and a wide variety of chemical substances.
5. Situational stresses from a variety of emotional traumas such as death or serious injury to a loved one.

While some of these factors are ongoing in nature, such as a psychiatric illness, the state of emotional upset or turmoil that has prompted an emergency response is an isolated event; thus it is often referred to simply as a **situational crisis**. The crisis is caused by a sudden disruptive event such as a physical illness, a traumatic injury, or the death of a loved one. Every emergency creates some form of situational crisis for the patient and those people close to the patient. You will often encounter this type of crisis as an EMR. Some of the concepts covered here are similar to the concepts covered in Chapter 2, *Workforce Safety and Wellness*.

Most situational crises are sudden and unexpected (such as a motor vehicle crash), cannot be handled by the person's usual coping mechanisms, last only a short time, and can cause socially unacceptable, self-destructive, or dangerous behavior.

Phases of a Situational Crisis

There are four emotional phases to each situational crisis. A person may not experience every phase during a crisis but will certainly experience one or more of the phases. If you understand what these phases are and why they occur, you can better understand how to help individuals experiencing a behavioral emergency.

High Anxiety or Emotional Shock

In the first phase of a situational crisis, a person exhibits high anxiety or emotional shock. High anxiety is characterized by rather obvious signs and symptoms: flushed (red) face, rapid breathing, rapid speech, increased activity, loud or screaming voice, and general agitation. **Emotional shock** (psychogenic shock) is often the result of a sudden illness or accident or the sudden death of a loved one. Like most other types of shock, emotional shock is characterized by signs and symptoms including cool, clammy skin; a rapid, weak pulse; vomiting and nausea; and general inactivity and weakness.

Denial

The next phase of a situational crisis may be denial or a refusal to accept the fact that an event has occurred. For example, a child who has just experienced the loss of a parent may refuse to accept the death by telling everyone that the parent is sleeping or has gone away.

Allow the patient to express denial. Do not argue with the patient, but try to understand the emotional and psychological trauma that the person is experiencing.

Anger

Anger is a normal human response to emotional overload or frustration. Anger may follow denial or, in some cases, may occur instead of denial. For example, the spouse of a patient may, for no apparent reason, begin screaming at you, calling you incompetent, or using foul language or racial slurs. Although it may be difficult, you should remain calm and not respond angrily as well.

In crisis situations, it is often easier to vent angry feelings on an unknown person (the EMR) or an authority figure (a law enforcement officer) than on a friend or family member. Anger is perhaps the most difficult emotion to deal with objectively because the angry person seems to be directing their anger at you. Do not take the person's anger personally, but acknowledge that it is a reaction to stress.

Frustration and a sense of helplessness can often build to anger. If these emotions are not released, the anger may be expressed by aggressive physical behavior. For example, in a serious crash involving a school bus, you may have to demonstrate to bystanders that you and other rescue personnel are indeed removing children from the bus. If little

YOU are the EMR **CASE 1**

In the middle of the night, you are dispatched for the report of a sick person at the bus stop at the corner of Pennsylvania Avenue and 6th Street. As you arrive on the scene, you find a middle-aged man pacing back and forth at the bus stop. He is shouting that he needs to get to Albuquerque tonight to stop his pain. He then asks you why you are there.

1. What types of conditions contribute to or cause a behavioral emergency?
2. What are the four phases of a situational crisis?
3. What are three communication tools that can help you communicate with this patient?

activity is apparent to the bystanders, leading them to believe that nothing is being done, they may become angry, hostile, and even violent. In such situations, you must show confidence. Demonstrate that you are making progress. Always be professional and do not react to anger by becoming angry yourself. Remain calm and deliberate in your actions to prevent the escalation of violence. If necessary, a member of the EMS team may have to explain the situation, including what is being done and why it appears to be taking so long. Acknowledge anger by saying something like, "Can you tell me what I can do to help?" Then allow the person to express their anger.

Treatment

Virtually every emergency call requires some degree of psychological intervention.

Remorse or Grief

An acceptance of the situation may lead to remorse or grief. People may feel guilty or sorry about their behavior or actions during an incident. They may also express grief about the incident itself.

Crisis Management

As an EMR, you should consider how you can best manage a patient's emotional concerns or crises. When you have a patient who is experiencing a behavioral or situational crisis, you need to approach the situation using the same general framework for patient assessment that applies to other types of patients.

In this section, you will learn about some additional skills that you can use for patients who are exhibiting situational crises or emotional stress.

Role of the Emergency Medical Responder

Remember, as an EMR, your approach to a patient who may be exhibiting abnormal behavior is to follow the steps of your patient assessment sequence:

1. Perform a scene assessment.
2. Perform a primary assessment.
3. Obtain the patient's medical history (SAMPLE).
4. Perform a secondary assessment.
5. Provide ongoing reassessment.

After you complete the primary assessment, you may need to obtain the patient's medical history or perform a physical examination, depending on the needs of that individual patient. As you perform these steps, it is important that you remain calm and reassure the patient.

Your most important assessment skill may be your ability to communicate with the patient. Your communication skills will help you obtain needed information from the patient as you calm and reassure the patient.

Communicating With the Patient

The first and most important step you can take in crisis management is to talk with the person. Talking lets the person know that someone cares. Introduce yourself to the patient, ask the patient's name, and ask what you can do to help. When you communicate with the patient, be honest, warm, caring, and understanding.

When you begin talking with the patient, your body language is as important as your words. Try to position yourself at eye level with the patient (**FIGURE 12-2**). If the person is lying down, kneel beside them. If the person is sitting, move down to their level. Do not stand above the person with your hands on your hips. This is a threatening position and communicates an uncaring attitude and indifference to the patient's problem (**FIGURE 12-3**).

When you establish eye contact, you are assuring the person that you are, indeed, interested in helping. Use a calm, steady voice when you talk to the person and provide honest reassurance. Avoid making false statements or giving false assurances. The patient does not want to be told that everything is all right when it obviously is not.

Do not let negative personal feelings about the person or about the person's behavior interfere with your attempt to assist. Your function is to help the person cope with the events that caused the crisis. You should remain neutral and avoid taking sides in any situation or argument.

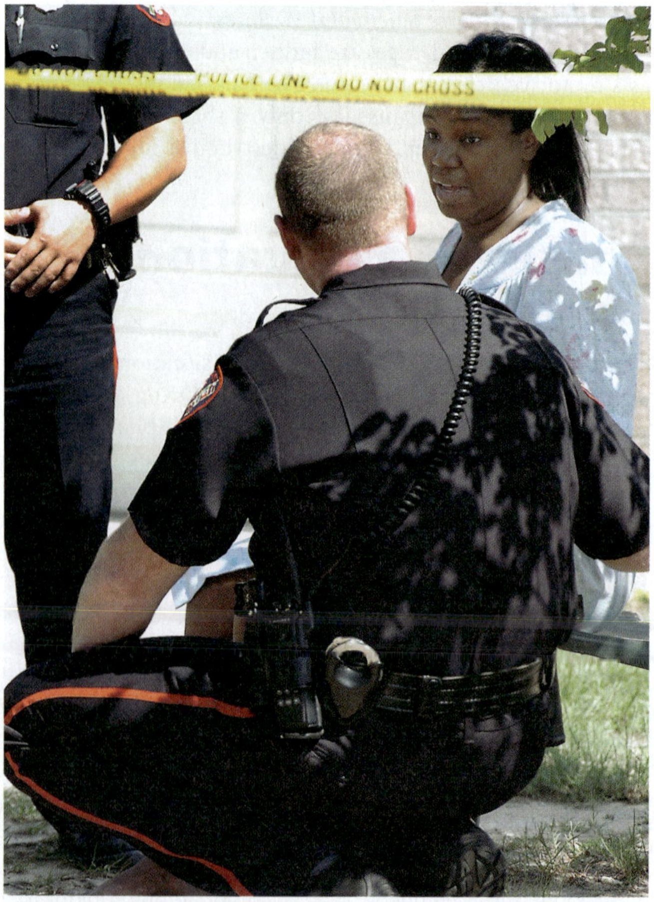

FIGURE 12-2 Crouch or seat yourself at the same level as the patient.
© The Daily Sentinel, Andrew D. Brosig/AP Photo

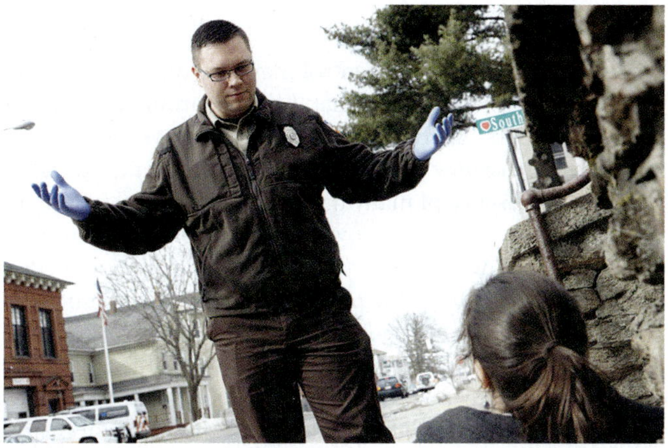

FIGURE 12-3 The body language shown here communicates an uncaring attitude.
© Jones & Bartlett Learning

Words of Wisdom

The following crisis intervention tips may help you at the scene of a behavioral emergency:

- Take your time.
- Remain calm.
- Reassure the patient.
- Use appropriate eye contact.
- Touch the patient reassuringly, if appropriate.
- Talk in a calm, steady voice.
- Demonstrate confidence.
- Do not take the patient's comments personally.

Sometimes a simple act, such as offering a tissue or a warm blanket, defuses the person's reaction to the immediate crisis. Simple acts of kindness can comfort and reassure the person that you are there to help. Some patients are comforted by your touch during an emergency. It provides a sense of presence, reassurance, and comfort to them. Other patients may find your touch offensive and may become upset or violent if you touch them without their permission. Be observant in determining when touch is appropriate.

Street Smarts

Often, the best thing you can do in a stressful situation is to offer to call someone, such as a family member, religious leader, or friend. This is especially true when there has been a death and the person is alone.

Restatement

To show that you understand what the person is saying, you can use a technique known as **restatement**. This means that you rephrase a person's own words and thoughts and repeat them back to the person. Here is one example of restatement:

Patient: "I just don't think I can go on anymore. Nobody cares."

EMR: "You sound like you are very discouraged. Why do you feel you can't go on and that nobody cares?"

These communication techniques can also be effective with patients who have sustained trauma or are experiencing a medical illness. Here is another example of restatement with an injured patient who is experiencing a crisis:

Patient with a broken arm: "I can't take any more of this pain!"
EMR: "The pain may seem unbearable to you right now, but it will ease up when we finish applying this splint."

It is not usually helpful to say, "I know what you mean" or "I know how you feel." You do not know exactly how the patient is feeling, even though you may have been through a similar experience. Be honest and give the patient hope, but do not give false hope.

Redirection

Sometimes a patient may be embarrassed about being the center of attention or may be concerned about others involved in the situation. **Redirection** helps focus a patient's attention on the immediate situation or crisis. You should use redirection in an attempt to lessen the concerns the patient expressed and draw their attention back to the immediate situation. An example of redirection follows:

Patient involved in a motor vehicle crash: "Oh my God! Where are my children? What's wrong with my children?"
EMR: "Your children are being taken care of by my partner; they are in good hands. Now, we must take care of you."

If the patient is in a public place such as on a sidewalk or in the lobby of a building, move the patient to a location that is quieter and more private, if the injury or illness permits.

Empathy

The ability to empathize involves the ability to sense someone else's emotions and to imagine what this individual might be thinking and feeling. **Empathy** helps you understand the emotional or psychological trauma the patient is experiencing. Ask yourself, "How would I feel if I was lying on the sidewalk with my clothes all torn and bloody and strangers were looking down at me?" Empathy is one of the most helpful traits you can demonstrate when caring for patients in crisis situations. To show empathy and to reassure the patient, you need to use a calm and caring approach.

Communication Skills

By using these various communication skills, you will be able to more effectively manage the patient's conditions. Practice these skills with another person until you are comfortable using them. Some principles you can use when assessing patients with a behavioral emergency are listed here:

1. Identify yourself and let the patient know you are there to help.
2. Inform the patient of what you are doing.

3. Ask questions in a calm, reassuring voice.
4. Allow the patient to tell you what happened. Do not be judgmental.
5. Show you are listening by using restatement and redirection.
6. Acknowledge the patient's feelings.
7. Assess the patient's mental status:
   - Appearance
   - Activity
   - Speech
   - Orientation to person, place, and time
   - Mood
   - Thought process
   - Memory

Special Populations

Communicating With Patients With Developmental Disabilities

Data from the Centers for Disease Control and Prevention indicate that one in six children has some type of developmental disability. Developmental disabilities range from learning disabilities and developmental delays to autism spectrum disorder. Some patients with developmental disabilities will present a challenge for you during an emergency. For example, patients with autism spectrum disorder might exhibit the following behaviors:

- Avoid eye contact and want to be alone.
- Not look at objects when another person points to them.
- Have trouble expressing their needs using typical words or motions.
- Appear to be unaware when people talk to them but respond to other sounds.
- Have trouble adapting when a routine changes.
- Prefer not to be held or touched.

Some of these behaviors may make it difficult for you to assess the patient, determine the patient's illness or injury, and provide needed treatment. A family member or caregiver, if available, is often helpful. This person can supply helpful information about the patient, can help you determine the patient's problem, and can often communicate more effectively with the patient. If no caregiver or relative is present, use the communication skills described in this chapter to help you. Remain calm, speak in a reassuring tone, and allow only one person to communicate with the patient.

Crowd Control

Performing simple crowd control may help reduce a patient's anxiety when there are too many people around, including family members. Encourage bystanders to leave. Sometimes too many emergency personnel have been dispatched to the scene. The presence of many uniformed personnel in a small apartment, for instance, is overwhelming or threatening to some people. Any emergency personnel who are not needed right away should leave the room or immediate area until the patient calms down.

During your initial overview of the emergency scene, look to see if there is a crowd that may become hostile. If you feel the potential exists, it is better to ask for assistance early on to deal with an unhappy crowd than it is to wait until the situation is unsafe for you and your patient.

Domestic Violence

Domestic violence is common in society. It takes on different forms, including elder abuse, child abuse, and spousal and domestic partner abuse. As an EMR, you need to recognize the signs and symptoms of abuse and to understand the cycle of abuse. Protecting yourself at the scene is the first priority. When you respond to a situation involving domestic violence, you need to know how to maintain safety for yourself and for the patient and how to conduct an effective assessment and treatment in what could be a volatile situation.

The signs of abuse include physical injuries, the emotional state of the patient, and the personality indicators of the abuser. Physical injuries from domestic violence include broken bones, cuts, head injuries, bruises, burns, and scars from old injuries. Internal injuries may also be caused by abuse. In some cases, injuries will be in varying stages of healing. The abused person's emotional scars and symptoms may include depression, suicide attempts, and misuse of alcohol or drugs. The patient may have feelings of anxiety, distress, and hopelessness. People who commit abuse may be paranoid, overly sensitive, obsessive, or threatening. They often misuse alcohol or drugs and have access to weapons.

If you suspect abuse, your responsibility is to maintain safety for yourself and for the patient. Interacting with a violent person is covered later in this chapter. To defuse a tense situation, try to separate the patient from the potential abuser. Doing so will create a safe place for the patient, give you a chance to gather needed information, and

YOU are the EMR **CASE 2**

It is 1600 hours when you are called to the local community center for the report of a 12-year-old girl who is having difficulty breathing. You arrive on scene and observe a young girl sitting on the ground, leaning against the wall. The girl is breathing rapidly. A counselor at the community center who is with the girl informs you that she became upset after being told her father was in a vehicle crash.

1. What actions should you take on arriving at the scene?
2. What care can you give to this patient?

allow you to treat the patient's injuries. As you question the patient, express your concern. Ask if the patient is all right. Avoid judging the patient. If the patient refuses to be transported, some agencies provide information about domestic abuse shelters. In some cases, the presence of law enforcement personnel will be helpful. Finally, learn the requirements for reporting cases of suspected abuse in your state.

Cycles of Abuse

Abuse has been described as a three-part cycle. In the tension-building phase, the abusive person becomes angry and often blames the victim. A victim who has been in the relationship for some time may recognize the tension buildup and react by trying to calm the abuser. The victim may also try to minimize or deny the abuse. The tension phase is usually the longest part of the abuse cycle.

The second stage is the explosive phase, or acute battery, when the abuser becomes enraged and loses control as well as the ability to think clearly. Most injuries to the victim occur during this stage.

The third phase is the honeymoon or makeup phase. During this stage, the abuser may make all sorts of promises, which are seldom kept. This phase helps keep the abused person in the relationship.

As an EMR, you may enter a domestic scene anywhere in this cycle. Understanding this cycle will help you to anticipate the actions of both the abuser and the person being abused.

Child Abuse

Child abuse is not limited to any ethnic, social, or economic group or to families with any particular level of education. Suspect child abuse if the child's injuries do not match the story you are told about how the injuries occurred. Child abuse is often masked as an accident. The abused or battered child may have many visible injuries, possibly at different stages of healing. The child may appear to be withdrawn, fearful, or even hostile. Signs and symptoms of child abuse include the following:

- Multiple fractures
- Bruises in various stages of healing (especially those clustered on the torso and buttocks) (**FIGURE 12-4A**)
- Human bites (**FIGURE 12-4B**)
- Burns (particularly cigarette burns and scalds from hot water) (**FIGURE 12-4C**)
- Reports of bizarre accidents that do not seem to have a logical explanation

Be concerned if the child refuses to discuss how an injury occurred. Occasionally, the child's parents or caretaker will reveal a history of several "accidents" in the past. Treat the child's injuries and, if you are suspicious that this may be a case of child abuse, ensure the safety of the child.

Make sure the child receives transport to an appropriate medical facility. If the parents object to having the child examined by a physician, summon law enforcement personnel

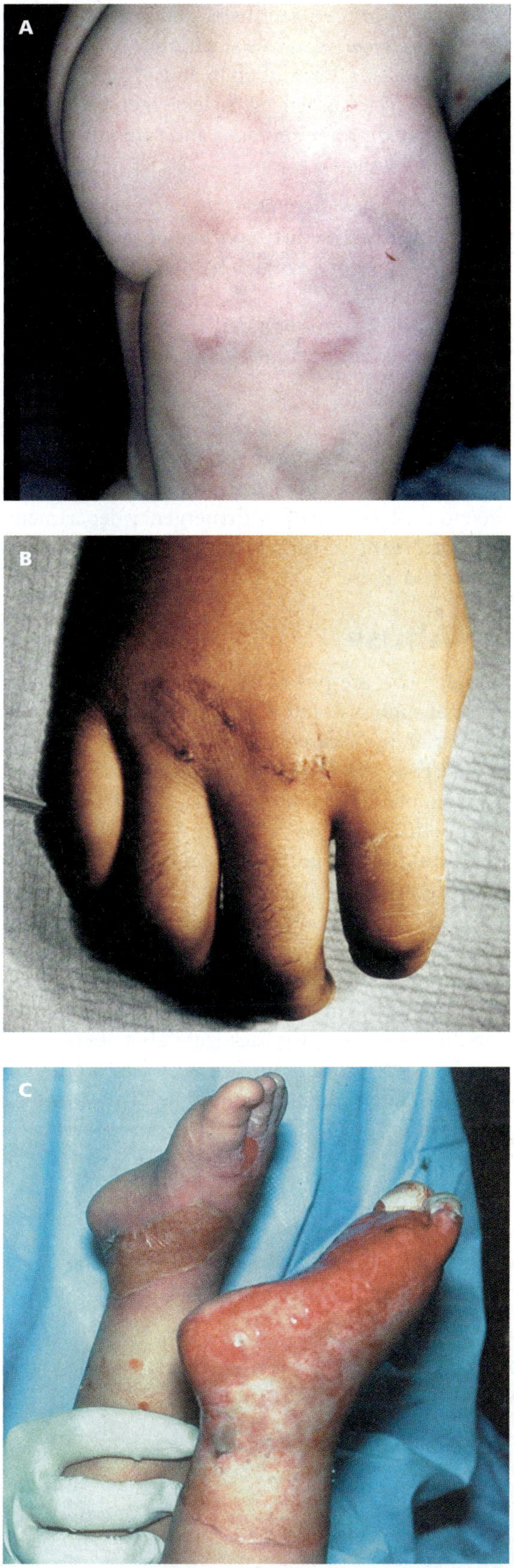

FIGURE 12-4 **A.** Bruises of different ages suggest physical maltreatment. New bruises are red or pink; over time, bruises turn blue, green, yellow-brown, and faded. **B.** A human bite wound has a characteristic appearance. **C.** Stocking/glove burns of the hands and feet in the infant or toddler are often inflicted injuries.

A & B: © American Academy of Orthopaedic Surgeons; **C:** Courtesy of Ronald Dieckmann, MD.

and explain your concerns to them. The safety of the child is your foremost concern in these situations.

Neglect is also a form of child abuse. You may observe children who have experienced neglect when you are making calls for unrelated problems. Signs and symptoms of neglect include the following:

- Lack of adult supervision
- Malnourished or dirty appearance
- Evident developmental delay due to lack of stimulation
- Unsafe living environment
- Untreated chronic illness or delay in seeking care for a serious injury

The parents of an abused child need help, and the child may need protection from the parents' future actions. Handle each situation in a nonjudgmental manner. Know whom you need to contact (usually the emergency department staff or law enforcement personnel), and report any instances of suspected child abuse.

Elder Abuse

Older adults who are physically weak or mentally compromised are at high risk for abuse by a spouse, other family members, friends, or caregivers. **Elder abuse** is hard to detect because those who are at the highest risk of abuse are also isolated from public view if they are confined to their homes or are living in an assisted care facility. As an EMR, you may be in a position to recognize physical or emotional abuse in geriatric patients. Elder abuse may occur in the form of physical abuse, sexual abuse, emotional abuse, financial abuse, or neglect (**FIGURE 12-5**). Patients with severe physical conditions or with dementia may not be able to report abuse.

The signs and symptoms of abuse include bruises, especially on the buttocks, lower back, genitals, cheeks, neck, and earlobes. Look for pressure bruises caused by a human hand grabbing the patient. Look for multiple bruises in different states of healing. Burns are another means of abuse. These may be caused by cigarettes or hot fluids. Suspect sexual abuse if there is trauma in the genital area. Finally, look for signs of neglect. Does the patient appear to be malnourished?

If you suspect abuse, you need to report it to the proper authorities. Learn the requirements for reporting elder abuse in your state and know how to follow the protocols for reporting within your department. Many community-based programs assist in supporting geriatric patients who need physical assistance, nutritional support, or emotional help. It is only by reporting signs and symptoms of abuse to the proper authorities that the condition can be improved.

Violent Patients

If you must treat an unarmed patient who is or may become violent, immediately attempt to establish verbal and eye contact with the patient. This begins the process of establishing rapport with the patient, which is important for communicating with a potentially violent person.

If family members or friends are present, ask them about the patient's history of violence. A patient with a history of violence is more likely to become violent again. Is the patient yelling or issuing verbal threats? Loud, obscene, or bizarre speech indicates emotional instability. Assess the patient's posture for indications of threatening behavior (**FIGURE 12-6**). A person who is pacing, cannot sit still, or tries to protect their personal space is more likely to become violent. Patients who have been using alcohol or drugs are also at a high risk of becoming violent. Do not force the patient into a corner, and do not allow yourself to be cut off from a route of retreat.

In these situations, it is usually best to have only one person talk with the patient. Having more than one rescuer attempt conversation is often very threatening. The communicator should be the rescuer with whom the patient seems to have the best initial rapport.

If all other means of approach and intervention fail, it may be necessary for you to summon law enforcement personnel to control a violent patient.

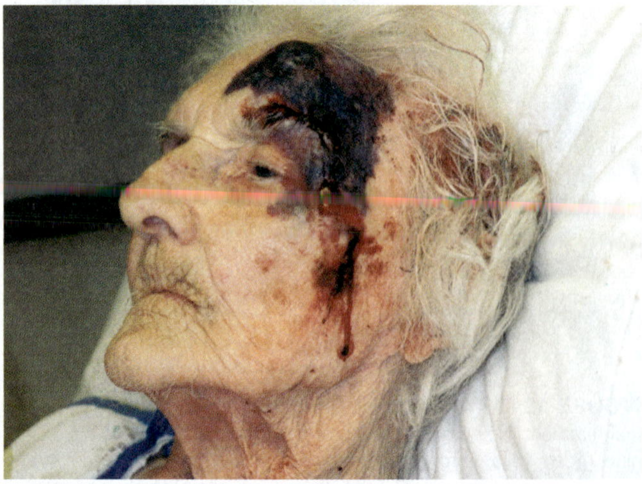

FIGURE 12-5 Physical abuse is one form of elder abuse.
Courtesy of Rhonda Hunt.

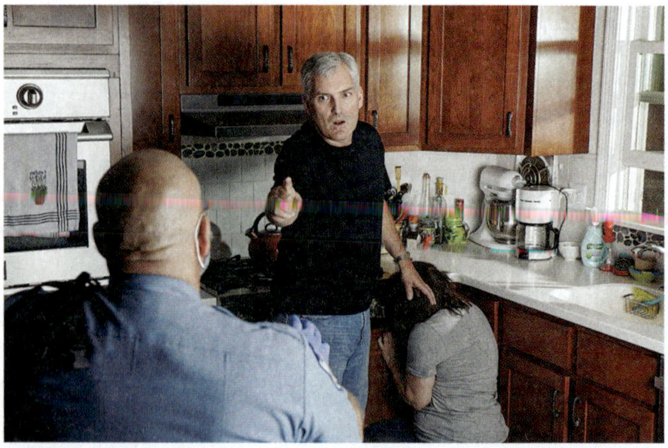

FIGURE 12-6 A patient's posture will indicate the potential for violent behavior.
© Jones & Bartlett Learning

Voices OF Experience

It was a slow afternoon when the call came in for a "sick person." Dispatch informed us that police officers were on scene and it was safe to move in, but otherwise we didn't have much to go on. We treated it as a routine response: no lights and siren, no adrenaline rush.

When we arrived at Santa Rita Park, a known gathering spot for the unsheltered community, a police officer was standing a few feet away from a man sitting on the curb. His shoulders were slumped forward, his arms resting on his knees, fingers absently tugging at the frayed edges of his weathered military jacket. He looked up briefly as we approached but didn't say anything. His face was lined with exhaustion, his boots damp from the recent drizzle.

"Sometimes offering medical care isn't the most important part of the job. So I did what I could: I listened."

The officer leaned in and discreetly said to me, "Concerned citizen called it in. Said he told them he's 'done with it all.' Just wants someone to talk to."

Seated next to him was the EMR, a member of the Community Assistance Program that was often dispatched alongside us for calls like this. She had arrived first and had already started building a connection, speaking to him in a calm, steady voice. As I stepped closer, I noticed she had taken out her blood pressure cuff, gently securing it around his arm while keeping the conversation going. "I just want to make sure you're doing okay physically while we chat, alright?" she said with an easy, practiced tone.

I crouched down next to them. "Hey, I'm Laura," I said, keeping my voice level. "Mind if I join you?"

He exhaled sharply, as if just the act of being seen had drained the last bit of energy from him. "I don't know," he muttered. "Feels like nothing ever changes. What's the point?"

The EMR gave me a small nod, as if to say, *We've made some progress*. She read off his vitals. There was nothing alarming, just the signs of someone who had been living a hard life outdoors for too long: dehydration, fatigue, stress. No acute medical emergency, but that didn't mean he didn't need help.

He told me his name and that he was a military veteran. He had served overseas, came home, and struggled to find his place again. One thing led to another—lost jobs, lost housing, and now he was here, sitting on a curb, unsure of his next move. He wasn't looking for a handout or a lecture, just for someone to acknowledge he was still here.

There wasn't much for me to do medically. His vitals were fine and he had no injuries. But sometimes offering medical care isn't the most important part of the job. So I did what I could: I listened. The EMR had already done a lot of the groundwork, treating him like a person instead of just another call. She reassured him that accepting help didn't mean he was weak, that there were options, even if they didn't seem obvious right now. Her presence had made all the difference. Instead of shutting down, he was engaging. And that gave us something to work with.

In the end, he agreed to come with us, not because he was being forced, but because the conversation had helped him see a different way forward. The transport wasn't for a medical emergency; it was a step toward something better—a warm meal, a caseworker, maybe even a chance to connect with veterans services.

That call didn't make the news. There was no dramatic rescue or heroics. But as we left the hospital that day, I was reminded of something important: not every call will be the high-speed, life-or-death moments we see on TV. Sometimes, it's the quiet ones, the ones that seem insignificant, where we make the biggest impact.

Laura Pieslewicz, BS Emergency Management, BS Fire Science
Instructional Faculty, Training Officer, Chaos Coordinator
Pima Community College
Tucson, Arizona

Adapted from the personal Medical Identification Symbol of the American Medical Association.

Violence Against EMRs

According to the National Institute for Occupational Safety and Health, the following factors increase the risk of violence in the workplace:

- Working alone or in small numbers
- Working late at night or early in the morning hours
- Working in high-crime areas
- Working in community settings

All of these factors describe your job as an EMR. You come in contact with all kinds of people at all hours of the day and night. You work in the community and may be called to high-crime areas. You should be alert when you respond to a call that has an increased chance for violence. These include crime scenes, incidents involving gangs, large gatherings of hostile or potentially hostile people, and domestic disputes (previously discussed). In these instances, request law enforcement to accompany you instead of waiting until a situation is out of control.

Even though you are more likely than the average citizen to be involved in potentially violent situations, there are steps you can take to minimize the chance of injury to you, other rescuers, and your patients. Remember, always keep an escape route between you and the patient at scenes that may become dangerous.

Prevention

Prevention is the best way to avoid violence. It is far better to avoid or prevent an incident of violence than to deal with an actual violent event. You may have several different opportunities for preventing violence. Can you learn anything from the dispatch information you received about the incident? As you arrive at the scene, use your personal antenna to pick up any signs that you may be approaching a violent situation. Make sure you have an escape route in mind as you approach any suspicious scene. Review the section on scene safety in Chapter 2, *Workforce Safety and Wellness*.

Your ability to use good interpersonal communication skills will help prevent many situations from becoming violent. Empathy can often defuse tense situations. Practice the communication skills discussed in this chapter. If you think you need backup or law enforcement personnel, request it early. If you are unable to handle a situation by yourself, remember your escape route. Learn your local protocols for violent situations and take part in additional training for handling this type of situation.

Safety

If you have any doubts about your safety at a scene, wait at a safe distance and request assistance from law enforcement officials.

The Armed Patient

You may encounter a person who is armed with a gun, knife, or other weapon. It is not your role to handle this situation unless you are a law enforcement officer. Be alert for potentially threatening situations and summon assistance if you think the person is armed. Do not proceed into an area where there may be an armed person without assistance from law enforcement personnel. If you must wait for law enforcement personnel to arrive, stay with your vehicle in a safe location. If, despite caution, you are confronted by an armed person, immediately attempt to withdraw. Your best defense is to avoid confronting a person who is armed! Work with the law enforcement personnel in your area to learn what your role is in cases that might involve an armed person.

Safety

If you cannot withdraw from a dangerous scene:

- Stay calm.
- Do not turn your back on the patient.
- Do not make threatening movements.
- Try to talk with the person and explain that you are there to give emergency medical assistance.

Other Types of Emotional Crises

Four other types of emotional crises—attempted suicide, posttraumatic stress disorder, sexual assault, and death and dying—also require you to have good communication skills. Each of these situations is difficult for the patient and for the EMR.

Attempted Suicide

Each year, thousands of people, from teenagers to older adults, attempt **suicide**. People attempt suicide by ingesting poisons, jumping from heights or in front of motor vehicles or trains, cutting their wrists or neck, and shooting or hanging themselves. Not all suicide attempts result in death, and many patients may repeat a suicide attempt. People

YOU are the EMR **CASE 3**

It is 2330 hours on a rainy Friday night and your unit is called to the scene of a motor vehicle crash where a vehicle has rolled over and crashed into a ditch. The driver is out of the car, walking with an unsteady gait, and not talking clearly.

The law enforcement officer says she thinks the driver may be intoxicated.

1. What actions should you take first with this patient?
2. What treatment do you need to give to this patient?

who attempt suicide often have a serious psychiatric illness, such as depression or alcohol or drug use disorder. Many people attempt suicide while under the influence of alcohol or drugs. The underlying psychiatric disease is usually treatable, however, and with proper treatment the patient will no longer have suicidal ideations. However, until that treatment is carried out, the patient must be considered at risk of experiencing further thoughts of suicide.

Words of Wisdom

Consider the following facts about suicide in the United States:

- In 2022, more than 49,000 people died by suicide.
- The suicide rate is highest among non-Hispanic American Indian/Alaska Natives and non-Hispanic White people.
- In 2022, men were four times more likely than women to die by suicide.
- In 2022, 13.2 million adults considered suicide, 3.8 million made a suicide plan, and 1.6 million attempted suicide.
- People 85 years and older have the highest rates of suicide.
- Firearms are used in more than one-half of all suicides.

Data from: Suicide data and statistics. Centers for Disease Control and Prevention. website. https://www.cdc.gov/suicide/facts/data.html. Published October 29, 2024. Accessed November 19, 2024.

All suicide attempts should be taken seriously. Do not be afraid to ask the patient questions about suicide such as: Do you feel depressed? Have you ever been prescribed medication for depression? Have you had thoughts about suicide? Do you have feelings of hopelessness?

Caring for a person who attempted suicide consists of the following steps:

1. Protect yourself and the patient from further harm.
2. Obtain a complete history of the incident.
3. Determine whether the patient is still in possession of a weapon or drugs.
4. Support the patient's ABCs as needed.
5. Dress open wounds.
6. Treat the patient for spinal injuries, if indicated.
7. Do not judge the patient. Treat the patient for the injuries or conditions you discover.
8. Provide emotional support for the patient and family.

Talk with the patient as you are providing treatment. Remember, many suicide attempts are cries for help. In addition to treating the patient, you should provide emotional support for the patient's family. It is not your role as an EMR to pass judgment on a patient; it is your role to provide a caring attitude and good medical care. **TABLE 12-1** lists risk factors and warning signs that indicate an increased likelihood that someone may consider or attempt to die by suicide. These suicide warning signs apply not only to your patients but also to your coworkers.

Street Smarts

9-8-8 Suicide and Crisis Lifeline

The 9-8-8 Lifeline provides free and confidential support for people in distress, and prevention and crisis resources for anyone needing them. It is available 24/7 by simply calling 9-8-8. This three-digit code routes callers to the 9-8-8 Suicide and Crisis Lifeline. The National Suicide Prevention Lifeline number is 1-800-273-8255 and is always available for people experiencing emotional distress or thoughts of suicide.

TABLE 12-1 Recognizing the Risk of Suicide

Risk Factors That Make It More Likely That Someone Will Consider or Attempt Suicide
• Excessive use of alcohol or other substance • Hopelessness • Impulsive and/or aggressive tendencies • History of trauma or abuse • Major physical illness • Previous suicide attempt • Family history of suicide • Job or financial loss • Loss of relationships • Easy access to lethal means • Local clusters of suicide • Lack of social support and sense of isolation • Stigma associated with asking for help • Lack of health care, especially treatment for mental health and substance use disorders • Cultural and religious beliefs, such as the belief that suicide is a noble resolution of a personal dilemma • Exposure to others who have died by suicide (in real life or via media and Internet)
Warning Signs of Increased Risk of Suicide
• Talking about wanting to die and making statements such as "I wish I were dead" • Looking for or obtaining a way to kill themselves, such as searching online for or buying a gun • Being preoccupied with death, dying, or violence • Talking about feeling hopeless or having no reason to live • Talking about feeling trapped or in unbearable pain • Talking about being a burden to others • Increasing use of alcohol or drugs • Acting anxious or agitated • Engaging in risky or self-destructive behavior, such as driving recklessly • Exhibiting changes in eating or sleeping patterns • Giving away belongings or getting affairs in order when there is no apparent explanation for doing so • Withdrawing from social contact, wanting to be left alone • Showing rage or talking about seeking revenge • Exhibiting extreme mood swings • Saying goodbye to people as if they won't be seen again

Adapted from National Suicide Prevention Lifeline. We can all prevent suicide. https://suicidepreventionlifeline.org/how-we-can-all-prevent-suicide/. Accessed November 19, 2024.

Posttraumatic Stress Disorder

Posttraumatic stress disorder (PTSD) is a mental health or behavioral condition triggered by experiencing or witnessing a

Special Populations

Understanding Suicide Risk in Children and Older Adults

One of the main causes of suicide in older adults is terminal disease. Individuals who know they will die from an incurable condition may choose suicide to avoid the final disability and pain associated with that disease. In these cases, the patient's family will be coping with the grief from the diagnosis of the terminal disease as well as the patient's suicide. This is a time when they need your comfort and understanding.

A second age group at high risk for attempted suicide is teenagers. For many, the teenage years are a difficult time of adjustment to growth and change. Stressors in this age group include school, interpersonal relationships, problems at home, and experimentation with drugs and alcohol. The rate of suicide among teenagers is high. Be especially alert for signs of depression and attempted suicide in teenage patients.

terrifying event. Although many people who experience traumatic events have difficulty coping and adjusting for a while, most get better with time and by taking care of themselves.

People experiencing PTSD, however, get worse with time and their anxiety often interferes with their normal day-to-day activities. General symptoms of posttraumatic stress disorder include severe anxiety, nightmares, flashbacks, and uncontrollable thoughts about the event. Symptoms may be broken into four different groups:

1. **Intrusive memories.** Includes unwanted distressing memories of the traumatic event, unsettling dreams, emotional distress when reminded of the event, or reliving the event.
2. **Avoidance.** People experiencing PTSD avoid places, activities, or people that remind them of the traumatic event.
3. **Negative feelings.** People with PTSD have negative changes in mood or thinking, such as the inability to experience positive emotions, experiencing negative feelings about themselves or others, a lack of interest in activities once enjoyed, difficulty maintaining close relationships, or feelings of hopelessness.
4. **Emotional reactions.** Being easily frightened, having difficulty sleeping, having trouble concentrating, engaging in self-destructive behavior, becoming irritable, or feeling overwhelmed with shame or grief.

Physicians are not sure why PTSD develops in some people and not in others. It may be caused by a mixture of multiple factors, and certain risk factors may make some people more likely to experience PTSD. These risk factors include having a job that increases the risk of being exposed to traumatic events (such as military personnel or first responders), having a preexisting mental health condition, lacking a good support system or coping mechanisms, or having experienced a trauma earlier in life. Traumatic events that may lead to PTSD include physical attack, sexual assault, childhood neglect, military combat exposure, or being threatened with a weapon.

People experiencing PTSD may experience self-destructive behaviors, including thoughts of suicide, eating disorders, or substance use disorders. They may also experience anxiety and depression or exhibit violent behaviors. Patients exhibiting any of these possible symptoms of PTSD need to receive appropriate medical care. PTSD is treated with a combination of psychotherapy and medications. It is important that these patients do not self-medicate and that they have a good support system to help them cope with their illness. As an EMR, you need to practice good communication skills when working with patients who have PTSD, ensure your safety and the safety of your partner and your patient, and make sure your patient is transported to a facility that can provide the necessary treatment.

Sexual Assault

Special consideration should be given to any person who has been sexually assaulted. These patients may be male or female, old or young. Because sexual assault creates an emotional crisis, the psychological aspects of treatment are important. The patient may have a hard time coping with a rescuer who is the same sex as the person who committed the assault. You may have to delay all but the most essential treatment until a responder of the same sex as the patient arrives. Your first priority is the medical well-being of the patient, so treat any injuries the person may have (knife wounds, gunshot wounds, and so forth). However, because sexual assault is a crime, you should not remove any of the patient's clothing except to give essential medical care. Try to convince the patient not to bathe or use the toilet. Keep the scene and any evidence as undisturbed and intact as

YOU are the EMR **CASE 4**

It has been a quiet Saturday night. Just after the bars close, you receive a report for an injured woman who has fallen. Your dispatcher reports she heard a man swearing loudly in the background while she was talking to the patient. As you and your partner approach the house, you are met by a 30-year-old man who appears to be agitated. He quickly tells you everything is all right and that there is no need for medical assistance. He tells you no one from this house called for assistance. As you glance in the front door you see a woman who has some abrasions on her face. She appears to be crying quietly. Her blouse appears torn.

1. What are your initial priorities in this case?
2. How should you proceed with treating the injured woman?

possible, and avoid aggressively questioning the patient as to what happened.

In addition to giving medical care, treat the patient with empathy. Maintain the patient's privacy by covering them with a sheet or blanket, and do not leave the patient alone. Contact your local law enforcement agency and the organization designated as the rape crisis center in your community.

Sexual abuse occurs in children as well as adults. It may occur in both male and female infants, young children, and adolescents. In addition to sexual assault, the child may have been beaten and may have other serious injuries. If you suspect sexual assault has occurred, obtain as much information as possible from the child and any witnesses. Realize that the child may be hysterical or unwilling to talk, especially if the abuser is a brother or sister, parent, or family friend. Providing a caring approach to these children is extremely important, and take appropriate action to shield them from onlookers.

All victims of sexual assault should receive transport to an appropriate medical facility. Sexual assault is a crime; cooperate with law enforcement officials during their investigation.

Death and Dying

As an EMR, you will encounter death and dying from natural, accidental, and intentional causes. How well you can help the dying patient and the person's family or friends largely depends on your own feelings about death. The material presented here expands on the material introduced in Chapter 2, *Workforce Safety and Wellness.*

In some situations, there is nothing you can do and the patient dies despite everyone's best efforts. In other situations, the patient's death is completely expected. In every case, you must do whatever you can to meet the patient's medical needs. Your attempts to save or give comfort to the patient help everyone (the patient, the family, and you) to cope emotionally with the patient's death.

Most people are afraid of dying. Witnessing the death of another person brings that fear to the forefront, if only for a brief time. You must work through your personal feelings about death so that you can confront it in the field. Although you may be somewhat uncomfortable bringing up the subject, it helps to discuss it with others in the emergency care field. If you are uncomfortable talking with your peers, talk to a member of your hospital's emergency department staff or an employee assistance counselor.

Once you have done everything you can to medically treat a patient, consider the psychological needs of the patient and family. Being there as an empathetic caregiver is helpful. Do not be afraid to offer a reassuring touch. Sometimes putting an arm around a shoulder or holding the hand of the patient or a member of the family helps everyone, including you (**FIGURE 12-7**). Do not make false statements about the situation, but it is just as important not to destroy hope. Even if, in your judgment, the situation is hopeless, try to give comfort by making such positive statements as, "We are here to help you and are doing everything we can. The ambulance is on its way, and you will be at the hospital as soon as possible."

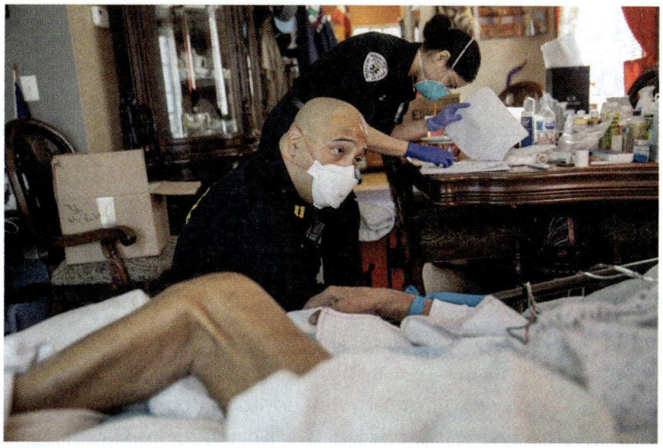

FIGURE 12-7 Do not be afraid to show empathy to patients and family members.

© John Moore/Getty Images News/Getty Images

As unfortunate as it may seem, coping with the deaths of others is a routine aspect of your job as an EMR. Therefore, you must constantly be on guard to prevent any callousness from entering your interactions with patients and their families. On every call you respond to, always deliver compassionate medical care.

Special Populations

Sudden Infant Death Syndrome

A condition that is frequently mistaken for child abuse is SIDS, also called crib death or sudden unexpected infant death. It is the sudden and unexpected death of an apparently healthy infant. SIDS usually occurs in infants between the ages of 3 weeks and 7 months. The infants are usually found dead in their cribs.

Currently, no adequate scientific explanation exists for SIDS. These deaths are not the result of smothering, choking, or strangulation. They are thought to result from a combination of factors, including vulnerability (eg, underlying medical conditions), developmental stage, and environmental stressors (eg, sleeping position, exposure to smoke, excessive warmth). SIDS deaths often remain unexplained, even after a complete and thorough autopsy.

You can imagine the shock and grief felt by parents who find their apparently healthy infant dead in bed. Your actions and words can be important in addressing their feelings of remorse and guilt.

If the infant is still warm, begin CPR and continue until help arrives. In many cases, the infant has been dead several hours and the body is cold and lifeless. Do not mistake the large, bruise-like blotches on the infant's body for signs of child abuse. The blotches are caused by the pooling of the infant's blood after death. Sometimes you may find a small amount of bloody foam on the infant's lips. If the child is obviously dead, follow the protocol in your community for the management of deceased patients.

Know your local guidelines for the management of SIDS. Remember that the parents could do nothing to prevent the death. Be compassionate and supportive during this tragic situation.

Mental Health Considerations in Geriatric Patients

Depression

Depression is a common mental health problem in the United States, affecting nearly 20% of adults. Although depression is less common in older adults, affecting approximately 14% of those 65 years and older, they are exposed to many causes of serious emotional distress. The recent loss of a spouse or close friend can contribute to depression. People with declining health, chronic health conditions, or terminal illnesses are especially likely to experience depression, as well as those who are socially isolated. Be aware of the high incidence of depression in older patients, and be alert for signs and symptoms of persistent feelings of sadness or despair. If you observe signs or symptoms of depression, bring this to the attention of other EMS clinicians or other medical professionals.

Do not overlook signs of mental health conditions in older patients. The symptoms of depression are the same in any age group and include, but are not limited to, the following:

- Sadness
- Feelings of worthlessness
- Irritability
- Fatigue
- Lack of concentration
- Withdrawal from social interactions and one's usual activities
- Sleep problems
- Changes in appetite
- Thoughts of suicide

Older men have the highest suicide rate of any age group in the United States. When older people attempt suicide, they choose more lethal means than younger people do. This factor results in more deaths from suicide than in some other age groups. Many factors contribute to the high suicide rate among older men, including physical illnesses (especially terminal illnesses), loss of a loved one, and alcohol use disorder. Listen carefully to the patient. Be alert for indications of hopelessness, depression, or attempts at suicide. If you think a patient may be considering suicide, arrange for transport to an appropriate medical facility. Be alert for your safety because weapons may be present on the scene. Contact law enforcement for assistance if needed. Know the protocols in your department for handling this type of situation.

Dementia

As people get older, some of them experience a pattern of decline in mental function called **dementia**. Dementia is a progressive and usually irreversible decline in mental functions. It is not considered a normal part of aging. It is marked by impairment in memory and may result in decreases in reasoning, judgment, comprehension, and ability to communicate verbally. An estimated one-third of people older than 85 years have some degree of dementia. You may hear people use the term **senile dementia** when referring to patients with decreased mental function. Senile dementia is a general term used to describe an abnormal decline in mental functioning seen in older patients. Dementia can be caused by many different conditions, including small strokes, hardening of the arteries, and/or heredity.

The most common type of dementia is **Alzheimer disease**. Alzheimer disease is a chronic degenerative disorder that attacks the brain and results in impaired memory, behavior, and thinking. According to the Alzheimer's Association, 6.9 million Americans aged 65 years or older are living with Alzheimer dementia as of 2024. This number is constantly rising; the population of Americans 65 years and older with Alzheimer and other forms of dementia is expected to be nearly 82 million by 2050. Patients with this illness may experience mood swings and feelings that people are plotting against them. Patients with Alzheimer disease may wander at night and are at increased risk for falls. In the terminal stages of this disease, patients may be unable to walk, control their bowels and bladder, and swallow.

When you care for patients with dementia, it is important to speak clearly to them and use their name. Let the patient know what you are doing at each step of your assessment and treatment. You will need to rely on family members or caregivers for a medical history. Because the patient's thought processes are impaired, communication may be difficult; therefore, inform the patient what you need to do. Be respectful and patient. Patients with dementia will pick up on your calm attitude and approach and respond accordingly. Use both verbal and nonverbal communication to connect with patients who are unable to communicate verbally. Your kind and caring approach will make the patient more comfortable and will make your job easier.

Medical and Legal Considerations

To protect the rights of the patient and to protect yourself from any possible legal action, you must understand the laws of your state and community that relate to caring for patients experiencing a behavioral emergency. If a patient agrees to be treated, there should be few legal issues. However, if a patient who appears to be disturbed refuses to accept treatment, it may be necessary to provide care against the patient's will. To do this, you must have a reasonable belief that the patient will harm self or others. Usually, if patients are a threat to themselves or to others, it is possible to treat and transport them without their consent. As an EMR, you usually will not be responsible for transporting the patient, but you should know what the laws in your state permit you to do. This direction should come from your medical director and from legal counsel.

There may be times when it is necessary for you to apply reasonable force to keep a patient from injuring themselves or others. If you are required to restrain a patient, you should consider the following factors: the patient's size and apparent strength, the sex of the patient, the type of abnormal behavior, the mental state of the patient, and the method of restraint. Whenever possible, you should avoid acts of physical force that may injure the patient. Be especially careful that you do not restrict the patient's ability to breathe. You may, however, use reasonable force to defend yourself against an attack by a behaviorally impaired patient.

To prevent legal issues if you must restrain a patient, seek assistance from law enforcement officials and from your medical director. It is also important to document the conditions present in cases where you must restrain or subdue a patient. To prevent accusations of sexual misconduct by behaviorally impaired patients, a caregiver of the same sex should take primary responsibility for the care of the patient, whenever possible.

Coping With Work-Related Stress

Providing emergency care is stressful for you as well as for the patient. As an EMR, you will encounter patients experiencing high levels of stress and anxiety. In emergency situations, there may be times when you cannot help patients. Some types of situations, such as rescue missions involving children or mass casualty incidents, tend to produce more stress than others. You may need counseling to cope with these stressors.

If you let stress build up without releasing it in healthy ways, it can begin to have negative effects on you and your performance.

Signs and Symptoms

Signs and symptoms of extreme stress include:

- Depression
- Inability to sleep
- Weight changes
- Increased consumption of alcohol or drugs
- Inability to get along with family and coworkers
- Lack of interest in food or sex

Critical Incident Stress Debriefing

To help prevent excess stress and to relieve stress caused by critical incidents, some departments use a process called **critical incident stress debriefing (CISD)**. CISD brings rescuers and a trained professional together to talk about the rescuers' feelings. CISD may help rescuers understand the signs and symptoms of stress and receive reassurance from the group leader. It also allows people to obtain more help from trained professionals, if needed. Some public safety agencies have set up CISD teams to handle stressful events. These teams may be helpful to rescuers who have been through an overwhelming or stressful event. Other departments have trained professionals available to counsel members who have experienced a highly stressful event. Check with your agency to see what types of counseling and CISD resources are available. Additional information about critical incident stress debriefing is presented in Chapter 2, *Workforce Safety and Wellness*.

Special Populations

Debriefing After Calls Involving Children

As an EMR, you will respond to many calls that involve children. These calls tend to produce strong emotional reactions. At times, you may experience a feeling of helplessness when a child is seriously injured or gravely ill. An ill or injured child may remind you of your own children. You may feel especially angry or helpless when you suspect the neglect or abuse of a child. After a major incident or an especially emotional incident involving children, it may be helpful for you to set up a CISD session. CISD can help you express your feelings, learn some coping strategies, and maintain a healthy approach to future calls.

Peer Support

Peer support is a process by which a properly trained member of your department provides confidential support to another member who is experiencing personal, emotional, or work-related problems and acts as a bridge to outside professional services. Many departments provide both CISD programs and peer support programs. Whereas CISD is especially valuable following stressful incidents that involve multiple members of a department, peer support is more appropriate for assisting individuals and for situations where ongoing follow-through is needed. Both programs provide valuable assistance for dealing with stressful situations.

One advantage of peer support is that it can build on the existing mutual trust and understanding between two members of the same department. Peer support provides a safe and nurturing environment for all affected members. Trained peer counselors understand the unique needs of public safety personnel. They are prepared to adjust to the irregular schedules and other logistical challenges of first responders. They understand the importance of confidentiality, and they understand the physical requirements and mental stressors of being a first responder. Peer counselors can respond in a moment of crisis. They can help to direct a member to self-care, or they can help to provide bridges to outside professional help when needed.

Peer support is voluntary. It can be initiated at the request of the member, a concerned coworker, or a supervisor. It may follow a potentially traumatic call. Your coworkers may be able to identify warning signs of stress early and reach out to other team members before these signs become significant problems. Peer counselors can follow up with members weeks or months after a troubling event.

Peer support is not limited to work-related problems. Family issues, financial difficulties, stress or anxiety, and substance use are all issues that may be helped through a peer support program. Properly trained peer support personnel can be available to the first responder's family members, too.

The effectiveness of peer support relies on confidentiality. This confidentiality is carefully maintained except in cases where there is a risk of harm to the member or to others, or where there is criminal activity. Check with your supervisor to see if a peer support program is available for members of your department.

Words of Wisdom

Some peer support programs use the acronym LOVE to describe the role of the peer counselor:

L Listen carefully.
O Offer assistance.
V Validate through understanding.
E Encourage the person to never give up and to seek assistance.

YOU are the EMR SUMMARY

You are the EMR: CASE 1

1. What types of conditions contribute to or cause a behavioral emergency?

As you begin your assessment of this situation, it is helpful to review the five types of conditions that can cause or contribute to a behavioral emergency:

- Medical conditions such as uncontrolled diabetes, low blood glucose level, and conditions that prevent the patient's brain from receiving enough oxygen
- Physical trauma such as head injuries and shock
- Psychiatric illnesses such as depression, panic disorders, and psychotic behaviors
- Alcohol and drug abuse
- Situational stressors such as serious injury or death of a loved one

By evaluating the patient for each of these conditions, you can get a better idea of what might be causing the behavior you are observing.

2. What are the four phases of a situational crisis?

The four phases of a situational crisis are high anxiety or emotional shock, denial, anger, and remorse or grief. Even though not all patients go through these phases in this order, learning about the phases will often give you some idea of why a patient is acting in a certain way.

3. What are three communication tools that can help you communicate with this patient?

Your ability to communicate with the patient will help you determine the cause of their problem, and often you can begin to defuse the patient's anger. Three tools that are useful in this communication process are restatement, redirection, and empathy.

You are the EMR: CASE 2

1. What actions should you take on arriving on the scene?

As you arrive on this scene, it is important for you to avoid getting tunnel vision regarding what is happening. Complete all the steps of the patient assessment sequence. Be sure to consider all the possibilities regarding what may be happening. Shortness of breath is a scary event for anyone. As you approach this patient, be sure to introduce yourself, and let the patient know you are there to help her. Ask her what the problem is. She may respond that she is having an asthma attack or is upset about a stressful event. Perform a careful patient assessment, including a thorough SAMPLE history. Ask additional questions to follow up on any problems she identifies. Remember, you cannot determine if the problem is purely emotional until all medical causes have been ruled out, and that is something only a physician can do. Many conditions can cause difficulty breathing, including asthma, pneumonia, head injuries, diabetic coma, imbalance of medications, and emotional crises. Do not be led into the trap of believing the problem is purely emotional just because a patient is upset.

2. What care can you give to this patient?

The care that you give to this patient should be based on her signs and symptoms and on any problems that you identify from performing a patient assessment. Because shortness of breath produces anxiety, anything you can do to calm this patient will help relieve her anxiety. Treat any medical problems you identify. It is often reassuring to have a family member or close friend for support. Try to determine where her family members are and see if it is possible to reunite her with one of them. If her condition is caused by a behavioral emergency, she may become calmer as you talk with her. You should arrange for her to be transported to an appropriate medical facility for further treatment.

You are the EMR: CASE 3

1. What actions should you take first with this patient?

As you arrive on this scene, you should understand that the mechanism of injury in this case leads to the high possibility that this patient has sustained serious injuries. This is complicated by the fact that there appear to be barriers to clear communication with this patient. Whether you smell alcohol or not, it is important to conduct a complete patient assessment to determine all injuries and illness that this patient has sustained. Talk with the patient to ensure that he knows you are there to help him. Help him to

YOU are the EMR SUMMARY

remember that he has experienced a vehicle crash. Take spinal precautions to prevent further injuries. Remember, if this patient is under the influence of alcohol or drugs, he is at high risk for traumatic injuries and may not realize that he is seriously injured.

2. What treatment do you need to give to this patient?

Your treatment should reflect the understanding that this type of incident places the patient at high risk for serious trauma to any part of the body. Consider the possibility of head injuries, spinal injuries, chest and abdominal injuries, and extremity injuries. Take spinal precautions. Consider whether this patient may have a serious medical condition, such as diabetes or heart disease, that contributed to this situation. Because this patient may not be able to communicate his history to you, see if there is a friend or family member with him. Provide the best treatment you can and arrange for transport to an appropriate medical facility as soon as possible. Remember, the odor of alcohol should serve as an indication for added caution and careful attention to assessment and treatment.

You are the EMR: CASE 4

1. What are your initial priorities in this case?

Your initial priorities in this case are to secure scene safety for yourself, for other rescuers, and for the patient. Unless you are a law enforcement officer trained to handle a situation such as this, you should not proceed into this residence. Back off to a safe location away from the house and call for immediate assistance from law enforcement personnel. It is their responsibility to secure the scene for you and for the patient. Only after they have secured the scene may you approach the injured woman and begin to examine and treat her. Domestic disputes can be some of the most explosive and dangerous situations you are called to manage.

2. How should you proceed with treating the injured woman?

Once the scene has been secured by law enforcement personnel, you can approach the injured woman and begin to examine and treat her. In situations such as this, it is important to separate the woman from any people who may be threatening her. This will give her some feeling of safety. Realize that she may be afraid to talk about her experience for fear of punishment from her significant other. Try to be supportive; be a good listener. Remember, you must report cases of suspected domestic abuse to the proper authorities.

Perform a complete patient assessment in a calm manner. Treat any physical injuries you find. Ask her about any other abuse. Document the results of your examination and treatment. Arrange for transportation of the woman to an appropriate medical facility for further examination and treatment.

Prep Kit

Ready for Review

- Only a small percentage of the patients you treat are severely mentally ill, but almost every patient you care for is experiencing some degree of emotional distress. No matter what type of incident or crisis is taking place, your response must be to help the patient.
- Behavioral emergencies are situations in which a person exhibits abnormal, unacceptable behavior that cannot be tolerated by the patients themselves or by family, friends, or the community.
- There are five major factors that contribute to behavioral emergencies: medical conditions, physical trauma conditions, psychiatric illnesses, mind-altering substances, and situational stresses.
- The four emotional phases to each crisis include high anxiety or emotional shock, denial, anger, and remorse or grief. A person may not experience every phase during a crisis but will certainly experience one or more of the phases.
- Your role as an EMR consists of assessing the patient and providing physical and emotional care. Your most important assessment skill may be your ability to communicate with the patient.
- You must understand the laws of your state and community that relate to caring for patients experiencing a behavioral emergency. If a patient who is experiencing a behavioral emergency agrees to be treated, there should be few legal issues. However, if a patient who appears to be disturbed refuses to accept treatment, it may be necessary to provide care against the patient's will. To do this, you must have a reasonable belief that the patient would harm self or others. Usually, if patients are a threat to themselves or to others, it is possible to treat and transport them without their consent.
- As an EMR, you need to recognize and respond appropriately to the different forms of abuse you may encounter, including elder abuse, child abuse, and spousal and domestic partner abuse.

Prep Kit

- It is helpful for you to have some understanding of the types of mental health conditions seen frequently in older people (depression, thoughts of suicide, and dementia or Alzheimer disease) so you will know how to help patients with these disorders.
- Even when you have thoroughly mastered the processes and tools for managing behavioral emergencies, it is important to remember that sometimes the best approach is to ask yourself, "How would I like to be treated if I were in this situation?"
- EMRs must also attend to their own emotional well-being. CISD and peer support can help prevent excess stress and relieve stress caused by critical incidents.

Vital Vocabulary

Alzheimer disease The most common subtype of dementia, characterized by confusion, memory failure, disorientation, speech disturbances, and inability to carry out purposeful movements.

behavioral emergency A situation in which the patient exhibits abnormal behavior that is unacceptable or cannot be tolerated by the patient or by family, friends, or the community.

critical incident stress debriefing (CISD) A system of psychological support designed to reduce stress on emergency personnel after a major stress-producing incident.

dementia A progressive, irreversible decline in mental functioning marked by memory impairment and decrease in reasoning, judgment, comprehension, and ability to communicate verbally.

depression A psychiatric disorder marked by persistent feelings of sadness, hopelessness, and decreased interest in daily activities. The person may have persistent thoughts of suicide.

elder abuse An action taken by a family member or caregiver that results in the physical, emotional, financial, or sexual harm to a person older than 65 years; also includes neglect.

emotional shock A state of shock caused by a sudden illness, an accident, or the death of a loved one; technically referred to as psychogenic shock.

empathy The ability to share another person's feelings or ideas.

posttraumatic stress disorder (PTSD) A mental health or behavioral condition triggered by experiencing or witnessing a terrifying event.

psychotic behavior Mental disturbance characterized by abnormal thought processes and/or the loss of contact with reality.

redirection A means of focusing the patient's attention on the immediate situation or crisis.

restatement The act of rephrasing a person's statement to demonstrate that the person is being heard and understood.

senile dementia A general term for dementia that occurs in older people.

situational crisis A state of emotional upset or turmoil caused by a sudden and disruptive event.

suicide The intentional causing of one's own death. It is especially common among older and chronically ill people.

References

Alzheimer's Association. 2024 Alzheimer's disease facts and figures. *Alzheimers Dement.* 2024;20(5):3708–3821.

Developmental disabilities. Centers for Disease Control and Prevention website. https://www.cdc.gov/environmental-health-tracking/php/data-research/developmental-disabilities.htm. Published February 9, 2024. Accessed November 19, 2024.

Lee B, Wang Y, Carlson SA, et al. National, state-level, and county-level prevalence estimates of adults aged ≥18 years self-reporting a lifetime diagnosis of depression—United States, 2020. *MMWR Morb Mortal Wkly Rep.* 2023;72(24):644–650.

National Institute of Occupational Safety and Health (NIOSH). *Violence in the Workplace* (DHHS NIOSH Publication No. 96–100). Cincinnati, OH: NIOSH; 1996.

Sudden infant death syndrome (SIDS). National Health Service website. https://www.nhs.uk/conditions/sudden-infant-death-syndrome-sids/. Reviewed October 27, 2021. Accessed

What is dementia? Symptoms, types, and diagnosis. National Institute on Aging website. https://www.nia.nih.gov/health/alzheimers-and-dementia/what-dementia-symptoms-types-and-diagnosis. Reviewed December 8, 2022. Accessed November 19, 2024.

Assessment IN ACTION

You and your partner are dispatched to a single-family home for a report of a possible overdose. On arrival, a man claiming to be the patient's husband opens the door and begins yelling at you, stating he arrived home and found his wife unresponsive on the floor of the bedroom with an empty bottle of diazepam (Valium). He thinks she took at least 40 pills. The husband is very agitated, flushed in the face, and obviously distraught. As your partner calms the man, you assess the woman and find her pulseless and not breathing. While you are performing CPR, the paramedics arrive and begin more advanced life support measures and provide transport to the hospital. The patient is pronounced dead on arrival at the hospital.

1. What emotional phase of a situational crisis is the husband exhibiting?

- **A.** High anxiety or emotional shock
- **B.** Denial
- **C.** Anger
- **D.** Remorse or grief

2. The signs and symptoms the husband is exhibiting are suggestive of:

- **A.** posttraumatic stress.
- **B.** high anxiety.
- **C.** hypovolemic shock.
- **D.** denial.

3. When performing your primary assessment of the woman, you should do all of the following EXCEPT:

- **A.** demonstrate confidence.
- **B.** provide emotional support for the family.
- **C.** allow personal feelings to influence your care.
- **D.** talk in a calm, steady voice.

4. What is the single most important personal history factor in an attempted suicide?

- **A.** Aggression
- **B.** Anxiety
- **C.** Excessive confidence
- **D.** Depression

5. All of the following skills are useful to you when communicating with patients in crisis EXCEPT:

- **A.** restatement.
- **B.** redirection.
- **C.** empathy.
- **D.** sympathy.

6. What is a behavioral emergency?

7. Describe the condition or conditions under which you could take a behaviorally disturbed patient to a medical facility against their will.

8. Explain how redirection might be used to improve your communication in this situation.

9. List the general symptoms of posttraumatic stress disorder.

10. Describe the risk factors that make a person more likely to develop posttraumatic stress disorder.

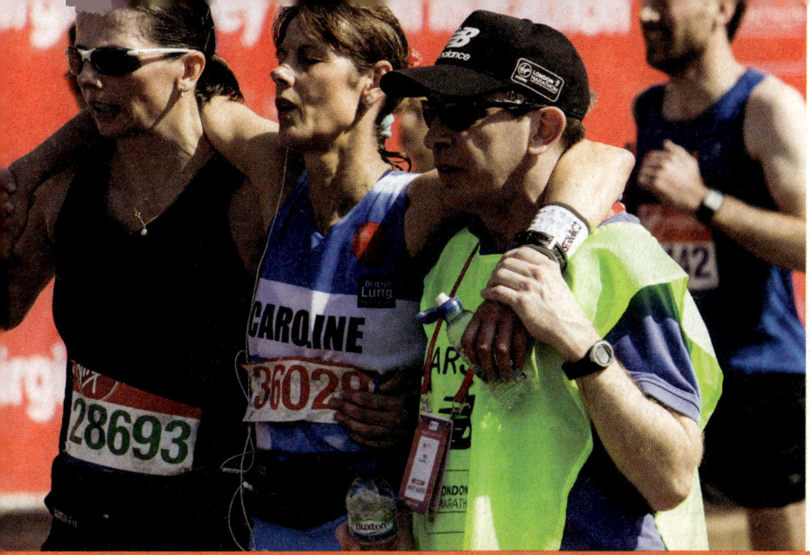

CHAPTER 13

Environmental Emergencies

National EMS Education Standard Competencies

Trauma

Uses knowledge to recognize and manage life threats based on assessment findings for an acutely injured patient while awaiting additional emergency medical response.

Environmental Emergencies

- Drowning (pp 285–287)
- Temperature-related illness (pp 280–285)
- Bites and envenomation (Chapter 11, *Poisoning and Substance Use*)
- Lightning injury (p 287)

Knowledge Objectives

1. Describe the signs and symptoms of a patient experiencing heat cramps. (p 281)
2. Describe the treatment of a patient experiencing heat cramps. (p 281)
3. Describe the signs and symptoms of a patient experiencing heat exhaustion. (p 281)
4. Describe the treatment of a patient experiencing heat exhaustion. (p 281)
5. Describe the signs and symptoms of a patient experiencing heatstroke. (p 281)
6. Describe the treatment of a patient experiencing heatstroke. (pp 281–282)
7. Describe the signs and symptoms of a patient experiencing frostbite. (p 282)
8. Describe the treatment of a patient experiencing frostbite. (pp 282–283)
9. Describe the signs and symptoms of a patient experiencing hypothermia. (p 284)
10. Describe the treatment of a patient experiencing hypothermia. (pp 284–285)
11. Discuss the relationship between hypothermia and cardiac arrest. (p 284)
12. Describe the signs and symptoms of a patient who sustained a submersion injury. (p 285)
13. Describe the treatment of a patient who sustained a submersion injury. (p 285)
14. Describe the signs and symptoms of a patient who has been struck by lightning. (p 287)
15. Describe the treatment of a patient who has been struck by lightning. (p 287)

Skills Objectives

1. Demonstrate patient assessment for a patient who has sustained an injury or illness from exposure to heat, exposure to cold, or submersion. (p 280)
2. Demonstrate cooling a patient who has experienced exposure to heat. (p 281)
3. Demonstrate treating a patient who has experienced exposure to cold. (pp 282–285)
4. Demonstrate treating a patient who has a submersion injury. (p 285)
5. Demonstrate treating a patient who has a lightning injury. (p 287)

© Bear Hench/Shutterstock

Introduction

This chapter describes medical conditions that are caused by environmental conditions such as excessive heat, humidity, and cold, and injuries and illnesses related to submersion in water. When a person is exposed to excessive heat, the body's mechanisms for controlling temperature can be overwhelmed, resulting in heat cramps, heat exhaustion, or heatstroke. Exposure to cold environments may result in conditions such as frostbite or hypothermia. You will learn about each of these conditions, including signs, symptoms, and common treatments. This chapter also discusses unintentional exposure to water leading to submersion injuries and drowning and the signs, symptoms, and treatment of these conditions. Special considerations for treating hypothermic patients in cardiac arrest are emphasized. Finally, this chapter outlines the injuries caused by lightning and emphasizes the importance of properly treating these patients.

Patient Assessment for Environmental Emergencies

Your approach to a patient who has signs and symptoms of an environmental emergency should follow the patient assessment sequence (**FIGURE 13-1**). Review your dispatch information and evaluate it to help you consider the possible conditions or injuries the patient may be experiencing. Carefully assess the scene to determine safety issues for you and your patient. As you perform the primary assessment, first try to form an impression of the patient's condition. Determine the patient's level of responsiveness as you introduce yourself. Then check the patient's Airway, Breathing, and Circulation (ABCs), and acknowledge the patient's chief complaint.

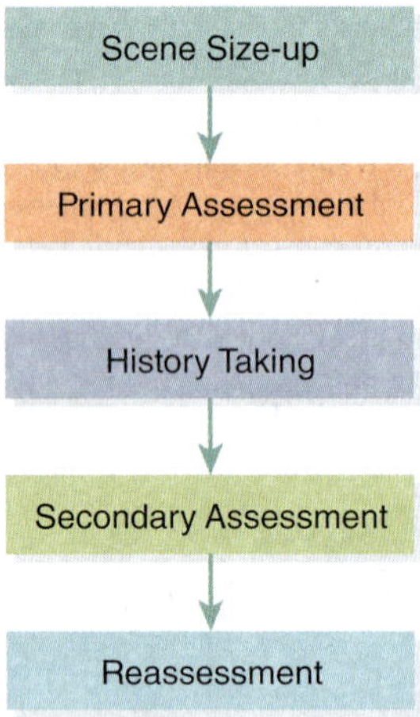

FIGURE 13-1 Patient assessment sequence.

© Jones & Bartlett Learning

Usually, it is best to collect a medical history on the patient experiencing a medical problem before you perform a secondary assessment. The medical history should be complete and include all factors that may relate to the patient's current illness.

Use the SAMPLE mnemonic to help you secure the medical history information you need:

- **S** Signs and symptoms
- **A** Allergies
- **M** Medications
- **P** Pertinent past medical history
- **L** Last oral intake
- **E** Events associated with or leading up to the illness or injury

Although the secondary patient assessment should focus on the areas related to the patient's current illness, you should also recognize that patients may not always be aware of all the various aspects of their condition. It is better to perform a complete patient assessment and find all the problems than to perform a partial assessment and miss an underlying problem. Obtain the patient's vital signs and do not forget to monitor your patient through the use of ongoing reassessment if the arrival of additional emergency medical services (EMS) personnel is delayed.

Safety

Environmental emergencies require you to evaluate the special hazards encountered by you and your patients. Take appropriate precautions against hazards, which include heat, cold, slippery surfaces, water hazards, darkness, insects, and animals. These precautions are covered throughout this textbook.

YOU are the EMR **CASE 1**

As you gather for the morning report at the beginning of your shift, you listen to your supervisor as she reviews the weather forecast for this July day. She reports the temperature is expected to reach 95°F to 97°F (35°C to 36°C), and the humidity is expected to be in excess of 80%. Just before ending her report, she encourages team members to monitor their fluid intake to avoid dehydration. After the report you are dispatched to stand by at an aid station for a local marathon. Soon after you arrive, a 38-year-old female runner is assisted to the aid station by two runners. She is sweating and her clothes are completely wet. You check her pulse and discover that it is weak and thready. She says she feels nauseous and was lightheaded during the last part of the race.

1. As you evaluate the patient's symptoms and the signs she exhibits, what condition do you think this patient may be experiencing?
2. What steps should you take to treat this patient?

Exposure to Heat

As an emergency medical responder (EMR), you will encounter patients who have been exposed to excessive heat. The following sections discuss the signs, symptoms, and treatment for patients experiencing heat cramps, heat exhaustion, and heatstroke to help you recognize and treat these patients.

Heat Cramps

Heat cramps are painful involuntary muscle spasms. They often occur after vigorous exercise, especially in hot weather. They can also occur in factory or construction workers and even in well-conditioned athletes. The exact cause of heat cramps is not known, but it is thought to be partly related to the change in the electrolytes that occurs during exercise, and partly a result of the dehydration that accompanies exercise or working in a hot environment. A large amount of water loss occurs during vigorous physical activity. This loss of water may affect muscles that are stressed and cause them to go into spasm. Heat cramps occur most often in the leg or calf muscles. They may also occur in the abdominal muscles. When abdominal cramps occur, it may appear that the patient is having an acute abdominal problem.

The first step in treating heat cramps is to move the patient to a cool place. Have the patient lie down in a comfortable position to rest the affected muscles. Give the patient water to drink. A diluted balanced electrolyte solution, such as Gatorade, can also be given if it is available. Usually, the cramps will go away with rest and fluid. Do not give anything by mouth if the patient is nauseated. Take measures to cool the patient and await the arrival of EMS. If the cramps do not go away, or if the patient is young, old, or has a chronic medical condition, you should arrange to have the patient transported to an appropriate medical facility for a thorough evaluation and treatment.

Heat Exhaustion

Heat exhaustion is a heat-related illness that occurs when a person is exposed to temperatures above 80°F (27°C), often in combination with high humidity. It may also occur as a result of vigorous exercise at lower temperatures, particularly in humid conditions that hinder sweat evaporation. A person experiencing heat exhaustion sweats profusely and becomes light-headed, dizzy, and nauseated.

Certain risk factors may make some people more susceptible to heat-related illnesses. Young children, older adults (age 65 years and older), and people who have preexisting medical conditions or who are taking certain medications are more likely to experience a heat-related illness. High air temperatures reduce the body's ability to cool itself by radiation. High humidity reduces the body's ability to lose heat through evaporation. Exercise results in greater production of sweat.

> **Signs and Symptoms**
>
> Signs and symptoms of heat exhaustion include the following:
>
> - Dizziness, light-headedness
> - Weak pulse
> - Profuse sweating
> - Nausea, vomiting

The patient's blood pressure may decrease (causing a weak pulse), and the patient may frequently report feeling weak. Body temperature is usually normal. The signs and symptoms of heat exhaustion are similar to the early signs of shock, and the treatments are similar as well.

When you encounter a patient who is experiencing heat exhaustion, complete a scene assessment and a primary assessment. Patients experiencing heat exhaustion sweat heavily and are in mild shock from fluid loss. To treat heat exhaustion, move the patient to a cooler place (for example, from a baseball diamond to a shady spot under a tree) and treat for shock. Unless the patient is unresponsive, nauseous, or vomiting, give fluids by mouth to replace fluid loss through sweating. Drinking cool water is excellent treatment for patients experiencing heat exhaustion. Monitor the ABCs and arrange for transport to a medical facility.

Heatstroke

Heatstroke is the most serious heat-related emergency. It occurs when the body is subjected to more heat than it can tolerate and the normal mechanisms for regulating body temperature, such as sweating, are overwhelmed. The patient's body temperature rises until it reaches a level at which brain damage occurs. Without prompt and proper treatment, a patient with heatstroke will die.

> **Special Populations**
>
> **Heatstroke in Pediatric Patients**
>
> The most dangerous heat-related illness in children is heatstroke. Any child who is in a closed, parked car on a hot day or in a poorly ventilated room and who has hot, dry skin may be experiencing heatstroke. To treat this serious and potentially fatal condition, you must work to quickly reduce the child's body temperature. Interventions for these patients include removing the clothing, sponging water over them, and fanning them. You may wrap the child in wet sheets (if they are available) to speed up the evaporation and cooling process, but do not let the child become chilled. Arrange for rapid transport to an appropriate medical facility.

The patient usually has flushed, dry skin that feels hot to the touch. Be aware that the patient's clothing may still be wet even though the person has stopped sweating. A person who is experiencing heatstroke may have an altered mental status; however, as the body temperature rises, the patient will rapidly become unresponsive. These patients may have body temperatures in excess of 104°F (40°C).

Maintain the patient's ABCs. Move the patient from the heat and into a cool place as soon as possible (**FIGURE 13-2**). Remove the patient's clothes, down to the underwear. Soak the patient with water. You should begin to aggressively cool the patient with water from a garden hose, a shower in the home or factory, or a low-pressure hose from a fire truck. Ice

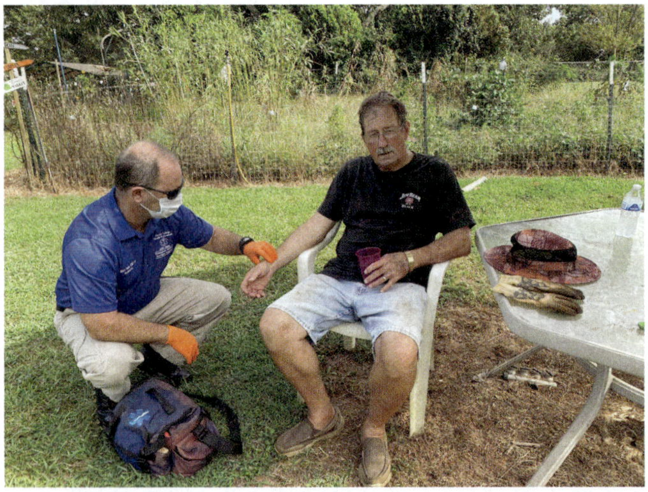

FIGURE 13-2 When caring for a person experiencing a heat-related emergency, move the patient from the heat as soon as possible.
Courtesy of Rhonda Hunt.

TABLE 13-1 Comparing Heat Exhaustion and Heatstroke

Heat Exhaustion	Heatstroke
Normal body temperature	High body temperature
Sweating	Dry skin (usually)
Cool and clammy skin	Hot and flushed skin
Dizziness and nausea	Altered mental status

© Jones & Bartlett Learning. Courtesy of MIEMSS.

packs can be placed on the groin and armpits. If the patient is alert and not nauseated, give small amounts of cool water. Arrange for rapid transport to an appropriate medical facility for further treatment. **TABLE 13-1** compares the signs and symptoms of heat exhaustion with those of heatstroke.

Treatment

Heatstroke is an emergency that requires immediate action. The patient's body temperature must be lowered quickly!

Safety

Firefighters are at high risk for heat exhaustion and heatstroke when wearing heavy turnout gear because, in addition to working in hot environments, the turnout gear does not allow body heat to escape. Law enforcement personnel are also at high risk for heat-related conditions because of the heavy ballistic vests they wear for protection. It is important to keep hydrated and to take breaks when operating in hot environments. Any protective gear that retains body heat should be removed during breaks to help reduce elevated body temperatures.

Exposure to Cold

As an EMR, you may encounter patients who are experiencing the adverse effects of exposure to excessive cold. When you assess these patients, you should follow the steps of the patient assessment sequence discussed earlier. The signs and symptoms exhibited by the patient will guide you in your treatment. To help you recognize and treat these patients, the signs, symptoms, and treatment for frostbite and hypothermia are discussed next.

Frostbite

Frostbite can result when parts of the body are exposed to a cold environment. It can occur outside on a winter day or in specific places, such as a walk-in food freezer or a cold-storage warehouse, in otherwise warm environments. It can also occur through contact with super-cooled gases, which will cause exposed body parts to freeze. The body parts most susceptible to frostbite are the face, ears, fingers, and toes (**FIGURE 13-3**). Depending on the temperature and wind speed, frostbite can occur in a short period.

Increases in wind speed have the same effect as decreases in temperature. Imagine holding your hand outside an automobile traveling at 55 mph on a cold winter day. The combination of wind speed and low temperature produces a windchill factor (**FIGURE 13-4**). When the temperature is relatively mild at 35°F (2°C), an accompanying 20-mph wind will produce a windchill equivalent to an actual temperature of 24°F (−4°C). If there is a combination of low temperature and high wind, the effect can be extreme. Protect yourself and your patient from the dangers of windchill.

YOU are the EMR **CASE 2**

It is now 1015 hours at the marathon when a runner is transported to the medical tent by the remote assistance team. The EMR handing off the patient to you indicates the runner is a 53-year-old man who collapsed at mile 18. He is responsive only to verbal stimuli and his skin is flushed and hot to the touch. Treatment was not initiated in the field; the patient was immediately transported to the medical tent.

1. What signs would indicate this runner is experiencing heat exhaustion or heatstroke?
2. After completing the primary assessment, what is the most appropriate treatment for this runner?

People weakened by old age, medical conditions, exhaustion, or hunger are the most susceptible to frostbite. In superficial frostbite, sometimes called frostnip, there may be a loss of feeling and sensation in the injured area. The area will appear flushed initially and eventually becomes pale. If the area is rewarmed, the patient may experience pain or a tingling feeling.

Warming a frostbitten area or body part must be done carefully. Usually, putting the fingers, toes, or ears next to a warm body part is enough. For example, place frostbitten fingers in the armpits. Do not try to warm a frostbitten area by rubbing it with your hands or a blanket, and never rub snow or ice onto a suspected frostbitten area. Doing so will only make the problem worse. Treat the frostbitten patient for shock.

A patient with frostbite who has been outside for an extended period may have deep frostbite. In this situation, the patient's skin will be white and waxy, and it may be firm or frozen. Swelling and blisters may be present. If the skin has thawed, it may appear flushed with areas of discolored skin, or it may be mottled and cyanotic. Follow the scene assessment, primary assessment, and secondary assessment sequence. Remove any jewelry the patient is wearing and cover the extremity with dry clothing or dry dressings. If possible, remove wet clothing and keep the patient warm to prevent hypothermia and further frostbite. Do not break blisters, rub the injured area, apply heat, or allow the patient to walk on an affected lower extremity. Patients with deep frostbite should receive prompt transport to a medical facility so they can be warmed under carefully controlled conditions. Remember, any patient with a frostbite injury may have been in the cold environment long enough to sustain hypothermia.

Treatment

Place 4 × 4–inch [10 × 10–cm] gauze pads between frostbitten fingers or toes to prevent the skin from sticking together.

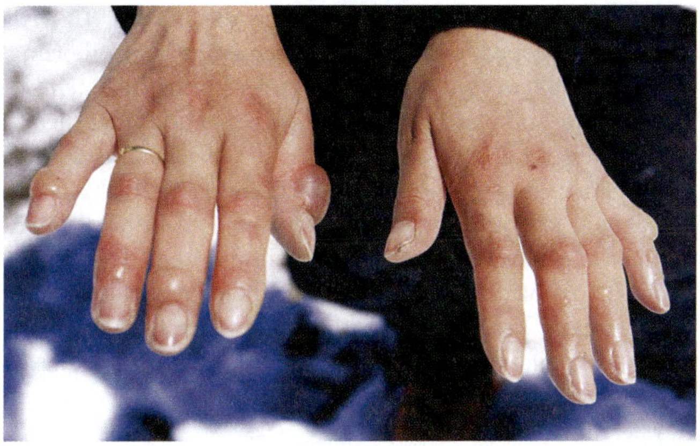

FIGURE 13-3 The fingers are among the most common areas affected by frostbite.
Courtesy of Neil Malcom Winkelmann.

Words of Wisdom

Remember that changes to skin color, whether pallor, cyanosis, flushing, or jaundice, will present differently among patients depending on their baseline skin tone. The EMR must consider what is normal for each patient and may need to look for signs of abnormal perfusion in places such as the oral mucosa, conjunctiva, or nail beds. The observations of friends and family members on scene may also provide valuable insights (eg, "My dad looks really pale.").

Wind Chill Chart

Wind (mph)	Temperature (°F)																	
Calm	40	35	30	25	20	15	10	5	0	-5	-10	-15	-20	-25	-30	-35	-40	-45
5	36	31	25	19	13	7	1	-5	-11	-16	-22	-28	-34	-40	-46	-52	-57	-63
10	34	27	21	15	9	3	-4	-10	-16	-22	-28	-35	-41	-47	-53	-59	-66	-72
15	32	25	19	13	6	0	-7	-13	-19	-26	-32	-39	-45	-51	-58	-64	-71	-77
20	30	24	17	11	4	-2	-9	-15	-22	-29	-35	-42	-48	-55	-61	-68	-74	-81
25	29	23	16	9	3	-4	-11	-17	-24	-31	-37	-44	-51	-58	-64	-71	-78	-84
30	28	22	15	8	1	-5	-12	-19	-26	-33	-39	-46	-53	-60	-67	-73	-80	-87
35	28	21	14	7	0	-7	-14	-21	-27	-34	-41	-48	-55	-62	-69	-76	-82	-89
40	27	20	13	6	-1	-8	-15	-22	-29	-36	-43	-50	-57	-64	-71	-78	-84	-91
45	26	19	12	5	-2	-9	-16	-23	-30	-37	-44	-51	-58	-65	-72	-79	-86	-93
50	26	19	12	4	-3	-10	-17	-24	-31	-38	-45	-52	-60	-67	-74	-81	-88	-95
55	25	18	11	4	-3	-11	-18	-25	-32	-39	-46	-54	-61	-68	-75	-82	-89	-97
60	25	17	10	3	-4	-11	-19	-26	-33	-40	-48	-55	-62	-69	-76	-84	-91	-98

Frostbite Times: 30 minutes; 10 minutes; 5 minutes

$$\text{Wind Chill (°F)} = 35.74 + 0.6215T - 35.75(V^{0.16}) + 0.4275T(V^{0.16})$$

Where, T= Air Temperature (°F) V= Wind Speed (mph)

Effective 11/01/01

FIGURE 13-4 Windchill table.
Courtesy of the National Weather Service/NOAA.

Safety

Prevention is the only defense against frostbite. If you are going outside in freezing weather, dress warmly and make sure the vulnerable parts of your body are well covered and protected.

Hypothermia

When a person's body temperature falls to a subnormal range of below approximately 95°F (35°C), the condition is called **hypothermia** (low temperature). Hypothermia occurs when the body is not able to produce enough energy to keep the internal (core) body temperature at a satisfactory level.

Special Populations

Risk of Temperature-Related Emergencies in Pediatric and Geriatric Patients

Infants and small children have poorly developed heat-regulating mechanisms. They sometimes spike a fever with a minor infection. They are also susceptible to both heat and cold injuries. They are more susceptible to cold injuries because they have a greater surface area relative to the mass of their body. This means they lose relatively more heat than adults. Also, their ability to generate or release heat is limited. Infants and very young children cannot tell you when they are cold or take steps to change their environment. Therefore, you need to keep the body temperature of children as close to normal as possible and warm them if they become chilled.

Older adults are also much more susceptible to heat and cold injuries. Many older adults have decreased sensation to heat and cold. Their bodies are not capable of generating heat as efficiently as younger adults. Some of the medications taken by many older adults reduce their ability to compensate for hot and cold conditions, and older adults generally tend to drink less fluids, which makes them more susceptible to dehydration. All of these factors make geriatric patients more susceptible to heat and cold injuries.

You should always be alert for the possibility of heat and cold injuries in infants, young children, and older adults.

Hypothermia does not occur only in the winter; it can occur in temperatures as high as 50°F (10°C). People who become cold because they do not have enough clothing or because their clothing is wet are likely to experience hypothermia, especially if they are weakened by illness. Patients under the influence of drugs or alcohol are at an especially high risk for experiencing hypothermia. The initial signs of hypothermia include feelings of being cold, shivering, decreasing level of consciousness, and sleepiness. Shivering is the body's attempt to produce more heat. As the body temperature drops and hypothermia progresses, shivering stops. Patients who are so cold that they cannot shiver cool down even faster. Signs of increasing hypothermia include a lack of coordination, decreased level of consciousness, mental confusion, and slowed reactions. As the body's temperature goes below approximately 90°F (32°C), the patient will become unresponsive. Patients experiencing hypothermia may have weak or very slow pulse rates. Therefore, it is important to carefully monitor their pulse for at least 30 seconds to accurately determine the underlying heart rate. Without treatment and warming to reverse the downward trend in body temperature, the patient will eventually die (**TABLE 13-2**).

If you suspect a patient is experiencing hypothermia, move the patient to a warm (or warmer) location. Remove wet clothing and place warm blankets over and under the patient to help retain body heat and begin the warming process. If the patient is alert, give them warm fluids to drink.

If you are outdoors and cannot easily take the patient inside a building, move the patient into a heated vehicle as soon as possible. If you cannot move the patient to a warmer environment, keep the patient dry and place as many blankets and insulating materials as possible around them. Any patient experiencing hypothermia must be examined by a physician.

Cardiac Arrest and Hypothermia

If the patient's body temperature falls below 83°F (28°C), the heart may stop and you will need to begin cardiopulmonary resuscitation (CPR). As odd as it may seem, hypothermia may protect patients from death in some cases. In the context of potential hypothermia, feel for a pulse for a full minute prior to starting chest compressions. Do not start

TABLE 13-2 Characteristics of Systemic Hypothermia

	Core Temperature			
	93° to 95°F (34° to 35°C)	89° to 92°F (32° to 33°C)	80° to 88°F (27° to 31°C)	<80°F (<27°C)
Signs and symptoms	Shivering, foot stamping	Loss of coordination, muscle stiffness	Coma	Apparent death
Cardiorespiratory response	Constricted blood vessels, rapid breathing	Slowing respirations, slow pulse	Weak pulse, dysrhythmias, very slow respirations	Cardiac arrest
Level of consciousness	Withdrawn	Confused, lethargic, sleepy	Unresponsive	Unresponsive

© Jones & Bartlett Learning. Courtesy of MIEMSS.

compressions if there is at least one heartbeat in a minute. If an automated external defibrillator (AED) is available, it should be used, but only one shock should be delivered. After the shock, continue with chest compressions and ventilations only, even if the AED indicates another shock is needed. Treat all hypothermic patients even if you believe they have been dead for several hours. Hypothermic patients should never be considered dead until they have been warmed in an appropriate medical facility.

Treatment

An example of hypothermia protecting a patient from death is an apparent drowning in water colder than 70°F (21°C). Many children who fell in cold water and apparently drowned have been resuscitated successfully. Always start CPR on apparent drowning victims pulled from cold water.

Words of Wisdom

The myocardium (heart muscle) of a hypothermic patient is very irritable. Chest compressions on a patient with even a very slow pulse can cause the patient to go into cardiac arrest. Feel for a carotid pulse for a full minute before starting compressions. Similarly, because of the irritability of a hypothermic heart, these patients should not be allowed to exert themselves; for example, clinicians should move them rather than having them move themselves.

Drowning and Submersion

Because EMRs are often the first trained people to arrive at the scene of a drowning, it is important for you to have some understanding of drowning and submersion injuries.

According to the Centers for Disease Control and Prevention, approximately 4,000 fatal unintentional drownings occur every year in the United States. Drowning is the leading cause of death for children 1 to 4 years and is the second-leading cause of death (after motor vehicle crashes) for children 5 to 14 years. Many cases of infant drowning occur in a bathtub. In children ages 1 to 4 years, most drownings occur in swimming pools. For children ages 5 to 14 years, most of the drownings occur in rivers and lakes. Alcohol consumption and drug use are contributing factors in many cases of drowning involving teenagers and adults.

Drowning is defined as the process of experiencing respiratory impairment from submersion or immersion in liquid. A **submersion injury** is any injury that results from being beneath the surface of water or another liquid.

Familiarize yourself with your emergency response area; consider the places a drowning could occur. Likely locations include streams, lakes, and swimming pools. Hot tubs, wading pools, public fountains, and storm drain ponds are also potential locations for drowning. For young children, ordinary water sources around the home can pose a drowning risk. Children left unattended in washbowls or bathtubs, even briefly, can drown. Buckets of water and toilet bowls also pose threats to young children who put their heads down to look into the water, lose their balance, fall in, and are unable to get out. Remember, young children can drown in liquids as shallow as 6 inches (15 cm).

The process of drowning progresses through several stages. Usually, the initial stage is panic as the person realizes that something is wrong, such as a strong current that is overpowering. In other instances, the person becomes fatigued, injured, and cold; becomes entangled in seaweed or kelp; experiences a loss of orientation; or becomes ill.

The feeling of panic produces an inefficient breathing pattern. If a swimmer is not able to take in full breaths, the ability to float is lost, and exhaustion sets in as the person struggles to stay on the surface of the water. Small quantities of water reaching the larynx (voice box) cause a spasm of the larynx (**laryngospasm**), which makes it hard or impossible to breathe. If this cycle of panic is not corrected, respiratory and cardiac arrest can result. Signs and symptoms of a submersion injury include coughing, vomiting, difficulty breathing, respiratory arrest, and cardiac arrest. Some patients who have sustained submersion injuries may have broken bones or spinal injuries from hitting a hard surface. Hypothermia is an added risk when a patient is wet, especially if the water is cold or if the air temperature is low.

YOU are the EMR **CASE 3**

On a cloudy cold day in November, you and your partner are restocking the rig when you are dispatched to assist a man who has collapsed. After a 4-minute response, you arrive at the scene at his apartment building. As you enter the apartment, you and your partner notice the temperature in the room is very chilly. As you enter the bedroom, you discover an older man lying on the floor between his bed and the wall. Your initial assessment reveals an older man in light clothing who is experiencing violent shivers. He has a shallow and thready pulse and slow respirations. His skin temperature is cold to the touch. Although he seems a bit withdrawn, the man knows his name and the date and is aware of his surroundings. As you complete your patient assessment, the patient does not indicate any areas of tenderness or pain. You are not able to obtain a good medical history because the patient is confused and does not remember what happened to him.

1. What is your initial treatment for this patient?
2. What other conditions might be causing these symptoms?

Voices OF Experience

Don and Margaret had been happily married for 52 years and, as with any couple, they had had their ups and downs. Recently, things had gotten harder for Don. It seemed Margaret's dementia was getting worse. Sometimes she did not recognize Don, and sometimes she did not know where she was. But throughout it all, Don always provided for all of Margaret's needs.

It was a cold, wintery night when Don got up around 0300 hours to use the bathroom. As he was getting back into bed, he looked over and realized Margaret was not in bed. Had she been there when he got up? He couldn't remember. He called her name, but heard nothing in the house. As he entered the living room, he found the worst: the front door was open. Frantically he called 9-1-1 and reported his wife missing.

As emergency medical responders and law enforcement officers arrived, they began searching the area. Looking for footprints was difficult due to the rapidly falling snow. After approximately 8 minutes, a police officer called saying he had found her, but she was not moving. As we got over to Margaret, we found her unresponsive, but she was breathing and had a pulse. We rapidly moved her into the ambulance, turned up the heat as high as possible, and removed all of her wet clothing. Drying Margaret as much as we could, we applied hot packs to the appropriate areas and covered her with all the blankets we could find. As we were shutting the doors of the ambulance, I heard Don say, "You're all I know, Margaret. I love you and don't want to lose you." Hearing this brought tears to my eyes. I looked at Don and told him we would do everything we could to help his wife.

"As we got over to Margaret, we found her unresponsive, but she was breathing and had a pulse."

As we were en route to the local, rural hospital, I called in a report and advised the physician that the patient was cold, really cold. Once we arrived at the emergency room, we turned over care to the waiting staff. There was a lot of frantic activity and I kept hearing, "Make sure the helicopter is coming." Just then we were dispatched to another call, so I could not follow up with the outcome of Margaret's care.

Almost a month later, my partner and I were sitting at our station watching television when there was a knock on the door. When I opened the door, I was met by Don and Margaret, along with a large plate of cookies. We invited our guests inside and Don immediately gave me a huge embrace and broke down in tears. He told us how the events surrounding that night unfolded. The doctors suspected that Margaret had become confused, had gone outside by herself, and had become disoriented. After a 2-week stay in the intensive care unit, Margaret was discharged and came home, with no lasting effects. Don is now working with a social worker to provide a safer home for Margaret.

As you study this material, consider the following: while you may not know the patients whose life you will impact, someone deeply cares about that individual, and you need to provide the best care possible.

Brian J. Williams
EMS Chief
Pembina Ambulance Service
Pembina, North Dakota

Adapted from the personal Medical Identification Symbol of the American Medical Association.

Follow the steps of the patient assessment sequence when examining and treating a patient who has sustained a submersion injury. Begin by assessing scene safety. If the patient is still in the water, do not exceed the limits of your training while attempting to rescue the patient. Keep yourself safe and attempt rescue only if you can do so safely. Use the reach, throw, row, and go sequence. Call for additional help if needed. If there is evidence of trauma and you need to move the patient, protect the spine from further injury. Chapter 18, *Vehicle Extrication and Special Rescue*, further discusses the EMR's role in these situations.

Perform a primary assessment. Correct any problems with airway, breathing, or circulation. You may need to carefully turn the patient onto the side to allow water to drain out of the mouth. Begin CPR if indicated, and consider the need to provide rescue breathing first in this instance, before compressions. If the patient is breathing adequately, administer high-flow oxygen as soon as it is available. As soon as the ABCs are stabilized, dry the patient, because wet skin results in a substantial loss of body heat. Then cover the patient with towels or blankets to help preserve body temperature. As soon as possible, perform a secondary assessment to check for other injuries. Obtain the patient's medical history from the patient if possible or from any family members present. Perform regular reassessments.

All patients who have sustained a submersion injury should be examined by a physician. These patients may appear to be uninjured immediately after submersion, but life-threatening respiratory problems can develop hours after the incident. You must arrange to have these patients transported to an appropriate medical facility for a complete examination by a physician.

Cold Water Drowning

You should begin CPR on a drowning victim as long as the patient does not show definitive signs of death. When a person is submerged in cold water, a protective mechanism called the mammalian diving reflex may be activated. This reflex slows the heart rate and metabolic rate and decreases the body's demand for oxygen. Because of the protection provided by the mammalian diving reflex, there have been cases in which a person has been in cold water for longer than 30 minutes and has been successfully resuscitated and recovered to a normal level of physical and mental functioning. Therefore, when you encounter a person who has been submerged in cold water even for an extended period, CPR should be started and continued until the person has been delivered to an appropriate medical facility. Resuscitating a cold water drowning patient often requires warming the patient in the hospital while continuing CPR.

Safety

Do not put your life at risk by exceeding the limits of your training.

Other Environmental Emergencies

Lightning Injuries

Lightning injuries are sometimes classified as environmental emergencies because they have an environmental cause. The electrical injury resulting from a lightning strike can cause cardiac irregularities or cardiac arrest. Treat patients who have been struck by lightning by supporting their ABCs. Oxygen administration, defibrillation, and CPR may be needed for some patients. Because there is a chance of cardiac problems occurring hours after the injury, it is important that patients who have been struck by lightning are transported to an appropriate medical facility for examination, treatment, and monitoring.

Lightning injuries also cause electrical burns. This type of burn is mainly internal, and the extent of burn damage will not be visible right after the injury occurs. For this reason, it is also important to transport all patients who have been struck by lightning to an appropriate medical facility. Electrical burns are discussed in Chapter 14, *Bleeding, Shock, and Soft-Tissue Injuries.*

Bites and Stings

Bites and stings are sometimes classified as environmental injuries. They are discussed in detail under the topic of poisoning in Chapter 11, *Poisoning and Substance Use.*

YOU are the EMR **CASE 4**

On one of the first warm days of the summer, you and your family are enjoying a restful day at a small lake close to your home. As you are finishing a picnic lunch, you hear cries for help coming from the lakefront. A woman shouts that her 11-year-old son has fallen off a small ledge 2 feet (less than 1 m) above the water. As you begin to run toward the cries for help, you can see a boy fighting to keep his head above the surface of the water. As you approach the scene, another bystander reaches out and grabs one of the boy's arms and pulls him to shore.

1. If the boy had still been in the water when you arrived at the lakefront, what steps would you have taken to rescue him from the water?
2. What steps should you take to provide care for this boy?

YOU are the EMR **SUMMARY**

You are the EMR: CASE 1

1. As you evaluate the patient's symptoms and the signs she exhibits, what condition do you think this patient may be experiencing?

The signs and symptoms of this patient seem to indicate that she may be experiencing heat exhaustion.

2. What steps should you take to treat this patient?

The first step in treating this patient is to perform the patient assessment sequence to determine what problems she is experiencing. Ensure that the scene is safe. Perform a primary assessment to determine the patient's level of responsiveness and assess the state of her ABCs. Obtain the patient's medical history and vital signs and complete the secondary assessment. The patient's signs and symptoms are consistent with heat exhaustion. Be alert for additional signs and symptoms that might indicate other conditions such as heart problems (for example, a heart attack or other medical conditions). Your treatment should include removing or drying wet clothing. Try to get the patient to a location that has a comfortable temperature and place the patient in a position of comfort (sitting or lying down). Slowly give water or other fluid with electrolytes, if available. Finally, reassess the condition of the patient and arrange for transport to an appropriate medical facility.

You are the EMR: CASE 2

1. What signs would indicate this runner is experiencing heat exhaustion or heatstroke?

This patient is showing signs and symptoms of a serious heat illness, heatstroke. The patient has an altered level of consciousness, and his skin is red, hot, and flushed compared with baseline. Because he was running prior to the illness, his skin may still be moist.

2. After completing the primary assessment, what is the most appropriate treatment for this runner?

This patient needs immediate medical treatment. You should initiate rapid cooling by removing the patient's clothing down to his underwear and placing ice bags around the groin and in the armpits. Fanning the patient may help if the humidity and temperature are not too high. Run cool water over the patient, if available. In the field it is very difficult to successfully cool a patient experiencing heatstroke. This patient needs continued assessment and immediate transport to a medical facility for more aggressive cooling.

You are the EMR: CASE 3

1. What is your initial treatment for this patient?

This patient needs to be warmed immediately to prevent further heat loss. After the primary assessment, the patient should be wrapped in blankets to help his body temperature return to a more normal level. Although he does not appear to have sustained any injuries, you cannot be sure given his current state of confusion. You should ask if anyone present is familiar with the medical history of the patient. Look for any medications that EMS might take to the hospital. When EMS arrives, the patient should be gently transported to the medical facility for more aggressive warming and monitoring. Handle the patient carefully to avoid causing cardiac dysrhythmias.

2. What other conditions might be causing these symptoms?

From the limited information available to you, it appears this patient is experiencing hypothermia. The actions described previously are helpful in beginning to warm the patient to a more normal body temperature. It is important that this patient be transported to an appropriate medical facility for further testing to determine the underlying cause of his condition. This patient may have experienced a stroke, a cardiac dysrhythmia, a diabetic emergency, or a seizure. He may have forgotten to take his prescribed medication, or he may have taken an incorrect dosage. As an EMR, you do not have sufficient training or equipment to determine the underlying cause of his hypothermia, but you must take the initial steps to rewarm this patient and arrange for his prompt transport to an appropriate medical facility for further warming and treatment.

You are the EMR: CASE 4

1. If the boy had still been in the water when you arrived at the lakefront, what steps would you have taken to rescue him from the water?

When you are on the scene of any emergency as it is happening, remember to call for assistance as soon as possible. In this instance, you might have another family member or a bystander call 9-1-1 as you rush to the scene. During water rescues, ensure your safety as well as the safety of the person in distress. Do not put your life in danger if there is little chance of saving a person. Also keep in mind your training and limitations. Follow the reach, throw, row, and go steps. Think first of reaching out to rescue the person. Extend your reach with any available object like a tree branch or ball bat. If you are not able to reach the person in distress, find a floatable object such as a ring buoy or improvise with any floatable object, such as an almost empty jug or a picnic cooler. If this is not possible, see if any type of small boat is available. Only as a final resort should you

YOU are the EMR SUMMARY

ever consider entering the water to rescue another person. In this case, an extended arm was enough to rescue this boy from the water. See Chapter 18, *Vehicle Extrication and Special Rescue*, for further discussion of the EMR's role in these situations.

2. What steps should you take to provide care for this boy?

As soon as the patient has been removed from the water, begin to assess his ABCs. If he has water in his mouth or throat, turn his head to the side to drain any retained water from his mouth. Support his ABCs, as necessary. Because it is early summer, the water in the lake is probably cold. Therefore, it is especially important to remove all his wet clothing as soon as possible and cover him with any available dry clothing, tablecloths, or blankets that are available. Examine the patient for any injuries and treat as necessary. Obtain a medical history from the patient or his mother. Confirm that EMS has been called and is responding to your location. Explain to the boy's mother that he may need to be transported to an appropriate medical facility for warming and for further treatment because of the possibility of delayed symptoms from his submersion into the cold water. Do not forget to always explain your actions to patients and their family members and to provide them with reassurance.

Prep Kit

Ready for Review

- Your approach to a patient who has experienced an environmental emergency should follow the patient assessment sequence.
- Heat cramps are thought to be caused by electrolyte imbalance and dehydration. They usually involve muscles in the calf, leg, or abdomen. Usually, the cramps disappear with rest and the administration of water.
- A person experiencing heat exhaustion sweats profusely and becomes light-headed, dizzy, and nauseated. Certain risk factors may make some people more susceptible to heat-related illnesses.
- Heatstroke results when a person has been in a hot environment for a long period, overwhelming the body's sweating mechanism. The patient's body temperature rises until it reaches a level at which brain damage occurs.
- The body parts most susceptible to frostbite are the face, ears, fingers, and toes. Warming the frostbitten part must be done quickly and carefully.
- Hypothermia occurs when a person's body is not able to produce enough heat to keep the internal (core) body temperature at a satisfactory level.
- The initial signs of hypothermia include feeling cold, shivering, decreasing level of consciousness, and sleepiness. Signs of increasing hypothermia include a lack of coordination, mental confusion, and slowed reactions.
- Hypothermic patients should never be considered dead until they have been warmed in an appropriate medical facility.
- Drowning can occur in a variety of settings around a home and outdoors. Signs and symptoms of a submersion injury include coughing, vomiting, difficulty breathing, respiratory arrest, and cardiac arrest.
- Lightning injuries are caused by a powerful jolt of electrical current that passes through part of the body. They may cause irregular heart rhythms or cardiac arrest. They also cause an electrical type of burn that damages tissue within the body.

Vital Vocabulary

drowning The process of experiencing respiratory impairment from submersion or immersion in liquid.

frostbite Partial or complete freezing of the skin and deeper tissues caused by exposure to the cold.

heat cramps Painful muscle spasms that usually occur after vigorous exercise in hot weather and are generally relieved by rest and drinking water.

heat exhaustion A form of shock that occurs from significant fluid loss and too many electrolytes through very heavy sweating after exposure to heat.

heatstroke A condition of rapidly rising internal body temperature that occurs when the body's mechanisms for releasing heat are overwhelmed. Can result in death if left untreated.

Prep Kit

hypothermia A condition in which the internal (or core) body temperature falls below 95°F (35°C) after prolonged exposure to cool or freezing temperatures.

laryngospasm A spasm of the muscles of the larynx or vocal cords resulting in an inability to breathe.

submersion injury An injury resulting from being beneath the surface of water or another liquid.

References

Casa DJ, DeMartini JK, Bergeron MF, et al. National Athletic Trainers' Association position statement: exertional heat illnesses [published correction appears in *J Athl Train.* 2017 Apr;52(4):401.]. *J Athl Train.* 2015;50(9):986–1000.

Dezfulian C, McCallin TE, Bierens J, et al. 2024 American Heart Association and American Academy of Pediatrics focused update on special circumstances: resuscitation following drowning: an update to the American Heart Association Guidelines for Cardiopulmonary Resuscitation and Emergency Cardiovascular Care. *Circulation.* 2024;150(23):e501–e516. doi:10.1161/CIR.0000000000001274

Drowning facts. Centers for Disease Control and Prevention website. https://www.cdc.gov/drowning/data-research/facts/. Published May 16, 2024. Accessed November 19, 2024.

Symptoms of heat-related illnesses. Centers for Disease Control and Prevention website. https://www.cdc.gov/extreme-heat/signs-symptoms/index.html. Published June 25, 2024. Accessed November 19, 2024.

Assessment IN ACTION

You are dispatched to a residence for the report of a possible drowning. As you are responding, your dispatcher reports that the patient is a 37-year-old man who has been removed from the backyard swimming pool. The dispatcher reports that the police were called to this residence earlier in the evening for the report of a noisy party. When you arrive at the scene, you find your patient lying on the pool deck. He is pale and unresponsive.

1. Which of the following contributing factors should you consider as you examine and treat this patient?

- **A.** Possible injuries
- **B.** Possible alcohol or drug use
- **C.** The patient's age and size
- **D.** Possible injuries and possible alcohol and/or drug use

2. What added step in clearing the airway is sometimes needed in drowning situations?

- **A.** Rinse out the patient's mouth.
- **B.** Place a towel under the patient's shoulders.
- **C.** Roll the patient onto one side to allow water to drain out of the mouth.
- **D.** Place a towel under the patient's head.

3. In submersion injuries, small quantities of water reaching the voice box cause a(n) ___________, which makes it hard or impossible to breathe.

- **A.** oropharynx block
- **B.** laryngospasm
- **C.** nasopharynx spasm
- **D.** tracheal spasm

4. Which of the following persons is at the highest risk for hypothermia?

- **A.** A person wearing cotton shorts and a T-shirt on a dry, windless 70°F (21°C) day
- **B.** A person sitting in the warm sun in a bathing suit
- **C.** A person wearing cotton jeans and a T-shirt on a rainy, windy 60°F (16°C) day
- **D.** A person running in a marathon on a 67°F (19°C) day

5. What environmental condition is of concern in a situation that involves drowning?

- **A.** Heatstroke
- **B.** Heat exhaustion
- **C.** Hyperthermia
- **D.** Hypothermia

6. The mammalian diving reflex is activated when:

- **A.** the person has been under the water for a long time.
- **B.** the person is young.
- **C.** the water is cold.
- **D.** the water is warmer than the body temperature.

7. Which of the following is NOT a sign of deep frostbite?

- **A.** Skin remains soft.
- **B.** Skin is white and waxy.
- **C.** Blisters are present.
- **D.** Swelling is present.

8. What are the typical stages in the drowning process?

9. Why should a person who has been submerged in cold water and is pulseless, not breathing, and cold *not* be pronounced dead at the scene?

10. Discuss the different signs and symptoms for early and late hypothermia.

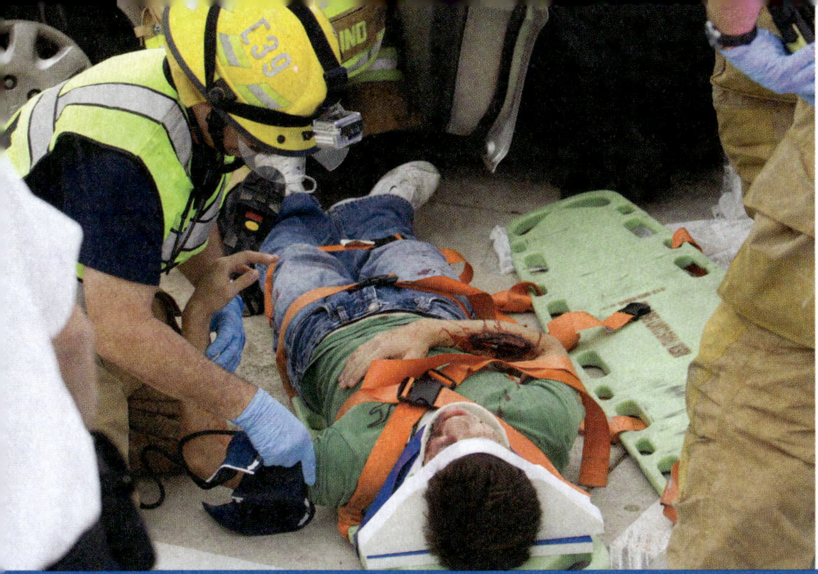

SECTION 5

Trauma

14 Bleeding, Shock, and Soft-Tissue Injuries

15 Injuries to Muscles and Bones

© Bob Daemmrich / Alamy Stock Photo

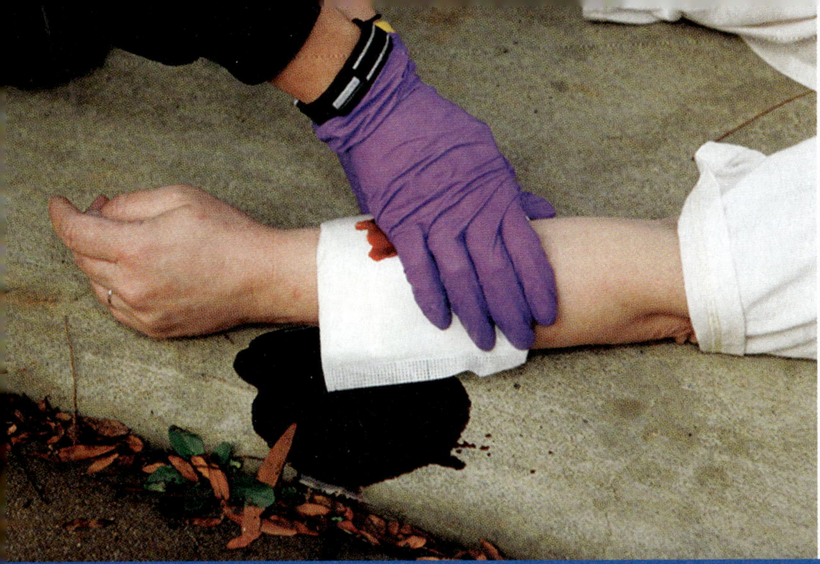

CHAPTER 14

Bleeding, Shock, and Soft-Tissue Injuries

National EMS Education Standard Competencies

Pathophysiology

Uses knowledge of shock and respiratory compromise to respond to life threats.

Shock and Resuscitation

Uses assessment information to recognize shock, respiratory failure or arrest, and cardiac arrest based on assessment findings and manages the emergency while awaiting additional emergency response.

Shock

- Definition (pp 299–304)
- Physiologic response (pp 299–304)

Trauma

Uses knowledge to recognize and manage life threats based on assessment findings for an acutely injured patient while awaiting additional emergency medical response.

Bleeding

- Bleeding (pp 304–309)

Head, Facial, Neck, and Spine Trauma

- Life threats (pp 314–320)
- Spine trauma (pp 314–320; Chapter 15, *Injuries to Muscles and Bones*)

Chest Trauma

- Blunt versus penetrating mechanisms (pp 314–318)
- Open chest wound (p 317)
- Impaled object (p 317)

Abdominal and Genitourinary Trauma

- Blunt versus penetrating mechanisms (pp 314–318)
- Evisceration (p 318)
- Impaled object (p 317)

© Jones & Bartlett Learning. Courtesy of MIEMSS.

Soft-Tissue Trauma

- Wounds (avulsion, bite, laceration, puncture, incision) (pp 310–320)
- Burns (electrical, chemical, thermal), including inhalational injury (pp 320–324)
- Chemicals in the eye and on the skin (p 323)

Multisystem Trauma

- Multisystem trauma (p 324)

Medicine

Recognizes and manages life threats based on assessment findings of a patient with a medical emergency while awaiting additional emergency response.

Immunology

- Anaphylactic reactions (p 300; p 303)

Disorders of the Eyes, Ears, Nose, and Throat

- Epistaxis (nosebleed) (p 314)

Knowledge Objectives

1. Describe the function and relationship among the following parts of the circulatory system:
   - Pump (heart) (p 298)
   - Pipes (blood vessels) (p 298)
   - Fluid (blood) (p 298)
2. Describe how and where to locate a patient's pulse. (pp 298–299)
3. Explain how shock is caused by pump failure, pipe failure, and fluid loss. (pp 299–301)
4. List four types of shock caused by pipe failure. (pp 299–301)
5. List signs and symptoms of shock. (p 301)
6. Describe the general treatment for shock. (pp 301–302)
7. Describe the treatment for shock caused by pump failure. (p 302)
8. Describe the treatment for shock caused by pipe failure. (p 303)

9. Describe the treatment for shock caused by fluid loss. (p 303)
10. Explain how to control external blood loss. (pp 304–309)
11. Describe the indications for use of a tourniquet. (pp 305–306)
12. Describe how to use the femoral and brachial artery pressure points to control bleeding. (pp 306–309)
13. List the four types of soft-tissue injuries. (pp 310–311)
14. Discuss the treatment of avulsions and amputations. (p 311)
15. Describe the principles of treatment for open soft-tissue injuries. (p 312)
16. Explain the functions of dressings and bandages. (pp 312–314)
17. Explain the relationship between standard precautions and soft-tissue injuries. (p 309)
18. Discuss the emergency medical care for patients with the following injuries:
    - Face and scalp wounds (p 314)
    - Nosebleeds (p 314)
    - Eye injuries (p 316)
    - Neck wounds (p 316)
    - Chest and back wounds (p 317)
    - Impaled objects (p 317)
    - Closed abdominal wounds (p 317)
    - Open abdominal wounds (p 318)
    - Genital wounds (p 318)
    - Extremity wounds (p 318)
    - Gunshot wounds (pp 318–320)
    - Bites (p 320)
19. Describe how the seriousness of a burn is related to the depth of the burn. (pp 320–321)
20. Describe how the seriousness of a burn is related to the extent of the burn. (p 321)
21. Describe the signs, symptoms, possible complications, and treatment associated with each of the following types of burns:
    - Thermal (p 322)
    - Respiratory (p 322)
    - Chemical (p 323)
    - Electrical (pp 323–324)
22. Explain the concept of multisystem trauma and how it affects your patient assessment and treatment. (p 324)

Skills Objectives

1. Demonstrate how and where to locate a patient's pulse. (pp 298–299)
2. Demonstrate the general treatment for shock. (pp 301–302)
3. Demonstrate the treatment for shock caused by pump failure. (p 302)
4. Demonstrate the treatment for shock caused by pipe failure. (p 303)
5. Demonstrate the treatment for shock caused by fluid loss. (p 303)
6. Demonstrate how to use the femoral and brachial pressure points to control blood loss. (pp 306–309)
7. Demonstrate how to use a tourniquet to control blood loss. (p 306; Skill Drill 14-1)
8. Demonstrate treatment of avulsions and amputations. (p 311)
9. Demonstrate treatment of soft-tissue injuries. (p 312)
10. Demonstrate the emergency medical care for patients with the following injuries:
    - Face and scalp wounds (p 314)
    - Nosebleeds (p 314)
    - Eye injuries (p 316)
    - Neck wounds (p 316)
    - Chest and back wounds (p 317)
    - Impaled objects (p 317)
    - Closed abdominal wounds (p 317)
    - Open abdominal wounds (p 318)
    - Genital wounds (p 318)
    - Extremity wounds (p 318)
    - Gunshot wounds (pp 318–320)
    - Bites (p 320)
11. Demonstrate treatment of the following types of burns:
    - Thermal (p 322)
    - Respiratory (p 322)
    - Chemical (p 323)
    - Electrical (pp 323–324)

Introduction

This chapter presents the skills you need to recognize and care for patients who are experiencing shock, are bleeding, or have soft-tissue injuries. Because most soft-tissue injuries result in bleeding, maintaining good standard precautions is important when you are caring for patients with these types of injuries. Soft-tissue wounds discussed in this chapter include abrasions, lacerations, punctures, and avulsions. Techniques for controlling external bleeding are discussed, and you will learn the various techniques for dressing and bandaging wounds.

Damage to internal soft tissues and organs can cause life-threatening conditions. Internal bleeding causes blood loss in the circulatory system and results in shock. **Shock** is a state of collapse of the cardiovascular system that results in inadequate delivery of oxygenated blood to the organs. More trauma patients die from shock than from any other condition. Your ability to recognize the signs and symptoms of shock and to take simple measures to aid shock patients will give them the best chance for survival. This chapter explains the causes and types of shock using an analogy of a pump, pipes, and fluid. You will learn how the failure of any part of the system can cause shock.

Burns are another type of soft-tissue injury. Burns may be caused by heat, chemicals, or electricity. They may damage any part of the body and are especially harmful if they occur inside the respiratory tract. This chapter examines the extent, depth, and cause of burns.

As you study this chapter, keep in mind the importance of maintaining standard precautions to prevent exposure to disease-carrying organisms.

Patient Assessment for Bleeding, Shock, and Soft-Tissue Injuries

It is important to follow the steps of the patient assessment sequence when caring for patients who are bleeding, are in shock, or have soft-tissue injuries. Your scene assessment needs to include all the steps you learned previously to ensure safety for you and your patient. When performing the primary assessment, you may need to temporarily halt the assessment if the patient is losing a significant amount of blood. However, once you have managed this problem, you should immediately return to completing the assessment sequence, performing all the remaining steps to ensure that no problems or injuries are overlooked.

Words of Wisdom

Remember that the ABC (Airway, Breathing, Circulation) sequence is adjusted if you are aware of life-threatening bleeding on arrival. In this situation, you must first control the bleeding (such as by applying a tourniquet); thus, the sequence becomes XABC, where the *X* stands for life-threatening eXternal bleeding (or eXsanguination). Once the bleeding is controlled, you will continue to airway and breathing assessments.

During your secondary assessment, be alert for any signs and symptoms of shock from internal or external blood loss. When obtaining a SAMPLE history (Signs and symptoms, Allergies, Medications, Pertinent past medical history, Last oral intake, Events leading up to the illness or injury), ask the patient whether they are taking a blood thinner, which may interfere with blood clotting. When performing a reassessment, watch the patient for signs and symptoms of shock such as skin that is pale compared with the patient's baseline color, increasing pulse rate, or decreasing blood pressure. (Note that in patients with darker skin, pallor may be easier to detect by checking the mucous membranes inside the lower eyelids or oral mucosa.)

For trauma patients, you will usually perform the secondary assessment before you obtain the SAMPLE history. Review the patient assessment sequence shown in **FIGURE 14-1**.

Standard Precautions and Soft-Tissue Injuries

The concept of standard precautions assumes that all body fluids are potentially infectious. Therefore, take appropriate measures to prevent contact with the patient's body fluids. Wear gloves to prevent contact with the patient's blood when caring for patients who have soft-tissue injuries. At times, you may also need to wear a surgical mask and eye protection if there is danger of blood splatter from a massive wound or if the patient is coughing or vomiting bloody material.

Safety

Most soft-tissue injuries involve some degree of bleeding and a mechanism that caused the injury. Always take standard precautions and ensure scene safety when you approach a patient with a potential soft-tissue injury.

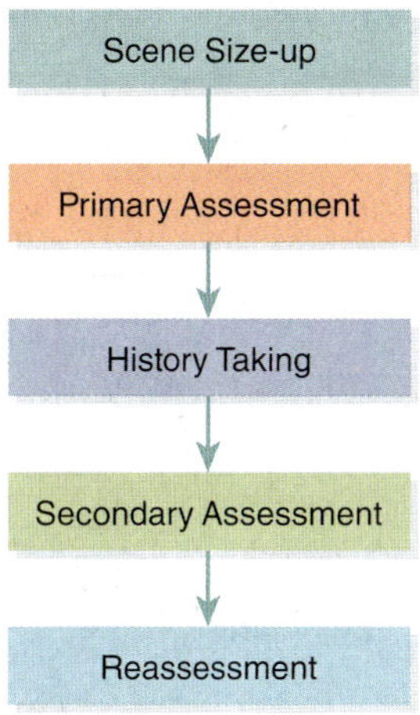

FIGURE 14-1 Patient assessment sequence. For trauma patients, you may perform the secondary assessment before obtaining a SAMPLE history.

© Jones & Bartlett Learning

YOU are the EMR **CASE 1**

On a crisp autumn day, you are dispatched for a report of an injured carpenter at the site of a new house under construction. As you are responding, the dispatcher informs you that your patient is a 38-year-old man who has cut his leg with a circular saw. He is actively bleeding from the wound.

1. What safety considerations should you keep in mind as you approach this situation?
2. What equipment and supplies do you want to take with you?
3. What are your treatment goals for this incident?

> **Safety**
>
> During an outbreak of an infectious disease that can spread through airborne or aerosolized particles, such as the coronavirus disease 2019 (COVID-19) pandemic, the concept of standard precautions is expanded. Standard precautions during these outbreaks include a face mask and protective eyewear for all patient encounters.

Parts and Function of the Circulatory System

The three parts of the circulatory system are the pump (heart), the pipes (arteries, veins, and capillaries), and the fluid (blood cells and other blood components). **FIGURE 14-2** presents a schematic illustration of the circulatory system.

The Pump

The heart functions as the human circulatory system's pump. The heart consists of four separate chambers: the two upper chambers on the top of the heart are called the left and right **atria** (a single chamber is called an atrium), and the two lower chambers on the bottom of the heart are called the left and right **ventricles**. The ventricles are the larger chambers and do most of the actual pumping. The atria are somewhat less muscular and serve as reservoirs for blood flowing into the heart from the body and the lungs (**FIGURE 14-3**).

The Pipes

The human body has three main types of blood vessels: arteries, capillaries, and veins. The arteries (big-flow, heavy-duty, high-pressure pipes) carry blood away from the heart. The capillaries (distribution pipes), the smallest of the blood vessels, form a network that distributes blood to all parts of the body. The smallest capillaries are so narrow that blood cells flow through them single file. The veins return the blood from the capillaries to the heart, where it is pumped to the lungs. There, the blood gives off carbon dioxide and absorbs oxygen (**FIGURE 14-4**).

The Fluid

Fluid in the circulatory system consists of blood cells and other blood components, each with a specific function. The liquid part of the blood is known as plasma. Plasma serves as the transporting medium for the solid parts of the blood, which are the red blood cells, white blood cells, and platelets. Red blood cells carry oxygen and carbon dioxide (**FIGURE 14-5**). White blood cells have a "search and destroy" function. They consume bacteria and viruses to combat infections in the body. Platelets interact with each other and with other substances in the blood to form clots that help stop bleeding.

Pulse

A pulse is the pressure wave generated by the pumping action of the heart. With each heartbeat, there is a surge of blood from the left ventricle as it contracts and pushes blood out

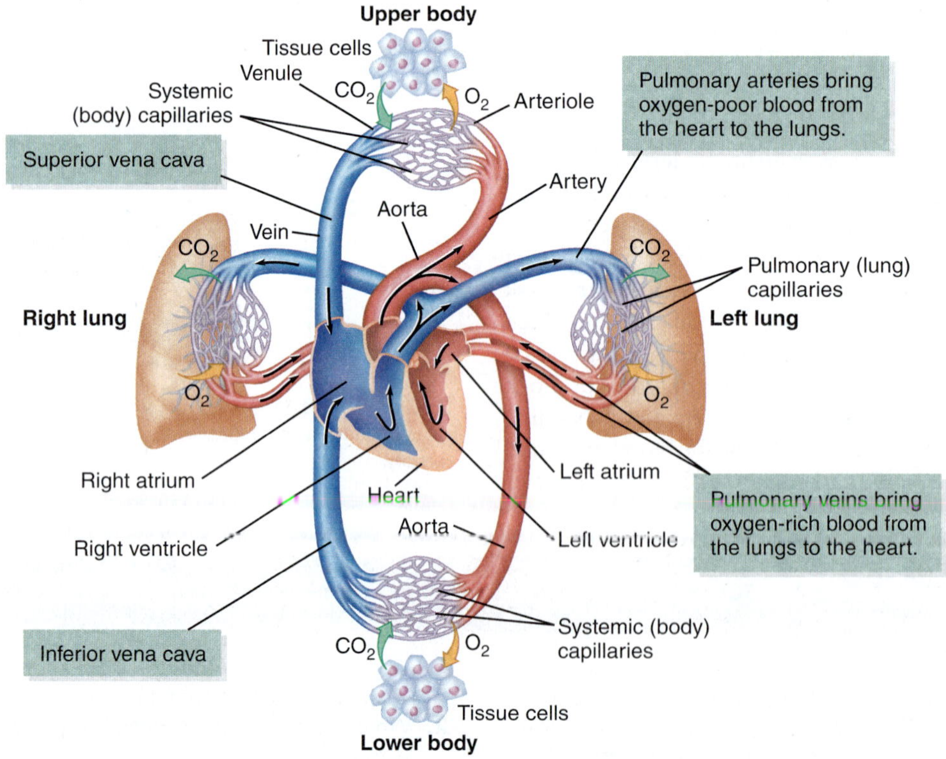

FIGURE 14-2 The circulatory system includes the heart, arteries, veins, and capillaries. At the center of the system is the heart, which pumps the blood.

© Jones & Bartlett Learning

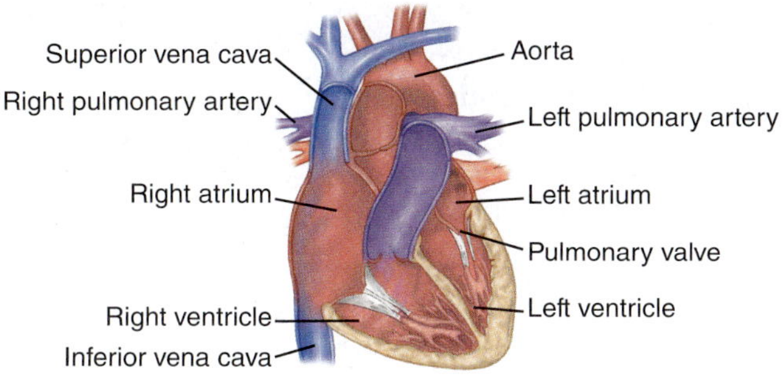

FIGURE 14-3 The heart functions as the pump of the human circulatory system.
© Jones & Bartlett Learning

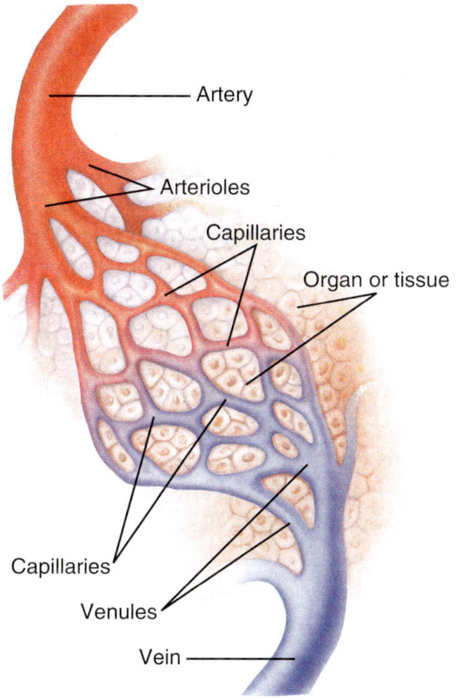

FIGURE 14-4 Blood enters an organ or tissue through the arteries and leaves through the veins.
© Jones & Bartlett Learning

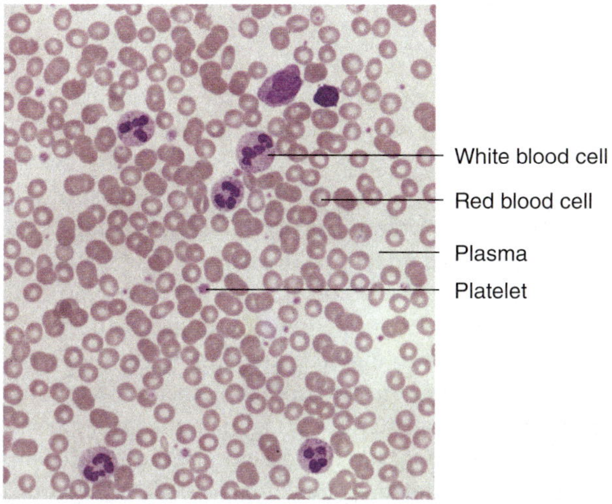

FIGURE 14-5 The components of blood.
© Donna Beer Stolz, PhD, Center for Biologic Imaging, University of Pittsburgh Medical School

into the main arteries of the body. When you are counting the number of pulsations per minute, you are counting each heartbeat per minute.

Usually you can feel a patient's radial and carotid pulses. In an alert patient, you can easily find the radial pulse on the inner wrist, just proximal to the base of the thumb. If the patient is unresponsive, experiencing shock, or both, it may be impossible for you to feel a radial pulse. Therefore, it is vital that you know how to locate the carotid (neck) pulse. If the patient is unresponsive, attempt to locate the carotid pulse first. In an infant, check the brachial (upper arm) pulse instead of the carotid pulse. See Chapter 8, *Professional Rescuer CPR*, and Chapter 9, *Patient Assessment*, for detailed discussions of pulse assessment.

Shock

Shock is inadequate tissue perfusion. There are many possible causes. The three primary causes are pump failure, pipe failure, and fluid loss (**TABLE 14-1**). These causes are explained next, followed by a discussion of the signs and symptoms of shock and the role of the emergency medical responder (EMR) in treating shock.

Primary Causes of Shock

Pump Failure

Cardiogenic shock occurs if the heart cannot pump enough blood to supply the needs of the body. Pump failure can result if the heart has been weakened by a heart attack or trauma. Inadequate pumping of the heart can cause blood to back up in the vessels of the lungs, resulting in a condition known as **heart failure**.

Pipe Failure

Pipe failure is caused by the expansion (dilation) of the vessels to as much as three or four times their normal size. This expansion causes blood to pool in the capillaries and seep out into the tissues, instead of circulating throughout the system. When vessels dilate and blood pools in the capillaries, the rest of the body, including the heart and other vital organs, is deprived of blood. Blood pressure falls and shock results.

TABLE 14-1 Causes of Shock

Cause	Type of Shock
Pump failure	Cardiogenic shock (heart failure)
Pipe failure	Psychogenic shock (fainting) Anaphylactic shock (allergic reaction) Septic shock (severe infection) Neurogenic shock (nerve injury)
Fluid failure	External bleeding Internal bleeding

Blood pressure is the pressure of the circulating blood against the walls of the arteries.

In shock caused by sudden expansion of the vessels, blood pressure may drop so rapidly that you are unable to feel either a radial or a carotid pulse.

The least serious type of shock caused by pipe failure is fainting. Fainting, a form of **psychogenic shock**, is the body's response to a major psychological or emotional stress. As the nervous system reacts, the vessels suddenly expand to three or four times their normal size. Blood then pools in the dilated vessels, resulting in reduced blood supply to the brain. Fainting is a short-term condition that corrects itself once the patient is placed in a horizontal position.

Anaphylactic shock is caused by an extreme allergic reaction to a foreign substance, such as venom from bee stings, penicillin, or certain foods. Shock may develop very quickly following exposure. The patient may suddenly start to sneeze or itch, a rash or hives may appear, the face and tongue may swell very quickly, and a blue color may appear around the mouth. The patient appears flushed (red, or for patients with dark skin, darker compared to baseline color). Breathing may quickly become difficult, with wheezing sounds coming from the chest. Blood pressure drops rapidly as the blood pools in the expanded capillaries. The pulse may be so weak that you cannot feel it. Pipe failure has occurred and death will result if prompt action to counteract the toxin is not taken. See Chapter 11, *Poisoning and Substance Use*, for a description of managing allergic reactions, including use of an epinephrine auto-injector.

Septic shock is a type of pipe failure that results from an overwhelming infection that has spread throughout the patient's body. A severe complication of infection is **sepsis**. Sepsis occurs when chemicals are released into the bloodstream as a result of infection and trigger an inflammatory response throughout the body. The most common types of infections that may cause sepsis include pneumonia, abdominal infections, bloodstream infections, kidney infections, and urinary tract infections. Sepsis is most common in older adults and people who have weakened immune systems. If untreated, sepsis can progress to septic shock and often results in death.

Septic shock causes the patient's blood vessels to dilate and become more porous, or leaky. These patients may have a weak and rapid pulse, rapid breathing, fever and chills, or a low body temperature. Organ damage may result from inadequate blood supply. These patients need to be transported promptly to a medical facility where the cause of their infection can be determined and where they can receive skilled medical care.

Neurogenic shock may occur in patients who have sustained a spinal cord injury. The injury to the spinal cord allows the vessels to expand, and blood pools below the level of the injury. The brain, heart, lungs, and other vital organs are deprived of blood, resulting in shock. This patient may present differently than other shock patients in that the skin does not appear cool and sweaty, as is common in other forms of shock, and the heart rate is not elevated and may even be decreased.

> **Special Populations**
>
> **Risk of Sepsis in Older Adults**
>
> Infectious diseases are illnesses caused by bacteria, viruses, or fungi. They may affect different body systems or different organs of the body. Because older people often have weakened immune systems, they are more susceptible to contracting infectious diseases.
>
> The most effective way to prevent complications and death from infection is to recognize and treat an infection as soon as possible. As an EMR, you do not have the training and tools to diagnose or treat patients who may have infections. Your job is to understand that older people are more likely to contract infections and experience sepsis than younger people and to recognize that older people often do not realize how sick they are. An older patient who shows signs or symptoms of an infection, such as fever, diarrhea, fatigue, muscle aches, or coughing, should be evaluated by a physician urgently to rule out the possibility of an infection or sepsis.

Note that with neurogenic shock, many other functions that are under the control of the same part of the nervous system are also lost. The most important of them, in an acute injury setting, is the ability to control body temperature. Body temperature in a patient experiencing neurogenic shock can rapidly fall to match that of the environment. In many situations, significant hypothermia occurs, severely complicating the situation. **Hypothermia** is a condition in which the internal body temperature falls below 95°F (35°C), usually after prolonged exposure to cool or freezing temperatures. Maintenance of body temperature is always an important element of treatment for a patient in shock.

> **Words of Wisdom**
>
> Four types of shock caused by vessel dilation are as follows:
>
> 1. Psychogenic shock
> 2. Anaphylactic shock
> 3. Septic shock
> 4. Neurogenic shock

Fluid Loss

The third general type of shock is caused by fluid loss. Causes of fluid loss include vomiting, diarrhea, excessive urination or sweating, and bleeding. Fluid loss caused by excessive bleeding (**hemorrhage**) is the most common cause of shock. Blood escapes from the normally closed circulatory system through an internal or external wound, and the system's total fluid level (blood volume) decreases until the pump cannot operate efficiently. To compensate for fluid loss, the heart begins to pump faster to maintain pressure in the pipes. However, as the fluid continues to drain out, the pump eventually stops pumping altogether, resulting in cardiac arrest.

External bleeding is easy to detect because you can see blood escaping from the circulatory system to the outside of the patient's body. With internal bleeding, blood escapes from the circulatory system, but the bleeding cannot be seen.

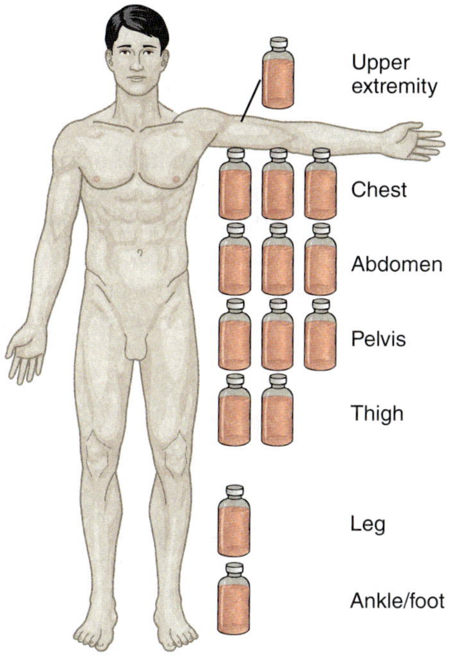

FIGURE 14-6 Depending on the injury location, a significant amount of blood can be lost within the body. The bottles suggest the relative proportion of circulating blood that can be lost within each area.
© Jones & Bartlett Learning

However, you may see signs of internal blood loss, such as bruising, swelling, and rigidity in the affected area. A patient who is alert may report severe pain in the immediate area. Even though the escaped blood remains inside the body, it cannot reenter the circulatory system, and it is not available to be pumped by the heart. Whether the bleeding is external or internal, if it remains unchecked, the result will be shock, eventual pump failure, and death.

A typical adult has approximately 10 pints (5 L) of blood circulating in the system. The loss of a single pint of blood will not produce shock in a healthy adult. In fact, 1 pint (0.5 L) per donor is the amount that blood banks collect. However, the loss of 2 or more pints (1 L or more) of blood can produce shock. This amount of blood loss can occur even within the body, such as from a fractured femur. **FIGURE 14-6** shows the amount of internal blood loss that can result from various injuries.

Signs and Symptoms of Shock

Shock deprives the body of enough blood to function normally. As shock progresses, the body alters some of its functions to maintain sufficient blood supply to its vital parts. A patient who is in shock may exhibit some or all of the signs and symptoms shown in the Signs and Symptoms box. Initially, the patient's breathing may be rapid and deep, but as shock progresses in severity, breathing becomes rapid and shallow. Remember that the signs and symptoms of neurogenic shock differ from those of other types of shock.

Changes in mental status may be the first signs of shock; therefore, monitoring the overall mental status of a patient can help you detect shock. Any change in mental status may be significant. In severe cases of shock, the patient becomes unresponsive. If a trauma patient who has been quiet suddenly becomes agitated, restless, and vocal, you should suspect shock. If a trauma patient who has been loud, vocal, and aggressive becomes quiet, you should also suspect shock and begin treatment. If the patient has dark skin, changes in skin color may be less obvious. Therefore, be especially alert for other signs of shock. The capillary refill test and the condition of the skin (cool and clammy) will help you recognize shock in patients who have dark skin.

Signs and Symptoms

Signs and symptoms of shock (except neurogenic shock) include:

- Confusion, agitation, restlessness, or anxiety
- Cold, clammy, sweaty, pale (compared with patient baseline) skin
- Rapid, shallow breathing
- Rapid, weak pulse
- Increased capillary refill time
- Nausea or vomiting
- Weakness or fainting
- Thirst

General Treatment for Shock

As an EMR, you can treat shock from any cause and keep it from getting worse by taking several simple but important steps. Remember that the protocols for use of these skills may vary. Always follow the protocols approved by your medical director.

Position the Patient Correctly

If the patient has no head injury, extreme discomfort, or difficulty breathing, place the patient flat on their back (supine) on a horizontal surface. Place a blanket, if available, under the patient and use another to cover them. Elevate the patient's legs according to local protocol. If the patient has a head injury, spine injury, or lower extremity injury, position the patient flat on their back. If the patient is having chest pain or difficulty breathing (which is likely to occur in cases of heart attack and emphysema) and no spinal injury is suspected, place the patient in a sitting or semireclining position.

Treatment

Follow these steps for the general treatment of shock:

1. Position the patient correctly.
2. Maintain the patient's ABCs.
3. Control any external hemorrhage.
4. Maintain the patient's body temperature by placing blankets under and over the patient.
5. Ensure that the patient does not eat or drink anything.
6. Assist with other treatments (such as administering oxygen, if available).
7. Arrange for immediate and prompt transport to an appropriate medical facility.

Treatment

Do not allow a patient in shock to stand.

Maintain the Patient's ABCs

Check the patient's ABCs at least every 5 minutes. If necessary, open the airway, perform rescue breathing, or begin cardiopulmonary resuscitation (CPR).

Control External Hemorrhage

Most patients who are in shock must be treated in the hospital, with care provided by specifically trained physicians. However, it is within your capabilities to treat one common cause of shock: external bleeding. By controlling external bleeding with direct pressure, elevation, a tourniquet, or pressure points, you can treat this cause of shock temporarily until the patient can be transported to an appropriate medical facility for more advanced treatment.

Maintain the Patient's Body Temperature

Attempt to keep the patient comfortably warm. A patient with cold, clammy skin should be covered. It is as important to place blankets under the patient to keep body heat from escaping into the surface beneath the patient as it is to cover the patient with blankets.

Treatment

In the summer or in hot environments, it is not necessary to cover every shock patient with blankets. You are trying to maintain body heat, not produce more.

Do Not Allow the Patient to Eat or Drink

Even though a patient in shock is often very thirsty, do not give liquids by mouth. There are two reasons for this rule:

1. A patient in shock may be nauseated, and eating or drinking may cause vomiting.
2. A patient in shock may need emergency surgery. Patients should not have anything in their stomachs before surgery to decrease the risk of aspiration while under anesthesia.

If you are working in an area where ambulance response time is more than 20 minutes, you may give patients a clean cloth or gauze pad that has been soaked in water to suck on. This relieves dryness of the mouth but does not quench thirst.

Assist With Other Treatments

When an advanced life support (ALS) unit arrives at the scene, be ready to assist them with further treatment. Patients may be given oxygen or **intravenous (IV) fluids**. If you are trained in the administration of oxygen and have it available, provide it to shock patients. Oxygen benefits shock patients by ensuring that the reduced number of red blood cells are as oxygen saturated as they can be. Advanced emergency medical technicians (AEMTs) or paramedics can administer IV fluids. Adding fluid to the body helps combat the loss of blood volume.

Arrange for Transport

As soon as you determine that you have a patient who is in shock, make sure an ambulance has been dispatched. When the ambulance arrives, give emergency medical services (EMS) personnel a concise handoff report, emphasizing the signs and symptoms of shock that you noted. The EMS personnel will then ensure that the patient is quickly prepared for prompt transport to an appropriate medical facility that can handle a patient with this type of condition. Usually, the most appropriate treatment for a patient who is in shock resulting from injury or bleeding is surgical repair, and the sooner the patient gets to the hospital, the better the chance of survival.

Words of Wisdom

A quiet patient may be a patient who is in shock. Conversely, a patient who suddenly becomes agitated may be going into shock. Watch all patients carefully for signs of shock!

Treatment for Shock Caused by Pump Failure

Patients experiencing pump failure may be confused, restless, anxious, or unresponsive. Their pulse is usually rapid and weak, and their skin is cold and clammy, sweaty, and pale. Their respirations are often rapid and shallow. Pump failure is a serious condition. Your treatment for signs and symptoms of shock and prompt transport by ambulance to an appropriate medical facility will give these patients their best chance for survival.

YOU are the EMR — CASE 2

At 1515 hours you are dispatched to a residential neighborhood for a report of a gunshot wound. As you are responding, your dispatcher reports the police are on the scene, and they report it appears to be an accidental discharge. As you arrive on the scene, a sheriff's deputy takes you to the basement where you find a 43-year-old man sitting in a chair. He is holding his hand on his right thigh. There is blood seeping around his hand and some blood on the floor. A police officer has taken possession of the gun and rendered it safe. There are no other weapons in sight. You cut off the patient's pants from around the gunshot wound. There is a small wound in the middle of his thigh that is bleeding moderately. You cannot locate an exit wound.

1. What are your initial steps in treating this patient?
2. How serious is an injury like this?

Treatment for Shock Caused by Pipe Failure

Patients who have fainted, who are experiencing anaphylactic shock or septic shock, or who have sustained a severe spinal cord injury will have pipe failure. Their capillaries may increase three or four times the normal size, causing signs and symptoms of shock.

Treatment for Anaphylactic Shock

The initial treatment for anaphylactic shock is similar to the treatment for any other type of shock. Anaphylactic shock is an extreme emergency, and the patient must be treated as soon as possible. AEMTs, paramedics, nurses, and physicians can administer medications that may reverse the allergic reaction. Some patients who have severe allergies may carry an epinephrine auto-injector. If the patient has a prescribed auto-injector, you can administer the epinephrine if you have been trained in its use and have permission from your local medical director. Be aware of and follow your local protocols. Support the patient's thigh and place the tip of the auto-injector lightly against the outer thigh at a location halfway between knee and hip; note that although it can be given through clothes, it is better to administer it directly to the skin. Using a quick motion, push the auto-injector firmly against the thigh and hold it in place for several seconds, allowing the medication to be fully injected. The detailed steps for administering epinephrine by auto-injector are outlined in Chapter 11, *Poisoning and Substance Use*.

Treatment for Neurogenic Shock and Septic Shock

Your treatment for neurogenic shock consists of keeping the spine supported in a neutral position, supporting the patient's ABCs, treating the symptoms of shock, and arranging for prompt transport to an appropriate medical facility. Remember, these patients are often unable to regulate their body temperature effectively. Therefore, maintaining body heat, particularly in cold weather, is even more important.

Your treatment of a patient who may be experiencing septic shock consists of supporting the patient's ABCs, treating the symptoms of shock, and arranging for prompt transport to an appropriate medical facility. Patients experiencing this type of shock need comprehensive medical care, including rapid administration of antibiotics, to treat their underlying conditions.

Treatment for Shock Caused by Blood Loss

Shock may be caused by internal blood loss (blood that escapes from damaged blood vessels and stays inside the body) or by external blood loss (blood that escapes from the body). While external blood loss is usually caused by trauma, internal blood loss can be caused by trauma or medical conditions.

The following section discusses control of internal bleeding. Control of external bleeding is discussed in greater detail in the sections that follow.

Shock Caused by Internal Blood Loss

Patients can die quickly and quietly from internal bleeding following abdominal injuries that rupture the spleen, liver, or large blood vessels. You must be alert to detect the earliest signs and symptoms of internal bleeding and to begin treatment for shock. If you are treating several injured patients, those with internal bleeding should be transported first to the medical facility because immediate surgery may be needed. Chapter 17, *Transport Operations*, discusses how to decide which patients should receive care first.

Bleeding from stomach ulcers, ruptured blood vessels, or tumors can cause internal bleeding and shock. This bleeding can be spontaneous, massive, and rapid, often leading to the loss of large quantities of blood by vomiting or bloody diarrhea.

It is important to recognize the signs and symptoms of internal bleeding and take prompt corrective action. In addition to the classic signs of shock (confusion, rapid pulse, cold and clammy skin, weak pulse, and rapid breathing), patients with internal bleeding may show additional signs and symptoms as provided in the Signs and Symptoms box.

Signs and Symptoms

Signs and symptoms of internal bleeding include the following:

- Coughing or vomiting of blood
- Abdominal tenderness, rigidity, bruising, or distention
- Rectal bleeding
- Vaginal bleeding in women
- Classic signs of shock

Treatment

You cannot stop internal bleeding. You can only treat its symptoms and arrange for the patient to be promptly transported to an appropriate medical facility.

Words of Wisdom

Patients who regularly consume large quantities of alcohol are at high risk for internal bleeding. Heavy alcohol consumption damages the liver and reduces the production of clotting factors and platelets. Because platelets are needed for blood coagulation and clotting, these patients can experience life-threatening internal bleeding from relatively minor injuries.

Alcohol also irritates the digestive system, which makes patients with alcohol use disorder more likely to experience life-threatening bleeding from the esophagus or stomach.

Traumatic Shock in Children

Signs and symptoms of shock are much slower to develop in children than in adults. However, once they appear, the child's condition will deteriorate rapidly. An injured child displaying obvious signs of shock, such as cool, clammy skin; a rapid, weak pulse; or rapid or shallow respirations, is already experiencing severe shock. It is vital that you learn to recognize and treat shock quickly.

Immediate treatment of an injured child experiencing shock includes controlling external bleeding, keeping the child warm, and administering oxygen if it is available. Children who show signs of shock should be transported as soon as possible to an emergency department. Seizures and vomiting are relatively common in children who have sustained a serious head injury. Be prepared to manage this condition by maintaining the airway and protecting the child from further injury.

The greatest dangers to any patient who has sustained trauma are hemorrhage and airway obstruction. When caring for an injured child, the most important actions you should perform are as follows:

- Control severe external hemorrhage, including application of a tourniquet if appropriate.
- Open and maintain the airway.
- Assist ventilations.
- Control less significant bleeding.
- Arrange for prompt transport to an appropriate medical facility.

Bleeding

Blood loss can occur through external bleeding, which is visible, or through internal bleeding, which can be hard to detect. It ranges from minor cuts to massive blood loss that can kill a person in a few minutes. As an EMR, it is important for you to recognize the signs and symptoms of external bleeding and internal bleeding. It is also important for you to know what steps to take to control bleeding and what care you can administer for patients who are experiencing internal blood loss and shock.

Controlling External Blood Loss

This section describes how to control external blood loss using direct pressure elevation, tourniquets, and pressure point technique. Follow your local protocols for the use of these bleeding control measures.

There are three types of external blood loss: capillary, venous, and arterial (**FIGURE 14-7**). The most common type of external blood loss is **capillary bleeding**. In capillary bleeding, the blood oozes out (such as from a cut finger). You can control capillary bleeding simply by applying direct pressure to the site.

The next most common type of bleeding is **venous bleeding**. This type of bleeding has a steady flow. Bleeding from a large vein may be profuse and life threatening. To control venous bleeding, apply direct pressure to the site for at least 5 minutes.

The most serious type of bleeding is **arterial bleeding**. Arterial blood spurts or surges from the laceration or wound with each heartbeat. Blood pressure in arteries is higher than in capillaries or veins, and unchecked arterial bleeding can result in death from loss of blood in a short time. To control arterial bleeding, exert and maintain sufficient direct

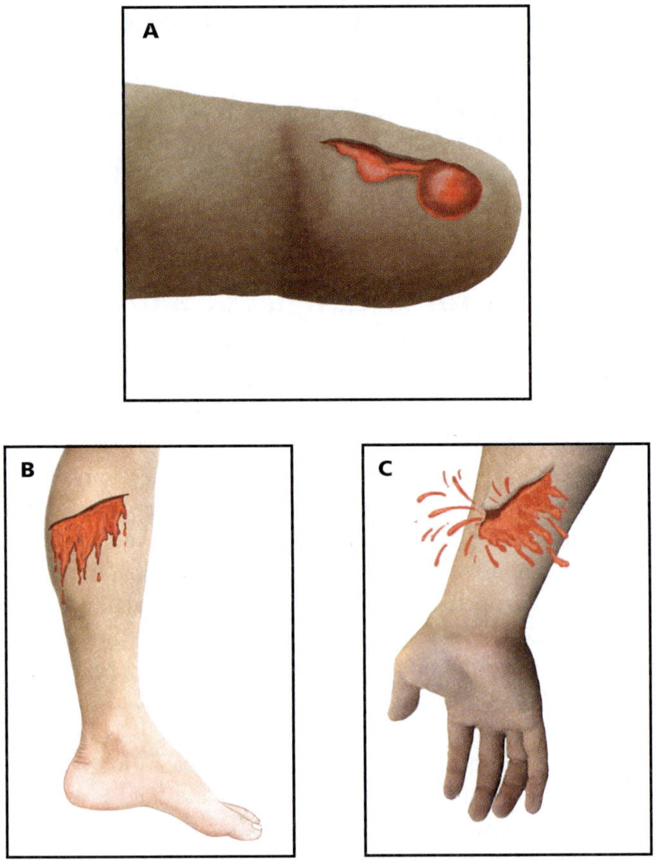

FIGURE 14-7 Recognizing the three types of external bleeding. **A.** Capillary. **B.** Venous. **C.** Arterial.

© Jones & Bartlett Learning

pressure on the site to stop the flow of blood. If the bleeding from an arm or leg wound does not stop with direct pressure, apply a tourniquet 2 to 3 inches (5 to 8 cm) proximal to the site of the bleeding (that is, between the wound and the heart). Place the tourniquet more proximally if necessary to avoid placement over a joint. When in doubt, place the tourniquet as proximally as possible. If a tourniquet is not available, you can use the pressure point technique to stop the flow of bleeding from an extremity wound.

Because many injured patients die from shock caused by blood loss, it is vital that you control external bleeding quickly.

Treatment

Methods of controlling external bleeding are as follows:

1. Apply direct pressure.
2. Elevation.
3. Apply a tourniquet.
4. Use pressure point technique.

Direct Pressure

The first method of controlling external bleeding is direct pressure on the wound. Most external bleeding can be controlled by applying direct pressure to the wound. Place a dry,

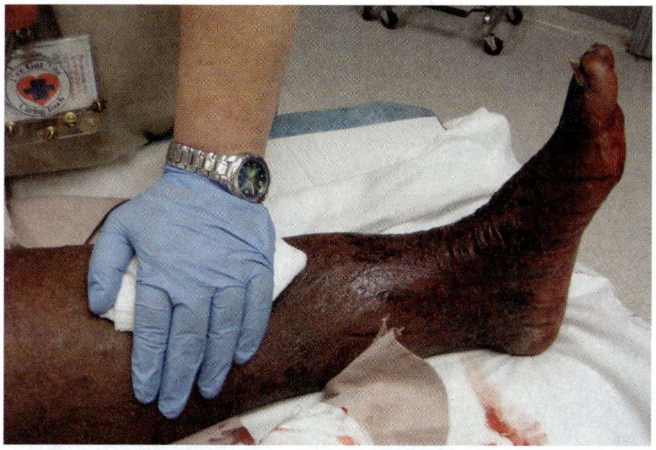

FIGURE 14-8 Applying direct pressure to a wound.
Courtesy of Rhonda Hunt.

sterile **dressing** directly on the wound and apply pressure to the wound with your gloved hand (**FIGURE 14-8**). If you do not have a sterile dressing or gauze bandage, use the cleanest cloth available. After applying a sterile dressing, wrap the dressing and wound snugly with a roller gauze bandage to maintain direct pressure on the wound. Do not remove a dressing after you have applied it. If the dressing becomes blood soaked, place another dressing on top of the first and keep them both in place.

Elevation

The second method of controlling external bleeding is elevation. Elevation as a method to control bleeding has limited usefulness. While raising the arm of a person with a minor cut may slow or stop minor bleeding, elevation should not be considered as a primary method to control bleeding. Elevating an arm or leg after bleeding control has been achieved with direct pressure, bandaging, pressure point technique, or tourniquet application may be more comfortable for a patient and may help to reduce swelling, but it will not stop bleeding that has not been controlled.

Tourniquet Application

The third method of controlling external bleeding is using a tourniquet. Use a tourniquet only when you cannot stop severe bleeding by other means. Certain types of trauma, such as wounds resulting from high-velocity firearms, explosive devices, and knives, can sever arteries in the arm or leg. These types of injuries result in rapid and profound blood loss and can lead to death in minutes.

Recent military experience in combat situations has resulted in the development of improved tourniquets that are easier to apply and are effective at controlling severe bleeding (**FIGURE 14-9**). These tourniquets can be applied rapidly. Some can even be applied with one hand.

As discussed, tourniquets should be applied 2 to 3 inches (5 to 8 cm) proximal to the wound, but not over a joint. Medical research has demonstrated that a tourniquet can be applied and left in place for up to 2 hours without causing additional damage to the injured limb. This means that the use of tourniquets has been proven to have great benefit to the patient without incurring a high risk of additional damage to the limb. However, you should use tourniquets only when there is severe, spurting bleeding from an artery. Use of a tourniquet for more minor bleeding can cause unnecessary injury to that limb.

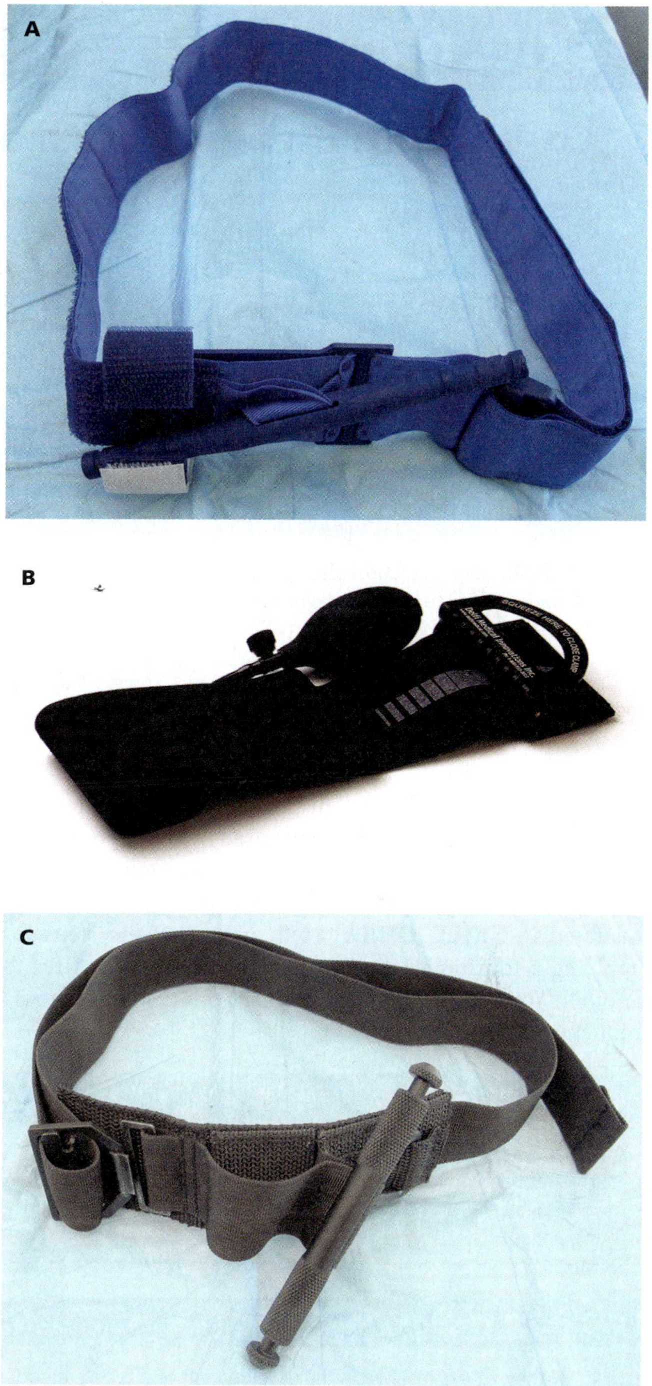

FIGURE 14-9 Different types of tourniquets used by EMS personnel. **A.** A CAT tourniquet. (This blue CAT tourniquet is used for training. CAT tourniquets intended for use in the field are black and are single use.). **B.** An EMT tourniquet. **C.** A SOF-T tourniquet.
A: Courtesy of Peter T. Pons, MD, FACEP; **B:** Courtesy of Delfi Medical Innovations, Inc.; **C:** Courtesy of Peter T. Pons, MD, FACEP.

A tourniquet usually consists of four parts. There is a flat strap that is wrapped around the limb, a buckle or clasp that secures the strap, a rod (windlass) that is used to tighten the tourniquet, and a clip that folds the windlass in place. There is some

SKILL DRILL 14-1

Controlling Bleeding With a Tourniquet

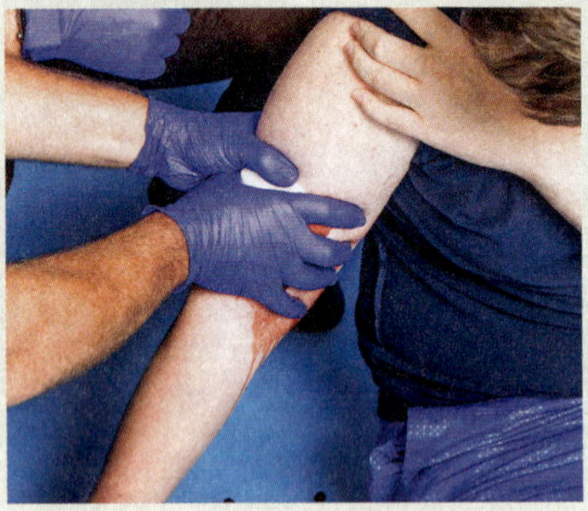

STEP 1 *Place* the tourniquet around the wounded extremity approximately 2 to 3 inches (5 to 8 cm) above (proximal to) the wound, but not over a joint.

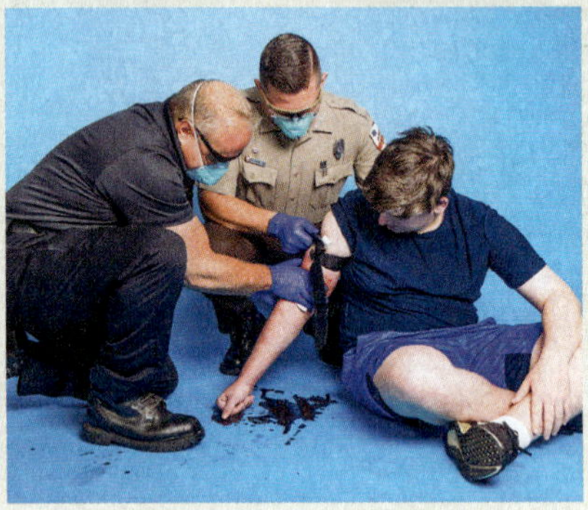

STEP 2 *Pull* the strap tight.

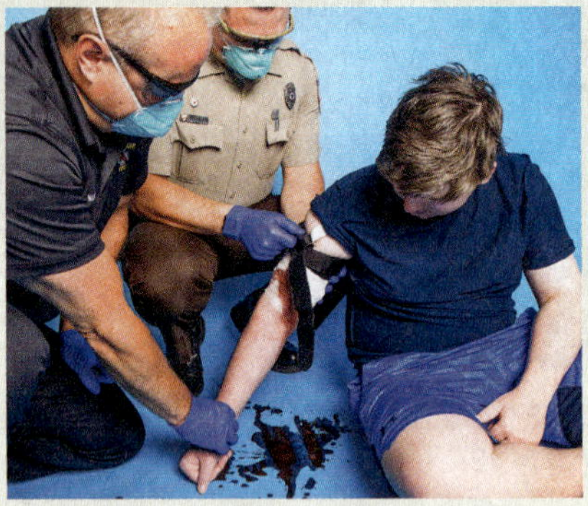

STEP 3 *Twist* the rod until the bleeding stops or until you cannot twist it any further.

STEP 4 *Clip* the rod in place.

© Jones & Bartlett Learning

variation between different tourniquets. You need to become familiar with the specific tourniquet used by your department.

The application of a tourniquet requires you to remember four steps: place, pull, twist, and clip. The process is illustrated in **SKILL DRILL 14-1**. Note that the steps for applying a tourniquet may vary from one manufacturer to another. You need to become familiar with the type of tourniquet used by your agency.

> **Words of Wisdom**
>
> After you have applied a tourniquet, write "TK" and the time the tourniquet was applied on the patient's forehead with a pen so all medical clinicians will be aware that a tourniquet has been applied to the patient.

> **Words of Wisdom**
>
> Military research has resulted in the development of effective blood clotting agents, or **hemostatic agents**. These are usually impregnated in gauze dressings or supplied as a powder. These agents can be packed into a wound and aid in the formation of a blood clot in less time. They are useful for extremity wounds and for wounds in junctional areas, such as the groin, shoulder and armpit, or neck, where a tourniquet cannot be applied. Hemostatic agents are carried by some EMS agencies and are carried in special kits by some law enforcement agencies for rapid treatment of gunshot wounds. Use these clotting agents only if you have received special training and are permitted by your local protocols.

Manual Pressure Point Technique

The fourth method of controlling external bleeding is the manual **pressure point** technique. In cases of severe bleeding, this technique can be lifesaving. Pressure point techniques work by compressing a major artery against the bone at a specific location. Use of this technique requires training and practice, but it offers key advantages in an emergency where resources and time are limited: it does not require any equipment, it can control bleeding within seconds, and it can be used to stop bleeding until a tourniquet can be applied. This technique should be considered for extremity wounds where direct pressure and elevation do not control the bleeding and a tourniquet is not available.

> **Words of Wisdom**
>
> In studies of the pressure point technique published in 2022 and 2023, nearly all participants were able to stop the flow of blood to both the lower and the upper extremities in a matter of seconds following proper instruction.

To stop bleeding in the upper extremity, the brachial artery pressure point (in the upper arm) is used. To stop bleeding in the lower extremity, the femoral artery pressure point (in the groin) is used.

Brachial Artery Pressure Point Technique. When you are applying pressure to the brachial artery, remember the words *slap*, *slide*, and *squeeze* while following these steps (**FIGURE 14-10**):

1. Position the patient's arm so the elbow is bent at a right angle (90°), and hold the upper arm away from the patient's body.
2. Gently "slap" the inside of the biceps with your fingers halfway between the shoulder and the elbow.
3. "Slide" your fingers upward to push the biceps away.

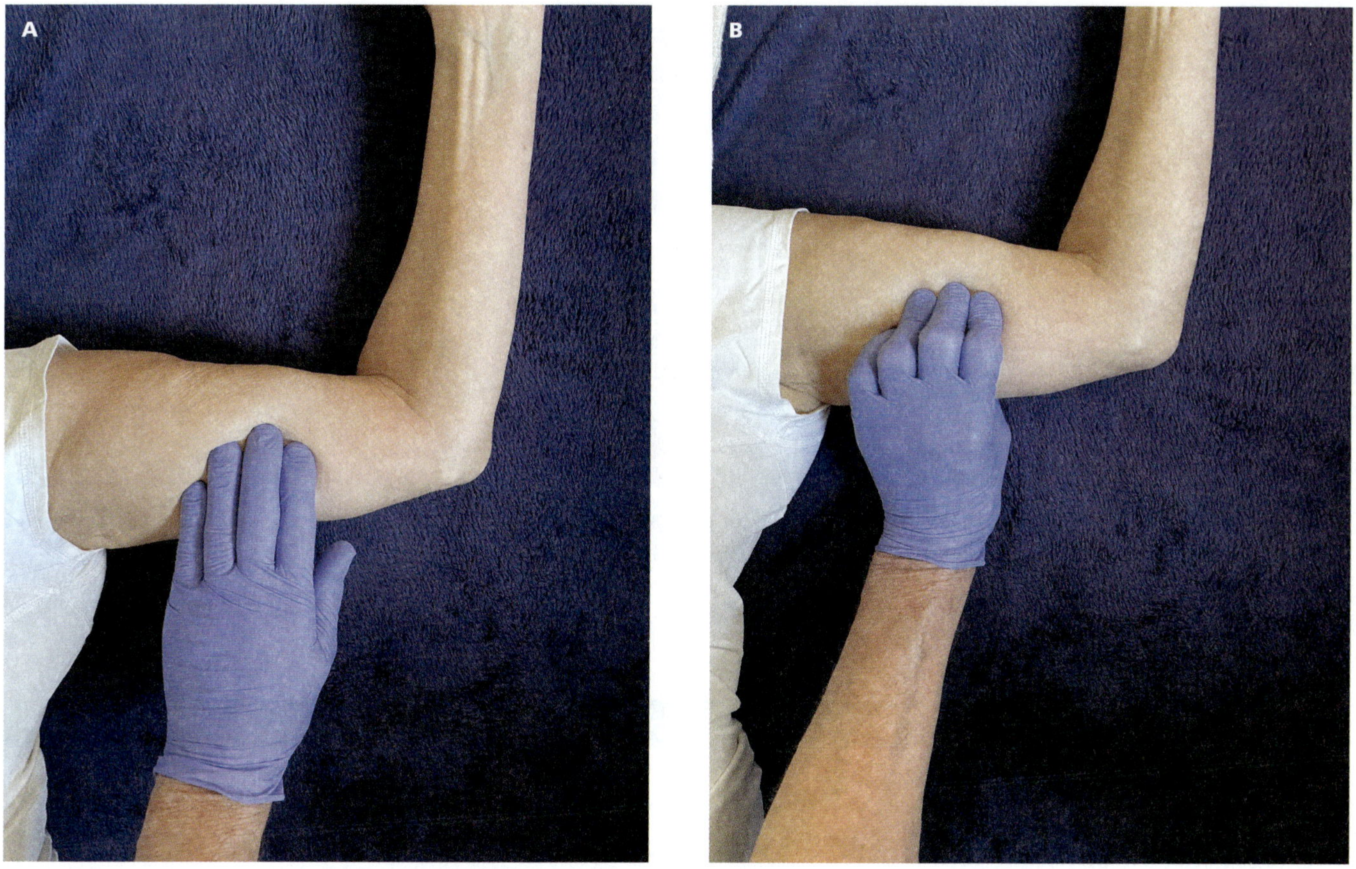

FIGURE 14-10 Brachial artery pressure point technique. **A.** "Slap" the inside of the biceps with your fingers halfway between the shoulder and the elbow. **B.** "Slide" your fingers upward and "squeeze" the humerus.
Courtesy of Maggie Daley.

4. "Squeeze" by pressing your hand down on the humerus (upper arm bone). You should be able to feel the pulse as you press down.

If the patient is sitting down, squeeze the arm by placing your fingers halfway between the shoulder and the elbow and your thumb on the opposite side of the patient's arm. When properly applied, this technique will quickly stop bleeding below (distal to) the point of application.

Femoral Artery Pressure Point Technique. Severe bleeding in the lower extremity can be stopped using the femoral artery pressure point technique by carefully following these steps (**FIGURE 14-11**):

1. Position the patient on their back and kneel next to the patient's hips while facing the patient's head. You should be on the side of the patient opposite the extremity that is bleeding.
2. Find the pelvis and place the little finger of your hand closest to the injured leg along the anterior crest on the injured side.
3. Rotate the palm of your hand downward firmly into the groin area between the genitals and the pelvic bone. This action compresses the femoral artery against the pelvic bone and stops the blood flow to the lower extremity.
4. If the bleeding does not slow immediately, reposition your hand and apply pressure again.

To effectively apply brachial and femoral pressure point techniques, you must learn these steps thoroughly and practice them regularly.

> **Words of Wisdom**
>
> Motivated by many tragedies throughout the country, in October 2015, the White House launched the Stop the Bleed campaign in an attempt to train, equip, and empower bystanders to act in an emergency situation prior to the arrival of professional help. The idea is that by providing bystanders and emergency responders such as law enforcement with the skills and basic tools needed to stop uncontrolled bleeding, many lives could be saved. The principles include three key actions, as shown in **FIGURE 14-12**.

Some public venues have placed bleeding-control kits in the same location as automated external defibrillators (AEDs). Items included in the kits range from nitrile gloves for personal protection, tourniquets, compression dressings, rolled gauze, and trauma shears. The key to the success of this initiative is widespread education of the public and having kits available for use. EMS clinicians can provide a vital link in this accomplishment.

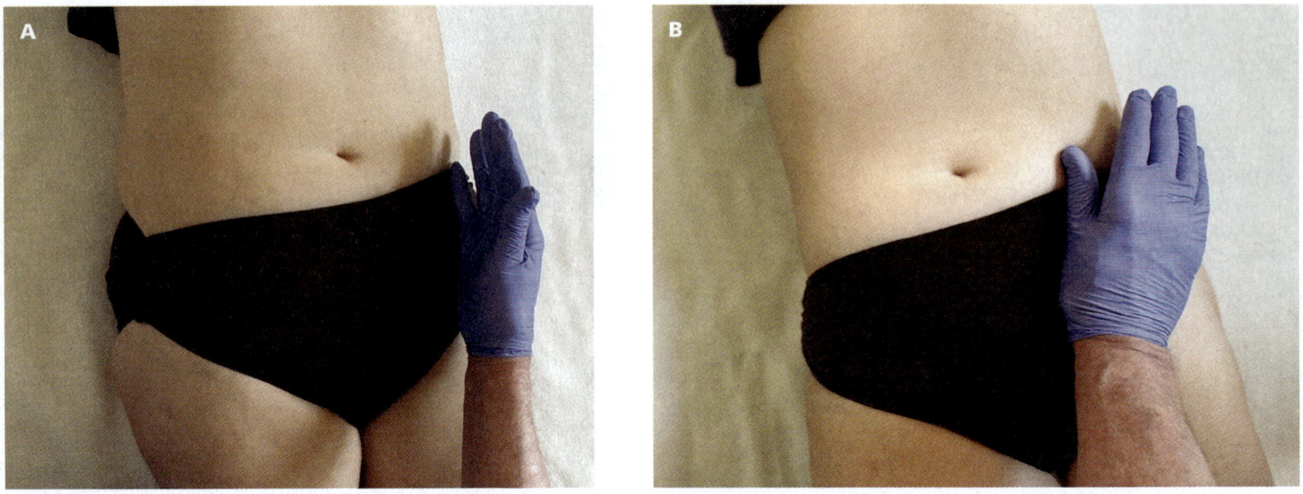

FIGURE 14-11 Femoral artery pressure point technique. **A.** Find the pelvis and place your little finger along the anterior crest. **B.** Rotate your palm downward firmly into the groin area between the genitals and the pelvic bone.
Courtesy of Maggie Daley.

Treatment

Follow these steps to treat shock caused by pump failure:

1. Keep the patient lying down unless the patient is able to breathe easier in a sitting position.
2. Maintain the patient's ABCs. Be prepared to perform CPR, if necessary.
3. Maintain the patient's normal body temperature.
4. Ensure that the patient does not eat or drink anything.
5. Keep the patient quiet, and limit their movement by performing tasks for them when possible.
6. Provide reassurance.
7. Arrange for prompt transport by ambulance to an appropriate medical facility.
8. Provide high-flow oxygen as soon as it is available.

Follow these steps to treat shock caused by pipe failure:

Fainting

1. Examine the patient to ensure there is no injury.
2. Keep the patient lying down.
3. Maintain the ABCs.
4. Maintain the patient's normal body temperature.
5. Provide reassurance.

Anaphylactic Shock

1. Keep the patient lying down, and elevate the legs if indicated by local protocol.
2. If the patient has an epinephrine auto-injector, help the patient use it if indicated by local protocol.
3. Maintain the patient's ABCs. Anaphylactic shock may cause airway swelling. In severe reactions, the patient may require mouth-to-mask breathing or full CPR.
4. Maintain the patient's normal body temperature.
5. Provide reassurance.
6. Arrange for rapid transport by ambulance to an appropriate medical facility.

Septic Shock

1. Maintain the ABCs.
2. Maintain the patient's normal body temperature.
3. Ensure that the patient does not eat or drink anything.
4. Provide reassurance.
5. Arrange for prompt transport by ambulance to an appropriate medical facility.

Neurogenic Shock

1. Place the patient on their back. Because the spine may be injured, keep the patient's head and neck stabilized to protect the spinal cord. See Chapter 15, *Injuries to Muscles and Bones*.
2. Maintain the patient's ABCs.
3. Maintain the patient's normal body temperature.
4. Ensure that the patient does not eat or drink anything.
5. Assist with other treatments. Help other medical clinicians place the patient on a backboard.

Follow these steps to treat shock caused by blood loss:

Internal Blood Loss

1. Keep the patient lying down.
2. Maintain the patient's ABCs.
3. Maintain the patient's normal body temperature.
4. Ensure that the patient does not eat or drink anything.
5. Provide reassurance.
6. Keep the patient quiet, and do any necessary moving for them.
7. Provide high-flow oxygen as soon as it is available.
8. Monitor the patient's vital signs at least every 5 minutes.
9. Arrange for prompt transport by ambulance to an appropriate medical facility.

External Blood Loss

1. Control external bleeding by applying direct pressure on the wound, elevating the wound, or applying a tourniquet; if the bleeding is from an arm or leg and these methods are not effective or possible, use the pressure point technique. Take standard precautions.
2. Ensure that the patient is lying down.
3. Maintain the patient's ABCs.
4. Maintain the patient's normal body temperature.
5. Ensure that the patient does not eat or drink anything.
6. Provide reassurance.
7. Provide high-flow oxygen as soon as it is available.
8. Arrange for prompt transport by ambulance to an appropriate medical facility.

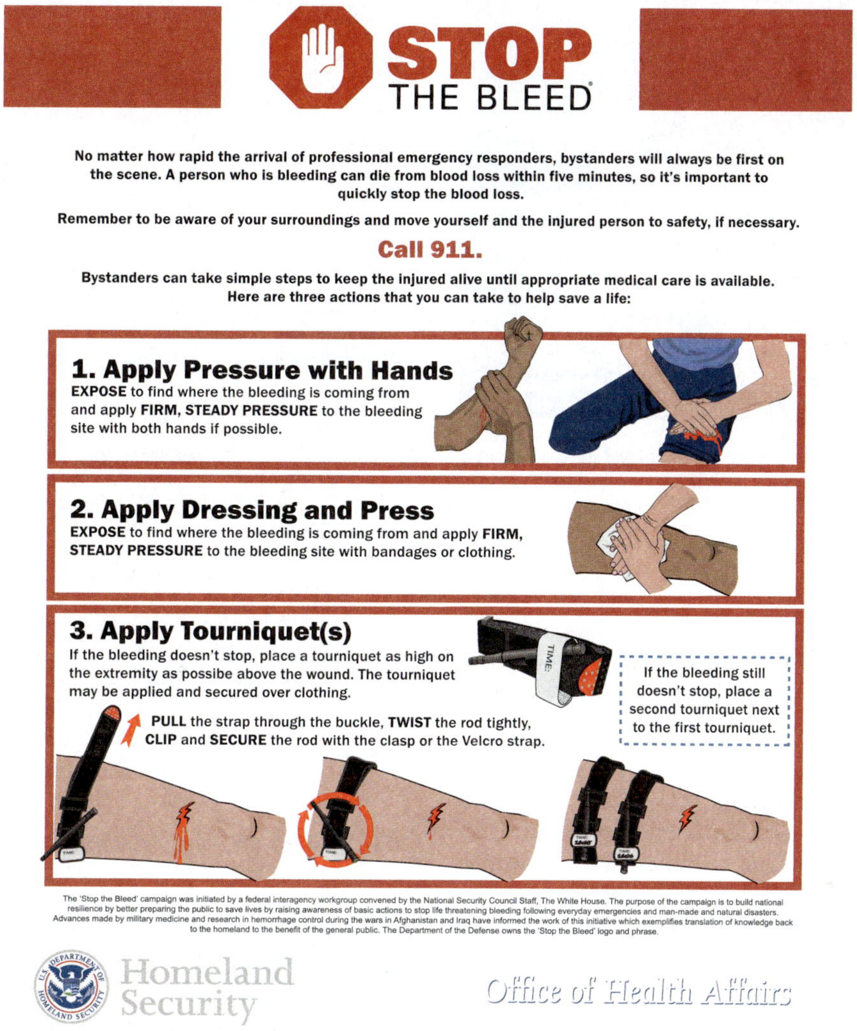

FIGURE 14-12 Three actions you can take to help save a life.
Courtesy of the United States Department of Defense and the United States Department of Homeland Security. STOP THE BLEED® is a registered trademark of the Department of Defense.

Standard Precautions and Bleeding Control

Certain communicable diseases such as hepatitis or human immunodeficiency virus (HIV) can be spread by contact with blood from an infected person. This risk is greatly increased when the infected blood comes into contact with a cut or an open sore on your skin. Although your risk of contracting hepatitis or HIV through intact skin is small, you should minimize this risk as much as possible by wearing nitrile or latex gloves whenever you might come in contact with a patient's blood or body fluids (**FIGURE 14-13**). Carry your gloves on top of your EMR jump kit or in a pouch on your belt for quick access (**FIGURE 14-14**). If you do get blood on your hands, wash it off as soon as possible with soap and water. If you are in the field and cannot wash your hands, use a waterless hand-cleaning solution that contains an effective germ-killing agent.

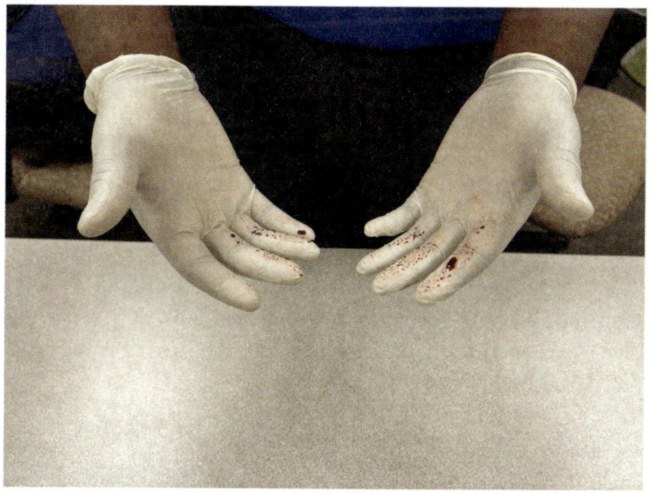

FIGURE 14-13 Wear gloves to minimize your risk of infection.
Courtesy of Rhonda Hunt.

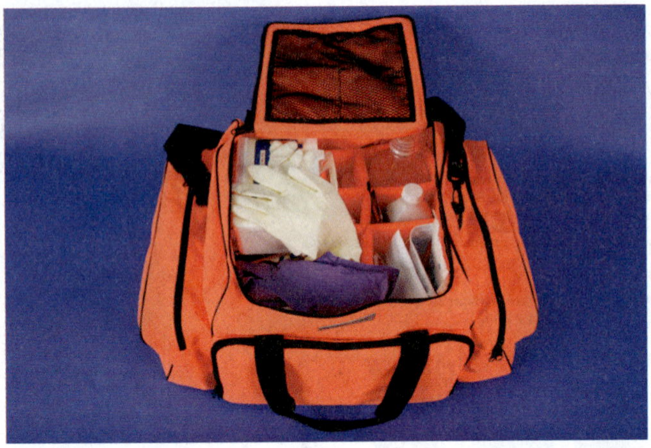

FIGURE 14-14 Keep your gloves on top in your EMR jump kit or in a pouch on your belt.
© Jones & Bartlett Learning

Wounds

A wound is an injury caused by any physical means that leads to damage of a body part. Wounds are classified as closed or open.

Closed Wounds

In a **closed wound**, the skin is not broken, meaning tissue beneath the skin is not exposed to the environment and external bleeding cannot occur. One example of a closed wound is a **bruise** (contusion). A bruise is an injury of the soft tissue beneath the skin. Because small blood vessels are broken, the injured area becomes discolored and swells. The severity of these closed soft-tissue injuries varies greatly. A simple bruise heals quickly.

In contrast, bruising and swelling following an injury may also be a sign of an underlying fracture. Whenever you encounter a significant amount of swelling or bruising, suspect the possibility of an underlying fracture.

Open Wounds

In an **open wound**, the skin is broken, exposing the tissue beneath the skin to the environment and allowing external bleeding. There are several types of open wounds, including abrasions, puncture wounds, lacerations, avulsions, and amputations. Each type is described in the following subsections.

Abrasion

Commonly called a scrape, **road rash**, or rug burn, an **abrasion** occurs when the skin is rubbed across a rough surface (**FIGURE 14-15**).

Puncture

Puncture wounds are caused by a sharp object that penetrates the skin (**FIGURE 14-16**). These wounds may cause a significant deep injury that is not immediately recognized. Puncture wounds do not bleed freely. If the object that caused the puncture wound remains sticking out of the skin, it is called an **impaled object**.

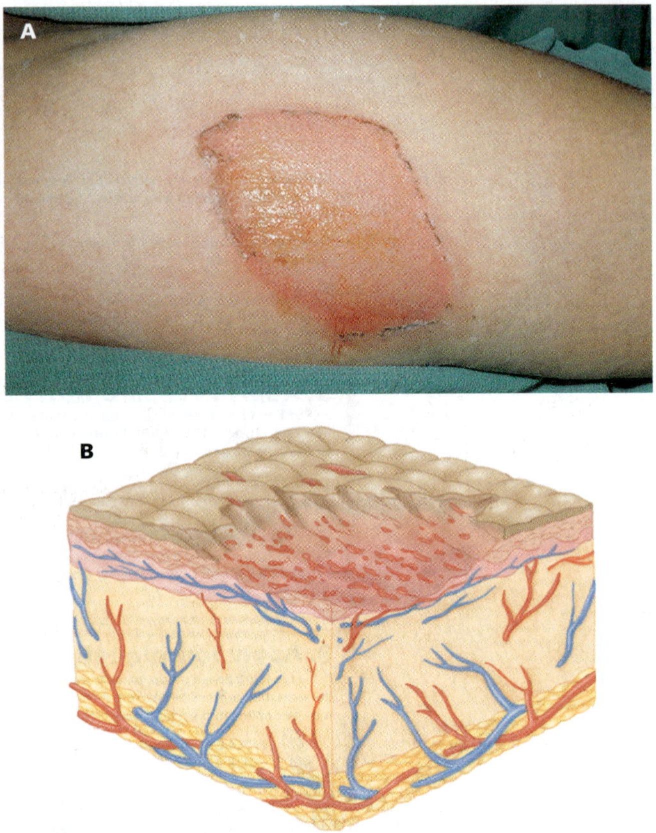

FIGURE 14-15 Abrasions involve variable depth of the skin.
A: © American Academy of Orthopaedic Surgeons; B: © Jones & Bartlett Learning

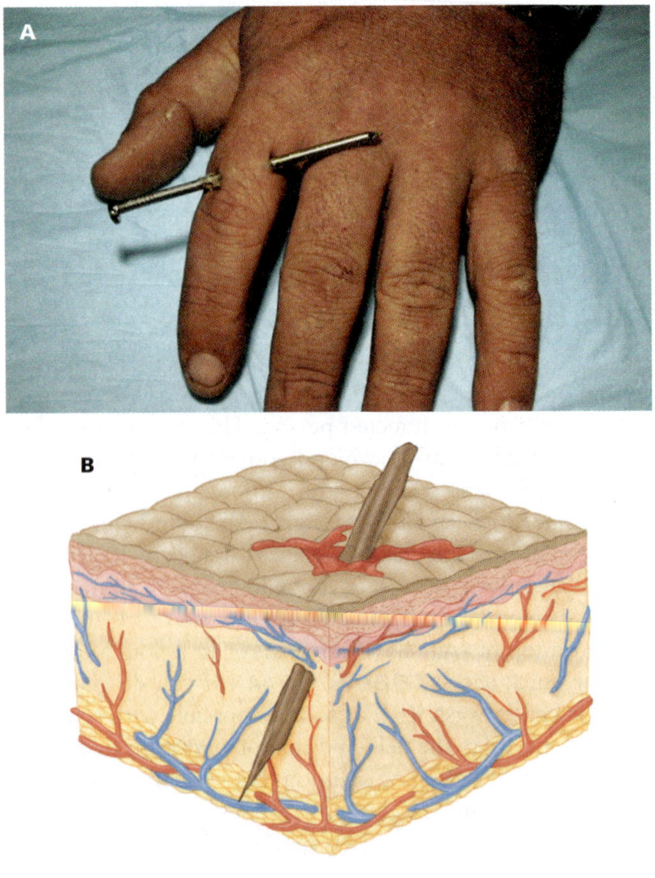

FIGURE 14-16 Puncture wounds may penetrate the skin to any depth.
A: © E. M. Singletary, MD. Used with permission; B: © Jones & Bartlett Learning

A **gunshot wound** is a special type of puncture wound. The amount of damage done by a gunshot depends on the type of gun used and the distance between the gun and the victim. A gunshot entry wound may appear as an insignificant hole, but the bullet can cause massive damage to internal organs. Some gunshot wounds are smaller than a dime, and some are large enough to destroy significant amounts of tissue. Gunshot wounds sometimes have both an **entrance wound** and an **exit wound**. The entrance wound is usually, but not always, smaller than the exit wound. Rather than referring to the wound as an exit or an entry wound, describe it by its size and location. Most deaths from gunshot wounds result from internal blood loss as well as damage to internal organs and major blood vessels as the bullet passes through the body. There may be more than one gunshot wound. It is important to conduct a thorough patient exam to ensure that you have discovered all entrance and exit wounds.

Laceration

A **laceration** is an open wound and is commonly referred to as a cut (**FIGURE 14-17**). It is the most common type of wound. Lacerations can be caused by a sharp object or by blunt force and can have ragged or sharp edges. An **incision** is a type of laceration that is made with a sharp object such as a knife. Lacerations range from small cuts to a large wounds. Minor lacerations may require little care, but large lacerations can cause extensive bleeding and can be life threatening.

Avulsions and Amputations

An **avulsion** is a tearing away of body tissue (**FIGURE 14-18**). The avulsed part may be totally severed from the body or it may be attached by a flap of skin. Avulsions may involve small or large amounts of tissue. If an entire body part is torn away, the wound is called a traumatic amputation (**FIGURE 14-19**). Any amputated body part should be located, placed in a clean plastic bag, kept cool, and taken with the patient to the hospital for possible reattachment (reimplantation). An effective method to keep the part cold without allowing it to freeze, which will damage the tissue

Treatment

Many older patients with heart conditions are on blood thinners (anticoagulants) to keep blood clots from forming in their body vessels. If they are taking blood thinners, it may take longer to control bleeding from an open wound. As part of your SAMPLE history, ask patients if they are taking any blood thinners.

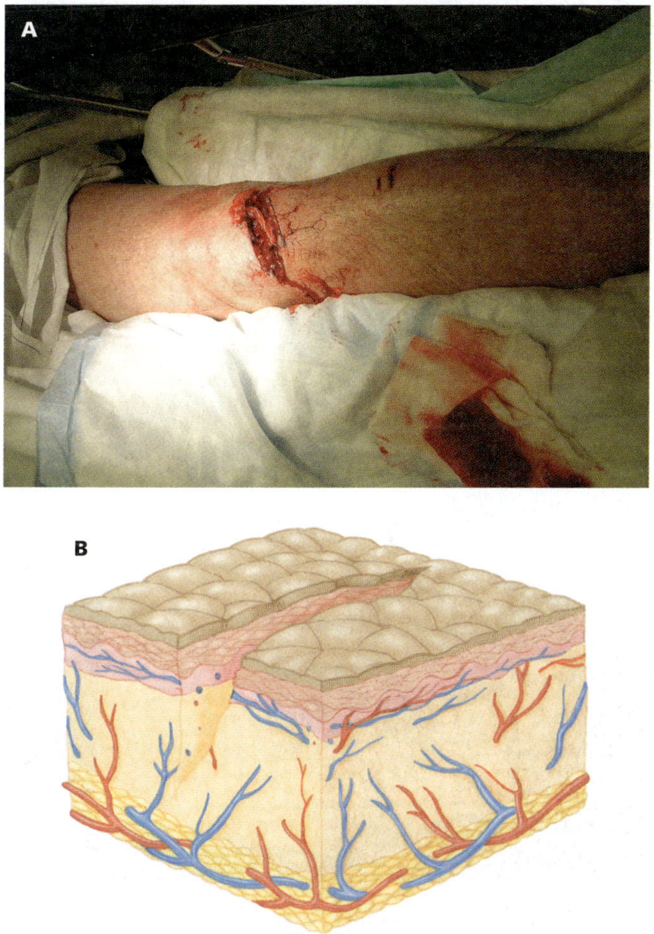

FIGURE 14-17 A laceration is an open wound caused by a sharp object or by blunt force.

A: © E. M. Singletary, MD. Used with permission; B: © Jones & Bartlett Learning

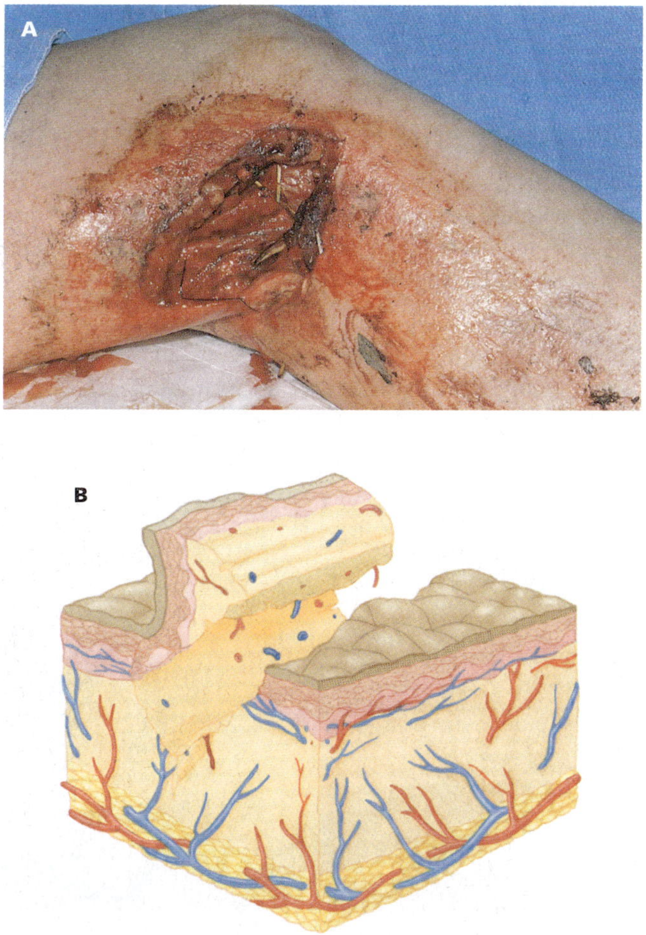

FIGURE 14-18 Avulsions raise flaps of tissue; significant bleeding is common.

A: © Jones & Bartlett Learning. Courtesy of MIEMSS; B: © Jones & Bartlett Learning

and make reattachment impossible, is to wrap the part in saline gauze, place it in a plastic bag, and float the bag in ice water. If the amputated part is small and a clean plastic bag is not available, use a surgical glove turned inside out.

Principles of Wound Treatment

Minor bruises need no treatment. Other closed wounds should be treated by applying an ice pack wrapped in a towel and gentle compression and by elevating the injured body part. Because extensive bruising may indicate an underlying fracture, **splint** all major contusions. Splinting involves using flexible or rigid support to prevent the movement of the injured body part. Splinting is discussed in greater detail in Chapter 15, *Injuries to Muscles and Bones.*

It is important to stop bleeding as quickly as possible using the cleanest dressing available. You can usually control bleeding by covering an open wound with a dry, clean, or sterile dressing and applying pressure to the dressing with your hand. If the first dressing does not control the bleeding, reinforce it with a second layer. If bleeding continues, apply a tourniquet.

A dressing should cover the entire wound to prevent further contamination. Do not attempt to clean the contaminated wound in the field because cleaning will only cause more bleeding. A thorough cleaning will be done at the hospital. All dressings should be secured in place by a compression bandage.

Learning to dress and bandage wounds requires practice. As a trained EMR, you should be able to bandage all parts of the body quickly and competently (**FIGURE 14-20**).

Dressing and Bandaging Wounds

All wounds require bandaging; therefore, you should be familiar with the general principles of applying dressings and bandages to effectively cover and protect wounds. Dressings and bandages are applied to achieve the following:

- Control bleeding
- Prevent further contamination
- Stabilize the injured area (reduce movement)
- Prevent movement of impaled objects

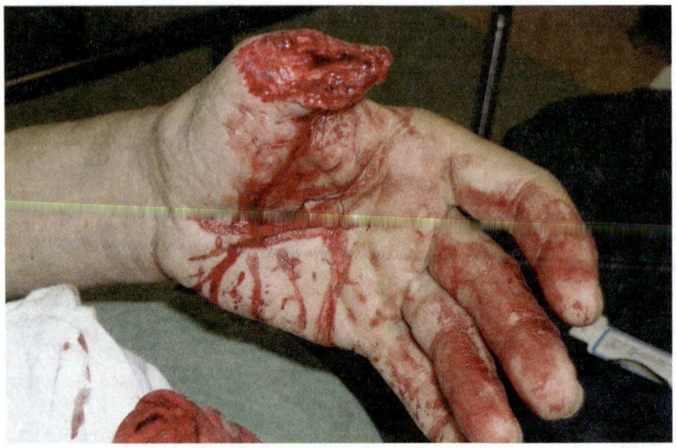

FIGURE 14-19 Amputated parts can often be reattached. Attempt to locate the body parts and transport them to the hospital with the patient.

© E. M. Singletary, MD. Used with permission.

Dressings

A dressing is an object placed directly on a wound to control bleeding and prevent further contamination. Once a dressing is in place, apply firm, direct manual pressure on it to stop any bleeding. It is important to stop severe bleeding as quickly as possible using the cleanest dressing available. If no dressing materials are available, you may have to apply direct pressure with your hand to a wound that is bleeding extensively; if this is the case, be sure to take standard precautions.

Sterile dressings come packaged in many different sizes. The three most common sizes are gauze squares that measure 4 × 4 inches (10 × 10 cm) (commonly known as 4 × 4s), heavier pads that measure 5 × 9 inches (13 × 23 cm) (known as 5 × 9s), and trauma dressings that are thick, sterile dressings that measure 10 × 30 inches (25 × 76 cm). Use a trauma dressing to cover a large wound on the abdomen, neck, thigh, or scalp or as padding for splints (**FIGURE 14-21**).

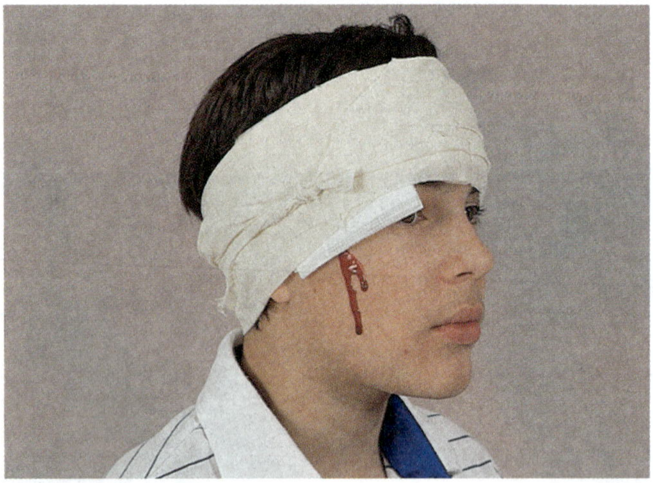

FIGURE 14-20 Head bandage.

© American Academy of Orthopaedic Surgeons

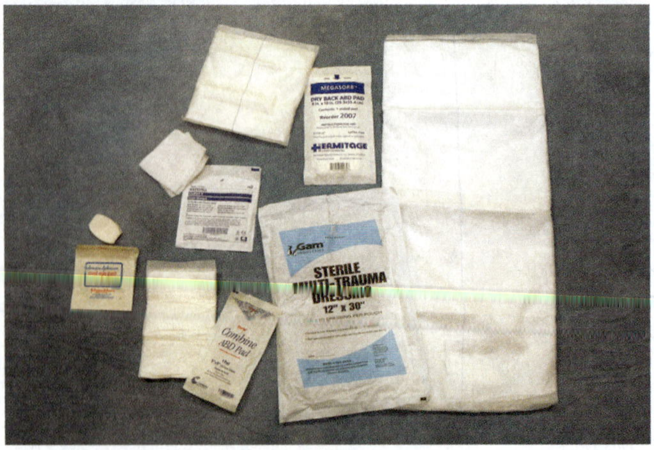

FIGURE 14-21 Common sizes of wound dressings are 10 × 30 inches (25 × 76 cm), 5 × 9 inches (13 × 23 cm), and 4 × 4 inches (10 × 10 cm). Open the package containing a sterile dressing carefully to avoid contaminating the dressing.

© Jones & Bartlett Learning. Courtesy of MIEMSS.

When you open a package containing a sterile dressing, touch only one corner of the dressing. Place it on the wound without touching the side of the dressing that will be next to the wound. If bleeding continues after you have applied a compression dressing to the wound, put additional gauze pads over the original dressing. Do not remove the original dressing because the blood-clotting process will have already started and should not be disrupted. When you are satisfied that the wound is sufficiently dressed, you can proceed to bandaging the wound.

Treatment

If commercially prepared dressings are not available, use the cleanest cloth object available, such as a clean handkerchief, washcloth, disposable diaper, or article of clothing.

Bandaging

A bandage is used to hold the dressing in place. Two types of bandages commonly used in the field are roller gauze and triangular bandages. The first type, conforming roller gauze, stretches slightly and is easy to wrap around the body part (**FIGURE 14-22**). Triangular bandages are usually 36 inches (91 cm) across (**FIGURE 14-23**). A triangular bandage can be folded and used as a wide **cravat**, or it can be used without folding (**FIGURE 14-24**). Roller gauze is easier to apply and stays in place better than a triangular bandage, but a triangular bandage is very useful for bandaging lacerations of the scalp, chest, abdomen, back, or thigh.

Before you apply a bandage, check that the dressing covers the wound completely and extends beyond all sides of the wound (**FIGURE 14-25**). Wrap the bandage just tightly enough to control bleeding. Do not apply it too tightly because it may cut off all circulation. It is important to regularly check circulation at a point farther away from the heart than the injury itself because swelling may make the bandage too tight. If this happens while the patient is under your care, remove the roller gauze or triangular bandage and reapply it, making sure that you do not disturb the dressing beneath.

Once you have applied the bandage, secure it so it cannot slip. Tape, tie, or tuck in any loose ends. Practice bandaging techniques for several types of wounds using both roller gauze

Treatment

Bandaging is a skill that requires practice. Apply bandages tight enough to stay in place, and apply sufficient pressure to stop the bleeding. However, do not apply bandages too tightly or they can occlude circulation to an extremity. Check bandages as part of your reassessment to ensure they are still applied correctly.

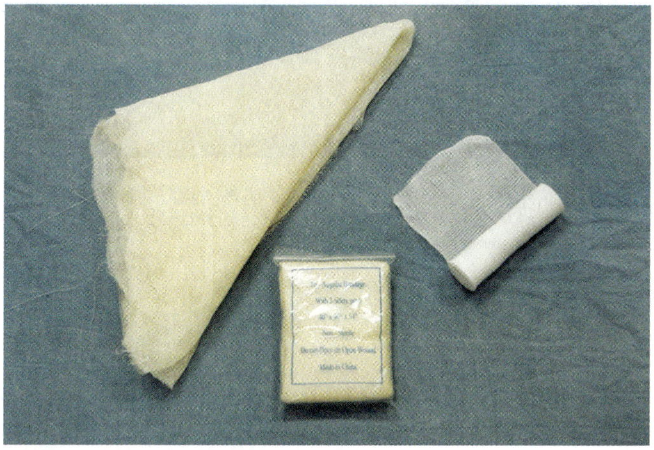

FIGURE 14-22 Roller gauze bandage.

© Jones & Bartlett Learning. Courtesy of MIEMSS.

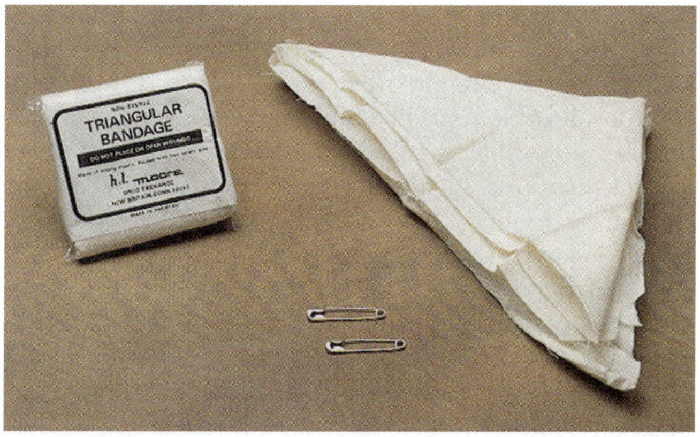

FIGURE 14-23 Triangular bandage.

© Jones & Bartlett Learning

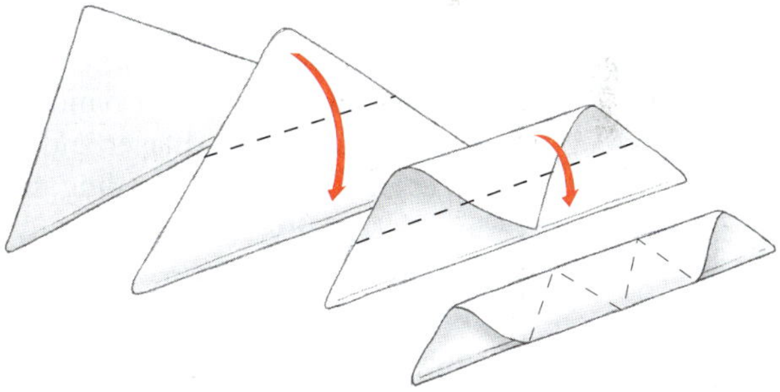

FIGURE 14-24 Folding a triangular bandage to make a cravat.

© Jones & Bartlett Learning

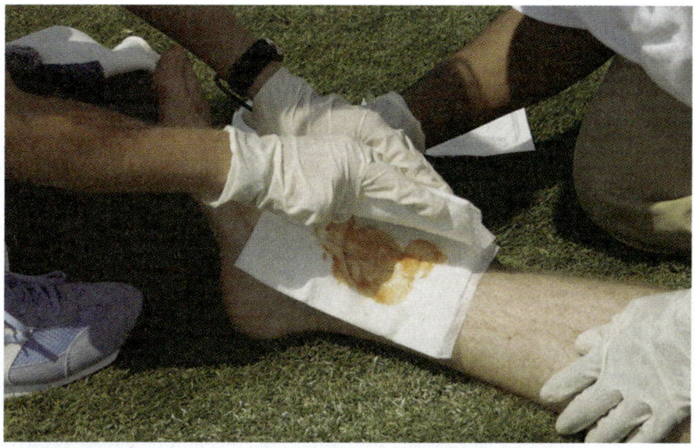

FIGURE 14-25 Ensure that the dressing covers the wound completely.

© Jones & Bartlett Learning

Safety

Providing for your own safety and that of the patient is always a high priority when you are examining and treating open wounds. Wear gloves to protect yourself against exposure to infectious diseases that may be present in the patient's blood and to avoid contaminating the patient's wound with dirt and infectious organisms that may be on your hands.

and triangular bandages. Although the principles of bandaging are simple, some parts of the body are difficult to bandage. It is important to practice bandaging different parts of the body to ensure competency in emergency medical care situations.

Specific Wound Treatment

The preceding material discussed the general principles of wound treatment. The next section discusses treatment for specific types of wounds on different parts of the body.

Face and Scalp Wounds

The face and scalp have many blood vessels. Because of this generous blood supply, a relatively small laceration can result in significant bleeding. Although face and scalp lacerations may not be life threatening, they are always bloody and cause much anxiety for the patient.

You can control almost all facial or scalp bleeding by applying direct manual pressure. Direct pressure is effective because the bones of the skull are so close to the skin. Direct pressure compresses the blood vessels against the skull and stops the bleeding. If bleeding continues, do not remove the dressing. Instead, reinforce it with a second layer and continue to apply manual pressure. After the bleeding stops, wrap the head with a bandage (**FIGURE 14-26**).

For wounds inside the cheek, hold a gauze pad inside the cheek (in the mouth). If necessary, apply a pad outside the cheek. Be careful not to block the airway or allow the patient to swallow gauze.

Severe scalp lacerations may be associated with skull fractures or even brain injury. If any brain tissue or bone fragments are visible, do not apply pressure to the wound. Instead, cover the wound loosely, being careful not to exert direct pressure on the brain or the bone fragments.

If the patient has a head injury, the neck and spine may also be injured. Move the head as little as possible and stabilize the neck. In patients with a head injury, always evaluate the patient's level of consciousness. Carefully monitor the patient's airway and breathing and protect the spine. Treatment of spinal injuries is discussed in Chapter 15, *Injuries to Muscles and Bones*.

Street Smarts

Patients who have injuries or are bleeding will likely be worried. It is your job to reassure them that you are doing everything you can to treat them. Do not forget to show your patients and their families that you care!

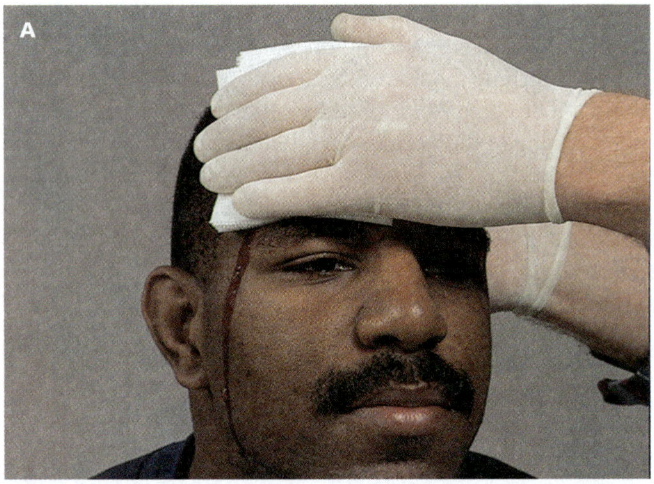

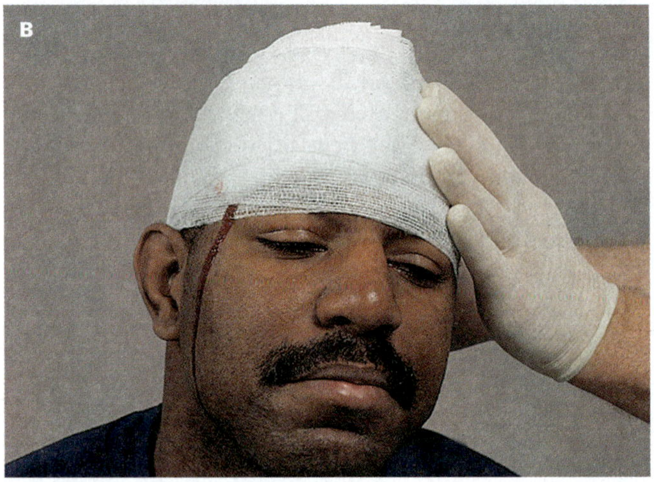

FIGURE 14-26 Bandaging a head wound. **A.** Apply direct pressure until bleeding stops. **B.** Wrap the head with a bandage.
© Jones & Bartlett Learning. Courtesy of MIEMSS.

Nosebleeds

A nosebleed (or epistaxis) can result from dry air, injury (including nose picking), use of certain medications and illegal drugs, high blood pressure, and other causes. In some cases, there is no apparent cause. A nosebleed with no apparent cause is called a **spontaneous nosebleed**. In a patient with high blood pressure, increased pressure in the small blood vessels of the nose may cause one to rupture, resulting in bleeding. A patient with high blood pressure should be seen and treated by a physician.

Most nosebleeds can be controlled easily. Unless the patient has a possible spinal injury, have the patient sit down and tilt their head slightly forward. This position keeps the blood from dripping down the throat. Swallowing blood may cause coughing or vomiting and make the nosebleed worse.

After the patient is seated correctly, pinch both nostrils together for at least 5 minutes. The patient may wish to do this without assistance. This treatment usually controls nosebleeds (**FIGURE 14-27**). If the nosebleed persists or is very severe, arrange for transport to an appropriate medical facility. Instruct the patient to avoid blowing their nose because doing so will often cause additional bleeding. If clots have formed inside the

Voices of Experience

We were called to assist the ambulance at an accident at the local paper manufacturing facility. An adult male had his gloved hand caught in a piece of machinery and several of his fingers had been amputated. After we made contact with our patient, we simultaneously determined he had an open airway, was breathing adequately, and was bleeding from his hand. We were able to successfully stop the bleeding with direct pressure, all the while reassuring our patient.

We radioed ahead to the ambulance to let them know the status of our patient and that four of his fingers had been amputated at the knuckle level. The ambulance, in turn, requested a helicopter flight meet them at the hospital for rapid transit to a larger, Level I trauma center, which could perform hand replant surgery.

I found all the fingers (sounds awful, but was not at all), wrapped them in gauze, put them in a plastic bag, and then placed the plastic bag into a container of ice water. The patient was transported to the hospital and on to the Level I trauma center.

About 6 months later, the patient made an unexpected visit to my place of business. He asked if I remembered him and I replied, "Of course!" He picked up his hand and waved at me, with all of his fingers intact and perfectly responding. He said, "I just wanted to say hi and say thank you."

He was back at work doing the same job, but being much more careful, and truly thankful for the quick action by the emergency medical responders.

> **"His gloved hand had gotten caught in a piece of machinery, and several of his fingers had been amputated."**

Ellen A. Mathein, EMT, CPA
Nicolet Area Technical College
Tripoli, Wisconsin

Adapted from the personal Medical Identification Symbol of the American Medical Association.

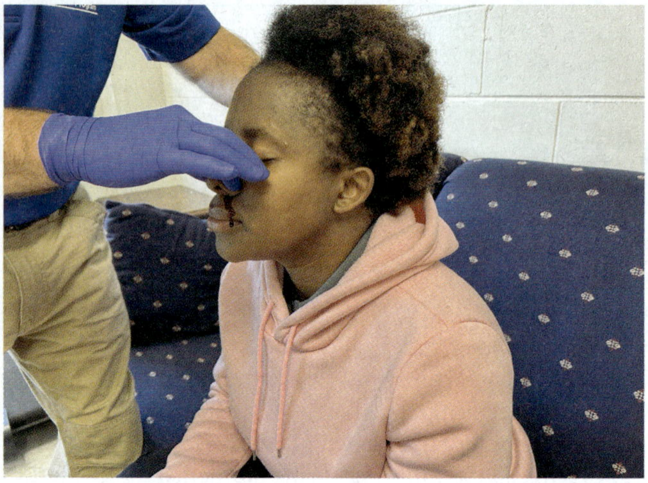

FIGURE 14-27 Pinch nostrils together to control a nosebleed.
Courtesy of Rhonda Hunt.

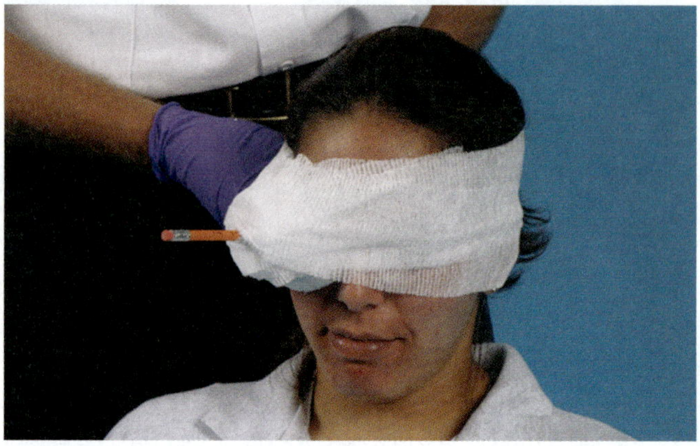

FIGURE 14-28 To bandage an eye impaled by an object, use a paper cup to cover the impaled object, then bandage both eyes to minimize eye movement.
© Jones & Bartlett Learning. Courtesy of MIEMSS.

nostril, advise the patient not to immediately remove them, as they may be helping to control the bleeding.

> **Treatment**
>
> If you suspect that a patient's blood pressure may be high, the patient should be evaluated by a physician.

Eye Injuries

All eye injuries are potentially serious and require medical evaluation. When an eye laceration is suspected, cover the entire eye with a dry gauze pad. Cover the other eye, too, because if the patient looks at something with the uninjured eye, the injured eye moves in conjunction, further aggravating the injury. Have the patient lie on their back and arrange for transport to an appropriate medical facility.

If a small foreign object is lying on the surface of the patient's eye, you can use a **saline** solution, when available, to gently flush the object from the eye. Clean water can also be used, but it tends to irritate the injured eye. Flush from the nose side toward the outside to avoid flushing the object into the other eye. Even small foreign objects can leave a small scratch on the surface of the eye. It is always a good idea to transport the patient to an appropriate medical facility for further assessment and possible treatment.

Occasionally an object will be impaled in the eye. Immediately place the patient on their back and cover the injured eye with a dressing and a paper cup so the impaled object cannot move. Again, remember to bandage both eyes (**FIGURE 14-28**). Arrange for transport of the patient to the hospital.

> **Treatment**
>
> Whenever you must bandage both eyes, explain to the patient why you are doing so. The eyes move in synchrony; bandaging both eyes helps ensure the injured eye remains still by preventing the patient from looking around with the uninjured eye. Keep in mind that having both eyes covered may be distressing to patients, especially children. Stay in contact with the patient to provide reassurance.

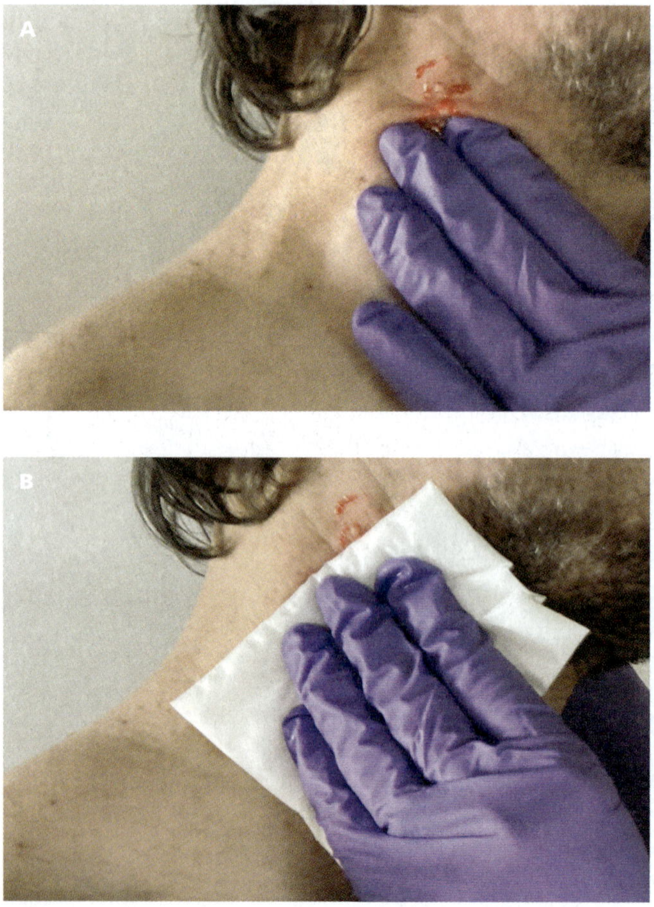

FIGURE 14-29 Dressing a neck wound. **A.** Apply direct pressure over the wound to control bleeding. **B.** Place a dressing over the wound.
© Jones & Bartlett Learning

Neck Wounds

The neck contains many important structures: the trachea, the esophagus, large arteries, veins, muscles, vertebrae, and the spinal cord. Because an injury to any of these structures may be life threatening, all neck injuries are considered serious.

Apply direct pressure to control bleeding neck wounds. Once bleeding is controlled, dress the neck (**FIGURE 14-29**).

In rare cases, you may have to exert finger pressure above and below the injury site to prevent further neck bleeding. Never wrap a dressing around the neck; doing so could affect the patient's breathing or circulation.

Always keep in mind that major trauma to the neck may be associated with airway problems and with neck fracture or spinal cord injury. Therefore, maintain the patient's airway and stabilize the head and neck.

If you see air bubbling or hear air movement into and out of a neck wound, you will need to apply an occlusive dressing (discussed in the next section).

Chest and Back Wounds

The major organs affected by chest wounds and back wounds are the lungs, large blood vessels, and heart. Any wound involving these organs is a life-threatening injury. Place the patient with a chest injury in a comfortable position (usually sitting).

If a lung is punctured, air can escape and the lung can collapse. The patient may cough up bright red blood. To help maintain air pressure in the lung, your first action should be to cover any open chest wound with an airtight material, thereby sealing the wound. This covering is called an **occlusive dressing**. Use a clear plastic cover from your medical supplies, aluminum foil, plastic wrap, gloves, a special dressing that has been impregnated with petroleum jelly (Vaseline), or a commercial chest seal. Any material that occludes (seals off) the wound is sufficient (**FIGURE 14-30**).

Administering oxygen is an important early treatment for a patient with an injured lung. It should be given by EMS personnel when they arrive or by EMRs who are trained and have the equipment available.

Chest wounds may also damage the heart. Seal the wound in the manner described and monitor the patient's ABCs. Treat the patient for shock and perform CPR, if necessary.

If the patient's breathing becomes more labored after you seal the chest wound, you may need to remove the seal briefly to allow excess air to escape and then reseal the wound.

Impaled Objects

If an object is impaled in the patient, apply a stabilizing dressing and arrange for the patient's prompt transport to an appropriate medical facility. Sometimes an impaled object is too long to permit the patient to be removed from the scene and transported to an appropriate medical facility. In these situations, it may be necessary to stabilize the impaled object and carefully cut it close to the patient's body. If you encounter a situation like this, stabilize the impaled object as well as you can and immediately request a specialized rescue team that has the tools and training to handle this type of incident.

Words of Wisdom

Do not remove an impaled object unless it is obstructing the airway or interfering with CPR.

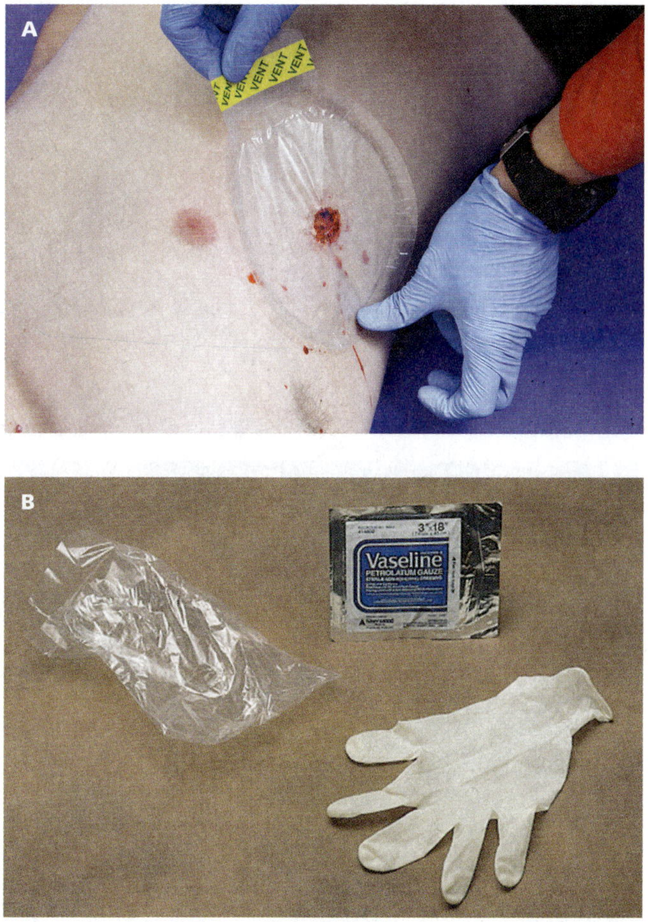

FIGURE 14-30 If a commercial chest seal (**A**) is not available, plastic wrap, a glove, or a dressing impregnated with Vaseline may serve as an occlusive dressing (**B**).

© Jones & Bartlett Learning

If your patient has a knife or other object protruding from the abdomen, do not attempt to remove it. Instead, support the impaled object so it cannot move. Place a large roll of gauze or towels on either side of the object and secure the rolls with additional gauze wrapped around the patient's body, or secure the rolls with wide tape. It is important to stabilize the object so it will not move while the patient is being transported to the hospital (**FIGURE 14-31**). Any movement of the object may cause further internal damage.

Closed Abdominal Wounds

Closed abdominal wounds commonly occur as the result of a direct blow from a blunt object. Check for a closed abdominal wound whenever force has been applied to the abdomen. Look for bruises or other marks on the abdomen that indicate blunt injury.

Any time an injured patient shows signs of shock, you should remember that there may be internal abdominal injuries accompanied by bleeding. When there is internal bleeding, the abdomen may become swollen, rigid, or hard like a board. Treat patients with closed abdominal injuries and signs of shock by placing them on their backs (unless they are having difficulty breathing). Use blankets to help conserve their body heat.

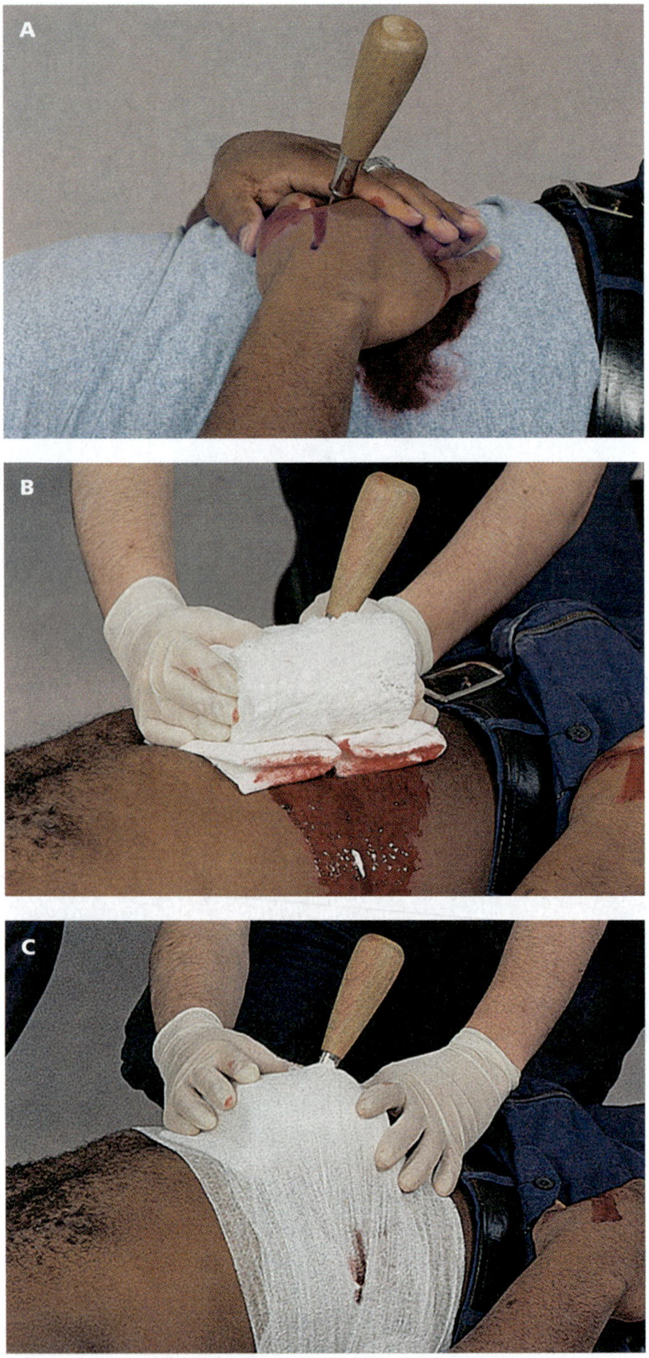

FIGURE 14-31 Bandaging an impaled object. **A.** Do not attempt to remove or move an impaled object. **B.** Stabilize the object in place using a large roll of gauze or towels. **C.** Place a gauze bandage over the dressings or tape the dressings to prevent further movement.

© Jones & Bartlett Learning. Courtesy of MIEMSS.

If the patient is vomiting blood (ranging in color from bright red to dark brown), it may be an indication of bleeding from the esophagus or stomach. Monitor the patient's airway and vital signs carefully because shock may result. Give the patient nothing by mouth. Arrange for prompt transport to an appropriate medical facility.

Open Abdominal Wounds

Open abdominal wounds usually result from slashing with a knife or other sharp object and are always serious injuries.

If the intestines are protruding from the abdomen (an evisceration), place the patient on their back with the knees bent to relax the abdominal muscles. Cover the injured area with a sterile dressing moistened with sterile saline (**FIGURE 14-32**). If sterile saline is not available, cover the injured area with a sterile dressing. Do not attempt to replace the intestines inside the abdomen.

You can make a bandage from a large trauma pad (10 × 30 inches [25 × 76 cm]) and several cravats to cover protruding intestines. Position the trauma pad to cover the whole area of the wound. Tie two or three wide cravats loosely over the trauma pad, just tightly enough to keep it firmly in place, but not tightly enough to push the intestines back into the abdomen. Tape can also be used to secure the trauma dressings in place.

Treatment

To treat an open abdominal wound, follow these steps:

1. Apply a sterile dressing moistened with sterile saline to the wound.
2. Maintain the patient's body temperature.
3. Place the patient on their back with the knees bent.
4. Place the patient who is having difficulty breathing in a semireclining position.
5. Administer oxygen if it is available and you are trained to use it.

Genital Wounds

Both male and female genitals have a rich blood supply. Injury to the genitals often results in severe bleeding. Apply direct pressure to any genital wound with a dry, sterile dressing. Direct pressure usually stops the bleeding. Although it may be awkward to examine the patient's genital area to determine the severity of the injury, you must do so if you suspect such injuries. The patient can experience a critical loss of blood if you do not find the injury and control the bleeding.

Extremity Wounds

To treat all open extremity wounds, apply a dry, sterile compression dressing and bandage it securely in place (**FIGURE 14-33** and **FIGURE 14-34**). Elevate the injured part to help decrease bleeding and swelling. Splint all injured extremities prior to transport because there may be an underlying fracture.

Gunshot Wounds

Some gunshot wounds are easy to miss unless you perform a thorough patient examination (**FIGURE 14-35**). Remember that a great deal of the blood loss and damage to the patient's body may be internal, and therefore not visible. Gunshot wounds of the trunk and neck can cause spinal cord injuries. Because you cannot see the bullet's path through the body, you should treat these patients for spinal cord injuries.

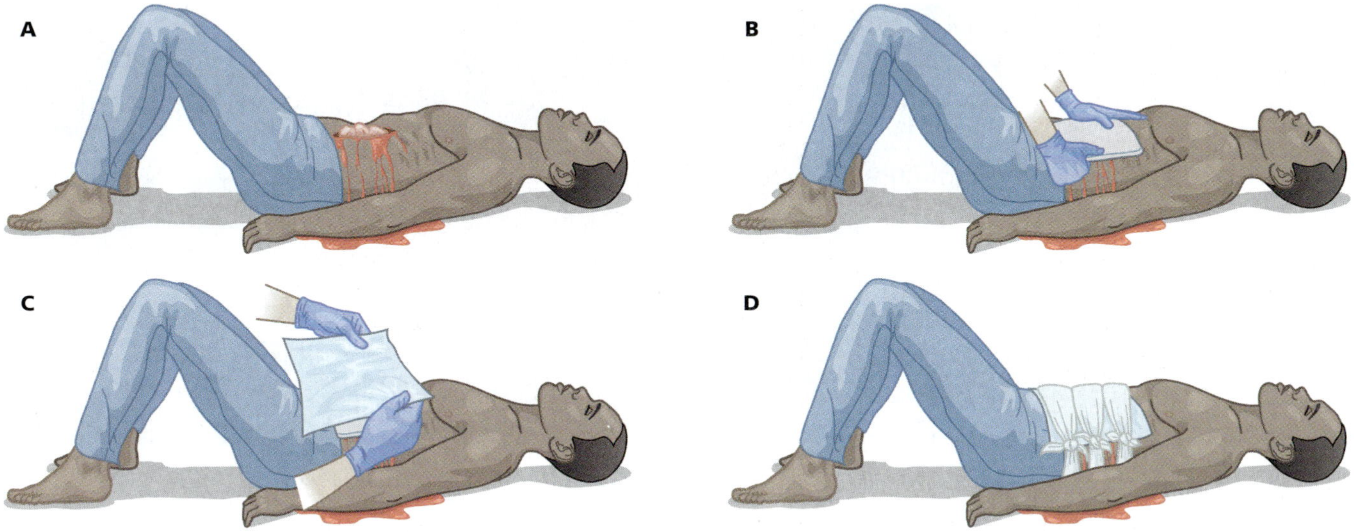

FIGURE 14-32 Bandaging an open abdominal wound. **A.** Place the patient on their back with the knees bent to relax the abdominal muscles. **B.** Cover the injured area with a sterile dressing that has been moistened with sterile saline, if available. Do not attempt to replace the intestines inside the abdomen. **C.** Place a large trauma pad over the wound. **D.** Tape the bandage in place by securing all sides.

© Jones & Bartlett Learning

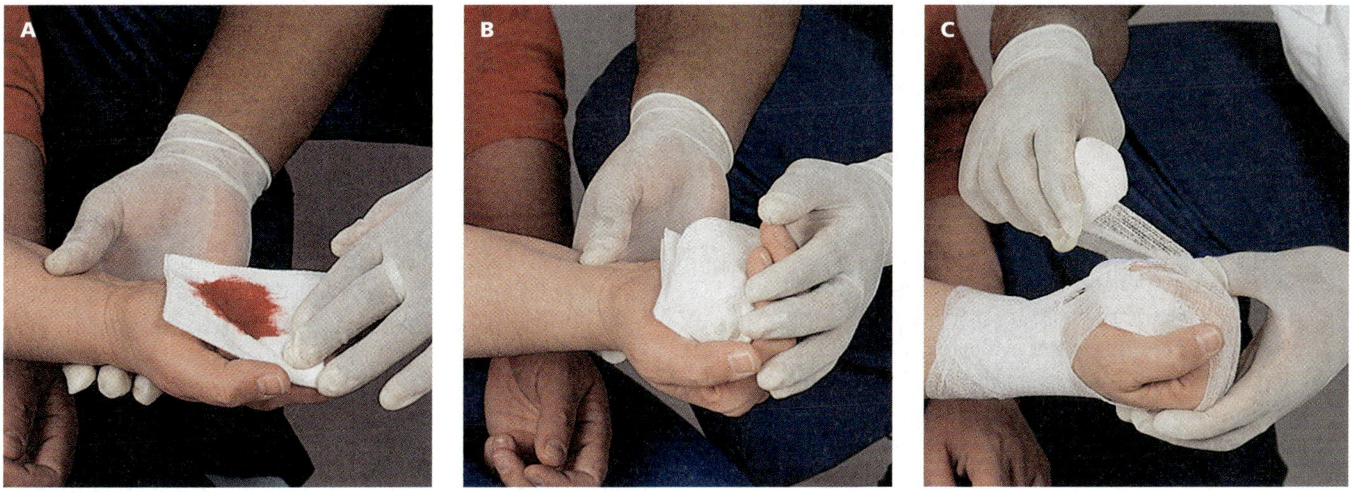

FIGURE 14-33 Bandaging a hand wound. **A.** Place a dressing over the wound. **B.** Place a gauze roll in the palm of the hand to apply pressure. **C.** Secure the dressing with a gauze roller bandage.

© Jones & Bartlett Learning

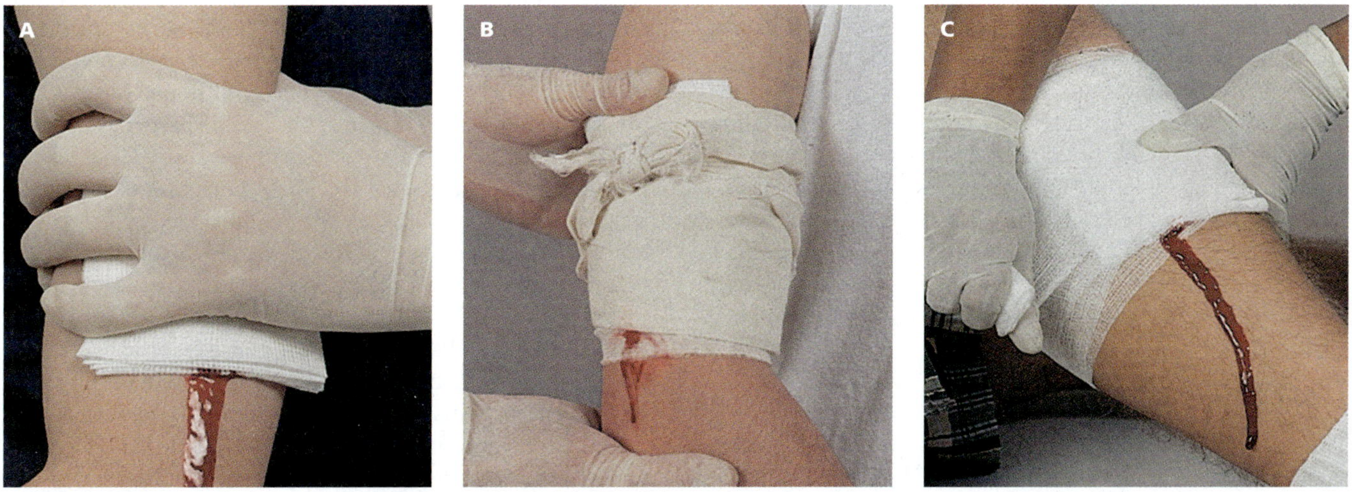

FIGURE 14-34 Bandaging an extremity wound. **A.** Place a dressing over the wound. Secure the dressing using either a cravat (**B**) or a roller bandage (**C**).

© Jones & Bartlett Learning

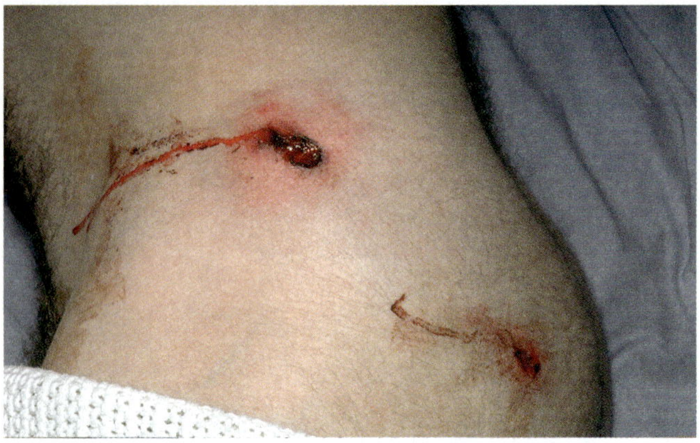

FIGURE 14-35 Bullet entry (smaller) and exit (larger) wounds.
© Mediscan/Alamy Stock Photo

Because gunshot wounds may be serious, prompt and effective treatment is important. To treat a patient with a gunshot wound, follow these steps:

1. Open the airway, and establish adequate ventilation.
2. Control any external bleeding by covering wounds with sterile dressings and applying pressure with your hand or a bandage.
3. Examine the patient thoroughly to ensure that you have discovered all entrance and exit wounds.
4. Treat for signs of shock by performing the following actions:
   - Maintain the patient's body temperature.
   - Place the patient on their back.
   - Place a patient who is having difficulty breathing in a semireclining position.
   - Administer oxygen, if available.
5. Arrange for prompt transport of the patient to an appropriate medical facility.
6. Perform CPR if the patient is pulseless and not breathing.

Bites

Bites from animals or humans may range from minor to severe. All bites carry a high risk of causing infection. **Rabies** can result from the bite of an unvaccinated or wild animal infected with the rabies virus; it is carried by mammals only, including bats, racoons, skunks, and foxes. Minor bites can be washed with soap and water, if they are available. Major bite wounds should be treated by controlling the bleeding and applying a suitable dressing and bandage.

All patients who have been bitten by an animal or another person must be treated by a physician. In most states, EMS or hospital personnel are required to report animal bites to the local health department or a law enforcement agency. Check the laws in your local area to determine requirements.

Burns

The skin serves as a barrier that prevents foreign substances, such as bacteria, from entering the body. It also prevents the loss of body fluids. When the skin is damaged, such as by a burn, it can no longer perform these essential functions.

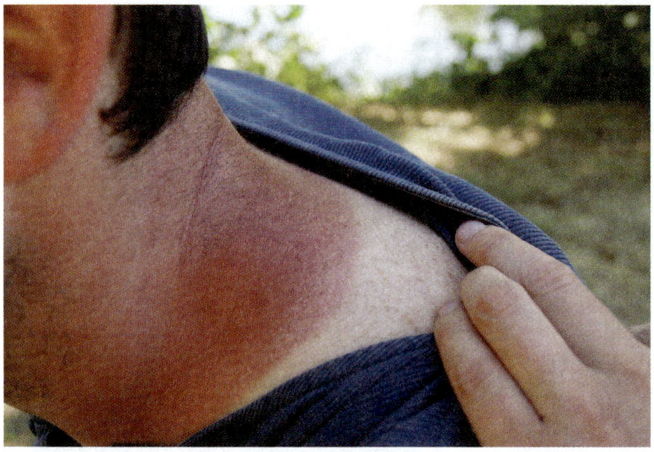

FIGURE 14-36 Superficial burn.
© iama_sing/Shutterstock

Words of Wisdom

Characteristics for burn classification include the following:

- Depth
- Extent (amount of the body injured by the burn)
- Cause or type

Burn Depth

Burns are categorized by depth as superficial burns, partial-thickness burns, and full-thickness burns. Although it is not always possible to determine the exact degree of a burn injury, it is important to understand this concept.

Superficial burns (sometimes called first-degree burns) are characterized by reddened and painful skin. The injury is confined to the outermost layers of skin, and the patient experiences minor to moderate pain. A superficial burn usually heals in about a week, with or without treatment (**FIGURE 14-36**).

Partial-thickness burns (second-degree burns) are further categorized as superficial partial-thickness burns and deep partial-thickness burns. These burns are somewhat deeper but do not damage the deepest layers of the skin (**FIGURE 14-37**). Blistering is present, although blisters may not form for several hours in some cases. There may be some fluid loss and moderate to severe pain because the nerve endings are damaged. Partial-thickness burns require medical treatment. They usually heal within 2 to 3 weeks.

Full-thickness burns (third-degree burns) damage all layers of the skin. In some cases, the damage is deep enough to injure and destroy underlying muscles and other tissues (**FIGURE 14-38**). Pain is often absent because the nerve endings have been destroyed. Without the protection provided by the skin, patients with extensive full-thickness burns lose large quantities of body fluids and are susceptible to shock and infection.

If the patient has injuries in addition to the burn, treat the injuries before transporting the patient. For example, if a

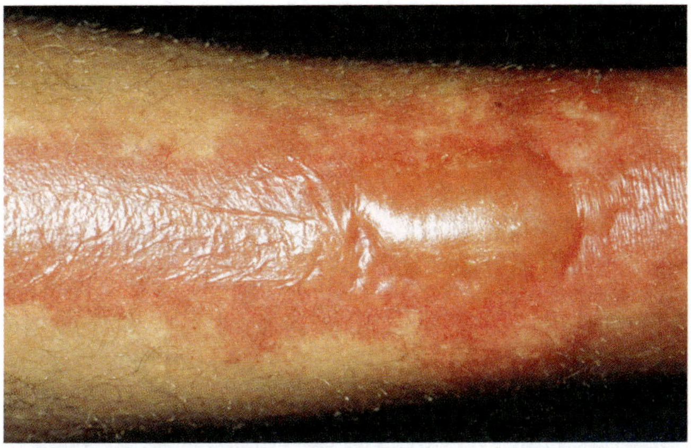

FIGURE 14-37 Partial-thickness burn.
© Dr. P. Marazzi/Science Source

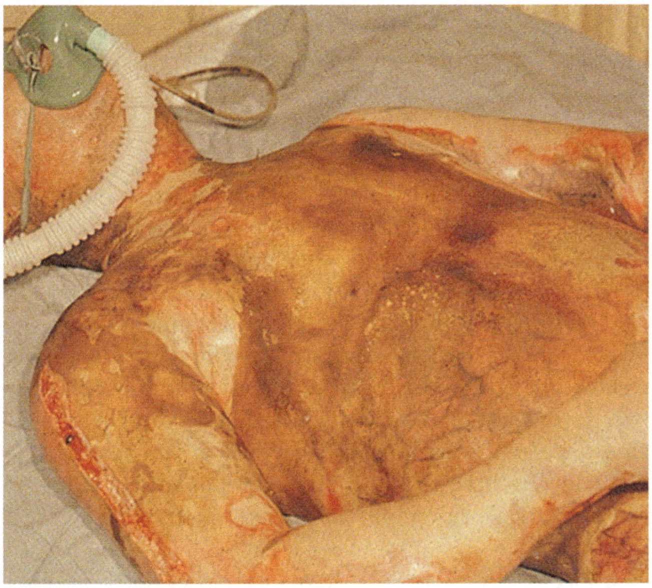

FIGURE 14-38 Full-thickness burn.
© American Academy of Orthopaedic Surgeons

patient who has a partial-thickness burn of the arm has also fallen off a ladder and fractured both legs, splint the fractures and place the patient on a backboard, in addition to treating the burn injury.

Extent of Burns

The **rule of nines** is a method used to determine what percentage of the body has been burned. Although this rule is most useful for EMTs and paramedics who report information to the hospital from the field, you should be able to roughly estimate the extent of a burn. **FIGURE 14-39** shows how the rule of nines divides the body. In an adult, the head and arms each equal 9% of the total body surface. The front and back of the trunk and each leg are equal to 18% of the total body surface. For example, if one-half of the back and the entire right arm of a patient are burned, the burn involves approximately 18% of the total body area. The rule of nines is slightly modified for young children, as shown in the figure.

Cause or Type of Burns

Burns are an injury to body cells caused by excess exposure to heat (thermal burns), chemicals, radiation, or electricity.

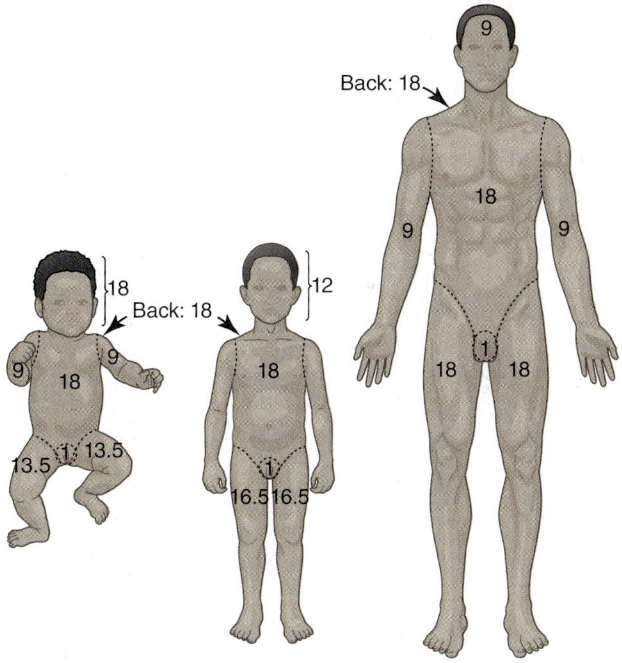

FIGURE 14-39 Use the rule of nines to determine the extent of burns.
© Jones & Bartlett Learning

YOU are the EMR — CASE 3

It is almost midnight on Saturday when you are dispatched to the Friendly Bar & Lounge for a report of a stabbing. Your dispatcher quickly announces that the police have been notified. On the way to the scene, you cannot help but think about scene safety. After a 4-minute response, you arrive at the scene. A quick glance at the parking lot reveals at least four police cars on the scene. An officer approaches your vehicle as you are getting out and tells you the scene is secure. She leads you to an outdoor bench where your patient is sitting. You find a 30- to 35-year-old man, Alex, who is holding his abdomen with both hands. He appears to be in a lot of pain. As you begin to question him, he tells you that he and Marco got into an argument and suddenly Marco pulled out a knife and stabbed him twice in the belly. Your patient exam reveals two small cuts on his stomach. Both cuts are seeping small amounts of blood. Your exam does not reveal additional injuries. Alex's pulse is 84 beats per minute, his blood pressure is 112/74 mm Hg, and his respirations are 22 breaths per minute. He is sweating. You detect a strong odor of alcohol on his breath.

1. What initial treatment can you give to this patient?
2. What additional care does this patient need?

They may involve a small area of the body or involve the entire body. Burns can cause minor injuries affecting only the top layers of the skin, or they can be deep, involving muscles, blood vessels, and nerves. Severe burns can involve damage to all the organs and systems of the body. This section covers the three major causes of burns: heat, chemicals, and electricity. It discusses the effect that the size and severity of the burn have on the patient, as well as the care and treatment you can provide to a burn patient.

Thermal Burns

Thermal burns are caused by heat. The first step in treating thermal burns is to cool the skin by putting out the fire (stop the burning process). Superficial burns can be quite painful, but if there is clean, cold water available, you can place the burned area in cold water to help reduce the pain. You can also wet a clean towel with cold water and put it on superficial burns. After the burned area is cooled, cover it with a dry, sterile dressing or a large sterile cloth called a burn sheet (found in your EMR jump kit).

Treatment

Do not apply burn ointments, butter, grease, or cream to any burn! Unless there is active burning, water or wet dressing should not be applied to any patient with a burn to more than 10% of their body surface area. Applying water can cause the patient to become hypothermic and reduce their chance of survival.

Partial-thickness burns should be cooled if the burn area is still burning. Cooling helps reduce pain, stops the heat from further injuring the skin, and helps stop the swelling caused by partial-thickness burns.

If blisters are present, be very careful not to break the blisters. Intact skin, even if blistered, provides an excellent barrier against infection. If the blisters break, the danger of infection increases. Cover partial-thickness burns with a dry, sterile dressing or burn sheet.

Full-thickness burns, if still burning, should also be cooled with water to keep the heat from damaging more skin and tissue. Cut any clothing away from the burned area, but leave any clothing that is stuck to the burn. Cover full-thickness burns with a dry, sterile dressing or burn sheet (**FIGURE 14-40**).

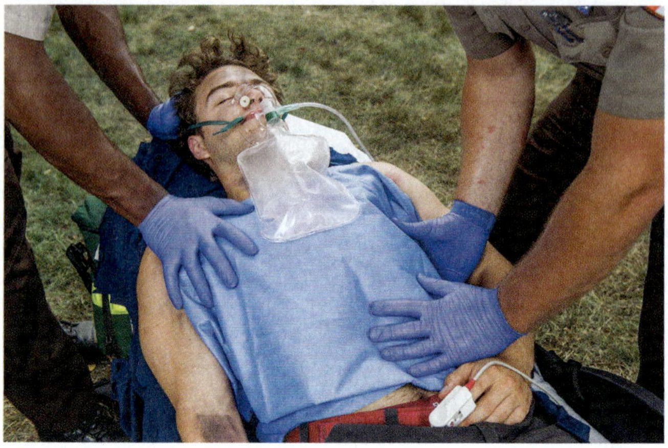

FIGURE 14-40 Applying a sterile burn sheet.
© Jones & Bartlett Learning

Patients with large superficial burns or any partial-thickness or full-thickness burns must be treated for shock and transported to a hospital.

Respiratory Burns

Respiratory burns, sometimes called inhalation burns, are burns to any part of the airway. If a patient has been burned around the head and face or while in a confined space (such as in a burning house), look for the signs and symptoms of respiratory burns listed in the Signs and Symptoms box.

Watch the patient carefully. Breathing problems that result from this type of burn can develop rapidly or slowly over several hours. Administer oxygen as soon as it is available, and be prepared to perform CPR. If you suspect that a patient has been exposed to fire or smoke in a confined space, arrange for prompt transport to a medical facility.

Signs and Symptoms

Signs and symptoms of a respiratory burn include the following:

- Burns around the face
- Singed nose hairs
- Soot in the mouth and nose
- Difficulty breathing
- Pain while breathing
- Noisy breathing (stridor)
- Unresponsiveness

YOU are the EMR — CASE 4

It is 2330 hours and you have been called to the local university for a report of a man who has burns as the result of a dormitory fire. You arrive at the scene to find a 20-year-old man with full-thickness burns to both forearms, from the wrist to the elbow. The patient indicates that while he was sleeping, his electric blanket caught fire. He attempted to put out the fire with his arms, which resulted in the severe burns on his arms. The fire department has extinguished the fire and removed the patient from the burned room.

1. What distinguishes a full-thickness burn from a partial-thickness burn?
2. Why is a person with full-thickness burns at an increased risk for shock?

Chemical Burns

Many strong substances can cause **chemical burns** to the skin, and chemicals are extremely dangerous to the eyes. These substances include strong acids such as battery acid or strong alkalis such as drain cleaners. Some chemicals are so strong or caustic that they can cause damage to the skin or eyes even if the exposure is very brief. The longer the chemical remains in contact with the skin, the more it damages the skin and underlying tissues, often resulting in superficial, partial-thickness, or full-thickness burns to the skin.

The initial treatment for chemical burns is to remove as much of the chemical as possible from the patient's skin. Brush away any dry chemical on the patient's clothes or skin, being careful not to get any on yourself. You may have to ask the patient to remove all clothing. Do not pull any clothing over the patient's head; doing so could cause chemicals on the shirt to be introduced into the eyes, nose, or mouth.

After you have removed as much of the dry chemical as possible, flush the contaminated skin with abundant quantities of water. Use water from a garden hose, a shower in the home or factory, or even the booster hose of a fire engine. It is essential that the chemical be washed off the skin quickly to avoid further injury. Flush the affected area of the body for at least 10 minutes, then cover the burned area with a dry, sterile dressing or a burn sheet and arrange for prompt transport to an appropriate medical facility.

> **Safety**
>
> Chemical burns are caused by hazardous materials. In situations like this, special protective equipment may be required. Follow your local protocols for these situations.

Chemical burns to the eyes cause extreme pain and severe injury. Gently flush the affected eye or eyes with water for at least 20 minutes (**FIGURE 14-41**). Hold the eye open to allow water to flow over its entire surface. Direct the water from the inner corner of the eye to the outward edge of the eye to avoid contaminating the unaffected eye. You may have to put the patient's face under a shower, garden hose, or faucet so the water flows across the patient's entire face. Continue flushing the eyes while the patient is being transported.

After flushing the eyes for 20 minutes, loosely cover the injured eye or eyes with gauze bandages and arrange for prompt transport to an appropriate medical facility. All chemical burns should be examined by a physician.

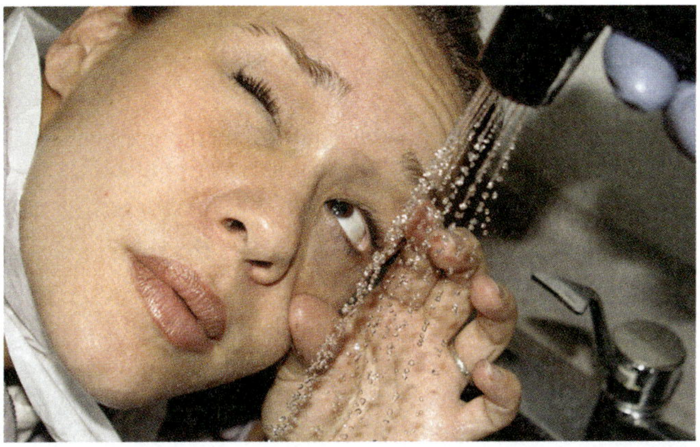

FIGURE 14-41 Flushing the eyes with water.

© American Academy of Orthopaedic Surgeons

Electrical Burns

Electrical burns can cause severe injuries or even death, but they leave little evidence of injury on the outside of the body. These burns are caused by an electrical current that enters the body at one point (for example, the hand that touches a live electrical wire), travels through the body tissues and organs, and exits from the body at the point of ground contact (**FIGURE 14-42**).

Electricity causes major internal damage, rather than external damage. A strong electrical current can actually "cook" muscles, nerves, blood vessels, and internal organs, resulting in major damage. Patients who have been subjected to a strong electrical current can also experience irregularities of cardiac rhythm or even full cardiac arrest and death. Children often sustain electrical burns by chewing on an electrical cord or by pushing something into an outlet. Although the burn may not look serious at first, it is often quite severe because of underlying tissue injury.

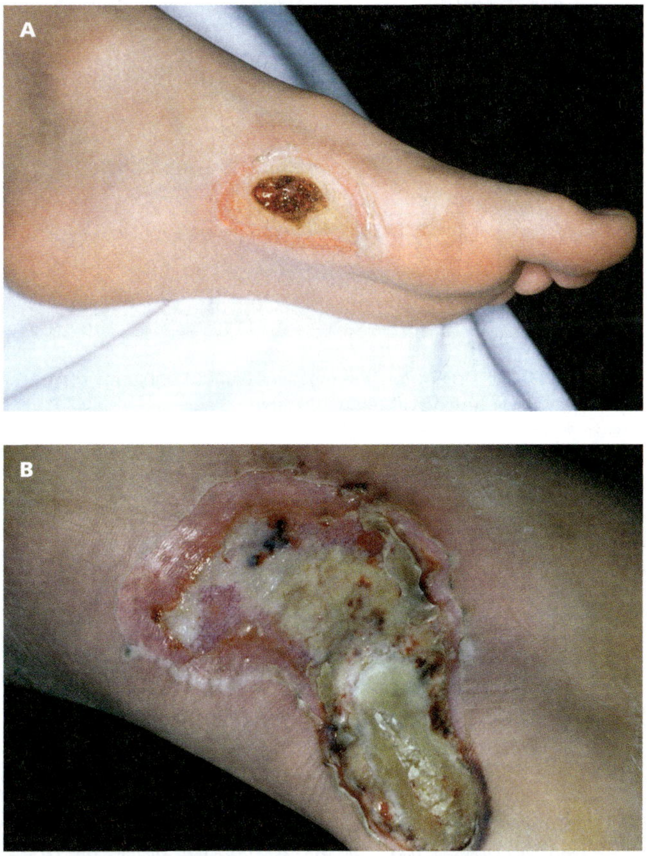

FIGURE 14-42 Electrical burns. **A.** An entrance wound is often small. **B.** An exit wound (as shown here, the other side of the foot shown in part A) can be extensive and deep.

© Charles Stewart, MD, EMDM, MPH

Persons who have been hit or nearly hit by lightning frequently sustain electrical burns. Treat these patients as you would electrical burn patients. Evaluate them carefully because they may also experience cardiac arrest. Arrange for prompt transport to an appropriate medical facility.

Safety

Avoid direct or indirect contact with live electrical wires. Direct contact occurs when you touch a live electrical wire. Indirect contact occurs when you touch a vehicle, a patient, a fence, a tree, or any other object that is in contact with a live electrical wire.

Before you touch or treat a person who has sustained an electrical burn, be certain the patient is not still in contact with the electrical power source that caused the burn. If the patient is still in contact with the power source, anyone who touches the patient may be electrocuted. If the patient is touching a live power source, your first act must be to unplug, disconnect, or turn off the power (**FIGURE 14-43**).

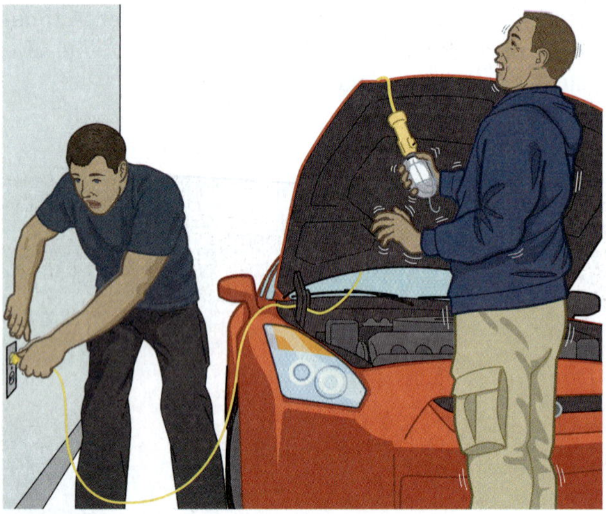

FIGURE 14-43 Do not touch the patient without unplugging, disconnecting, or turning off the power first.
© Jones & Bartlett Learning

If you cannot do this alone, call for assistance from the power company or from a qualified rescue squad or fire department.

After ensuring that the power has been disconnected, examine each electrical burn patient carefully, assess the ABCs, and treat the patient for visible, external burns. Cover these external burns with a dry, sterile dressing and arrange for prompt transport to an appropriate medical facility.

Monitor the ABCs of patients with an electrical burn closely, and arrange to have these patients transported promptly to an appropriate medical facility for further treatment.

Safety

When a power line falls across a vehicle, the occupants inside are safe from electrocution as long as the rubber tires are in contact with the ground and the occupants stay inside the vehicle. Stay away from the scene and use a public address system or yell to instruct the vehicle occupants to stay inside until the electric company arrives and ensures the line is no longer charged.

Multisystem Trauma

Multisystem trauma is an injury that affects more than one body system. The injuries in multisystem trauma can occur in one part of the body but involve different body systems. For example, an unrestrained patient who hits the steering wheel in a motor vehicle crash can sustain trauma to the chest. This trauma could result in injuries to the ribs (the musculoskeletal system), the heart (the circulatory system), and the lungs (the respiratory system). Another patient in a vehicle crash might have injuries to different parts of body, for example, to the abdomen and to the head. Both patients have sustained multisystem trauma. As an EMR, you are not expected to diagnose a patient's injuries. However, it is important to remember that several body systems may be injured in situations that involve significant trauma. As you assess your patients, be alert for signs and symptoms of injury to each part of the body.

YOU are the EMR SUMMARY

You are the EMR: CASE 1

1. **What safety considerations should you keep in mind as you approach this situation?**

   Ensure that the scene is safe for you, the patient, and bystanders. As you approach the scene, ensure that there are no objects that can fall from above. Be certain that all power tools are turned off and unplugged. Be certain the saw blade and other sharp objects are out of the way. Take standard precautions to prevent the spread of bloodborne diseases. Remember to wear gloves to protect yourself from contact with blood. If there is a chance of blood splatter, consider the need for eye protection.

2. **What equipment and supplies do you want to take with you?**

   For an incident such as this, there are three types of equipment you should take with you: equipment to maintain standard precautions, supplies for wound treatment, and equipment to treat the patient for shock. The equipment for standard precautions includes latex or nitrile gloves,

YOU are the EMR **SUMMARY**

mask, and eye protection for any possible blood splatter. Wound treatment equipment should include an adequate supply of dressings and bandages to treat the wound and supplies to stabilize the affected extremity. Equipment to treat for shock should include blankets to preserve body heat, a blood pressure cuff to assess blood pressure, and oxygen administration equipment if it is available and you have been trained in its use.

3. What are your treatment goals for this incident?

The goals for this incident include maintaining standard precautions, treating soft-tissue injuries by controlling external bleeding, preventing further contamination of the wound site, stabilizing the affected extremity, and treating the patient for shock.

You are the EMR: CASE 2

1. What are your initial steps in treating this patient?

Your initial treatment steps should include the following: ensure scene safety; look for any additional hidden weapons as you approach to examine the patient; take standard precautions to prevent contact with blood; control the external bleeding by placing a dressing over the wound, applying direct pressure, and then applying a pressure dressing; treat the patient for shock by placing him either in a supine position or a reclining position if he is having difficulty breathing and maintaining body temperature; take an initial set of vital signs; and ensure that an EMS transport unit is responding.

2. How serious is an injury like this?

A gunshot wound to the thigh is a serious injury. You cannot determine the pathway of the bullet or the parts of the leg that have been damaged. There is the possibility that the bullet may have traveled into the abdomen and caused additional damage. This type of injury often causes a significant amount of internal blood loss. There are no good ways for you to measure this blood loss. It is important for you to take repeat vital signs every 5 minutes to monitor the patient for signs of shock. The initial signs and symptoms of shock include: skin that is cool, clammy, or pale compared with patient baseline; increased heart rate and respiratory rate; and a sense of anxiety. It is also important to arrange for prompt transport to an appropriate medical facility as soon as possible.

You are the EMR: CASE 3

1. What initial treatment can you give to this patient?

After you have completed your assessment of this patient, you need to put the pieces together to determine what type of injury you have found and then develop a treatment plan. This patient has two small wounds in his abdomen, reportedly from a knife. There is no way for you to determine how deep these wounds are, what organs have been damaged, or the amount of internal blood loss he has sustained. You need to understand that this type of wound can result in profound shock from internal blood loss; therefore, your actions are to treat the patient for shock by placing him in a comfortable position—often for this type of injury, it will be lying supine with his legs drawn up or reclining—and maintaining his body temperature. Monitor his ABCs. Monitor his vital signs every 5 minutes and be alert for the possibility that his vital signs may change rapidly. Apply a dressing to the abdominal wounds. Maintain standard precautions. Finally, ensure that this patient is promptly transported to a trauma center that can provide evaluation and needed treatment.

2. What additional care does this patient need?

ALS clinicians can provide additional treatment for shock by administering IV fluids. However, the care most needed by this patient can be provided only by a surgeon in an operating room. In the hospital, this patient will need to be taken into surgery to determine the extent of the damage to his abdominal organs and to stop the internal bleeding by surgically repairing the damaged organs. If not treated promptly and properly, life-threatening infections can develop in this patient. Therefore, it is important for you to arrange for prompt transport of this patient to a trauma center as soon as possible while continuing to monitor his vital signs and treating him for shock. If internal blood loss continues, his condition may deteriorate quickly.

You are the EMR: CASE 4

1. What distinguishes a full-thickness burn from a partial-thickness burn?

In partial-thickness burns, the burned area is very painful, the skin will be red, and blisters will form within a few hours. Full-thickness burns penetrate down through the dermis and epidermis, often into the underlying subcutaneous tissue, muscle, and bone. Full-thickness burns are usually blackened or charred. Pain in the burned area may be absent or diminished because of damage to the nerve endings. Often, it will not be possible to determine the thickness of burns immediately after they occur.

2. Why is a person with full-thickness burns at an increased risk for shock?

The integrity of the skin has been compromised in a full-thickness burn, allowing fluids to escape. The loss of body fluids can lead to hypovolemic shock. Severe infections can also develop in these patients if they do not receive proper and timely treatment.

Prep Kit

Ready for Review

- When caring for a patient who is bleeding or has sustained a soft-tissue injury, take standard precautions to prevent contact with the patient's body fluids.
- The three parts of the circulatory system are the pump (heart), the pipes (arteries, veins, and capillaries), and the fluid (blood cells and other blood components).
- Shock is a state of collapse of the cardiovascular system that results in inadequate delivery of blood to the organs. The three primary causes of shock are pump failure, pipe failure, and fluid loss. The general treatment for shock is positioning the patient correctly, maintaining the patient's ABCs, and treating the cause of shock, if possible.
- There are three types of external blood loss: capillary (blood oozes out), venous (bleeds at a steady flow), and arterial (blood spurts or surges). Most external bleeding can be controlled by applying direct pressure to the wound.
- A wound is an injury caused by any physical means that leads to damage of a body part. Wounds are classified as closed (skin is not broken) or open (skin is broken). Open wounds are classified as abrasions, punctures, lacerations, and avulsions or amputations.
- Control bleeding by covering an open wound with a dry, clean, or sterile dressing and apply pressure to the dressing with your hand. Additional ways to control bleeding include elevating an extremity, applying a tourniquet, and using pressure points.
- Burns are categorized by depth as superficial (first-degree) burns, partial-thickness (second-degree) burns, and full-thickness (third-degree) burns. Burns may be caused by heat, chemicals, or electricity.
- By learning to recognize and provide initial emergency treatment for patients experiencing shock, bleeding, and soft-tissue injuries, you will be able to provide physical and emotional assistance to these patients in their time of need. Your prompt recognition and treatment can significantly improve the patient's outcome.
- Injuries that affect more than one body system are called multisystem trauma. Multisystem trauma may be a result of an injury to one part of the body or may be caused by injuries to different parts of the body.

Vital Vocabulary

abrasion Loss or damage of skin as a result of a body part being rubbed or scraped across a rough or hard surface.

anaphylactic shock A type of shock caused by an extreme allergic reaction to certain foods, medications, or insect bites and stings.

arterial bleeding Serious bleeding from an artery in which blood frequently pulses or spurts from an open wound.

atria The two upper chambers of the heart.

avulsion An injury in which a piece of skin is torn completely loose or is left hanging as a flap.

blood pressure The pressure of the circulating blood against the walls of the arteries.

bruise Injury caused by a blunt object striking the body and crushing the tissue beneath the skin; also called a contusion.

capillary bleeding Bleeding from the capillaries in which blood oozes from the open wound.

cardiogenic shock A type of shock resulting from inadequate functioning of the heart.

chemical burns Burns that occur when any toxic substance comes in contact with the skin. Most chemical burns are caused by strong acids or alkalis.

closed wound Injury in which soft-tissue damage occurs beneath the skin but there is no break in the surface of the skin.

cravat A swathe of cloth made by folding a triangular bandage; applied around the injured body part to stabilize the injury or secure other dressing/bandaging materials over a wound.

dressing Any of various materials placed directly on a wound to control bleeding and prevent further contamination.

electrical burns Burns caused by an electrical current that enters the body at one point (producing an entrance wound), travels through the body tissues and organs, and exits the body (producing an exit wound).

entrance wound The point where an object such as a bullet enters the body.

exit wound The point where an object such as a bullet passes out of the body.

full-thickness burns Burns that extend through the skin and into the underlying tissues; the most serious class of burns.

gunshot wound A puncture wound caused by a bullet or shotgun pellets.

Prep Kit

heart failure Heart disease characterized by breathlessness, fluid retention in the lungs, and generalized swelling of the body.

hemorrhage Excessive bleeding.

hemostatic agents Chemical compounds that slow or stop bleeding by assisting with clot formation.

hypothermia A condition in which the internal (or core) body temperature falls below 95°F (35°C) after prolonged exposure to cool or freezing temperatures.

impaled object An object such as a knife, splinter of wood, or glass that penetrates the skin and remains in the body.

incision A type of laceration that is made with a sharp object such as a knife.

intravenous (IV) fluids Fluids other than blood or blood products infused into the vascular system to maintain an adequate circulatory blood volume.

laceration An open wound caused by a sharp object or by blunt force; can have ragged or sharp edges.

multisystem trauma An injury that affects more than one body system.

neurogenic shock A type of shock in which injury to the spinal cord allows the vessels to expand, causing blood to pool below the level of the injury. The brain, heart, lungs, and other vital organs are deprived of blood.

occlusive dressing An airtight dressing or bandage for a wound.

open wound Injury that breaks open the skin or mucous membrane.

partial-thickness burns Burns in which the outer layers of skin are burned; these burns are characterized by blister formation.

pressure point An anatomic location where a blood vessel lies near a bone; pressure can be applied to this point to help control bleeding.

psychogenic shock A type of shock caused by a temporary reduction in blood supply to the brain; commonly referred to as fainting.

puncture A wound resulting from a bullet, knife, ice pick, splinter, or any other pointed object.

rabies An acute viral infection of the central nervous system transmitted by the bite of an infected animal.

respiratory burns Burns to the respiratory system that result from inhaling superheated air.

road rash An abrasion caused by sliding on pavement. Usually seen after motorcycle or bicycle accidents.

rule of nines A means of calculating the amount of body surface burned; for adults, the body is divided into sections, each of which constitutes approximately 9% or 18% of the total body surface area; these percentages vary slightly for children.

saline Salt water.

sepsis A severe complication of infection that occurs when chemicals are released into the bloodstream and trigger an inflammatory response throughout the body.

septic shock A type of shock in which the blood pressure drops dramatically as a result of severe infection; often results in death.

shock A state of collapse of the cardiovascular system; the state of inadequate delivery of blood to the organs of the body.

splint A means of stabilizing an injured body part by using a rigid or soft support.

spontaneous nosebleed A nosebleed with no apparent cause.

superficial burns Burns in which only the outermost layers of skin are injured.

thermal burns Burns caused by heat; the most common type of burn.

venous bleeding External bleeding from a vein, characterized by steady flow; the bleeding may be profuse and life threatening.

ventricles The two lower chambers of the heart.

References

American Heart Association (AHA). *2020 Handbook of Emergency Cardiovascular Care*. Dallas, TX: AHA; 2020.

American Heart Association (AHA). *Pediatric Advanced Life Support Provider Manual*. Dallas, TX: AHA; 2020.

Guidelines for burn patient referral. American Burn Association website. https://ameriburn.org/resources/burnreferral/. Published 2022. Accessed March 26, 2025.

How to stop the bleeding in small and deep cuts. Cleveland Clinic website. https://health.clevelandclinic.org/how-to-stop-bleeding. Published October 27, 2021. Accessed January 23, 2024.

National Association of Emergency Medical Technicians. *PHTLS: Prehospital Trauma Life Support*. 10th ed. Burlington, MA: Jones & Bartlett Learning; 2023.

Prep Kit

Nosebleed (epistaxis). Cleveland Clinic website. https://my.clevelandclinic.org/health/diseases/13464-nosebleed-epistaxis. Reviewed December 18, 2024. Accessed January 23, 2024.

Pikman Gavriely R, Lior Y, Gelikas S, et al. Manual pressure points technique for massive hemorrhage control: a prospective human volunteer study. *Prehosp Emerg Care*. 2023;27(5):586–591.

Shock first aid treatment. Cleveland Clinic website. https://my.clevelandclinic.org/health/treatments/24055-shock-first-aid-treatment. Reviewed August 24, 2022. Accessed January 23, 2024.

Thompson P, Glassberg E, Alon Y, et al. The effectiveness of the manual pressure points technique for hemorrhage control: the 2022 THOR pre-conference meeting experience. *Transfusion*. 2023;63 Suppl 3:S222–S229.

Wang EN, Chan C, Anand S, et al. Considerations in the management of shock in the pediatric trauma patient. *Pediatr Emerg Med Rep*. 2006;11(11):129–144.

Assessment IN ACTION

You are dispatched to a lumberyard for a report of a log falling on a person. On arrival, you find a 21-year-old man lying in the supine position on the floor, holding his abdomen and reporting severe pain. He is also holding a blood-soaked T-shirt to his right forearm. Your primary assessment reveals a bruise approximately 3 inches (8 cm) in diameter to the right upper quadrant of the abdomen and a 1.5-inch (4-cm) flap of skin and fat that is loosely attached on his right arm, 2 inches (5 cm) below the elbow. Physical exam reveals a rigid abdomen. The patient has no pain in his head, neck, or spine. (Questions 1–5 relate to this scenario.)

1. What is your first concern as you arrive at the scene?

- **A.** The patient is bleeding profusely.
- **B.** How many patients are there?
- **C.** Do I have all the resources I need?
- **D.** Is the scene safe?

2. What is your primary concern about this patient?

- **A.** His back may be injured.
- **B.** He is bleeding into the abdomen and may go into shock.
- **C.** The cut on his arm may need a tourniquet.
- **D.** He is in a significant amount of pain.

3. What type of standard precaution is NOT needed when treating this patient?

- **A.** Gloves
- **B.** Eye protection
- **C.** Gown
- **D.** Steel-toed shoes

4. Which of the following is NOT a major principle of open wound treatment?

- **A.** Apply ice.
- **B.** Prevent further contamination of the wound.
- **C.** Stabilize the injured part.
- **D.** Stabilize any impaled object.

5. What type of wound does this patient have on his arm?

- **A.** Avulsion
- **B.** Amputation
- **C.** Laceration
- **D.** Impaled object

6. In which type of burn is the outer layer of skin burned, resulting in a blister formation?

- **A.** Superficial burn
- **B.** Partial-thickness burn
- **C.** Third-degree burn
- **D.** Full-thickness burn

7. Neck injuries may be life threatening because:

- **A.** they are close to the brain.
- **B.** they may result in injury to the parasympathetic nervous system.
- **C.** the neck contains many important structures.
- **D.** they result in shock.

8. Put the following steps for treating an impaled object in the proper order.

1. Stabilize the object in place with dressings.
2. Provide prompt transport to an appropriate medical facility.
3. Do not attempt to remove the impaled object.
4. Place a bandage over the dressings.

- **A.** 1, 4, 2, 3
- **B.** 3, 1, 4, 2
- **C.** 2, 3, 4, 1
- **D.** 3, 2, 1, 4

9. Which of the following is NOT a recommended treatment for an open abdominal wound?

- **A.** Bandage the abdomen with a large trauma pad and several cravats.
- **B.** Place the patient on their back with the knees drawn up.
- **C.** Cover the intestines with a sterile dressing.
- **D.** Attempt to replace the intestines back in the abdomen.

10. Which of the following statements is NOT true about a patient who has come in contact with an electrical current?

- **A.** Electrical current often produces severe burns.
- **B.** Contact with an electrical current leaves little evidence of injury on the outside of the body.
- **C.** Electrical current may produce entrance and exit wounds.
- **D.** Most of the injury from electricity is to the skin.

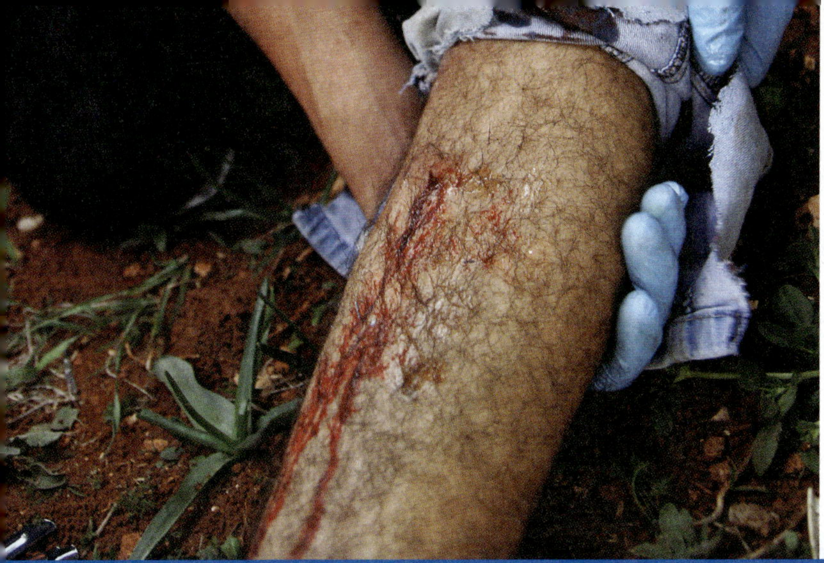

CHAPTER 15

Injuries to Muscles and Bones

National EMS Education Standard Competencies

Trauma

Uses knowledge to recognize and manage life threats based on assessment findings for an acutely injured patient while awaiting additional emergency medical response.

Orthopaedic Trauma

- Open fractures (pp 336–337)
- Closed fractures (pp 336–337)
- Dislocations (p 337; pp 343–344; pp 347–348)
- Amputations (p 311; Chapter 14, *Bleeding, Shock, and Soft-Tissue Injuries*)

Head, Facial, Neck, and Spine Trauma

- Life threats (pp 353–360)
- Spine trauma (pp 356–360)

Nervous System Trauma

- Traumatic brain injury (pp 353–356)

Medicine

Recognizes and manages life threats based on assessment findings of a patient with a medical emergency while awaiting additional emergency response.

Nontraumatic Musculoskeletal Disorders

- Nontraumatic fractures (pp 337–351)

Knowledge Objectives

1. Discuss the anatomy and function of the musculoskeletal system. (pp 333–335)
2. Describe the mechanisms of injury for musculoskeletal injuries. (pp 335–336)
3. Explain the characteristics of the following types of injuries:
   - Fractures (p 336)
   - Dislocations (pp 336–337)
   - Sprains and strains (p 337)
4. Explain the need for standard precautions when assessing or treating patients with musculoskeletal injuries. (pp 337–340)
5. Explain how to assess a patient with a musculoskeletal injury. (p 337)
6. Explain how to check circulation, sensation, and movement in an injured extremity. (pp 338–340)
7. Describe how a properly applied splint secures both the fractured bone and the joints above and below the fracture site. (p 340)
8. List the signs and symptoms of open and closed head injuries. (pp 354–355)
9. Describe the treatment of head injuries. (pp 354–355)
10. Describe the treatment of facial injuries. (p 356)
11. Discuss the mechanism of spinal injuries. (pp 356–357)
12. List the signs and symptoms of spinal injury. (p 357)
13. Describe the treatment of spinal injury. (p 357)
14. Explain how to remove the mask on a sports helmet. (pp 357–359)
15. Explain how to remove a helmet. (pp 358–360)
16. Describe the signs, symptoms, and treatment of the following injuries:
    - Fractured ribs (p 360)
    - Flail chest (pp 360–361)
    - Penetrating chest wound (pp 361–362)

Skills Objectives

1. Demonstrate use of standard precautions when assessing or treating patients with musculoskeletal injuries. (p 337)
2. Demonstrate assessment of a patient with a musculoskeletal injury. (pp 337–340)

© Abdalkarim Museitef/Pacific Press/AP Photo

3. Demonstrate how to check circulation, sensation, and movement in an injured extremity. (pp 338–340; Skill Drill 15-1)
4. Demonstrate how to apply various types of splints. (pp 342–349; Skill Drills 15-2, 15-4, 15-5, and 15-6)
5. Demonstrate how to splint the following injuries:
   - Shoulder girdle injury (p 343)
   - Shoulder dislocation (pp 343–344)
   - Elbow injury (p 344)
   - Forearm injury (pp 344–345; Skill Drill 15-3)
   - Hand, wrist, or finger injury (pp 344–345)
   - Pelvic fracture (pp 345–346)
   - Hip injury (p 347)
   - Thigh injury (pp 348–349)
   - Knee injury (pp 348–350)
   - Leg injury (p 350; Skill Drill 15-7)
   - Ankle or foot injury (pp 350–351; Skill Drill 15-8)
6. Demonstrate the treatment of head injuries. (p 355)
7. Demonstrate the treatment of facial injuries. (p 356)
8. Demonstrate the treatment of spinal injury. (pp 357–358; Skill Drill 15-9)
9. Demonstrate how to remove the mask on a sports helmet. (p 359; Skill Drill 15-10)
10. Demonstrate how to remove a helmet. (pp 359–360; Skill Drill 15-11)
11. Demonstrate treatment of the following injuries:
    - Fractured ribs (p 360)
    - Flail chest (pp 360–361)
    - Penetrating chest wound (pp 361–362)

Introduction

As an emergency medical responder (EMR), you will encounter many types of musculoskeletal injuries, including fractures, dislocations, sprains, strains, head injuries, spinal cord injuries, and chest injuries. Providing proper care at the scene can prevent additional injury or disability; however, before you can treat musculoskeletal injuries, you must be able to identify the problem and the appropriate care. Doing so requires an understanding of the basic anatomy and functioning of the musculoskeletal system as well as the causes, or mechanisms, of injury. Finally, it requires a familiarity with the signs and symptoms of specific injuries.

This chapter describes how to manage injuries to the upper and lower extremities, the head, the spinal cord, and the chest. It also provides information on standard precautions and the steps you must take to protect yourself when caring for patients with musculoskeletal injuries.

Patient Assessment of Injuries to Muscles and Bones

When assessing a patient who has sustained an injury to the muscles and bones, you need to complete all five of the parts of the patient assessment sequence (**FIGURE 15-1**). Begin with a thorough overview of the scene. This can often give you valuable information about the intensity and force of the incident. Do not get tunnel vision because the patient has an obvious injury. You need to complete all parts of the scene assessment to render the scene safe and to gain as much information as you can about the mechanism of injury. Be especially careful about taking standard precautions to protect yourself and the patient from infectious diseases. When a patient has sustained a traumatic injury, there is a high chance that blood will be present.

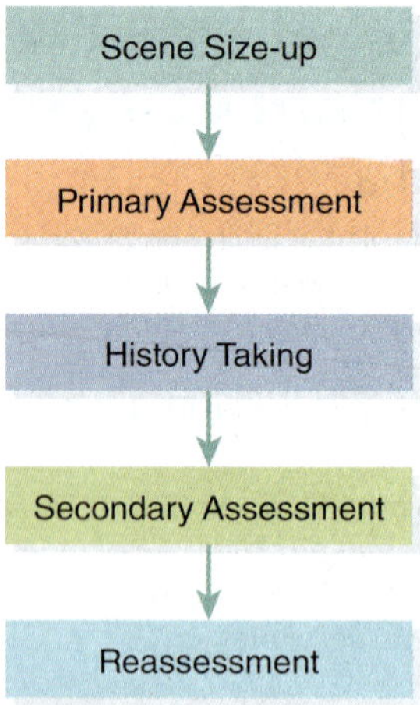

FIGURE 15-1 Patient assessment sequence.
© Jones & Bartlett Learning

Perform a complete primary assessment to determine whether the patient has any life-threatening conditions related to the airway, breathing, or circulation (ABCs), including serious blood loss. Remember, if the patient is experiencing life-threatening bleeding, the ABC sequence is adjusted to XABC, where *X* (for eXsanguination) becomes the first priority. Regardless of the abbreviation used, EMRs must check for and control *any* serious bleeding as part of the primary assessment.

A patient who has an obvious soft-tissue injury or deformity of a limb may focus on that single injury and not be aware of additional conditions. These additional conditions may be more serious than the presenting problem (the chief complaint).

When performing a patient assessment on a trauma patient, it is often more efficient and helpful to perform the primary assessment and then immediately follow with the secondary assessment, holding off on obtaining the patient's medical history. Reordering the steps in this manner will give you a complete picture of all the physical findings about the patient. While you perform the secondary assessment, be thorough and systematic in examining all parts of the patient. However, do not get tunnel vision and assume that a trauma patient has no medical conditions. Heart conditions and low blood glucose levels in patients with diabetes can result in traumatic events. Be sure to perform a thorough SAMPLE (Signs and symptoms, Allergies, Medications, Pertinent past medical history, Last oral intake, Events leading up to the illness or injury) medical history to determine whether the patient has any medical conditions that require attention. Finally, continue to reassess the patient every 15 minutes if the patient's condition is stable and every 5 minutes if the condition is unstable until other medical clinicians take over the care of the patient.

The Anatomy and Function of the Musculoskeletal System

The musculoskeletal system has two parts: the skeletal system, which provides support and form for the body, and the muscular system, which provides both support and movement.

The Skeletal System

The skeletal system consists of 206 bones and is the supporting framework for the body. The four functions of the skeletal system are:

1. To support the body
2. To protect vital structures
3. To assist in body movement
4. To manufacture red blood cells

The skeletal system is divided into seven areas (**FIGURE 15-2**):

1. Head, skull, and face
2. Spinal column
3. Shoulder girdle
4. Upper extremities
5. Rib cage (thorax)
6. Pelvis
7. Lower extremities

The bones of the head include the skull and the lower jawbone. The skull consists of many bones fused together to form a hollow sphere. It contains and protects the brain. The jawbone is a movable bone attached to the skull that completes the structure of the face.

The spine consists of a series of separate bones called vertebrae. The spinal vertebrae are stacked on top of each other. Muscles, tendons, disks, and ligaments hold them together. The spinal cord, a group of nerves that carry messages to and from the brain, passes through a hole in the center of each vertebra. In addition to protecting the spinal cord, the spine is the primary support structure for the entire body.

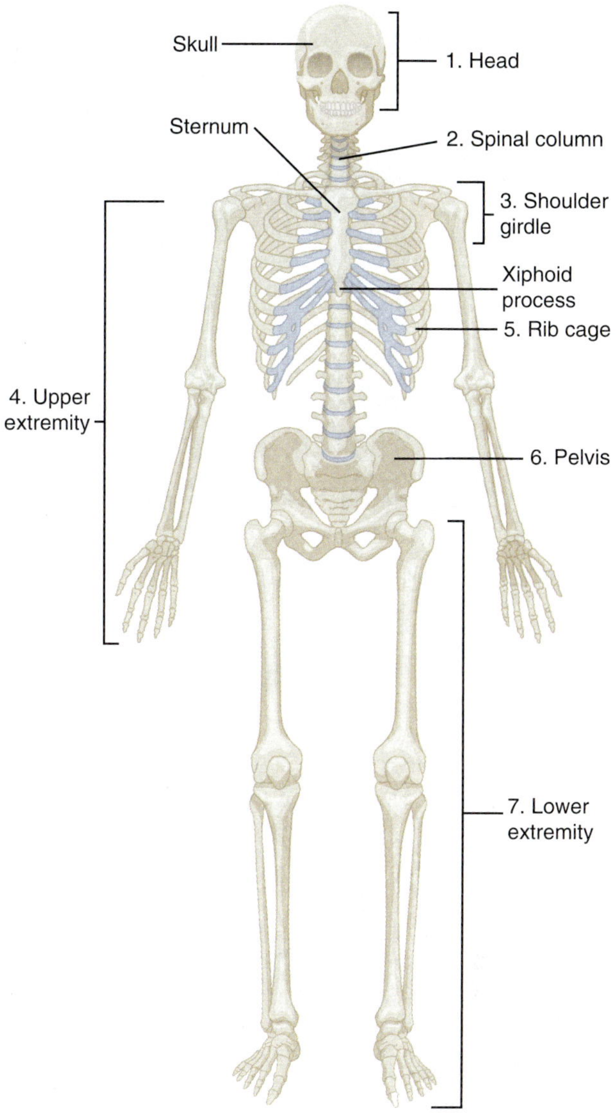

FIGURE 15-2 The seven major areas of the human skeleton.

© Jones & Bartlett Learning

The spine has five sections (**FIGURE 15-3**):

1. Cervical spine (neck), which contains 7 vertebrae
2. Thoracic spine (upper back), with 12 vertebrae
3. Lumbar spine (lower back), with 5 vertebrae
4. Sacrum, with 5 vertebrae
5. Coccyx (tailbone), typically with 4 vertebrae

The shoulder girdles form the third area of the skeletal system. Each shoulder girdle supports an arm and consists of the collarbone (clavicle) and the shoulder blade (scapula). The fourth area of the skeletal system, the upper extremities, consists of three major bones as well as the wrist and hand. The **arm** has one bone (the humerus), and the forearm has two bones (the radius and the ulna). The radius is located on the thumb side of the arm; the ulna is located on the side

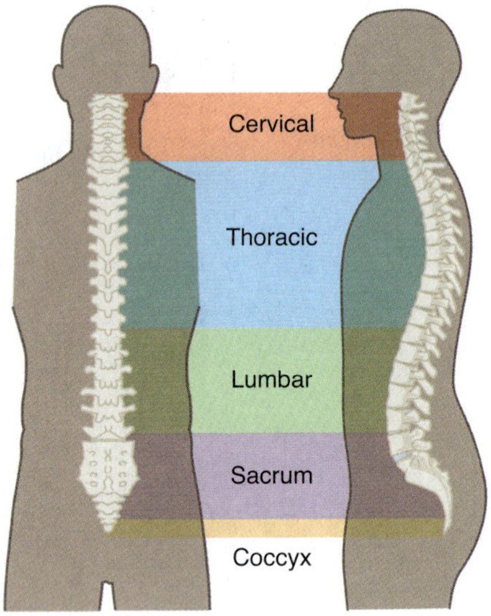

FIGURE 15-3 The five sections of the spine.

© Jones & Bartlett Learning

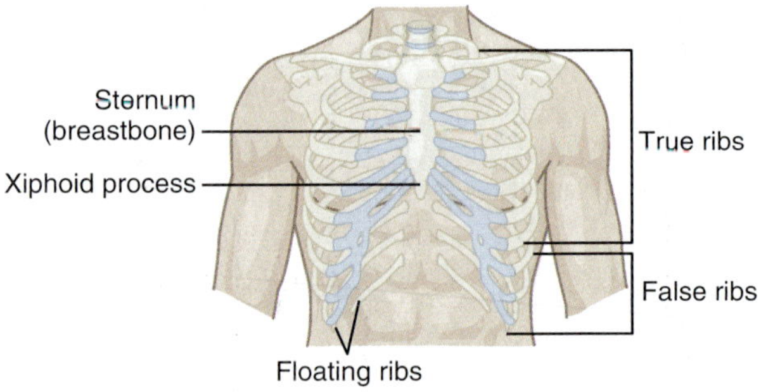

FIGURE 15-4 The rib cage.

© Jones & Bartlett Learning

of the little finger. There are several bones in the wrist and hand; however, you do not need to learn their names at this time and can consider them as one unit for the purposes of emergency treatment.

The fifth area of the skeletal system is the rib cage or chest (thorax). The 12 sets of ribs protect the heart, lungs, liver, and spleen. All of the ribs are attached to the spine (**FIGURE 15-4**). The upper five rib sets connect directly to the sternum (breastbone). A bridge of cartilage connects the ends of the 6th through 10th rib sets to each other and to the sternum. The 11th and 12th rib sets are called floating ribs because they are not attached to the sternum. The sternum is located in the front of the chest. The pointed structure at the bottom of the sternum is called the xiphoid process.

The sixth area of the skeletal system is the pelvis, which links the body and the lower extremities. The pelvis also protects the reproductive organs and the other organs located in the lower abdominal cavity.

The lower extremities (the thigh and the leg) form the seventh area of the skeletal system. The **thighbone** (femur) is the longest and strongest bone in the entire body. The **leg** consists of two major bones, the tibia and fibula, as well as the ankle and foot. The kneecap (patella) is a small, relatively flat bone that enhances knee extension and protects the front of the knee **joint**. Like the wrist and hand, the ankle and foot contain many smaller bones that can be considered as one unit.

A protective bony structure surrounds each of the body's essential organs. The skull protects the brain. The vertebrae protect the spinal cord. The ribs protect the heart and lungs. The pelvis protects the lower abdominal and reproductive organs.

A vital but often overlooked function of the skeletal system is to produce red blood cells. Red blood cells are manufactured primarily within the spaces inside the bone called the marrow.

The Muscular System

The muscles of the body provide both support and movement. Muscles are attached to bones by tendons and cause movement by alternately contracting (shortening) and relaxing (lengthening). Muscles are usually paired in opposition: As one member of the pair contracts, the other relaxes. This mechanical opposition moves bones and enables you to open and close your hand, turn your head, and bend and straighten your knee or other joints. To straighten the elbow, for example, the biceps muscle relaxes and an opposing muscle on the back of the arm contracts.

The musculoskeletal system gets its name from the coordination between the muscular system and the skeletal system to produce movement. Movement occurs at joints, where bones come together. Ligaments hold the bones together. Ligaments are thick bands that arise from one bone, span the joint, and insert into an adjacent bone.

YOU are the EMR — CASE 1

In late afternoon on a clear, brisk autumn day, you are dispatched to a nearby park for the report of an injured person. Dispatch information reveals that your patient is a 14-year-old boy who has been injured while skateboarding. When you arrive at the scene, you find your patient lying on his side, complaining of severe pain in his left arm and elbow. He states that he was trying to skate along a ledge that was 2 inches (5 cm) high when he fell and landed on the parking lot. There appears to be significant deformity between his shoulder and elbow.

1. How should you conduct an assessment of this patient?
2. What type of injuries should you suspect with this patient?
3. Under what circumstances should you move this patient?

Special Populations

Musculoskeletal Changes That Affect Mobility in Older Adults

As a person ages, several changes occur to the musculoskeletal system. Muscles decrease in strength. Part of this loss is the result of decreased physical activity, which can be offset by a good exercise program, and part is an inevitable outcome of the aging process. The disks between the vertebrae narrow; this change can cause a loss of height, curvature of the spine, and a loss of flexibility. The bones in the skeletal system decrease in strength because of a loss of calcium, leading to a risk of **osteoporosis**. Osteoporosis is a bone disease in which reduced bone density results in an increased risk of fracture. It affects both women and men but is especially prevalent in postmenopausal women. Many older people also experience some loss of balance caused by a variety of issues. Together, the loss of muscular strength, weakened bones, and decreased balance result in an increased incidence of falls among older patients.

The body has three types of muscles: voluntary, involuntary, and cardiac. Voluntary, or skeletal, muscles are attached to bones and can be contracted and relaxed by a person at will. They are responsible for the movement of the body. Involuntary, or smooth, muscles are found on the inside of the digestive tract and other internal organs of the body. They are not under conscious control and function automatically. Cardiac muscle is found only in the heart (**FIGURE 15-5**). Most musculoskeletal injuries involve skeletal muscles.

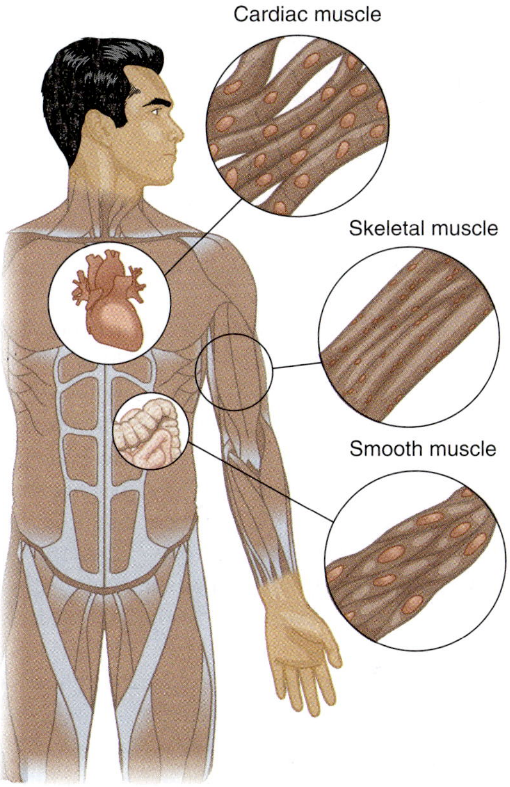

FIGURE 15-5 Three types of muscle in the human body.
© Jones & Bartlett Learning

Mechanism of Injury

As an EMR, you must understand the **mechanism of injury (MOI)**, or how injuries occur. Three types of MOIs cause musculoskeletal injuries: direct force, indirect force, and twisting force (**FIGURE 15-6**).

Examples of each mechanism and the type of injury it causes are as follows:

- **Direct force.** A car strikes a pedestrian on the leg. The pedestrian sustains a broken leg.
- **Indirect force.** A woman falls on her shoulder. The force of the fall transmits energy to the middle of the collarbone and the excess force breaks the bone.
- **Twisting force.** A football player is tackled while turning. As the leg twists, the knee sustains a severe injury. Injuries can be caused by direct force at the site of impact or by indirect force at an impact site removed from the site of the injury.

As an EMR, you will see many different types of traumatic injuries. Some of these injuries will be the result of motor vehicle crashes involving one or more motor vehicles or a motor vehicle and a pedestrian; others will be the result of

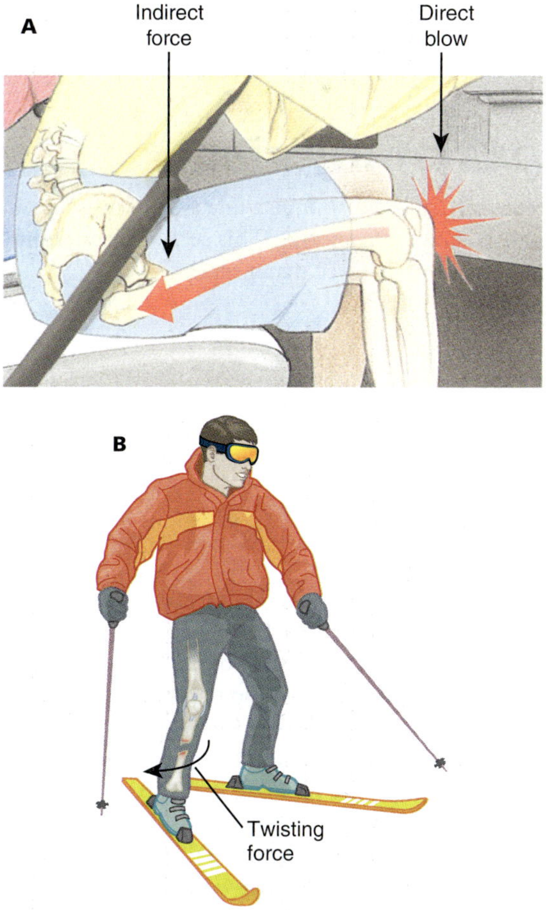

FIGURE 15-6 Three types of mechanisms of injury cause musculoskeletal injuries. **A.** Direct force and indirect force. **B.** Twisting force.
© Jones & Bartlett Learning

athletic activities, work-related accidents, falls, or violence. You will see injuries in people of all ages, from very young children to older people. Use the information provided by your dispatcher and gathered from your overview of the scene to identify the possible MOIs. You will gain additional information from examining and questioning the patient. By understanding the MOI (how the injury occurred), you will be better able to assess the patient and provide the needed treatment.

A Word About Terminology

A patient's injuries can be described in different ways. You must rely on your senses of sight and touch to determine the type of injury the patient has experienced. You must also listen to the information that the patient gives you. However, keep in mind that, as an EMR, you do not have the training or tools to diagnose an injury as a physician can.

The next section defines fractures, dislocations, and sprains/strains. Although you are not expected to diagnose these injuries, the patient's signs and symptoms will lead you to suspect that a certain injury is most probable. Some instructors and medical directors may choose to identify musculoskeletal injuries strictly in terms of the signs and symptoms present, such as a painful, swollen, deformed extremity. Others may choose to use terms such as suspected or possible fracture, dislocation, or sprain. Regardless of the terminology used, the most important part of your job is to provide the best assessment and treatment for the patient.

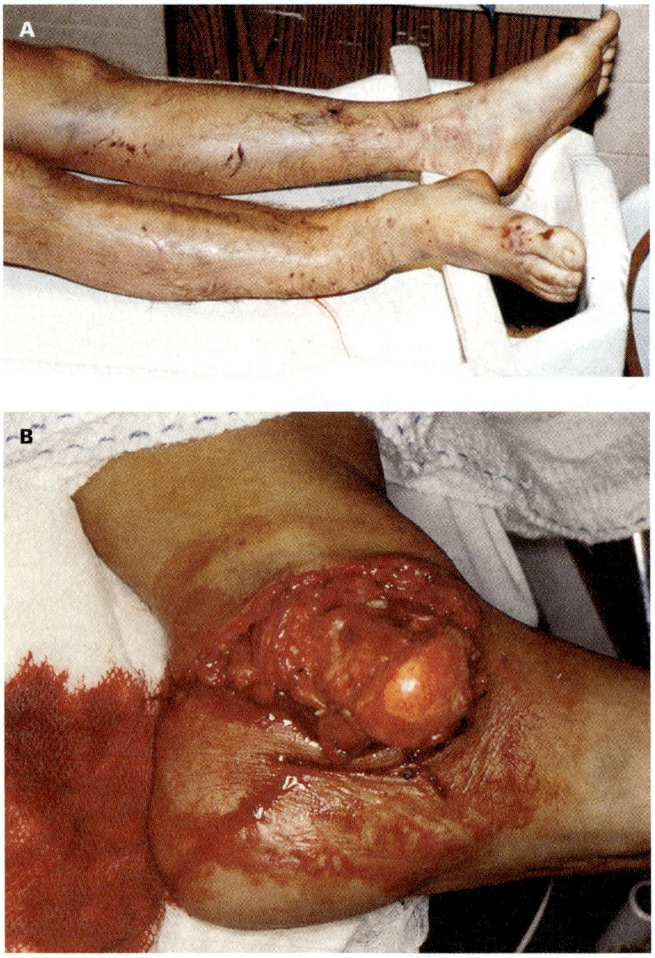

FIGURE 15-7 A. Closed fracture. **B.** Open fracture.
© Charles Stewart, MD, EMDM, MPH

Types of Injuries

It is often difficult to distinguish one type of musculoskeletal extremity injury from another. This section classifies musculoskeletal injuries by three major types:

- Fractures
- Dislocations
- Sprains and strains

All three types are serious, and all extremity injuries must be identified so that appropriate medical treatment can be provided.

Fractures

A fracture is a broken bone. The break may be significant enough to visibly displace the bone from its normal position or may be less apparent. A variety of mechanisms can cause a fracture, but a fracture most often occurs as a result of a significant force, unless the bone is weakened by a disease such as osteoporosis or cancer. Fractures are generally classified as closed or open (**FIGURE 15-7**). In the more common **closed fracture**, the bone is broken but there is no break in the skin.

In an **open fracture**, the bone is broken and the overlying skin is lacerated. The open wound can be caused by a penetrating object or by the fractured bone end itself protruding through the skin. Open fractures are likely contaminated by dirt and bacteria that may lead to infection. A patient with an open fracture requires more extensive care in the hospital to ensure that the associated wound is properly cleaned and the fracture properly treated to reduce the risk of a serious infection developing. Both open and closed fractures injure adjacent soft tissues, resulting in bleeding at the fracture site. Fractures can also injure nearby nerves and blood vessels, causing severe nerve injury and excessive internal or external bleeding.

Fractures occur frequently in the geriatric population because of osteoporosis and the increased risk of falling due to worsened balance, vision loss, and muscle weakness. Be aware that a simple fall at home can result in multiple severe fractures in an older patient who has weakened bones. Fractures of the wrist, spine, and hip are particularly common. Some of these fractures, even fractures of the vertebrae, can occur with little trauma. Geriatric patients may also have a reduced awareness of pain. They may experience little pain, even with a major fracture, and may not realize the seriousness of their injury. Splinting and **spinal motion restriction** of a geriatric patient can be a challenge when a spinal curvature (kyphosis) or osteoporosis is present. Handle these patients carefully.

Dislocations

A **dislocation** is a disruption that tears the supporting ligaments of the joint. The bone ends that make up the joint separate completely from each other and can lock in one position. Any attempt to move a dislocated joint is very painful. Because many nerves and blood vessels lie near joints, a dislocation can damage these structures as well.

Sprains and Strains

A **sprain** is a joint injury caused by excessive stretching of the supporting ligaments. Think of it as a partial dislocation. Strains are caused by stretching or tearing of a muscle.

Signs and Symptoms

Signs and symptoms of extremity injuries include the following:

- Pain at the injury site
- An open wound
- Swelling and discoloration (bruising)
- The patient's inability or unwillingness to move the extremity
- Deformity or angulation
- Tenderness at the injury site

Standard Precautions and Musculoskeletal Injuries

When you examine and treat patients with musculoskeletal injuries, you need to take standard precautions. These patients may have open wounds related to the musculoskeletal injury or to a separate, open soft-tissue injury. Assume that trauma patients have open wounds that pose a threat of infection. Always wear approved gloves. When you are responding to motor vehicle crashes or to other situations that may present a hazard from broken glass or other sharp objects, it is wise to wear heavy rescue gloves that provide protection from sharp objects. Some EMRs wear latex or nitrile gloves under the heavy rescue gloves for added protection from infectious body fluids. If the patient has active bleeding that may splatter, wear protection for your eyes, nose, and mouth as well. In the context of a pandemic involving community transmission of a viral respiratory illness, standard precautions should be expanded to include protection from aerosolized or airborne particulate matter. Thus, standard precautions in such circumstances should include at minimum a simple face mask and eye protection for all patient encounters.

Safety

Standard precautions are for *your* protection.

Examination of Musculoskeletal Injuries

The three essential steps in examining a patient with a limb injury are as follows:

1. General assessment of the patient according to the patient assessment sequence
2. Examination of the injured part
3. Evaluation of the circulation, sensation, and movement in the injured limb

General Patient Assessment

When caring for an injured patient, you must carry out all the steps in the patient assessment process before focusing your attention on any injured limb. Once you have controlled any life-threatening hemorrhage and checked and stabilized the patient's ABCs, you can then direct your attention to the injured limb identified during the physical examination.

Limb injuries are not life threatening unless there is excessive bleeding from an open wound. Therefore, it is essential that you first stabilize the patient's ABCs before you focus on a limb injury, regardless of the pain or deformity that may be present at that injury site.

As you examine and treat patients with musculoskeletal injuries, remember that this is a frightening and painful experience for them. Explain what you are doing as you conduct your examination and stabilize the patient. Treat the patient with the same care and consideration that you would give to a close member of your own family.

Street Smarts

Listen to the patient. The patient is usually right about the location and type of injury.

Examination of the Injured Limb

As an EMR, you should initially inspect the injured limb and compare it to the opposite, uninjured limb. To do this, gently and carefully cut away any clothing covering the wound, if necessary.

When you examine the limb, you may find any of the following:

- An open wound
- Deformity
- Swelling
- Bruising

After you uncover and look at the injured limb, gently feel for any points of tenderness. Tenderness is the best indicator of an underlying fracture, dislocation, or sprain.

To detect limb injury, start at the top of each limb (where it connects to the body) and using both hands, squeeze the entire limb in a systematic, firm (yet gentle) manner, moving down the limb and away from the body (**FIGURE 15-8**). Make sure you examine the entire extremity.

As you carry out your hands-on examination, it is important to ask the patient where it hurts most; the location of greatest pain is probably the injury site. Also ask if the patient feels tingling or numbness in the extremity because this may indicate nerve damage or lack of circulation.

Careful inspection and a gentle hands-on examination will identify most musculoskeletal injuries. After you have made a careful visual and hands-on examination, and if the patient shows no sign of injury, ask the patient to move the limb carefully. If there is an injury, the patient will report pain and refuse to move the limb.

The signs and symptoms described earlier (deformity, swelling, bruising, tenderness, or pain with motion) indicate the presence of a limb injury. Only one sign is necessary to indicate an injury to the limb. Manage all limb injuries, regardless of type or severity, in the same way.

Treatment

If even the slightest motion causes the patient to report pain, *no* further motion should be attempted.

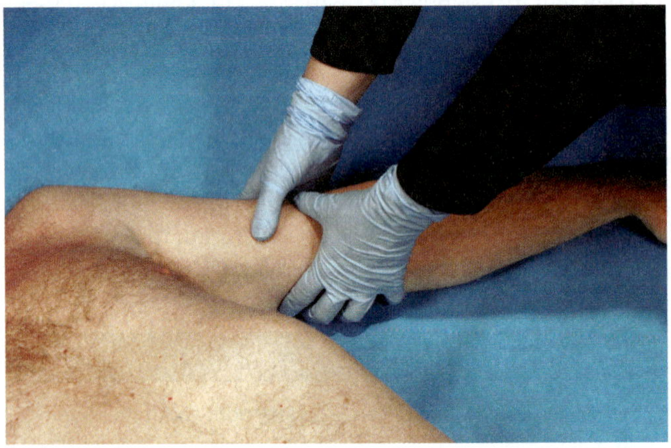

FIGURE 15-8 Examine the extremities by gently squeezing from the end closest to the body to the end farthest from the body.
© Jones & Bartlett Learning. Courtesy of MIEMSS.

Evaluation of Circulation, Sensation, and Movement

Once you suspect limb injury, you must evaluate the circulation and sensation in that limb. Many important blood vessels and nerves lie close to the bones, especially around major joints. Therefore, any injury may have associated blood vessel or nerve damage. It is also essential to check circulation and sensation after any movement of the limb (such as for splinting). Moving the limb during splinting may cause a bone fragment to press against or even cut a blood vessel or nerve. Consider any open wound, deformity, swelling, or bruising of a limb to be evidence of a possible limb injury and treat it as such. Try to keep the extremity in a position of comfort for the patient.

Treatment

Examine the following factors for each injured limb:

- Pulse
- Capillary refill
- Sensation
- Movement

SKILL DRILL 15-1 describes how to check circulation, sensation, and movement in an injured extremity.

SKILL DRILL 15-1

Checking Circulation, Sensation, and Movement in an Injured Extremity

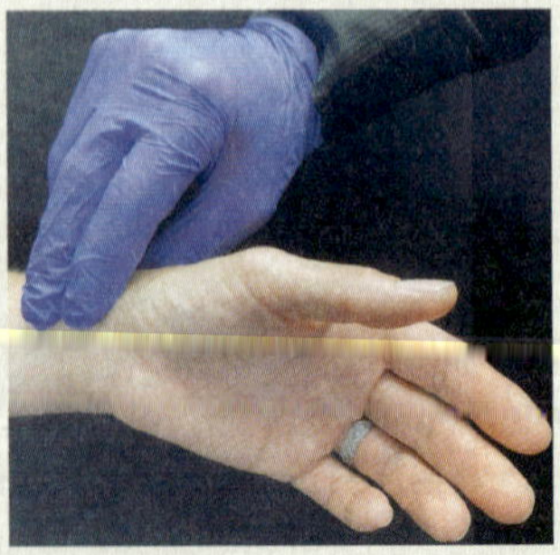

STEP 1 Pulse. Feel the pulse distal to the point of injury. If the patient has an upper extremity injury, check the radial (wrist) pulse.

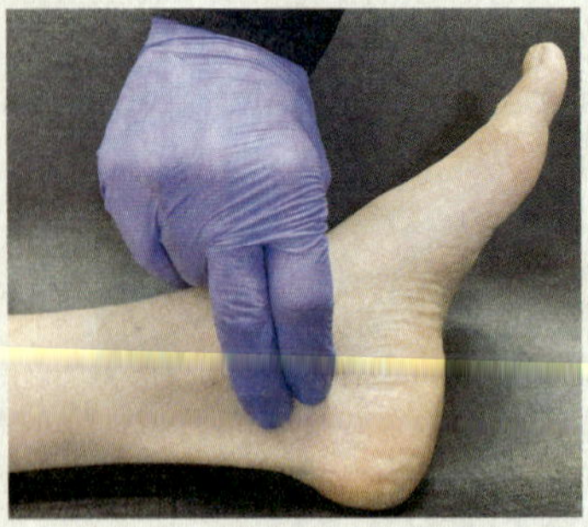

STEP 2 If the patient has a lower extremity injury, check the tibial (posterior ankle) pulse.

SKILL DRILL 15-1 *(continued)*

Checking Circulation, Sensation, and Movement in an Injured Extremity

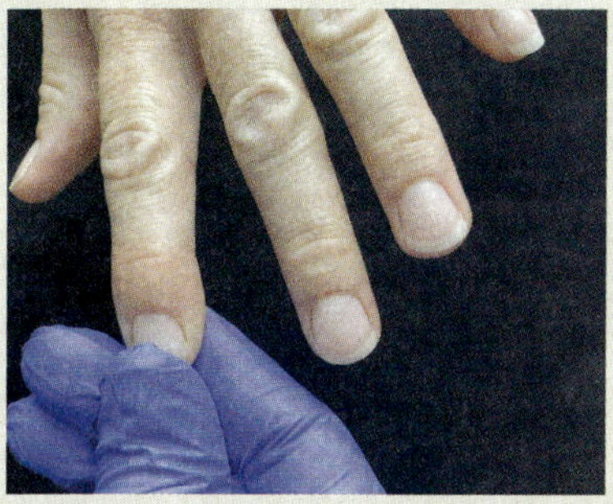

STEP 3 Capillary refill. Test the capillary refill in a finger or toe of any injured limb. Firm pressure on the tip of the nail causes the nail bed to blanch (turn a lighter color).

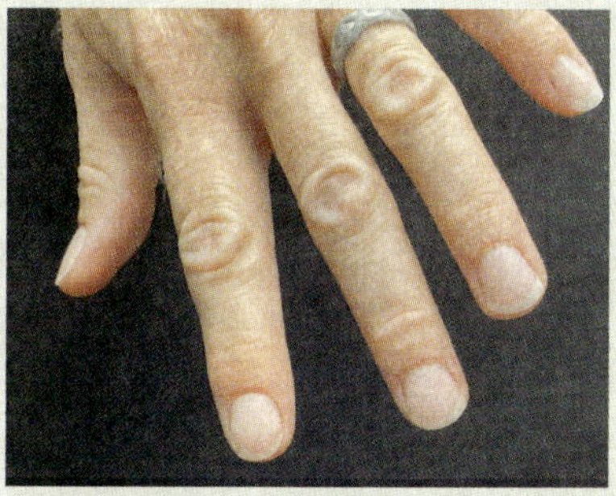

STEP 4 Release the pressure on the tip of the nail. The nail tip should return to its original darker color. If the nail remains blanched after 2 seconds, capillary refill is considered delayed or absent, which indicates a circulation condition in the limb. A cold environment will naturally delay capillary refill, so do not use capillary refill to assess an injured limb in that situation. The absence of a pulse or capillary refill indicates that a limb is in immediate danger. Impaired circulation demands prompt transport and medical treatment at an appropriate medical facility.

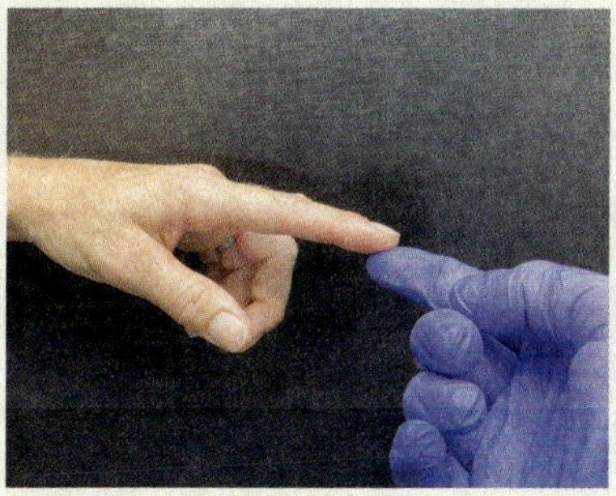

STEP 5 Sensation. The patient's ability to feel your light touch on the fingers or toes is a good indication that the nerve supply is intact. In the hand, check sensation by lightly touching the tips of the index and little fingers.

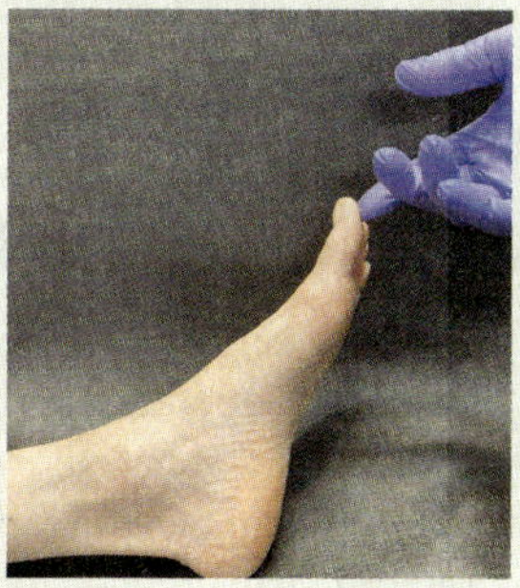

STEP 6 In the foot, check the tip of the big toe and the top of the foot for sensation.

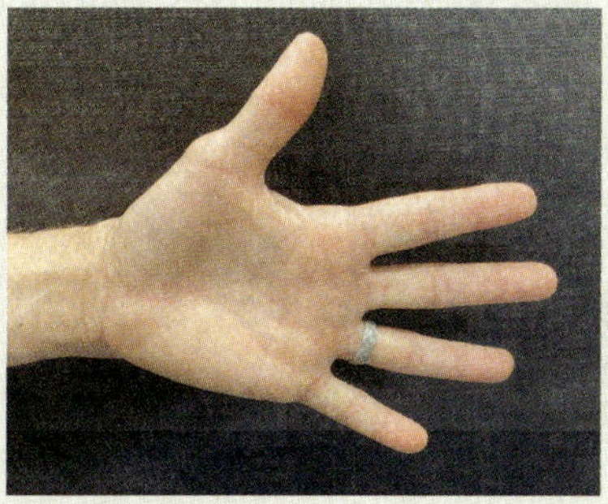

STEP 7A Movement. The simple movements performed during steps 7 and 8 indicate whether the nerves to the muscles are working. If an attempt at motion produces pain, do not ask the patient to move the limb any further.

Upper extremity assessment: If the hand is injured, do not have the patient perform step 7. Check for movement of the upper extremities by asking the patient to open (7A) and close (7B) the fist.

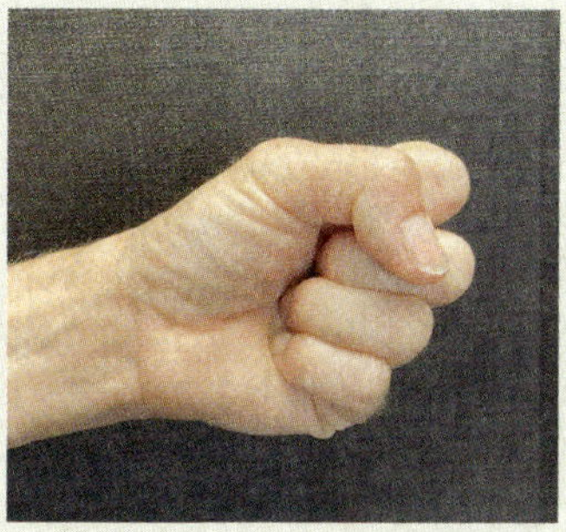

STEP 7B

(continues)

SKILL DRILL 15-1 *(continued)*

Checking Circulation, Sensation, and Movement in an Injured Extremity

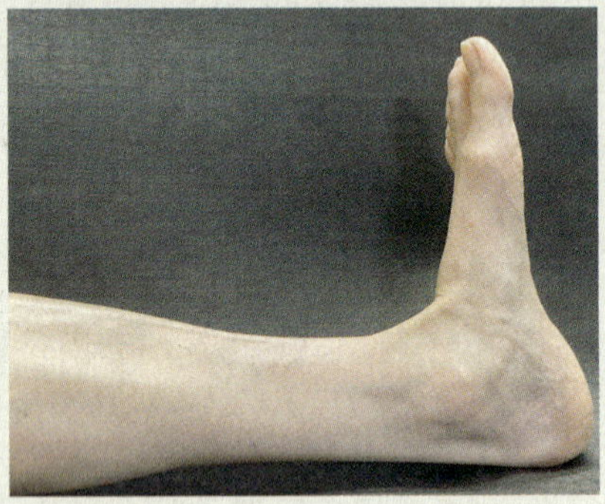

STEP 8A **Lower extremity assessment:** If the foot is injured, do not have the patient perform step 8. Check for movement of the lower extremities by asking the patient to flex (8A) and extend (8B) the ankle.

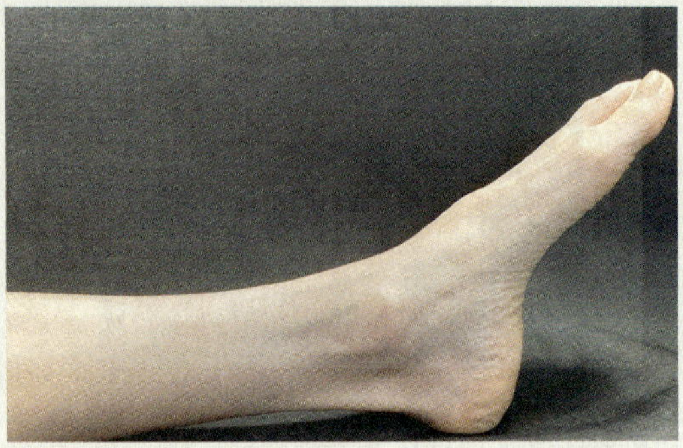

STEP 8B

© Jones & Bartlett Learning

Treatment of Musculoskeletal Injuries

Regardless of their extent or severity, treat all limb injuries in the same way in the field. For all open extremity wounds, first cover the entire wound with a dry, sterile dressing, then apply firm but gentle pressure to control bleeding, if necessary. The sterile compression dressing protects the wound and underlying tissues from further contamination. Apply a cold pack (making sure to place bandaging or a cloth between the pack and the skin) to painful, swollen, or deformed extremities. Then splint the injured limb.

General Principles of Splinting

Splint all limb injuries before moving a patient, unless the environment prevents effective splinting or threatens the patient's life (or your life). Splinting prevents the movement of broken bone ends, a dislocated joint, or damaged soft tissues and thereby reduces pain. With less pain, the patient relaxes and the trip to the medical facility is easier. Splinting also helps to control bleeding and decreases the risk of damage to the nearby nerves and vessels by sharp bone fragments. Splinting prevents closed fractures from becoming open fractures during movement or transport.

All EMRs should know the following general principles of splinting:

1. In most situations, remove clothing from the injured limb to inspect the limb for open wounds, deformity, swelling, bruising, and capillary refill.
2. Note and record the pulse, capillary refill, sensation, and movement distal to the point of injury, both before and after splinting.
3. Cover all open wounds with a dry, sterile dressing before applying the splint.
4. Do not move the patient before splinting, unless there is an immediate danger to the patient or to you.
5. Stabilize the joint above and the joint below the injury site. If the injury involves a joint, stabilize the bone above and the bone below the injury.
6. Pad all rigid splints.
7. When applying the splint, use your hands to support the injury site and minimize movement of the limb until splinting is completed.
8. Splint the limb without moving it unnecessarily.
9. When in doubt, splint.

Materials Used for Splinting

Many different materials can be used as splints, if necessary. There are three basic types of splints.

- Rigid
- Soft
- Traction

Note that even when standard splints are not available, you can still stabilize an injured extremity. For example, you can bind an injured arm to a patient's chest and secure an injured leg to the other, uninjured lower extremity for temporary stability.

Rigid Splints

A **rigid splint** is made from firm material and is applied to the sides, front, or back of an injured extremity. Common types of rigid splints include padded board splints, molded plastic or aluminum splints, padded wire ladder splints, structured aluminum malleable (SAM) splints, and folded cardboard splints (**FIGURE 15-9**). Padded wire ladder or SAM splints can be molded to the shape of the limb to splint it in the position found.

Soft Splints

A **soft splint**, also called a formable splint, is flexible and easy to place around an injured limb (**FIGURE 15-10**). The most commonly used soft splints are the **vacuum splint** and inflatable, clear plastic air splints. Vacuum splints become rigid when air is removed from the splint. Air splints become rigid when they are inflated with air.

Vacuum splints consist of an airtight covering that is shaped to fit around an arm or a leg. They are constructed with an inner layer of airtight fabric and an outer layer of the same fabric. Located between these two layers of fabric are small beads of a hard foam material surrounded by air. This makes the splint flexible and easy to mold to the contours of the patient's injured limb. When you remove air from inside the vacuum splint, it becomes more rigid and provides support for the injured limb. A vacuum pump to remove the air is included with the splint. Most vacuum splints have Velcro fasteners to make it easier to apply the splint. Vacuum splints come in a variety of sizes, including large vacuum mattresses that can be used for spinal stabilization.

Vacuum splints are not transparent, so it is not possible to observe the limb once the splint is applied. Protect vacuum splints from damage from sharp objects. If they are punctured, the splint will become flexible and no longer effective. When using vacuum splints, you must monitor the pulse, movement, and sensation of the injured limb and the status of the vacuum splint itself. Changes in altitude and temperature can affect the rigidity of a vacuum splint. The steps for applying a vacuum splint are illustrated in **SKILL DRILL 15-2**.

Air splints are constructed of a clear, flexible, plastic material. They are manufactured in a variety of sizes and shapes, with or without a zipper that runs the length of the splint (**FIGURE 15-11**). Air splints are applied around the limb and then inflated by blowing into a specially constructed valve. Do not use a pump to inflate an air splint. The pressure from the air forms the air splint around the injured limb in a manner opposite from the way a vacuum splint works. Air splints are largely transparent, so it is possible to monitor the appearance of the injured limb after you apply one. Air splints provide support and are comfortable for the patient. Because they provide uniform pressure, you can use an air splint to apply pressure on a bleeding wound.

Protect air splints from sharp objects that could puncture them. When using air splints, monitor the pulse, motor function, and sensation of the injured limb. Also monitor the level of inflation of the air splint. Swelling of the injured limb and changes in altitude and temperature can affect the rigidity of an air splint.

> **Safety**
>
> *Never* use anything but the air from your mouth to inflate an air splint!

Traction Splints

A **traction splint** holds a femur fracture in alignment by applying a constant, steady pull on the extremity. Properly applying a traction splint requires two well-trained emergency medical

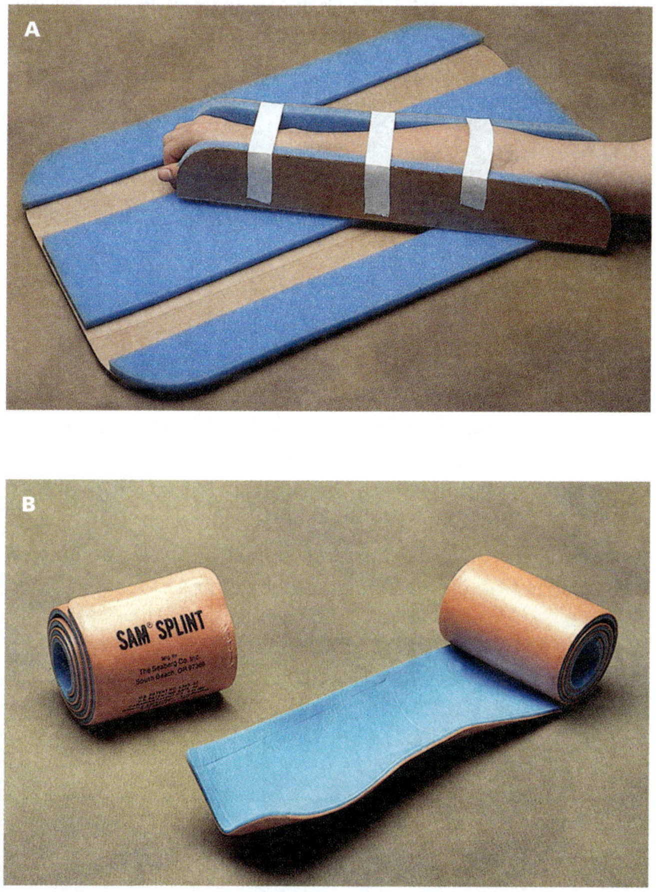

FIGURE 15-9 A. Rigid cardboard splints. **B.** SAM splints.

© American Academy of Orthopaedic Surgeons

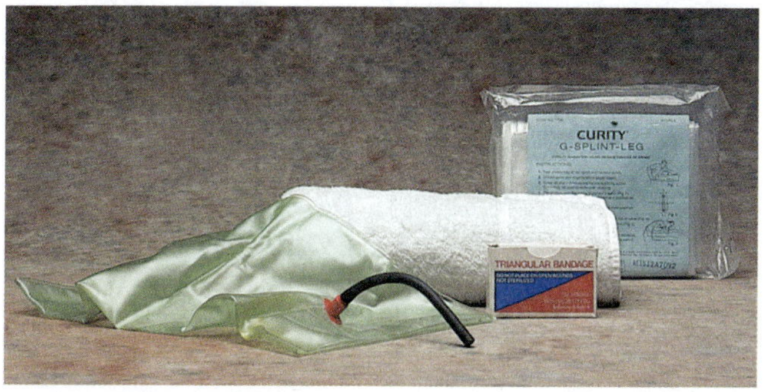

FIGURE 15-10 Soft splints.

© American Academy of Orthopaedic Surgeons

SKILL DRILL 15-2

Applying a Vacuum Splint

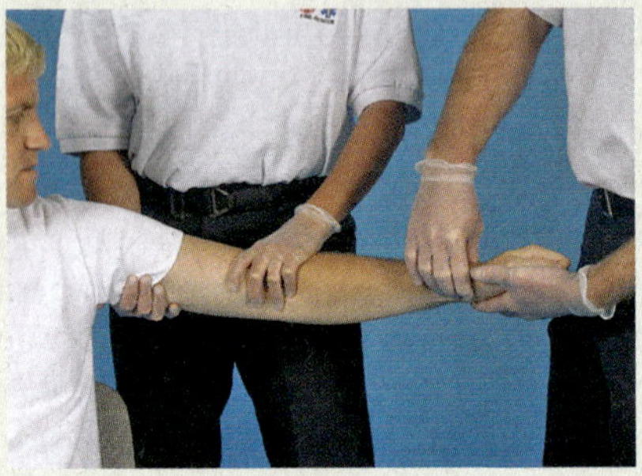

STEP 1 Assess distal pulse and motor and sensory function. Your partner supports and stabilizes the injured limb, applying traction if needed.

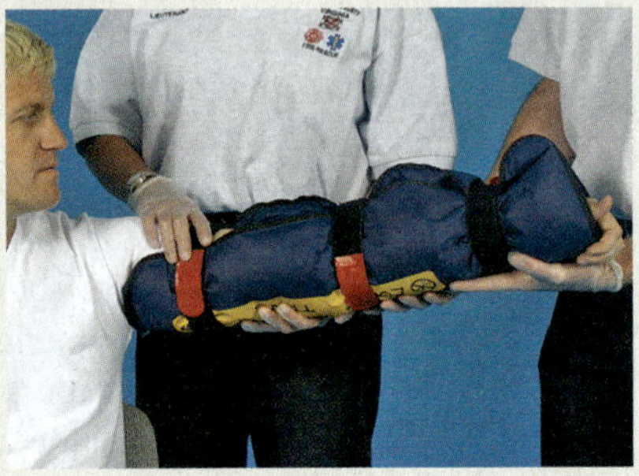

STEP 2 Gently place the injured limb onto the vacuum splint, and wrap the splint around the limb.

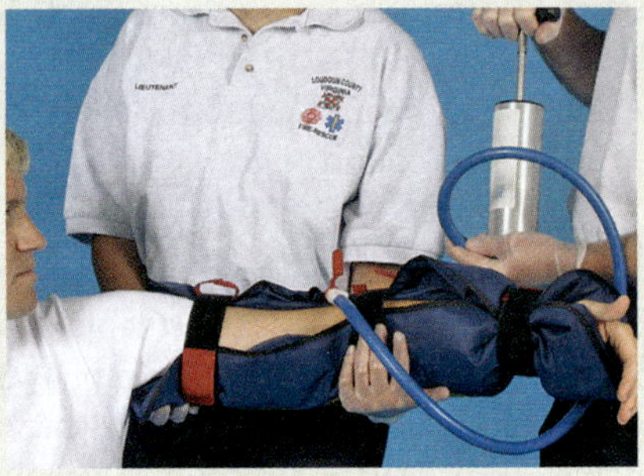

STEP 3 Open the valve and suction air from the splint until it becomes rigid and supports the limb deformity. Close the valve to maintain stability and secure the splint (if needed). Monitor distal circulation and nervous function for any change.

© Jones & Bartlett Learning. Courtesy of MIEMSS.

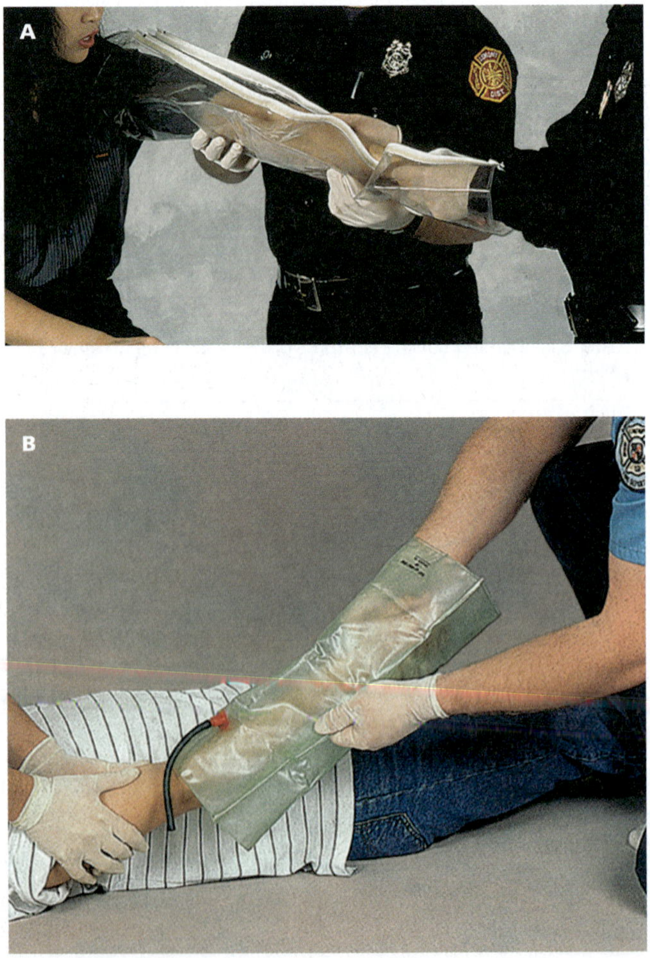

FIGURE 15-11 **A.** A zippered air splint. **B.** An unzippered air splint.

© Jones & Bartlett Learning. Courtesy of MIEMSS.

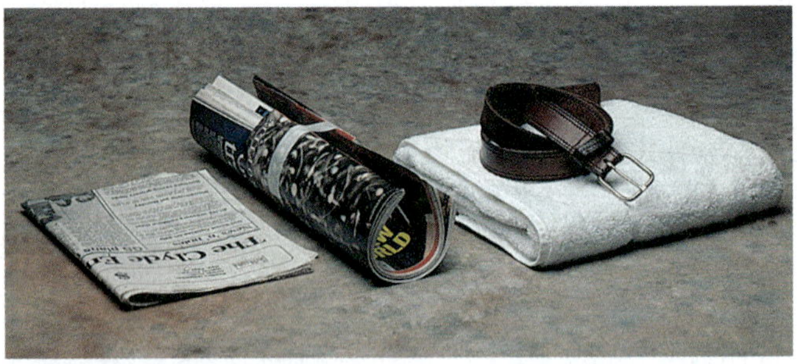

FIGURE 15-12 Improvised splints.

© American Academy of Orthopaedic Surgeons

services (EMS) clinicians working together; one person cannot do it alone. While most EMRs do not learn the skills necessary to apply this type of splint, you may be asked to assist trained medical personnel in the placement of a traction splint, and you should be familiar with the general techniques, as shown later in Skill Drill 15-6. There are several different types of traction splints. If you will be helping to apply a traction splint, you need instruction on the device used by your service.

Treatment

Improvised splints can be made from rolled newspapers, magazines, towels, or belts (**FIGURE 15-12**). Pillows make excellent splints for ankle injuries.

Splinting Specific Injury Sites

A person with EMR training and with materials readily available can carry out the treatment techniques described here.

Most splinting techniques are two-person operations. One person stabilizes and supports the injured limb while the other person applies the splint.

Shoulder Girdle Injuries

The easiest way to splint most shoulder injuries is to apply a **sling** made of a triangular bandage and to secure the sling (and arm) to the patient's body with swathes around the arm and chest. Apply the sling by tying a knot in the point of the triangular bandage, placing the elbow into the cup formed by the knot, and passing the two ends of the bandage up and around the patient's neck. Tie the sling so the wrist is slightly higher than the elbow (**FIGURE 15-13**).

To keep the arm from moving, fold another triangular bandage until you have a long swathe that is 3 to 4 inches (8 to 10 cm) wide (**FIGURE 15-14**). Tie one or two swathes around the upper arm and chest of the patient. This easily applied splint adequately stabilizes fractures of the collarbone, most shoulder injuries, and fractures of the arm.

Shoulder Dislocation

The dislocated shoulder is the only shoulder girdle injury that is difficult to stabilize with a sling and swathe. In a shoulder dislocation, there is often a space between the upper arm and the chest wall. Fill this space with a pillow or a rolled blanket before applying a sling and swathe as for other shoulder injuries (**FIGURE 15-15**).

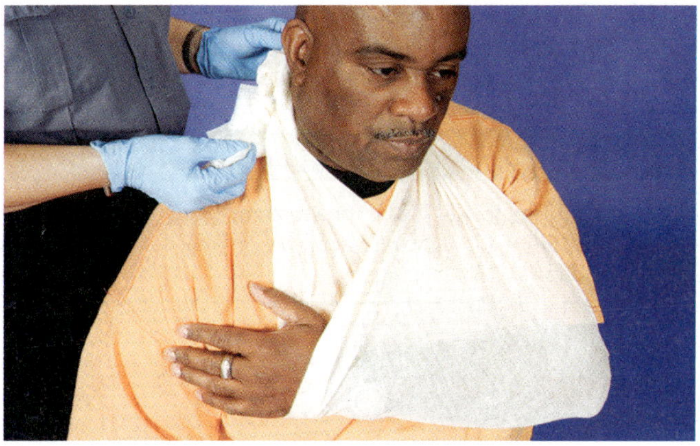

FIGURE 15-13 Sling.
© Jones & Bartlett Learning. Courtesy of MIEMSS.

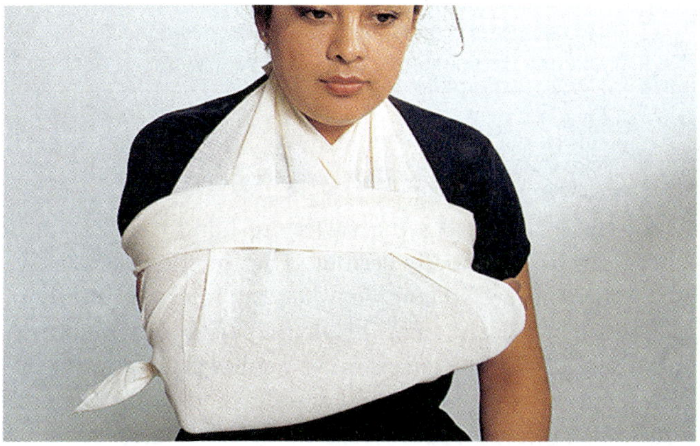

FIGURE 15-14 Sling and swathe.
© Jones & Bartlett Learning. Courtesy of MIEMSS.

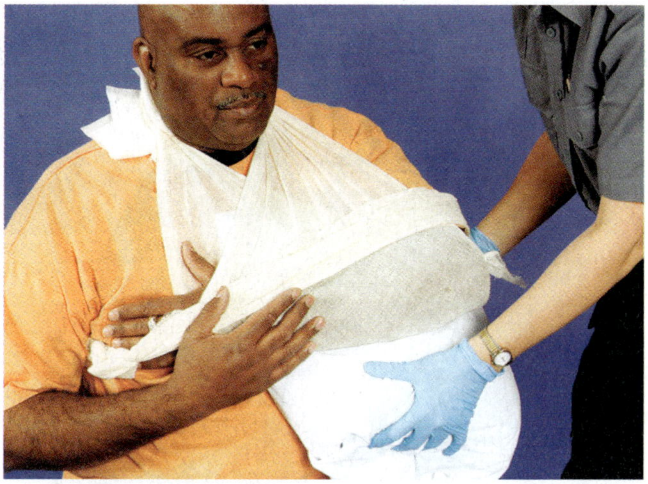

FIGURE 15-15 Splint the dislocated shoulder in a position of comfort by placing a pillow or towel between the arm and the chest before applying a sling and swathe.
© Jones & Bartlett Learning. Courtesy of MIEMSS.

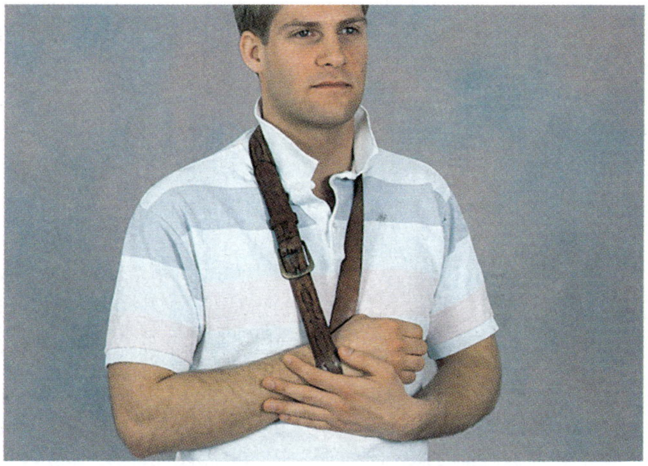

FIGURE 15-16 Improvised sling using a belt.
© American Academy of Orthopaedic Surgeons

Words of Wisdom

When triangular bandages are not available, loop a length of gauze (or even a belt) around the patient's wrist and suspend the limb from the neck (**FIGURE 15-16**). Secure the arm gently, but firmly, to the chest wall with another length of gauze or belt. If you have not cut away the coat a patient is wearing, you can also pin a coat sleeve to the front of the patient's coat as a temporary splint (**FIGURE 15-17**). This technique is less secure than a sling and swathe, but it may be of use in cold weather areas.

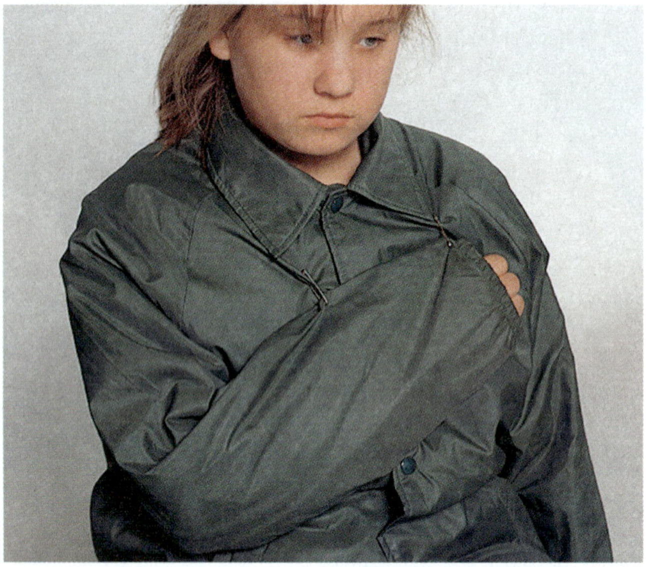

FIGURE 15-17 Improvised sling using safety pins.
© American Academy of Orthopaedic Surgeons

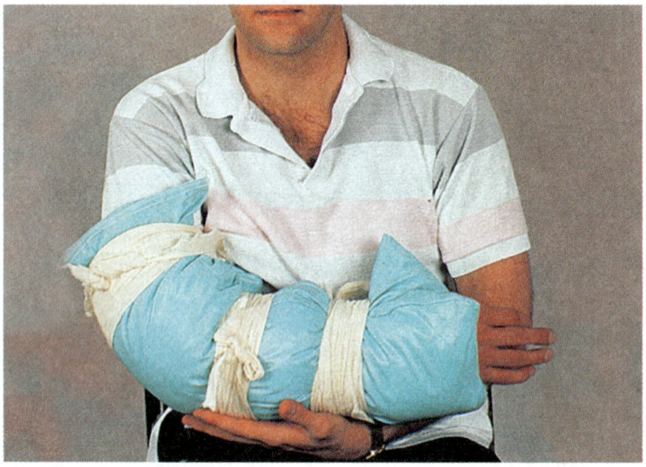

FIGURE 15-18 Pillow splint.
© American Academy of Orthopaedic Surgeons

Elbow Injuries

Do not move an injured elbow from the position in which you find it. You must splint the elbow as it lies because any movement can cause nerve or blood vessel damage. If the elbow is straight, splint it straight. If the elbow is bent at an unusual angle, splint it in that position.

After splinting the injured elbow of a patient who does not have a significant shoulder injury (and only if it does not cause pain), gently move the splinted injury to the patient's side for comfort and ease of transport. An effective splint for an injured elbow is a pillow splint. Wrap the elbow in a pillow, add additional padding to keep the elbow in the position found, and secure the pillow as shown in **FIGURE 15-18**.

The patient is usually transported in a sitting position with the splinted elbow resting on their lap. A padded wire ladder or SAM splint is also effective for splinting elbows that are found in severely deformed positions (**FIGURE 15-19**).

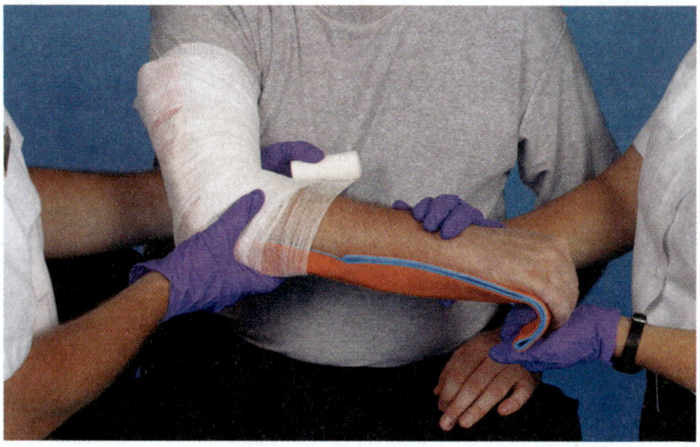

FIGURE 15-19 SAM splint.
© Jones & Bartlett Learning. Courtesy of MIEMSS.

Forearm Injuries

Several splints can be used to stabilize the **forearm**: the air splint, the cardboard splint, the SAM splint (**SKILL DRILL 15-3**), and even rolled newspapers and magazines. Be sure to pad all rigid splints adequately.

An air splint can be applied quickly, and it stabilizes the forearm quite well. Of the several types of air splints available, the one with a full-length zipper is easiest to use (**SKILL DRILL 15-4**). The steps for applying an air splint without a zipper are illustrated in **SKILL DRILL 15-5**.

Treatment

If you have to improvise a splint for a forearm injury, **FIGURE 15-20** shows how to apply a splint made of magazines and newspapers.

Safety

In the context of active community transmission of an aerosolized disease, such as the coronavirus disease 2019 (COVID-19) pandemic, it is important to ensure that all types of patient care equipment, including splints, are properly cleaned, disinfected, or disposed of. Follow your department's guidelines and the latest recommendations from the Centers for Disease Control and Prevention and the Occupational Safety and Health Administration.

Hand, Wrist, and Finger Injuries

As an EMR, you will see a variety of hand injuries, all of which can be potentially serious. The functions of the fingers and hand are so complex that any injury, if poorly or inadequately treated, may result in permanent deformity and disability. Treat even seemingly simple lacerations carefully. You can use a bulky hand dressing and a short splint to stabilize all injuries of the wrist, hand, and fingers. Send any amputated parts to the hospital with the patient by placing them in a sealed plastic bag. Cool the plastic bag by placing

SKILL DRILL 15-3

Stabilizing the Forearm

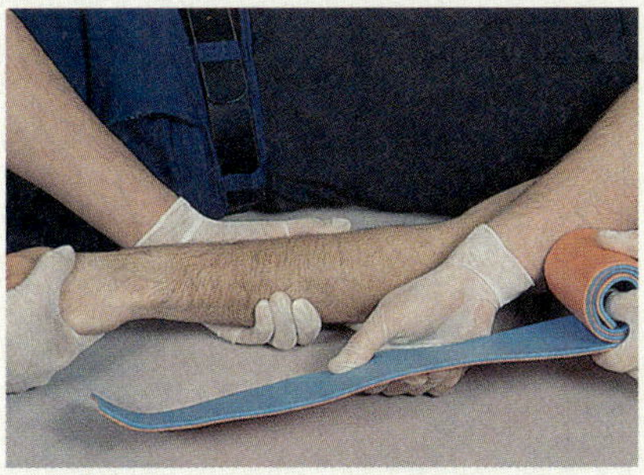

STEP 1 Support and stabilize the injured limb. Form the SAM splint to the injured forearm.

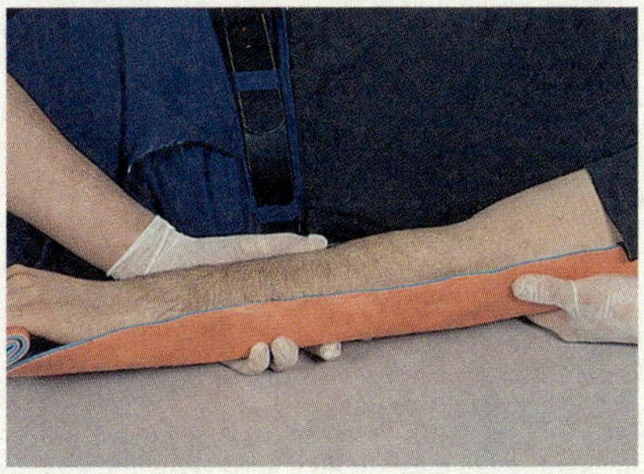

STEP 2 Place the splint under the injured limb.

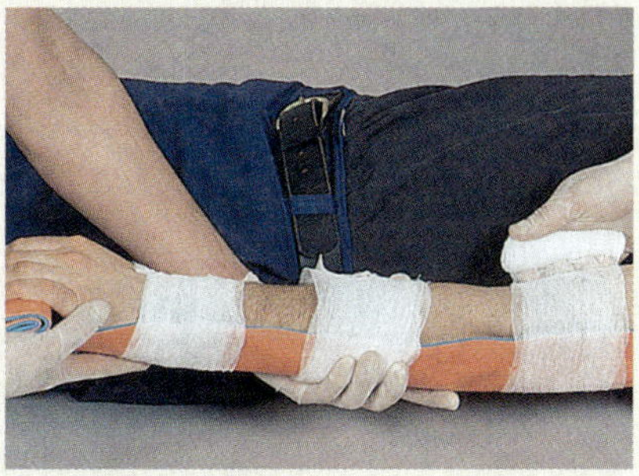

STEP 3 Secure the splint in place with gauze. Recheck the pulse, capillary refill, and sensation of the injured forearm.

© Jones & Bartlett Learning. Courtesy of MIEMSS.

SKILL DRILL 15-4

Applying a Zippered Air Splint

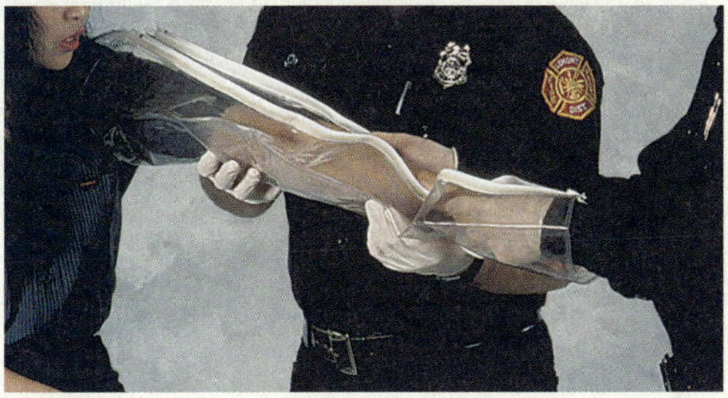

STEP 1 Apply gentle traction to the limb and support the site of injury. Have your partner place the open, deflated splint around the limb.

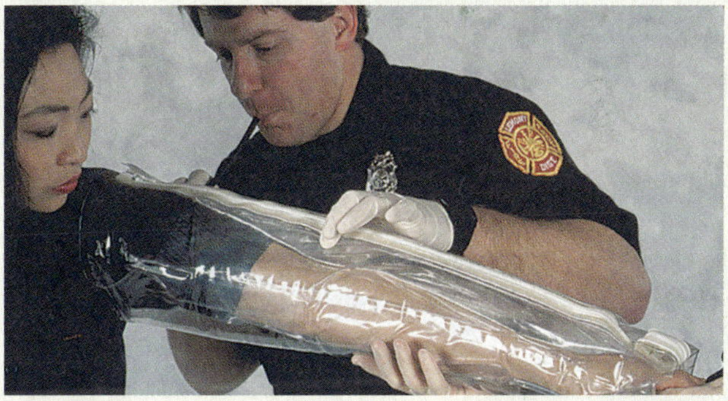

STEP 2 Zip up the splint and inflate it by mouth. Then test the pressure in the splint. With proper inflation, you should just be able to compress the walls of the splint together with a firm pinch between the thumb and index finger near the edge of the splint. Check and record pulse and motor and sensory functions, and monitor them periodically until the patient reaches the hospital.

© Jones & Bartlett Learning. Courtesy of MIEMSS.

it in a cold-water bath; never place the amputated part directly on ice.

To treat injuries of the hand, wrist, or fingers, first cover all wounds with a dry, sterile dressing. Then place the injured hand and wrist into the position of function (**FIGURE 15-21**). Place one or two soft roller dressings into the palm of the patient's hand. Apply a splint to hold the wrist, hand, and fingers in the position of function and secure the splint with a soft roller bandage.

Pelvic Fractures

Fractures of the pelvis often involve severe blood loss because the broken bones can easily lacerate the large blood vessels that run directly beside the pelvis. These vessels can release a large amount of blood into the pelvic area. Pelvic fractures commonly cause shock. Therefore, you must always treat the patient for shock.

The most definite sign of a pelvic fracture is tenderness when you use both your hands to firmly compress the patient's pelvis (**FIGURE 15-22**). Stabilize fractures of the pelvis

SKILL DRILL 15-5

Applying an Unzippered Air Splint

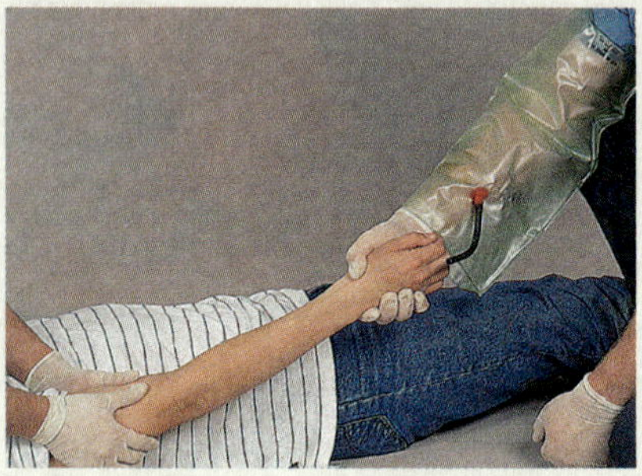

STEP 1 Assess distal pulse and motor and sensory functions. Your partner supports the patient's injured limb until splinting is complete. Place your arm through the splint. Extend your hand beyond the splint, and grasp the hand or foot of the injured limb.

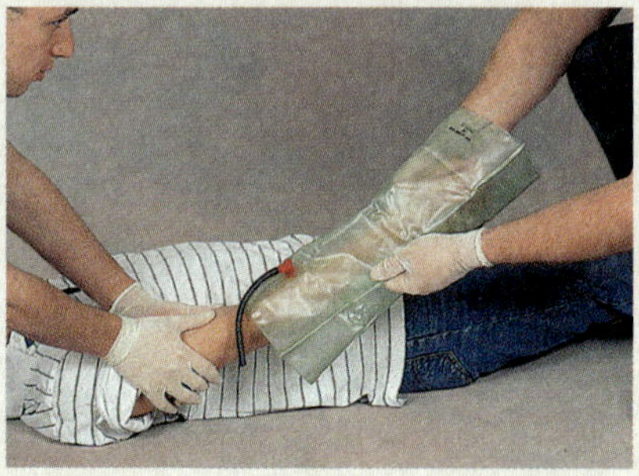

STEP 2 Apply gentle traction to the hand or foot while sliding the splint onto the injured limb. The hand or foot of the injured limb should always be included in the splint.

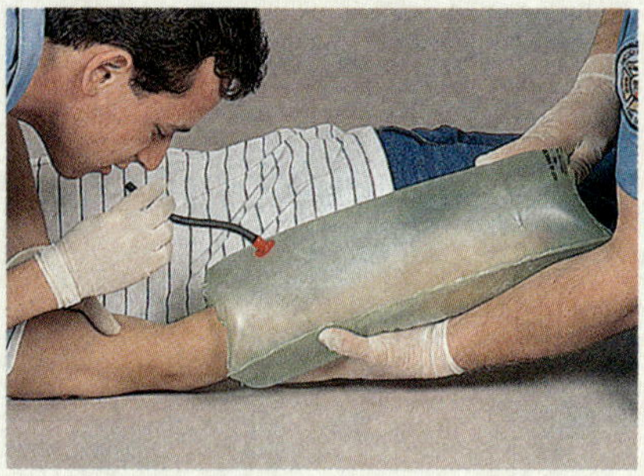

STEP 3 Your partner inflates the splint by mouth. Test the pressure in the splint. Check and record pulse and motor and sensory functions, and monitor them en route.

© Jones & Bartlett Learning. Courtesy of MIEMSS.

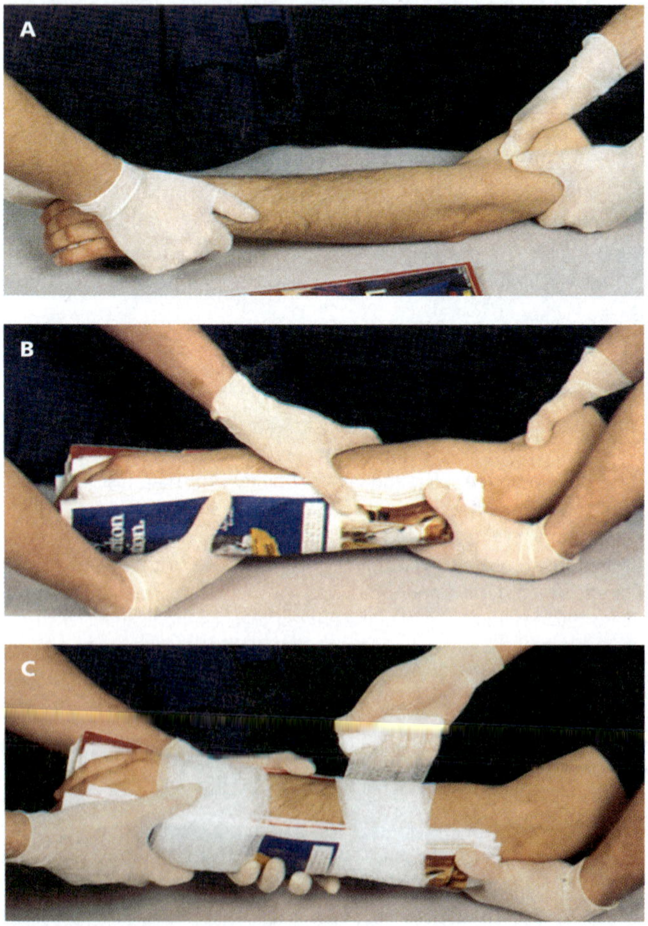

FIGURE 15-20 Applying an improvised splint using magazines. **A.** Stabilize the fracture above and below the fracture site. **B.** Place improvised splinting material around injured extremity. **C.** Secure in place with gauze, cravats, or other available material.

© American Academy of Orthopaedic Surgeons

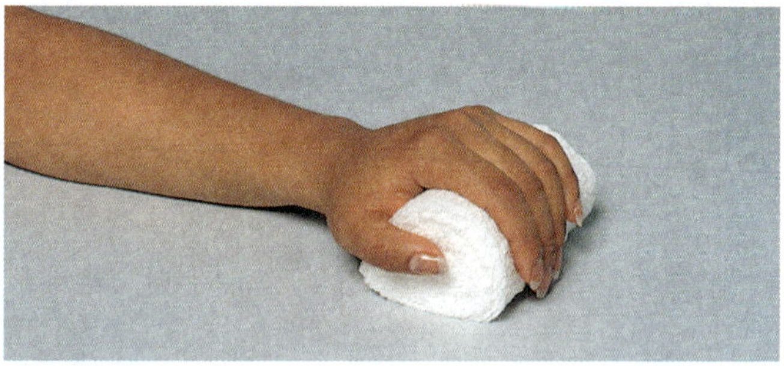

FIGURE 15-21 Position of function for the hand and wrist.

© American Academy of Orthopaedic Surgeons

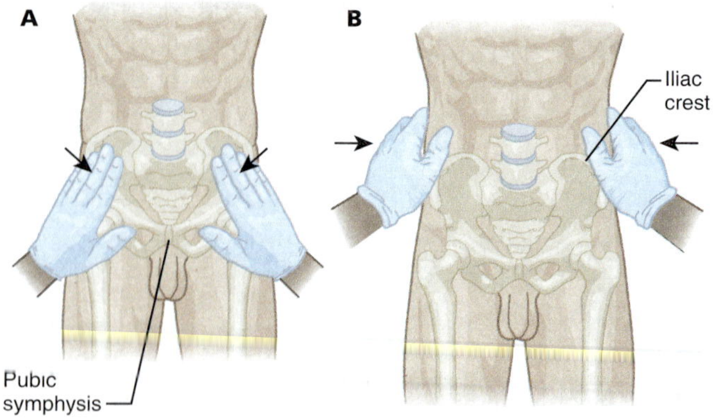

FIGURE 15-22 Examining the patient for pelvic fracture. **A.** Push down. **B.** Push in.

© Jones & Bartlett Learning

with a long backboard, as illustrated in **FIGURE 15-23**. EMTs may apply a pelvic compression binder to stabilize the fracture and treat shock.

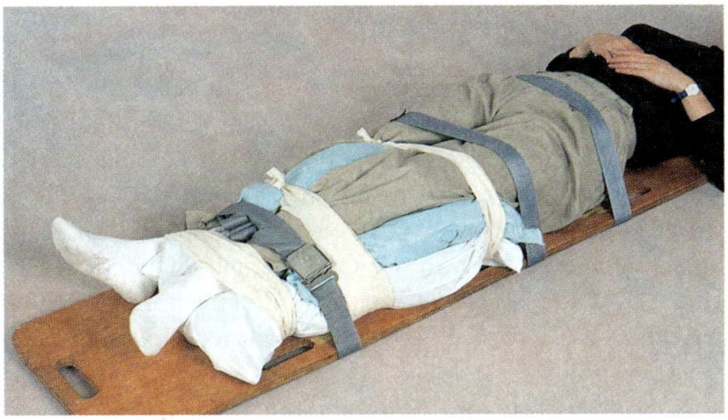

FIGURE 15-23 Stabilization of hip or pelvic injuries using a backboard.

© American Academy of Orthopaedic Surgeons

Hip Injuries

Two types of hip injuries are common: dislocations and fractures. Both injuries may result from high-energy **trauma**. When a passenger in the front seat of a motor vehicle is not wearing a seat belt and the vehicle crashes, the person is thrown forward and crashes against the dashboard. The impact of the knee against the dashboard is transmitted up the shaft of the thighbone (femur), injuring the hip and often producing either a dislocation or a fracture, or both (see Figure 15-6A).

Hip fractures occur at the upper end of the femur, rather than in the hip joint itself. Fractures of the hip region usually cause the injured limb to become shortened and externally (outwardly) rotated (**FIGURE 15-24**).

High-energy trauma is not the only cause of hip fractures. They can occur in older adults after only minimal trauma (such as when falling down). As mentioned previously, older adults, particularly women, are at an increased risk of osteoporosis. Patients with osteoporosis may sustain major fractures from minor falls. As you conduct your primary assessment, remember that other conditions may have contributed to the fall. Patients may have experienced a minor stroke, heart attack, or confusion before the fall, or they may not have seen an obstacle that caused them to trip.

A dislocated hip is extremely painful, especially when any movement is attempted. The joint is usually locked with the thigh flexed and rotated inward across the midline of the body. The knee joint is often flexed as well.

Treat all hip injuries by stabilizing the hip in the position found. Use several pillows and/or rolled blankets, especially under the flexed knee. The patient should be placed on a backboard for transport. The patient and the limb should be well stabilized to eliminate all motion in the hip region (see Figure 15-23).

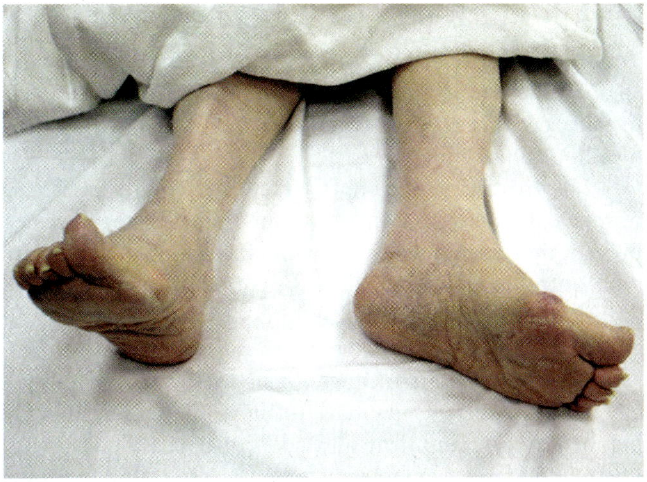

FIGURE 15-24 Signs of a hip fracture may include external rotation and shortening of the injured leg.

© E. M. Singletary, MD. Used with permission.

Because fractures of the upper end of the femur are so common in older patients, any older person who has fallen and reports pain in the hip, thigh, or knee should be splinted and transported to the hospital for radiographic evaluation, even if there is no deformity.

Special Populations

Nervous System Changes That Affect Mobility in Older Adults

Some conditions that affect balance and mobility may occur as the result of changes in the nervous system. One example is Parkinson disease. This condition affects the nerves' ability to properly conduct impulses and results in impaired mobility. Signs of Parkinson disease include slowed movements, shuffling, tremors, unsteady balance, trouble rising from a chair, abnormal stiffness, and light-headedness or fainting when standing.

When you assist an older patient, remember that as a person ages, physical movements become slower. Lend a helping hand or supporting arm. Many older patients are afraid of falling and your support will help them overcome this fear. Allow enough time for patients to move safely; do not rush them.

YOU are the EMR — CASE 2

On one of your days off from the station, you volunteer as an EMR at the local community college during events. Today you are working the softball tournament when one of the women slides safely into home plate with her right arm and hand outstretched. After making impact with the home plate, she immediately stands up, yelling in pain and cradling and protecting her right hand. Examination reveals considerable deformity on the palm side of the right hand. The patient reports significant pain in the hand and wrist and does not want to move the hand.

1. What type of examination should you perform on the patient's right arm?
2. Describe how you should splint this patient's injury.

Thigh Injuries

Trauma to the thigh can bruise the muscles or fracture the shaft of the femur. A fractured femur is very unstable and usually produces significant thigh deformity, with much bleeding and swelling.

The treatment of femoral fractures requires skill and proper equipment. As an EMR, you can take measures to prevent the onset of shock by maintaining body temperature and controlling bleeding. Place the patient in as comfortable a position as possible, and call for additional personnel and equipment.

However, there are times, such as after a motor vehicle crash, when you may have to move the patient quickly before proper equipment and additional personnel arrive. Learn and practice emergency temporary splinting for lower extremity injuries. Secure both legs together with several swathes, cravats, or bandages so they function as one unit. This technique will allow you to remove the patient from a dangerous environment quickly.

A traction splint is the most effective way to splint a unilateral isolated fractured femur. You cannot use a traction splint if there are injuries to the pelvis, knee, lower leg, ankle, or foot. Although you most likely do not have a traction splint in your EMR life support kit, you should learn this technique so that you can assist other EMS personnel if needed.

Before applying a traction splint, trained EMTs align deformed fractures by applying manual longitudinal traction. Once manual traction is applied, it must be maintained until the traction splint is fully in place (**FIGURE 15-25**). Because many different types of traction splints are available, you should learn to use the one that your department uses. Most are applied using basically the same method. **SKILL DRILL 15-6** illustrates the steps for applying a Hare traction splint.

To apply proper traction using this type of splint, it is essential that the foot end of the traction splint be elevated 6 to 8 inches (15 to 20 cm) off the ground. If the heel of the injured leg touches the ground, you will lose traction and have to reapply the splint. Most traction splints include a foot stand that elevates the limb. Check and recheck the pulse, capillary refill, and nerve function before and after a splint is applied (**FIGURE 15-26**). If your department uses a different type of traction splint, you will need to be instructed in how to apply it properly.

Knee Injuries

Always stabilize an injured knee in the same position that you find it. If it is straight, use long, padded board splints or a

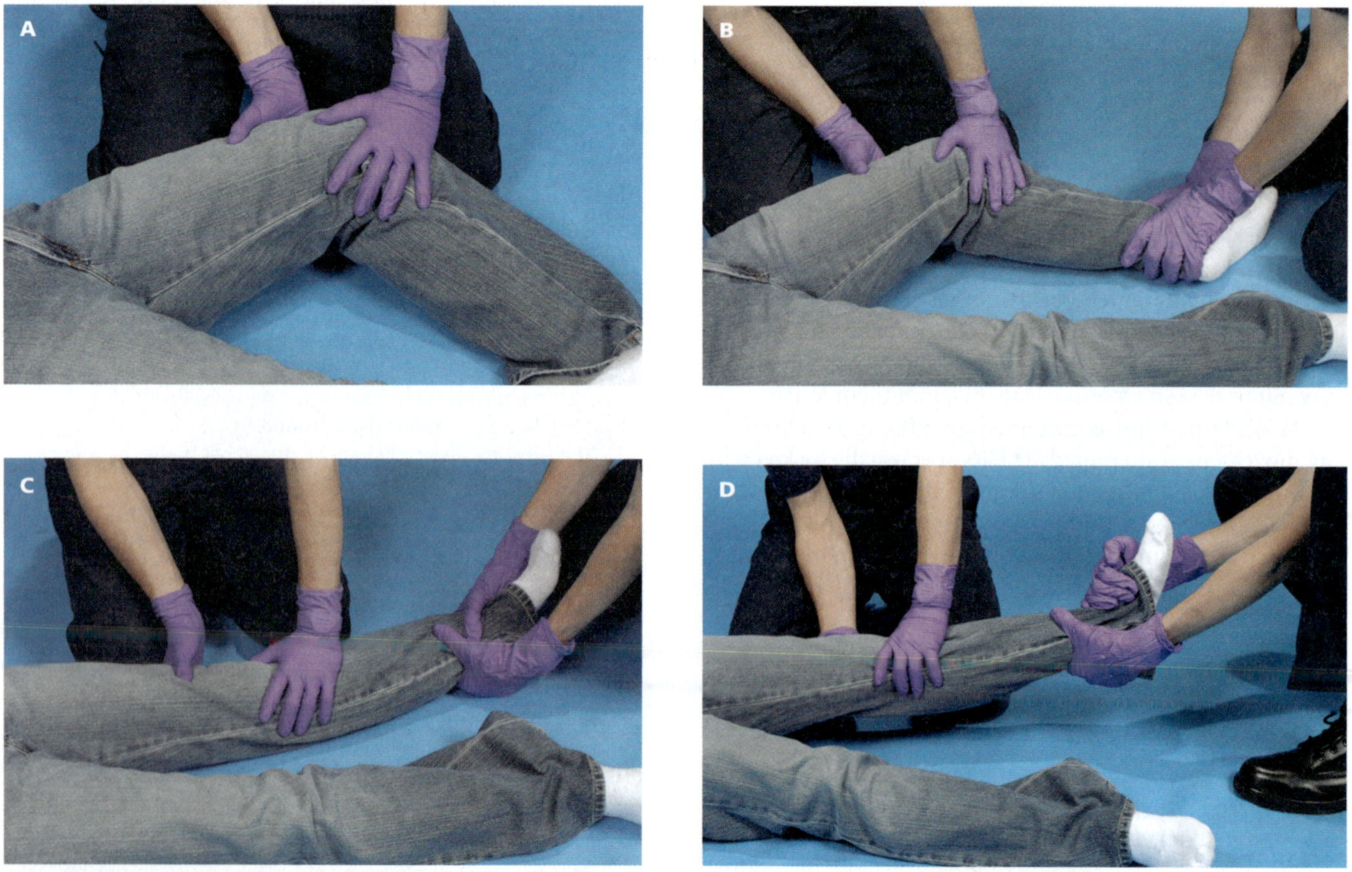

FIGURE 15-25 Straightening an injured leg for splinting. **A.** The first rescuer grasps the injured leg at the knee and applies traction in the long axis of the body. **B.** The second rescuer grasps the ankle. **C.** The second rescuer straightens the leg. **D.** The second rescuer maintains traction by leaning back.

© Jones & Bartlett Learning. Courtesy of MIEMSS.

SKILL DRILL 15-6

Applying a Traction Splint

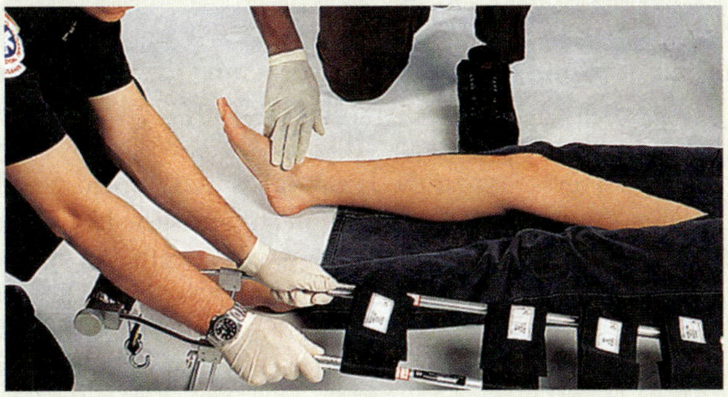

STEP 1 Place the splint beside the patient's uninjured leg and adjust it to the proper length. Open and adjust the four support straps. Position the support straps at the midthigh, above the knee, below the knee, and above the ankle.

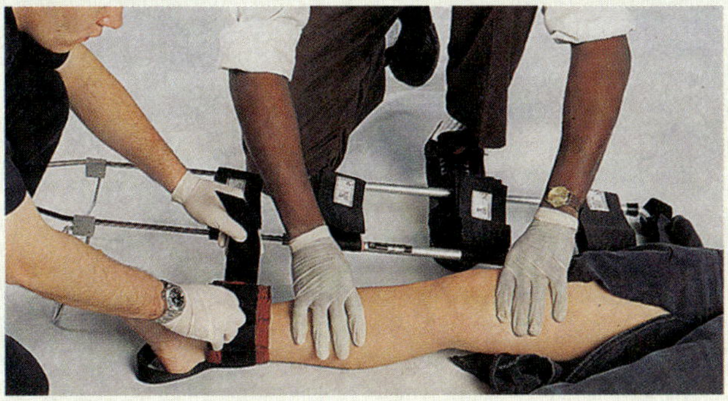

STEP 2 The first rescuer supports and stabilizes the injured limb while the second rescuer fastens the ankle hitch about the patient's ankle and foot.

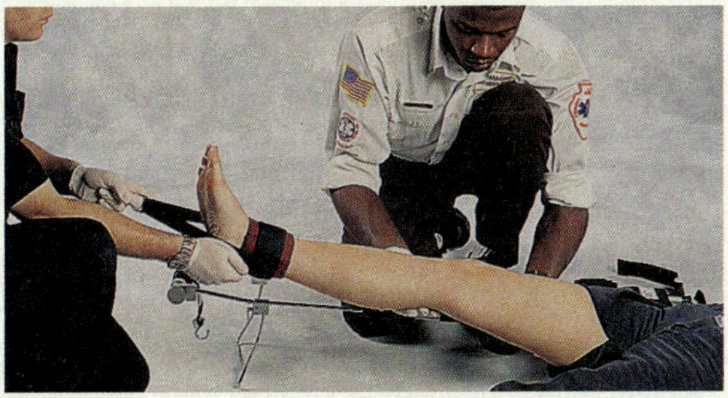

STEP 3 The first rescuer supports the leg at the site of the suspected injury while the second rescuer manually applies gentle traction to the ankle hitch and foot. Use only enough force to reposition the limb so it will fit into the splint.

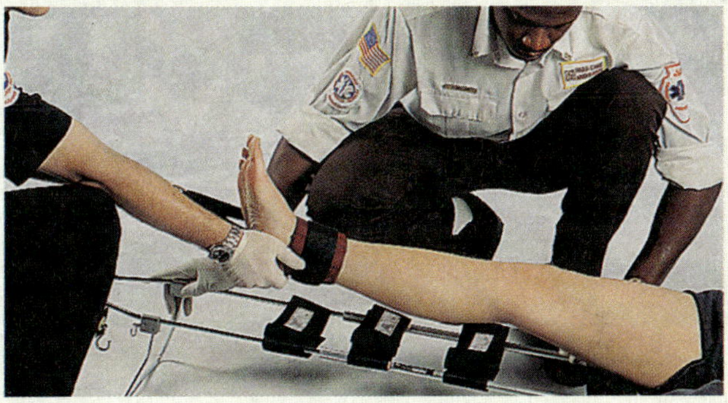

STEP 4 The first rescuer slides the splint into position under the patient's injured limb.

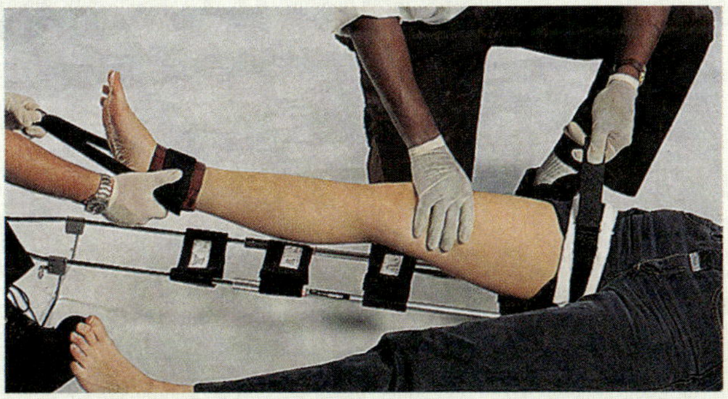

STEP 5 Pad the groin area and gently apply the strap around the midthigh.

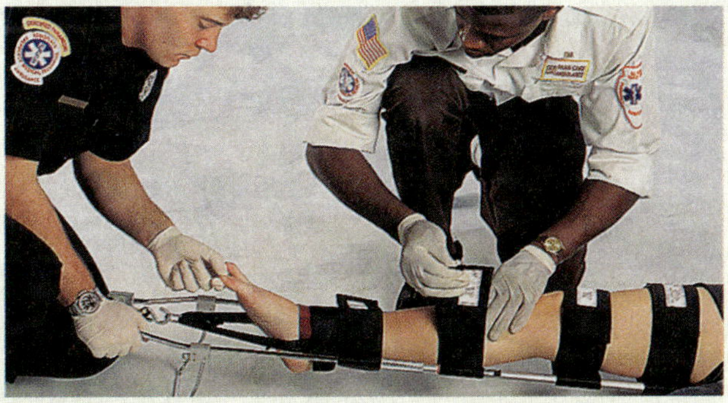

STEP 6 The first rescuer connects the loops of the ankle hitch to the end of the splint while the second rescuer continues to maintain traction. Apply gentle traction to the connecting strap between the ankle hitch and the splint until pain is relieved or the injured leg is the same length as the uninjured leg. Once the proper traction is applied, fasten the support straps to hold the limb securely in the splint. Check all support straps to make sure they are secure, and reassess pulse, capillary refill, and sensation.

© American Academy of Orthopaedic Surgeons

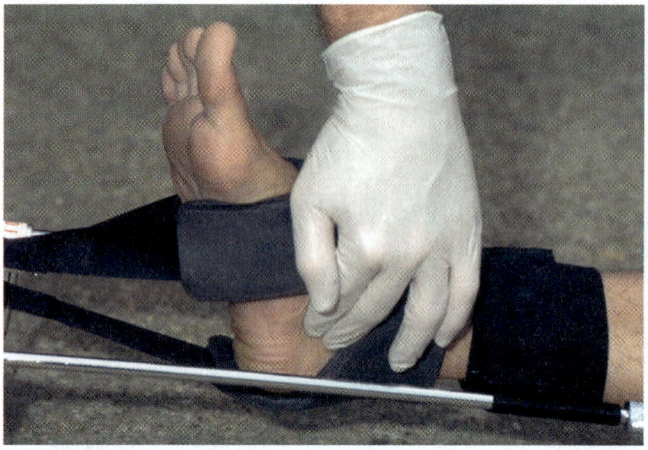

FIGURE 15-26 Checking the ankle pulse.
© Jones & Bartlett Learning. Courtesy of MIEMSS.

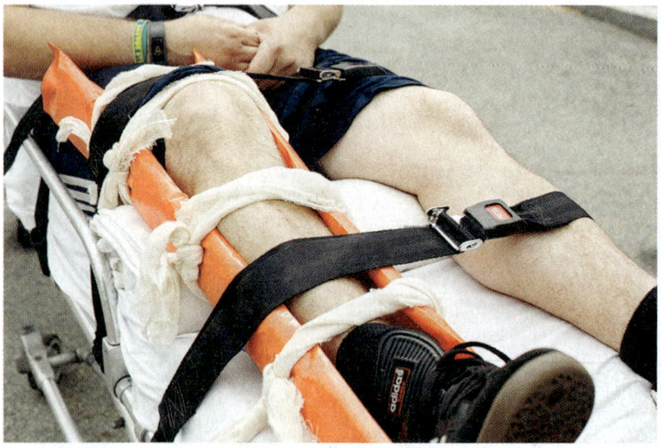

FIGURE 15-27 Stabilizing an injured knee.
© Jones & Bartlett Learning

long-leg air splint. If there is a significant deformity, place pillows, blankets, or clothing beneath the knee (**FIGURE 15-27**), secure the splint materials to the leg with bandages, swathes, or cravats, and secure the injured leg to the uninjured leg. Then place the patient on a backboard.

Leg Injuries

Like fractures of the forearm, fractures of the leg can be splinted with air splints, cardboard splints, and even magazines and newspapers. **SKILL DRILL 15-7** shows how to apply an air splint to the leg. It takes two trained people to splint an injured leg. One person supports the leg with both hands (above and below the injury site), while the other person applies the splint.

Ankle and Foot Injuries

You can splint fractures of the ankle and foot with a pillow or an air splint. Place the pillow splint around the injured ankle and foot, and tie or pin it in place (**SKILL DRILL 15-8**).

Additional Considerations

Remember that extremity injuries are not, in themselves, life threatening unless excessive bleeding is present. You may not always have the equipment or help you need to manage all types of extremity injuries. You may not even have time to splint an injury before additional EMS personnel arrive. However, there will be times when you are the only trained person at the scene of an incident. To prepare for such situations, practice splinting until you can quickly and competently apply the principles in any situation. Because you may find patients in a variety of positions and locations, practice splinting both a sitting and a prone volunteer.

SKILL DRILL 15-7

Applying an Air Splint to the Leg

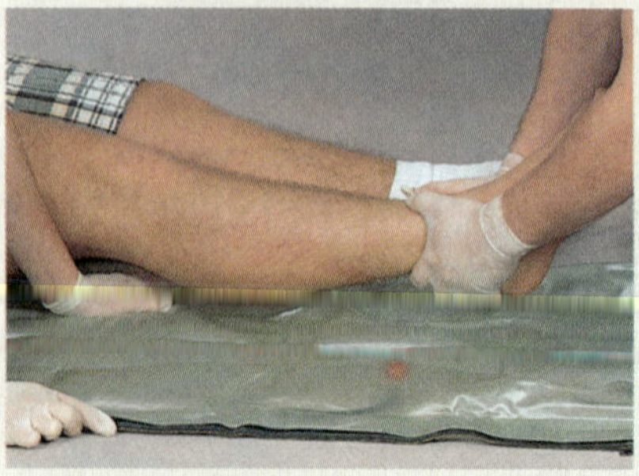

STEP 1 The first rescuer supports the injured limb. The second rescuer slides the splint under the limb.

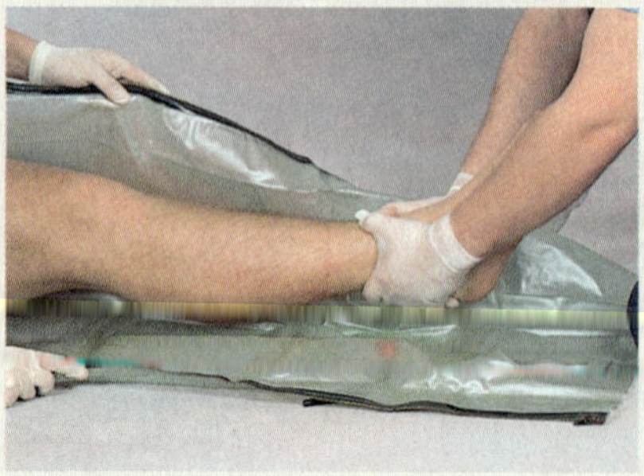

STEP 2 The second rescuer places the splint around the limb.

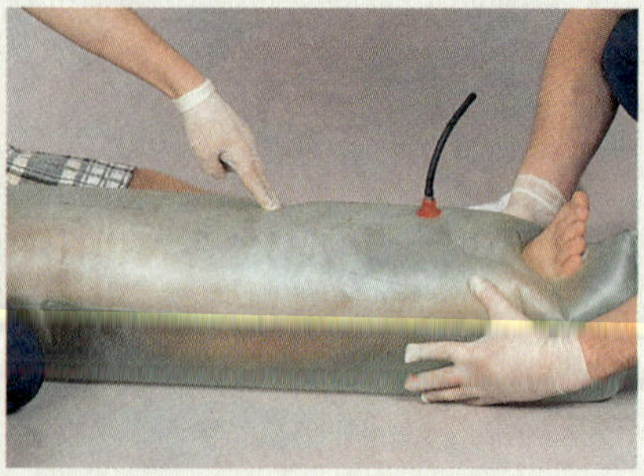

STEP 3 The first rescuer slides their hands out of the splint while the second rescuer inflates the splint. Either rescuer rechecks the pulse, capillary refill, and sensation of the injured leg.

© Jones & Bartlett Learning. Courtesy of MIEMSS.

SKILL DRILL 15-8

Applying a Pillow Splint for Ankle or Foot Injury

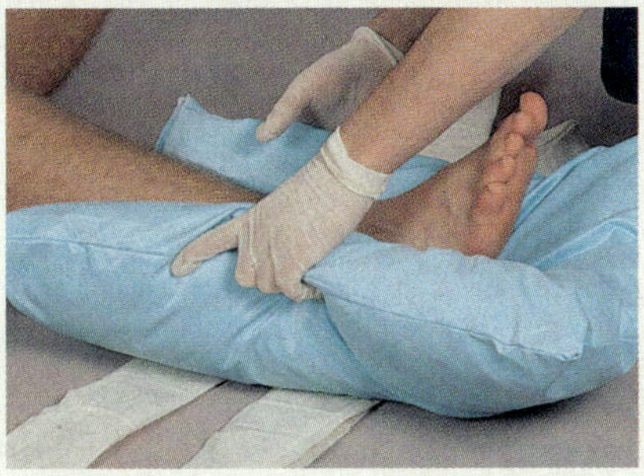

STEP 1 Place a pillow under the injured limb. Mold the pillow around the foot and ankle, keeping the foot in the position of function.

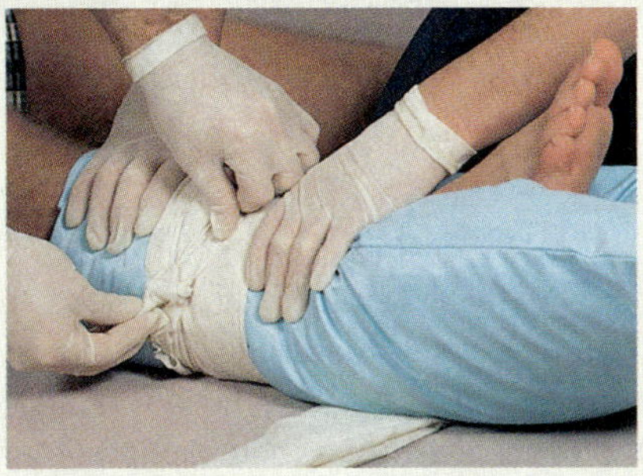

STEP 2 Secure the pillow with cravats, swathes, or bandages.

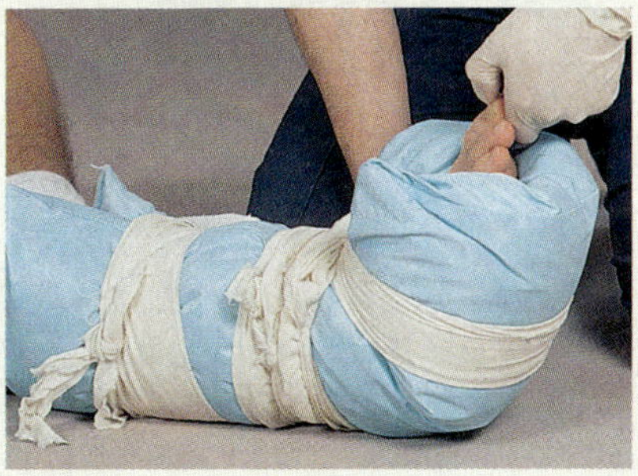

STEP 3 Recheck the pulse, capillary refill, and sensation.

© Jones & Bartlett Learning. Courtesy of MIEMSS.

Treatment

Pad all rigid splints to provide the best stabilization and pain relief. Do not apply any splint too tightly. Recheck the pulse, capillary refill, and sensation after applying the splint to make sure that no damage has been done (**FIGURE 15-28**).

It takes two people to splint most limb injuries adequately: one person to stabilize and support the extremity and one person to apply the splint. Most of the principles and techniques of splinting covered in this chapter require that you work with another member of the EMS team. Learn how the team functions as a unit during stressful situations and be prepared to work with any member of the EMS team who arrives to assist you.

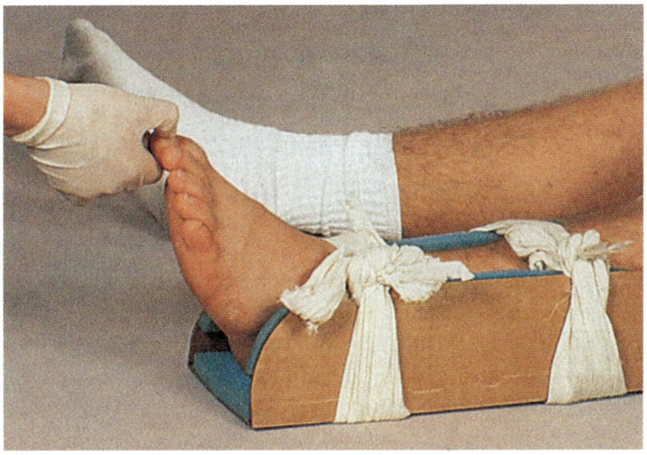

FIGURE 15-28 Checking capillary refill on splinted injured leg.

© Jones & Bartlett Learning. Courtesy of MIEMSS.

YOU are the EMR — CASE 3

It is a quiet Sunday morning. At 1043 hours, you are dispatched to a local church for a report of a woman who has fallen in a religious education room. When you arrive at the scene, an usher takes you to your patient. The woman is lying on her back and has her left leg pulled up in an abnormal position. She complains of pain in her left hip area. In response to your questions, she tells you that she is 73 years old and that she takes medication for high blood pressure and diabetes and also takes calcium supplements. She tells you that she got up from her chair and tripped on a loose piece of carpeting. She thinks she heard a snap when she fell. Your assessment reveals moderate pain in her left hip area and an externally rotated and shortened left leg.

1. What type of injury do you believe is most likely based on her pain and on your patient assessment?
2. Because the patient did not experience significant trauma, what underlying factors may have contributed to this injury?
3. How should you prepare this patient for transport?

Voices of Experience

Early in my career, when faced with a patient who had a painful, bruised, or swollen injury, I would complete a full primary and secondary assessment. On completion of my assessment, and after realizing that the patient had only an isolated musculoskeletal injury, I would put my splinting and immobilizing knowledge and skills to use. Many times, we would splint extremities with padded boards or padded metal splints, then tape or use cravats to secure the splint to the extremity to prevent continued movement and pain.

Looking back, I believe many times we manipulated the injury more than necessary by applying the splint at the scene and then removing it at the emergency department. In many cases, we caused more movement and pain than if we had used simple splinting material or had the patient self-splint their injury. When delivering the patient to the hospital after completing a detailed splint, we would often get funny looks from the hospital staff as they were removing our splint. Over the years, I have realized that a fancy splint, especially if it required manipulating the injured extremity, was not necessary.

"A fancy splint, especially if it required manipulating the injured extremity, was not necessary."

On one occasion, we moved a patient with a chief complaint of hip pain from her couch onto a scoop stretcher. We then secured her to a backboard, making sure we did not move her excessively. We then put her on the ambulance cot and transported her to the hospital, which was a 45-minute transport. Really!

With the experience I have now gained, I would do a three-person lift, placing her directly on the soft ambulance cot with blankets and pillows under her knees and her head raised for comfort. Not only can you stabilize the hip on the stretcher with pillows and straps, but you can avoid making your patient lie on a hard, flat backboard where bed sores can start forming, as long as there is no reason to suspect a spinal injury.

You've probably heard the phrase "keep it simple" many times, and in EMS, this holds true most of the time. Use simple equipment that minimizes movement and pain and that can be applied and removed easily. Vacuum splints make splinting very easy. Don't forget to put a cold compress and a gauze or towel on the injury to decrease swelling. Keep it simple, and have a great career in EMS.

Mark Weber
EMS Director
Golden Heart Services
Heart of America Medical Center
Rugby, North Dakota

Adapted from the personal Medical Identification Symbol of the American Medical Association.

Special Populations

Pediatric Trauma Patients

Trauma remains the number one killer of children. Treat an injured child as you would treat an injured adult, but remember the following differences:

1. A child cannot communicate symptoms as well as an adult.
2. A child may be shy and overwhelmed by adult rescuers (especially those in uniform), so it is important to develop a good relationship quickly to reduce the child's fear and anxiety.
3. You may have to adapt materials and equipment to the child's size.
4. A child does not show signs of shock as early as an adult but can progress into severe shock quickly.

The type of trauma a child experiences, the type of activity causing the injury, and the child's anatomy affect the pattern of injuries sustained by the child. Motor vehicle crashes produce different patterns of injuries depending on whether the patient was using a seat belt, whether the patient was strapped into a car seat, and whether an airbag inflated in the crash. Unrestrained patients tend to have more head and neck injuries. Restrained passengers often sustain head injuries, spinal injuries, and abdominal injuries. Children struck while riding a bicycle often have head, spinal, abdominal, and extremity injuries. The use of bicycle helmets greatly reduces the number and severity of head injuries. Pedestrians who are struck by a vehicle often sustain chest and abdominal injuries with internal bleeding, injuries to the thighs, and head injuries. Falls from a height or diving accidents tend to cause head and spinal injuries and extremity injuries. Burns are a major cause of injuries to children. Sports activities cause a wide variety of injuries depending on the type of sports activity. By learning some of the basic patterns of injury, you can anticipate the injuries you may find when carefully examining pediatric patients.

If the child has been struck by a motor vehicle, look for the common types of injuries shown in **FIGURE 15-29**. Major trauma in children usually results in multiple system injuries. No matter what the cause of injury, your first priority is always to check the patient's ABCs, perform lifesaving interventions, and proceed with the full-body assessment to determine the extent of any other injuries. The full-body assessment is a hands-on procedure. A complete examination is especially important because a child cannot always communicate symptoms. It should proceed from toe to head, starting with noninjured areas before moving to painful ones. Involve the child in the physical examination as much as possible. Ask the child simple questions. Complete the full-body assessment even if the patient is too young to understand what is happening. Then stabilize all injuries you find. Splint suspected fractures, bandage wounds, and initiate spinal motion restriction when appropriate.

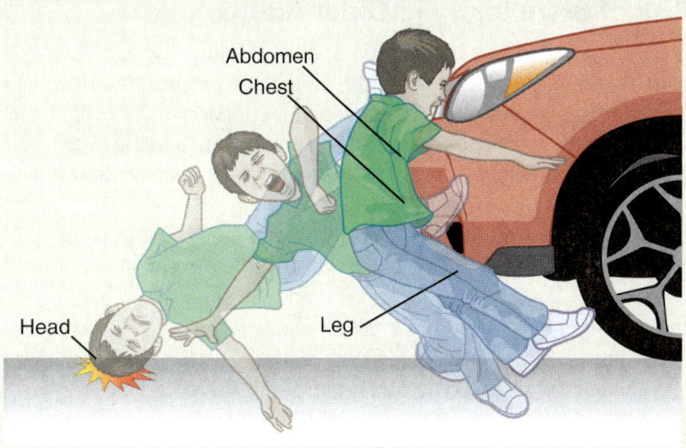

FIGURE 15-29 Look for these typical injuries when a child has been hit by a motor vehicle.
© Jones & Bartlett Learning

Injuries of the Head (Skull and Brain)

Severe head and spinal cord injuries can result from many different types of trauma. These injuries are common causes of death and can lead to irreversible **paralysis** and permanent brain damage. Improperly handling a patient after an incident can cause further injury or death. For example, well-intentioned citizens pulling a patient from a wrecked car or poor treatment from inadequately trained emergency personnel can cause spinal injuries. As an EMR, you must know what to do to provide prompt treatment and avoid errors that may make the injury worse.

The human skull has two primary parts (**FIGURE 15-30**):

1. The top of the skull, or vault, is formed by a tough four-bone shell that protects the brain.
2. The facial bones, which give form to the face and supply frontal protection for the brain.

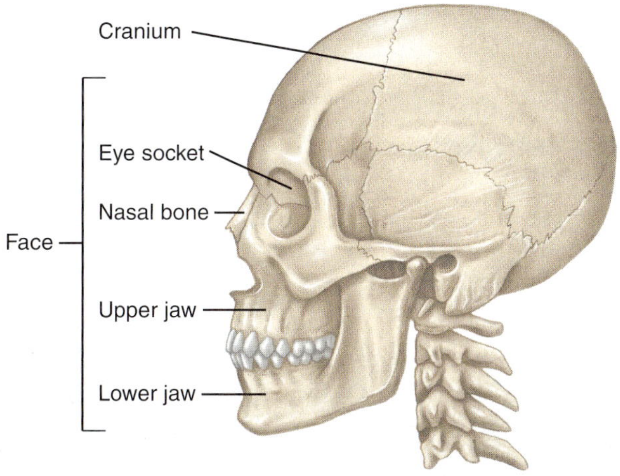

FIGURE 15-30 Cranium and face of the human skull.
© Jones & Bartlett Learning

Mechanisms of Injury

Head injuries are common with certain types of trauma. Of patients involved in motor vehicle crashes, 70% sustain some degree of head injury. Imagine the cranium as a rigid bowl, containing the delicate brain (**FIGURE 15-31**). Between the skull and brain, a fluid called **cerebrospinal fluid (CSF)** cushions the brain from direct blows. A direct force such as a hammer blow can injure the skull and the brain inside. Indirect forces can also cause injury, such as in a motor vehicle

Special Populations

Risk of Brain Injury in Older Adults

The older adult's brain is more susceptible to injury during falls because the blood vessels are more fragile and because the brain becomes smaller with advanced age. The reduction in the brain's size results in greater space in the cranium, which increases the potential force with which the brain may impact the skull during a traumatic event.

Spinal injury is often associated with head injury. The force of direct blows to the head is often transmitted to the spine, producing a fracture or dislocation. The injuries may damage the spinal cord or at least put it at risk for injury. Any time you suspect or identify an injury to the head or skull, suspect injury to the neck and spinal cord as well. Therefore, perform spinal motion restriction for all patients with head injuries to protect the spinal cord.

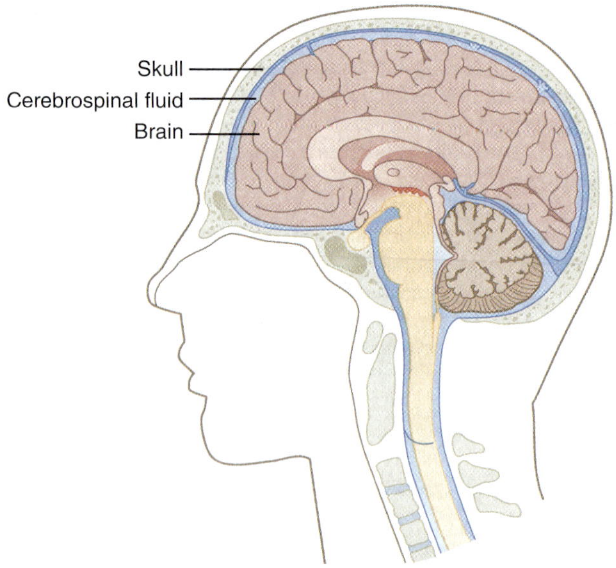

FIGURE 15-31 The brain.
© Jones & Bartlett Learning

Words of Wisdom

In many cities, electronic bikes and scooters are set out in public areas for rental, offering tourists and commuters a convenient, inexpensive way to get around. Unfortunately, their popularity has come with an increase in traumatic injuries relating to their use. In the United States, hospitalizations from scooter crashes nearly tripled from 2016 to 2020. Compared to individuals involved in conventional bicycle or scooter crashes, these patients are more likely to sustain injuries requiring surgery, particularly head injuries and long bone fractures or paralysis. As an EMR, you should understand the unique risks in your community and be prepared to provide the necessary care. As a public health advocate, you may also have the opportunity to participate in legislative or educational efforts (such as helmet use) to reduce injuries.

crash when the head strikes the windshield and causes the brain to bounce against the inside of the skull.

Types of Head Injuries

Injuries of the head are classified as open or closed (**FIGURE 15-32**). In a **closed head injury**, bleeding and swelling within the skull may increase pressure on the brain, leading to irreversible brain damage and death if it is not relieved. An open injury of the head usually bleeds profusely. Severe open head injuries are serious but not always fatal.

Examine the nose, eyes, and the wound itself to see if any blood or CSF is seeping out. The CSF is clear, watery, and straw colored. In severe cases of open head injury, brain tissue or bone may be visible.

Signs and Symptoms of Head Injuries

A patient who sustained a head injury may exhibit some or all of the signs and symptoms shown in the Signs and Symptoms box. A serious head injury may also produce raccoon eyes and Battle sign. Raccoon eyes look like the black eyes that develop after a fistfight. Battle sign appears as a bruise behind one or both ears (**FIGURE 15-33**).

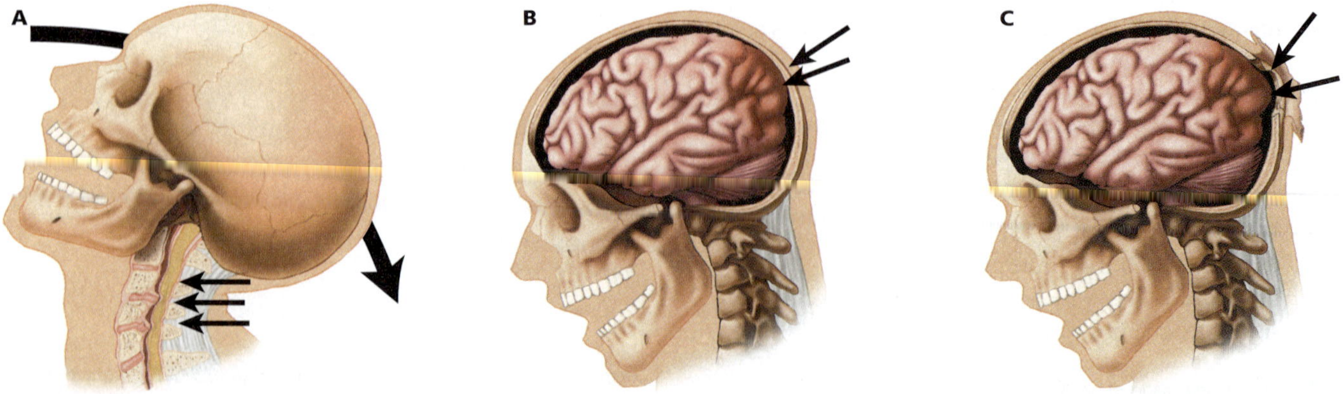

FIGURE 15-32 Open and closed head injuries. **A.** A head injury may occur in conjunction with a cervical spine injury. **B.** A closed head injury. **C.** An open head injury.
© Jones & Bartlett Learning

Signs and Symptoms

Signs and symptoms of head injuries include the following:

- Confusion
- Unusual behavior
- Unresponsiveness
- Nausea or vomiting
- Blood from an ear
- Decreasing responsiveness
- Unequal pupils
- Paralysis
- Seizure
- External head trauma: bleeding, bumps, and contusions

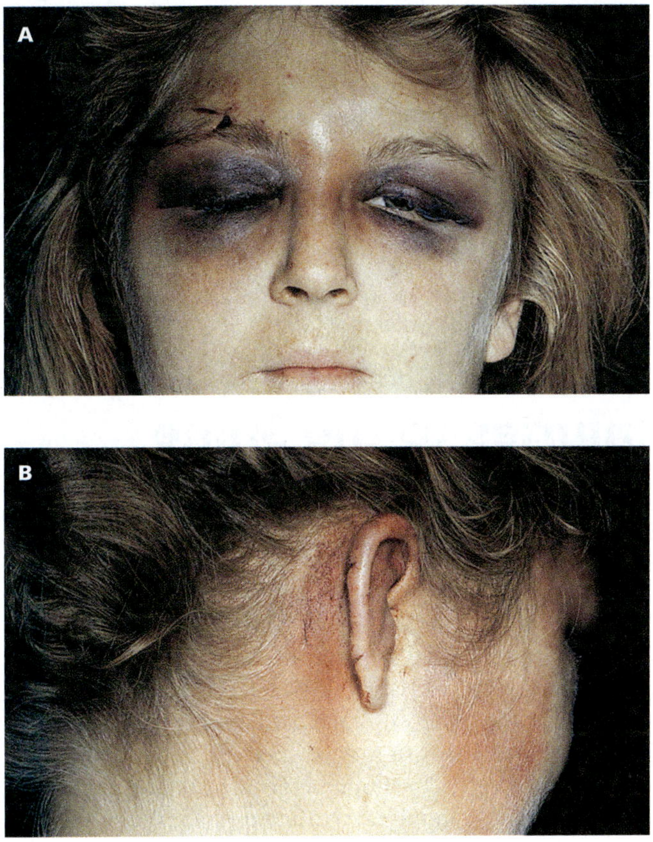

FIGURE 15-33 Signs of head injury. **A.** Raccoon eyes. **B.** Battle sign.

© American Academy of Orthopaedic Surgeons

A **concussion**, or mild **traumatic brain injury (TBI)**, is a closed brain injury caused by a blow, a bump, or a jolt that disrupts the normal function of the brain. Children and older people are at high risk for these injuries. The severity of concussions may range from a mild injury that causes a brief change in mental status to a severe injury that causes an extended period of unresponsiveness or memory loss after the injury. The leading causes of concussions are falls, motor vehicle crashes, and impact by or against an object (such as sports injuries or blast injuries). These injuries can occur without visible signs of trauma. The signs and symptoms of a concussion can be subtle and may not be immediately apparent. Symptoms may be immediate or may not appear until hours or days after the injury. They may include the following:

- Temporary loss of responsiveness
- Headache or feeling of pressure in the head
- Confusion or seeming to be dazed
- Inability to remember the traumatic event
- Dizziness or seeing stars
- Nausea and vomiting

Any time you see that a patient has experienced a traumatic event and exhibits these signs and symptoms, assess the patient and then prepare for transport to an appropriate medical facility for evaluation by a physician.

Treatment of Head Injuries

When one sign or symptom of head injury is present, proceed as follows:

1. With the head in a neutral in-line position, stabilize the patient's neck and prevent movement of the head. If returning the head to a neutral position is met with resistance, leave it in the position found.
2. Maintain an open airway. To avoid extending the patient's neck, use the jaw-thrust maneuver to open the airway. Be prepared to suction if the patient vomits. Avoid movement of the head and neck.
3. Support the patient's breathing. Be sure that the patient is breathing adequately on their own. If not, institute bag-mask ventilation. Administer oxygen as soon as it is available if you are trained to use it. Oxygen helps reduce the severity of brain injury.
4. Monitor circulation. Be prepared to support circulation by performing full cardiopulmonary resuscitation (CPR) if the patient's heart stops.
5. Check to see if CSF or blood is seeping from a wound or from the nose or ears (**FIGURE 15-34**). Do not try to stop leakage of CSF from a wound or any other opening because leakage from inside the skull relieves internal pressure. Instead, tape a dressing loosely over the ear to prevent other debris from entering through the opening.
6. Control bleeding from all head wounds with dry, sterile dressings. Use enough direct pressure with the palm of your hand to control the bleeding without disturbing the underlying tissue. Never use your fingers to apply pressure. They may actually penetrate the brain tissue.
7. Examine and treat other serious injuries.
8. Arrange for prompt transport to an appropriate medical facility.

Safety

If a patient has a head injury, assume that an associated neck or spinal cord injury is also present. Do nothing that would cause undue movement of the head and spine. Always restrict motion throughout the entire spine before moving the patient. If you are alone and need to ventilate the patient with a bag-mask device, use your knees to maintain the head in a neutral in-line position.

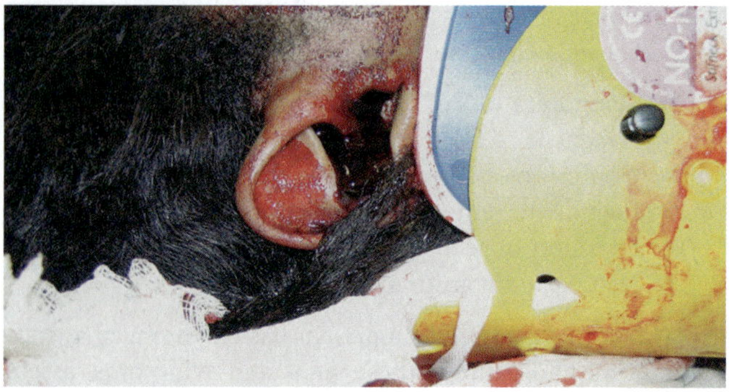

FIGURE 15-34 Blood or cerebrospinal fluid draining from the ear indicates head injury.
© E. M. Singletary, MD. Used with permission.

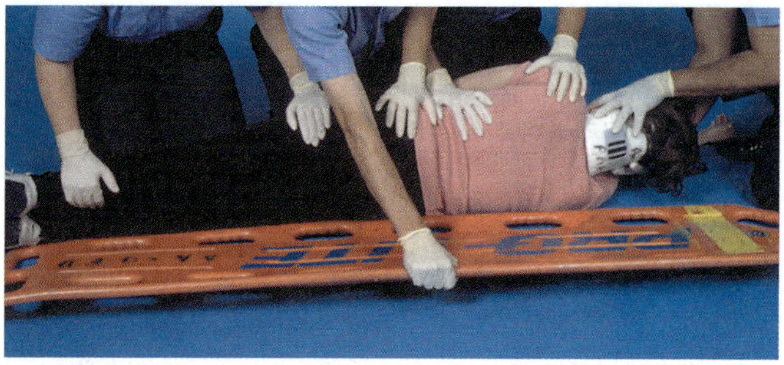

FIGURE 15-35 Keep the head and spine in alignment by using the log roll technique.
© Jones & Bartlett Learning

Injuries of the Face

Facial injuries commonly result from the following types of incidents:

- Motor vehicle crashes in which the patient's face hits the steering wheel or windshield
- Assaults
- Falls

Airway obstruction is the primary immediate danger in severe facial injuries. Severe damage to the face and facial bones can cause bleeding and the collapse of the facial bones, leading to airway conditions. If the patient has facial injuries, also suspect a spinal injury. Although facial injuries may bleed considerably, they are rarely life threatening unless the airway is obstructed.

Treatment of Facial Injuries

When facial injuries are present, proceed as follows to care for the patient:

1. With the head in a neutral in-line position, stabilize it to prevent further movement of the neck.
2. Maintain an open airway. Use the jaw-thrust maneuver to open the airway. Clear any blood or vomitus from the patient's mouth with your gloved fingers or a suction device if available.
3. Support breathing. Be prepared to ventilate the patient, if necessary.
4. Monitor circulation.
5. Control bleeding by covering any wound with a dry, sterile dressing and applying direct pressure. Be sure to check for wounds inside the mouth. Try to prevent the patient from swallowing blood because this can cause vomiting. Have suction ready for use.
6. Look for and stabilize other serious injuries.
7. Arrange for prompt transport to an appropriate medical facility.

If these measures do not keep the airway clear or if you are unable to control severe facial bleeding, log roll the patient onto a side, keeping the head and spine stable and rolling the whole body as a unit. Turn the head and body at the same time. Do not allow the neck to twist (**FIGURE 15-35**).

Bandage facial injuries. If possible, leave the patient's eyes clear of bandages so they can see what is happening. Being able to see reduces the patient's tendency to panic. Bandaging facial injuries is discussed in Chapter 14, *Bleeding, Shock, and Soft-Tissue Injuries*.

Safety

If a patient has head or spine injuries, use a log roll to move the patient onto their side. Do not place these patients in the recovery position. Provide support for the head and neck.

Injuries to the Spine

Spinal injuries can cause irreversible paralysis. As an EMR, you must know how to handle a patient properly and provide prompt treatment. Errors may make the injury worse.

Mechanisms of Injury

If one or more vertebrae are injured, the spinal cord may also be injured. A displaced vertebra, swelling, or bleeding may put pressure on the spinal cord and damage it (**FIGURE 15-36**). In severe cases, the cord may be severed. If all or part of the spinal cord is cut, nerve impulses (which are like signals in a telephone cable) cannot travel to and from the brain. Without the conduction of these nerve impulses, the patient is paralyzed below the point of injury. Injury to the spinal cord high in the neck paralyzes the diaphragm as well as the chest wall and results in complete loss of the patient's ability to breathe on their own. Gunshot wounds to the chest or abdomen may produce spinal cord injury at that level. Falls, motor vehicle crashes, and stabbings are other common causes of spinal injuries. Consider the possibility of a spinal injury if the patient has sustained high-energy trauma.

Some common causes of spinal cord injuries are as follows:

- Athletic collisions
- Diving injuries
- Gunshot wounds and stabbings to the chest or neck
- Falls of greater than three times the patient's height
- Hangings

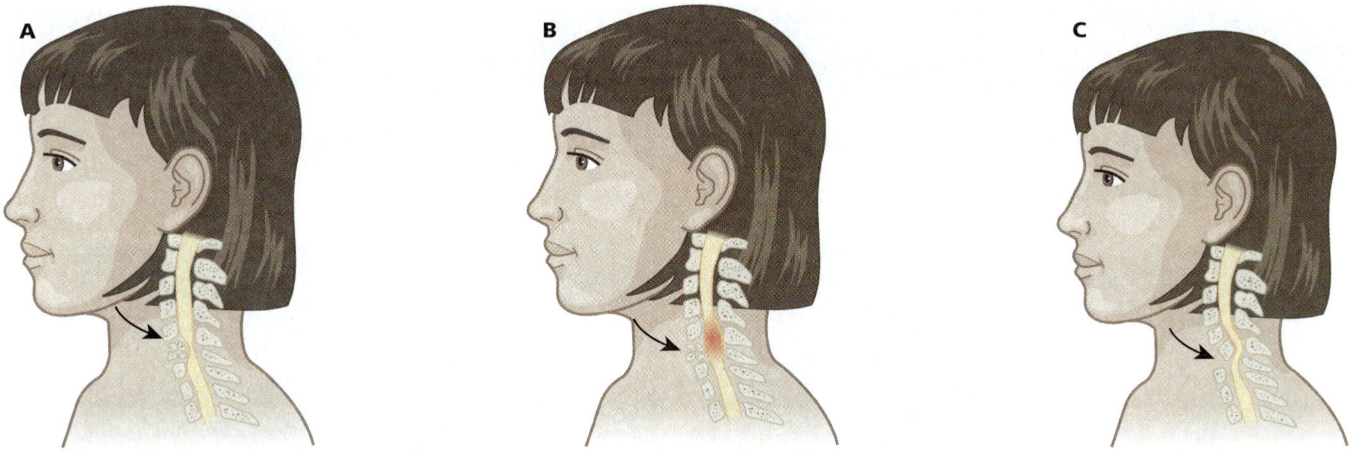

FIGURE 15-36 Types of spinal cord injuries. **A.** Pressure on the spinal cord from swelling or fracture. **B.** Bruising of the spinal cord by broken vertebrae. **C.** Injury by displacement and fractured vertebrae.
© Jones & Bartlett Learning

- Motorcycle crashes at speeds of over 20 mph
- Motor vehicle crashes with the following conditions:
  - Patient is ejected from vehicle.
  - Patient is unrestrained.
  - Speed is more than 40 mph.
  - There is at least 12 inches (30 cm) of intrusion into the passenger compartment.

Signs and Symptoms of Spinal Cord Injury

To determine whether a patient has sustained an injury to the spinal cord, talk to the patient and perform a careful examination to help determine the MOI. Gently conduct a hands-on examination to detect paralysis or weakness. Ask the patient to describe any points of tenderness or pain. Do not move the patient during your examination, and ask the patient to keep still. The key signs and symptoms of a spinal injury are noted in the Signs and Symptoms box. During your examination, be extremely careful and take your time. Position yourself so that the patient will not need to move their head to communicate with you. Do not move patients unless they are in a hazardous area.

Signs and Symptoms

Signs and symptoms of spinal injuries include:

- Tenderness over any point on the spine or neck
- Pain in the neck or spine or pain radiating to an extremity
- Extremity weakness, numbness, paralysis, or loss of movement
- Loss of sensation or movement, or tingling or burning sensation, in any part of the body below the neck
- Loss of bowel or bladder control

Treatment of Spinal Injuries

If any sign or symptom of spinal injury is present, proceed as follows:

1. Place the head and neck in a neutral in-line position. Avoid unnecessary movement of the head.
2. Stabilize the head and prevent movement of the neck (**SKILL DRILL 15-9**).
3. Maintain an open airway. Use the jaw-thrust maneuver to open the airway to avoid movement of the head and neck. Clear any blood or vomitus from the mouth with your gloved fingers or suction if it is available.
4. Support the patient's breathing. A spinal cord injury may paralyze some or all of the respiratory muscles, resulting in abnormal breathing patterns. In some cases, only the diaphragm may be working. Breathing using the diaphragm only is called **abdominal breathing**. The abdomen (not the lungs) swells and collapses with each breath. Help the patient breathe by administering oxygen (if available) and by keeping the airway open.
5. Monitor circulation.
6. Assess the pulse, movement, and sensation in all extremities.
7. Examine and treat other serious injuries.
8. Do not move the patient unless it is necessary to perform CPR or to remove the patient from a dangerous environment.
9. Assist with spinal motion restriction using an appropriate device.
10. Arrange for prompt transport to an appropriate medical facility.

Safety

If you suspect the presence of a spinal injury, it is essential to establish spinal motion restriction and protect the injury until hospital tests rule out a spinal cord injury. Do not move patients unless it is necessary to perform CPR or remove them from a dangerous environment.

Motorcycle and Sports Helmets

Many patients with neck injuries are motorcyclists or sports players who are wearing protective helmets. In almost all instances, it is not necessary to remove a helmet. Helmets are

SKILL DRILL 15-9

Stabilizing the Cervical Spine and Maintaining an Open Airway

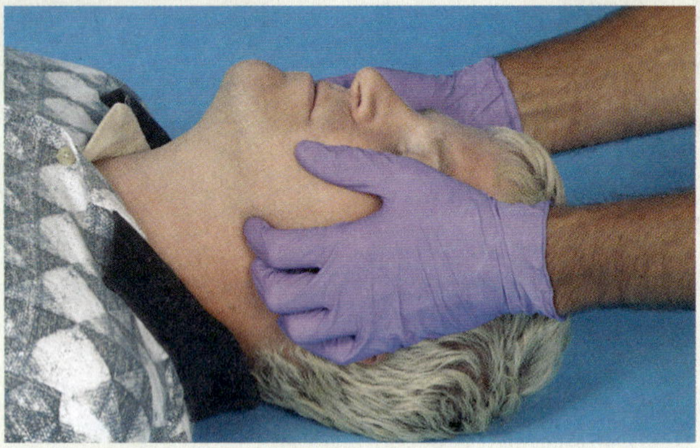

STEP 1 Stabilize the head and prevent movement of the neck. Place the head and neck in a neutral in-line position with the ears directly over the shoulders.

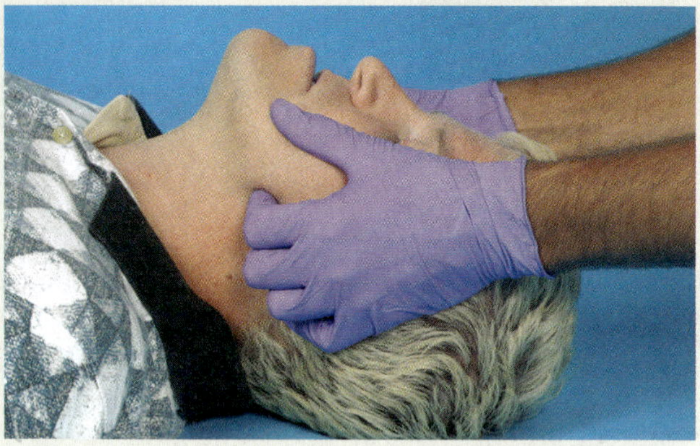

STEP 2 In this position, the rescuer can maintain an open airway with the jaw-thrust maneuver. Do not manipulate or twist the head and neck. After you have manually stabilized the head and neck, you must maintain support until spinal motion restriction is complete. Use a rigid collar and a long or short backboard. Review the steps for applying a cervical collar and a short backboard device, which are covered in Chapter 3, *Lifting and Moving Patients*.

© Jones & Bartlett Learning. Courtesy of MIEMSS.

frequently snug and cradle the head; therefore, they can be secured directly to the transport device. However, if helmets are not removed, you may need to pad under the shoulders to maintain the head in a neutral in-line position. If the patient is a football player and wearing shoulder pads, this may not be necessary.

Remove part or all of a helmet under only two circumstances:

1. **The face mask or visor interferes with adequate ventilation or with your ability to restore an adequate airway.** In this situation, lift the visor away from the face. In the case of a football helmet, remove the face guard. Some newer football helmets have a tough plastic strap fixing the face guard to the mask. Trainers and coaches should have a special tool readily available that can remove the face guard. Also, loosen the chin strap to facilitate the jaw-thrust maneuver. In most instances, exposing the face and jaw allows you access to the airway to secure adequate ventilation. Most football face guards are fastened to the helmet by four plastic clips, which can be cut with a sharp knife or unscrewed with a screwdriver to remove the face guard, as shown in **SKILL DRILL 15-10**.
2. **The helmet is so loose that securing it to the transport device will not provide adequate stabilization of the head.** Most motorcycle helmets fall into this category, whereas most football helmets fit snugly. A loose helmet can be removed easily while the head and neck are being stabilized manually. The procedure for helmet removal in this circumstance is shown in **SKILL DRILL 15-11**. Note that this procedure requires two experienced people.

Words of Wisdom

Once you have established spinal motion restriction, maintain it until the care of the patient is turned over to more highly trained prehospital EMS personnel or hospital-based personnel. Measures taken to protect the spine may be removed in the hospital after a physician evaluates the patient and often after radiographs or other diagnostic tests are conducted. Some EMS systems have adopted specific protocols that permit EMTs and paramedics to remove spinal motion restriction in certain specific situations after they have completed a thorough patient assessment process that follows a specific protocol approved by their medical director.

The steps for evaluating a patient to determine if spinal motion restriction can be removed are not taught in this course. Continue to maintain spinal motion restriction until you turn the care of the patient over to more highly trained EMS or hospital personnel, but be aware that they may use a process that results in discontinuation of the procedures that you appropriately initiated.

SKILL DRILL 15-10

Removing the Mask on a Sports Helmet

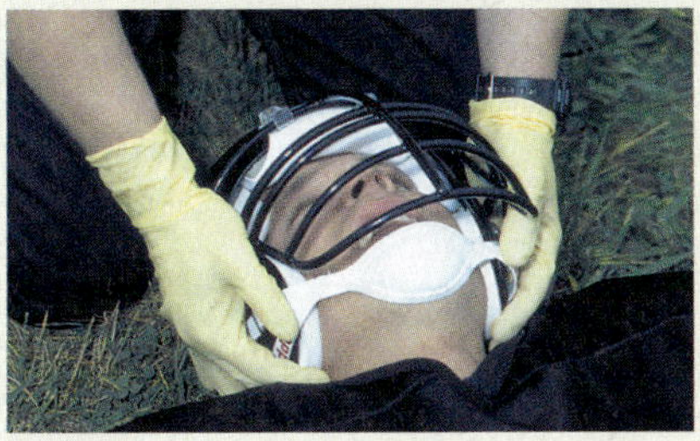

STEP 1 Stabilize the patient's head and helmet in a neutral, in-line position. Then remove the mask in one of two ways.

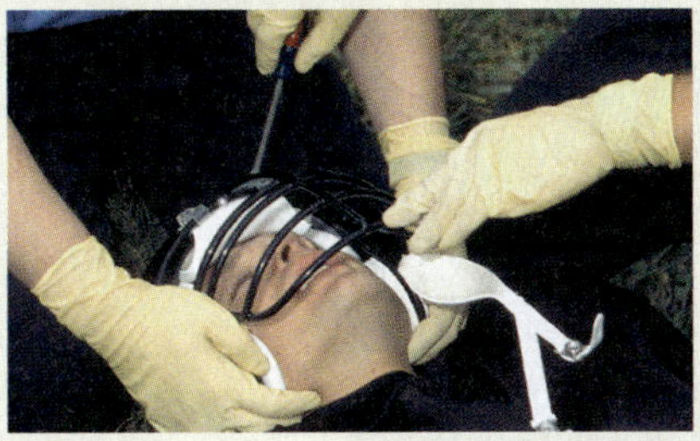

STEP 2 **Method 1.** If a trainer's tool designed for cutting retaining clips is not available, or if using it is unfamiliar, unscrew the retaining clips from the face mask. Assess the patient's airway.

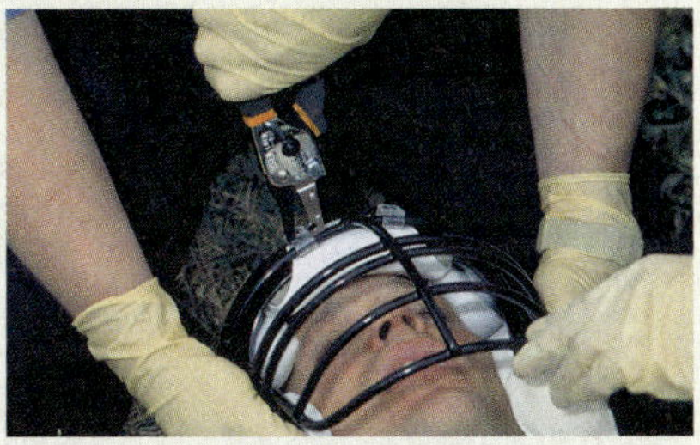

STEP 2 **Method 2.** If a trainer's tool designed for cutting retaining clips is available, and you are comfortable using it, use this tool to cut the clips. Assess the patient's airway.

© Jones & Bartlett Learning. Courtesy of MIEMSS.

SKILL DRILL 15-11

Removing a Helmet

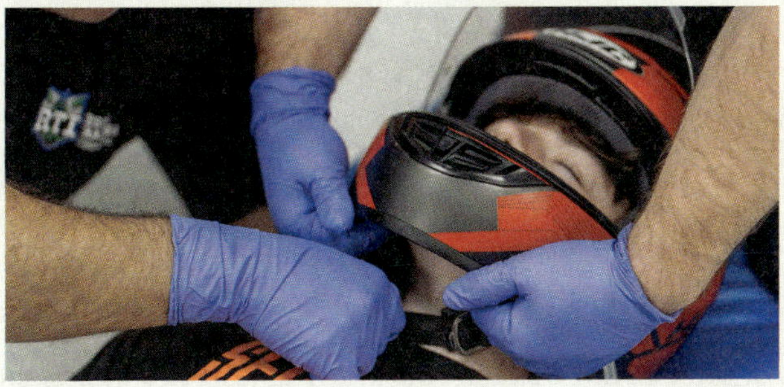

STEP 1 Kneel down at the patient's head and open the face shield so that you can assess the airway and breathing. Remove the eyeglasses if the patient is wearing them. Stabilize the helmet by placing your hands on either side of it, ensuring that your fingers are on the patient's lower jaw to prevent movement of the head. Your partner can then loosen the strap.

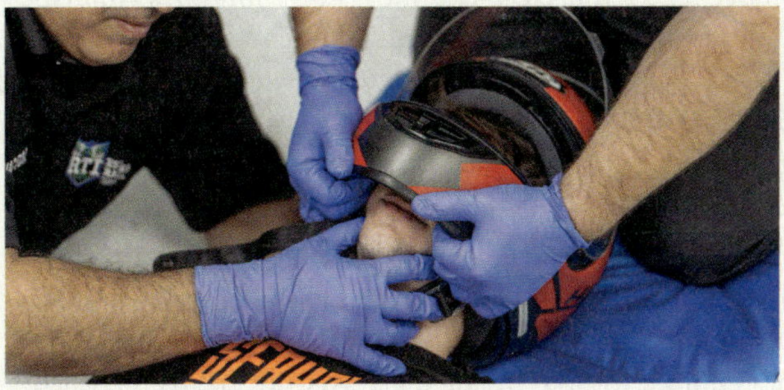

STEP 2 After the strap is loosened, your partner should place one hand on the patient's lower jaw and the other behind the head at the occiput.

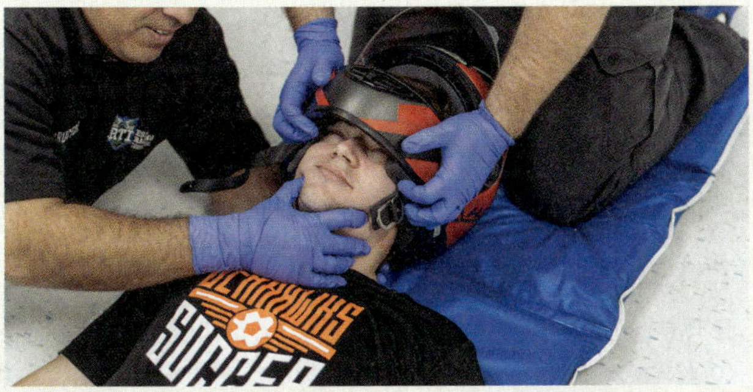

STEP 3 Once your partner's hands are in position, gently slip the helmet off about halfway and then stop.

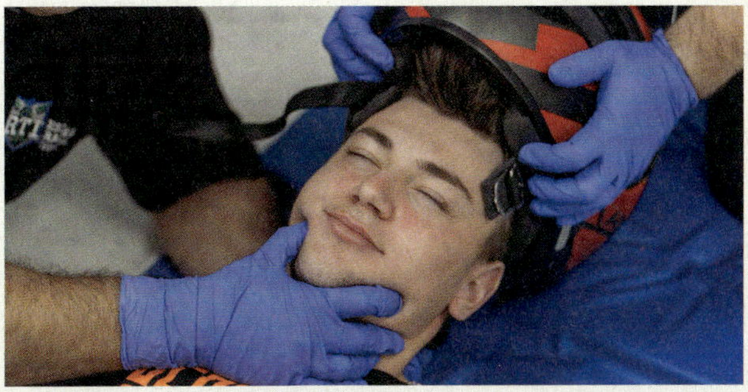

STEP 4 Have your partner slide a hand from the occiput to the back of the head to prevent the head from snapping back once the helmet is removed.

(continues)

SKILL DRILL 15-11 *(continued)*

Removing a Helmet

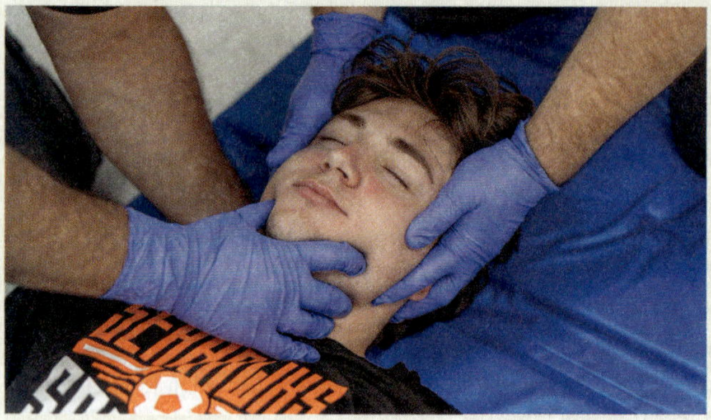

© Jones & Bartlett Learning

STEP 5 With your partner's hand in place, remove the helmet and stabilize the cervical spine. Apply a cervical collar and then secure the patient to a long backboard. Note: With large helmets or small patients, you may need to pad under the shoulders.

Injuries of the Chest

The chest cavity contains the lungs, the heart, and several major blood vessels. The cavity is surrounded and protected by the chest wall, which is made up of the ribs, cartilage, and associated chest muscles. The most common chest injuries are fractures of the ribs, flail chest, and penetrating wounds.

Fractures of the Ribs

Injury may produce fracture of one or more ribs. Even a simple fracture of one rib produces pain at the site of the fracture and difficulty breathing (**FIGURE 15-37**). Multiple rib fractures result in significant breathing difficulty. The pain may be so intense that the patient cannot breathe deeply enough to take in adequate amounts of oxygen. Rib fractures may be associated with injury to the underlying organs.

To determine whether a rib is bruised or broken, apply some pressure to another part of the rib. Pain in the injured area indicates a bruise or possible fracture. If the injury is to the side of the chest, place one hand on the front of the chest and the other on the back and gently press. To check an injury to the front or back of the rib cage, put your hands on either side of the chest and gently press inward. If there is no pain and you do not feel any movement, the rib is probably not broken. In patients with rib fractures, be alert for signs and symptoms of internal injury, particularly shock.

Treatment of Rib Fractures

Try to reassure and make a patient with rib fractures more comfortable. Prevent excessive movement of the patient as you prepare for transport to an appropriate medical facility. Administer oxygen if it is available and you are trained to use it.

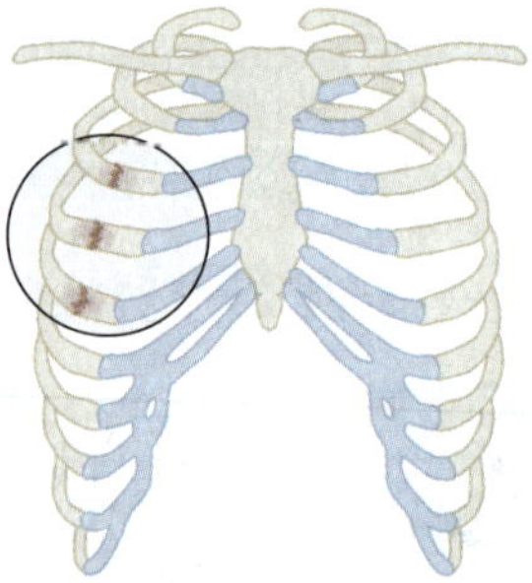

FIGURE 15-37 Broken or fractured ribs.
© Jones & Bartlett Learning

Flail Chest

If three or more ribs are broken in at least two places, the injured portion of the chest wall does not move at the same time as the rest of the chest. The injured part bulges outward when the patient exhales and moves inward when the patient inhales. This condition is called a **flail chest** (**FIGURE 15-38**). A flail chest decreases the amount of oxygen and carbon dioxide exchanged in the lungs, and it causes breathing problems that will progressively worsen.

You can identify a flail chest by examining the chest wall and observing chest movements during breathing. If the injured portion of the chest moves inward as the rest of the chest moves outward (and vice versa), the patient has a flail chest (**FIGURE 15-39**).

Treatment of Flail Chest

If the patient is having difficulty breathing, do not attempt to restrict the movement of the chest while the patient is inhaling. It may be helpful to support the patient's breathing with positive-pressure ventilation. This can be done by using a bag-mask device and supplemental oxygen. If alert, the patient may also be given a pillow to hold against the ribs.

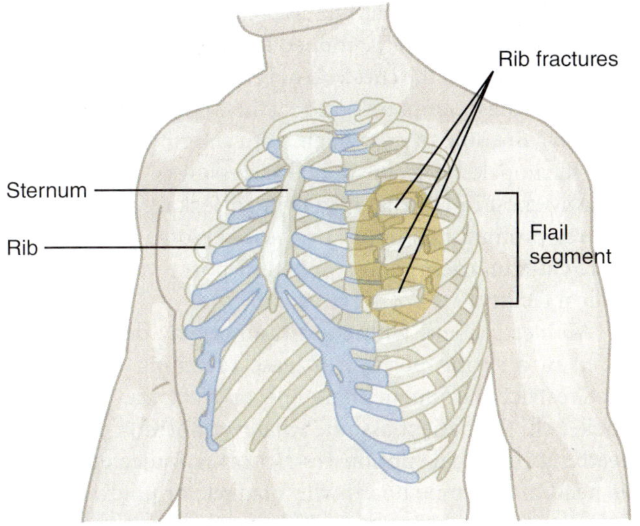

FIGURE 15-38 A flail chest occurs when three or more ribs are broken in at least two places.
© Jones & Bartlett Learning

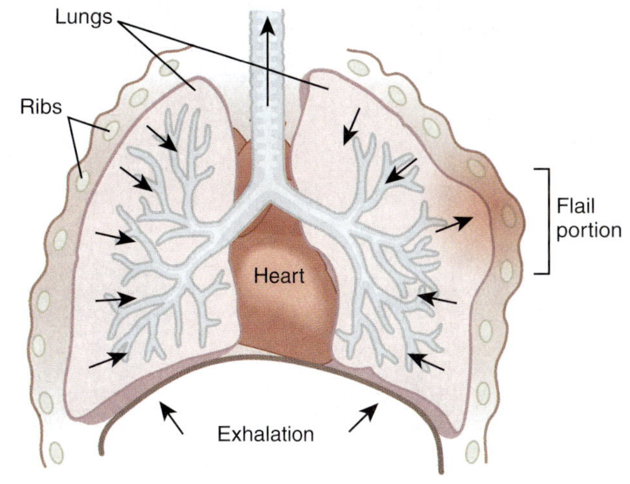

FIGURE 15-39 As the patient breathes, the flail portion of the chest moves in the opposite direction.
© Jones & Bartlett Learning

Monitor and support the patient's ABCs and arrange for prompt transport to an appropriate medical facility.

Penetrating Chest Wounds

If an object (usually a knife or bullet) penetrates the chest wall, air and blood escape into the space between the lungs and the chest wall (**FIGURE 15-40**). The air and blood cause the lung to collapse. Lung collapse greatly reduces the amount of oxygen and carbon dioxide that is exchanged and can result in shock and death. Blood loss into the chest cavity can produce shock.

Treatment of Penetrating Chest Wounds

Quickly seal an open chest wound with a material that will prevent more air from entering the chest cavity. A commercial occlusive dressing is shown in **FIGURE 15-41**. If you do not have a commercial dressing, you can use petroleum jelly–impregnated gauze, aluminum foil, plastic wrap, or a latex

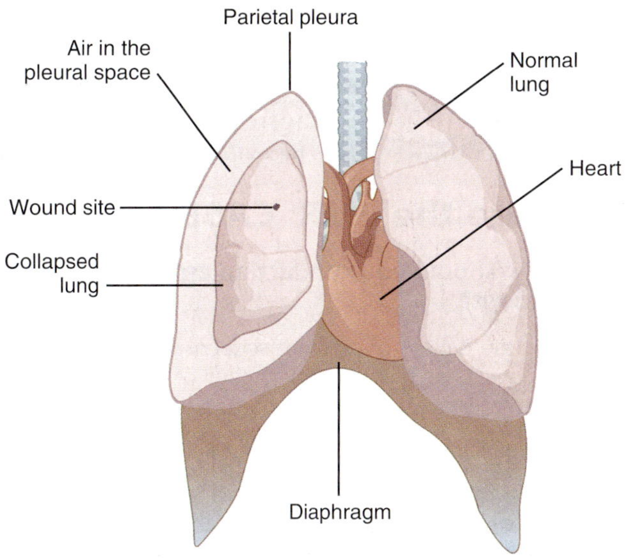

FIGURE 15-40 A penetrating chest wound may cause the patient's lung to collapse.
© Jones & Bartlett Learning

YOU are the EMR — CASE 4

At 0727 hours, you are dispatched to a residence in a part of town where most houses were built approximately 50 years ago. After a 5-minute response, you arrive at the scene. The first thing you notice is that there are three trucks parked on the street and in the driveway. They all display the logo of the J&D Roofing Company. Before you can get out of your vehicle, an excited roofer directs you to follow him to the side of the house. While you are walking to the side of the house, he tells you that Alex was on the roof and slipped on a wet spot on the tin roof. He fell approximately 25 feet (8 m) and landed on a small walkway on the side of the house. As you approach, you find Alex lying on the sidewalk. He says he is not sure why he fell. He seems to be alert and oriented. You examine him and note some bruises and scrapes on his back and one spot that is very painful when you touch the back of his neck. When you ask him to squeeze your hands, you note that his right hand is much weaker than his left hand. You examine his lower extremities, and you ask Alex to move his toes. You do not detect any movement in his feet or toes.

1. What signs and symptoms of injuries does this patient exhibit?
2. How would you treat this patient?

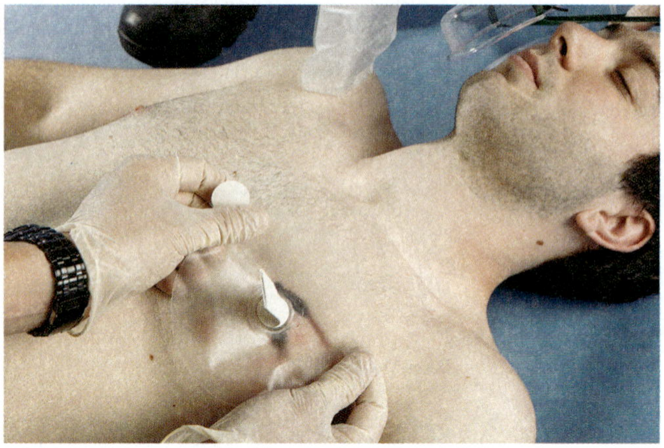

FIGURE 15-41 A commercial occlusive dressing.
© Jones & Bartlett Learning. Courtesy of Glen Ellman.

glove. In rare cases, sealing the wound may increase the patient's breathing difficulty. If it is harder for a patient to breathe after you seal the wound, uncover one corner of the occlusive dressing to see if the breathing improves. Administer oxygen if it is available and you are trained to use it. If a knife or other object is impaled in the chest, do not remove it unless you need to perform chest compressions. Seal the wound around the object with a dressing to prevent air from entering the chest. Stabilize the impaled object with bulky dressings.

Any chest injury that results in air leakage and bleeding requires prompt attention. For these reasons, patients with severe chest injuries require rapid transport to an appropriate medical facility.

An alert patient with chest trauma may demand to be placed in a sitting position to ease breathing. Unless you must restrict motion in the spine or treat the patient for shock, help the patient assume whatever position eases their breathing. If spinal motion restriction is indicated, elevate the head of the spine board with blankets or pillows. If oxygen is available, administer it. If the patient's respirations are excessively slow or absent, support breathing. A bag-mask device may also be used by trained personnel. If the patient's heart stops, begin chest compressions, regardless of whether there are chest injuries.

YOU are the EMR SUMMARY

You are the EMR: CASE 1

1. How should you conduct an assessment of this patient?

Use the patient assessment sequence to conduct a systematic and complete assessment of this patient. Start with a scene assessment to be sure that you and the patient are safe. Perform a primary assessment to evaluate the ABCs and correct any problems. Acknowledge the painful injury to the patient's arm and then perform a secondary assessment by examining the patient from head to toe for additional injuries. As you examine the extremities, remember to check for circulation by checking pulses and capillary refill. Check for sensation and movement in each limb. Be especially aware of the potential for head and spinal injuries from the trauma of falling from the wall and landing on the hard surface of the parking lot. Look for open wounds. Perform a complete SAMPLE history to determine whether any medical conditions contributed to this fall. Finally, reassess the patient to ensure that he is stable.

2. What type of injuries should you suspect with this patient?

In any fall or trauma of this type, examine the patient for signs and symptoms of a head injury. This is especially important if the skateboarder was not wearing a helmet. Stabilize the head and neck as well as you can with the personnel and equipment available to prevent any further damage to the patient's spine. Examine the patient thoroughly for additional injuries to bones and joints besides the obvious injuries to his arm and elbow. Check for soft-tissue injuries. Do not forget to treat the patient for shock, especially because it is a cool autumn day.

3. Under what circumstances should you move this patient?

Do not move the patient unless a dangerous situation exists or you need to start lifesaving treatment. If the patient is in a place where there is uncontrolled traffic or other danger, you need to consider moving him. If you are unable to open the patient's airway, it may be necessary to move the patient to secure an open airway. However, if you can safely leave the patient in the location found, this is generally the best solution because you will need three or four people and a backboard to safely move this patient. Wait until you have adequate equipment and a sufficient number of trained personnel.

You are the EMR: CASE 2

1. What type of examination should you perform on the patient's right arm?

After completing a full primary assessment, expose the patient's right arm. Cut away any clothing that may interfere with a complete examination of the injured area. Confirm circulation in the arm, including checking for pulses and testing capillary refill in the fingers. Evaluate the patient for normal movement and sensation in the affected arm and compare the findings with the uninjured limb. Palpate the arm to determine the extent of the injury from the hand to the elbow.

YOU are the EMR **SUMMARY**

2. Describe how you should splint this patient's injury.

Stabilize the lower part of the right arm using a rigid splint extending from the hand to the elbow. Pad the splint to fill any voids between the limb and the splint. Stabilize the hand in the position of function by placing one or two roller bandages in the hand. Secure the limb to the splint using roller gauze. Then secure the entire arm using a sling to minimize movement and a swathe to secure it to the body. Recheck circulation, sensation, and motion after the sling is in place.

You are the EMR: CASE 3

1. What type of injury do you believe is most likely based on her pain and on your patient assessment?

The full-body assessment revealed moderate pain in the left hip area. The patient's left leg is bent at an abnormal angle, and her left leg appears to be shorter than her right leg. These signs and symptoms are consistent with a hip fracture.

2. Because the patient did not experience significant trauma, what underlying factors may have contributed to this injury?

Osteoporosis is a chronic health condition that affects older people, more commonly women. Osteoporosis results in a weakening of bone. In people with osteoporosis, fractures can occur with a low-force MOI. Based on the MOI and the fact that this woman takes calcium, it is likely that she has osteoporosis, which contributed to the hip fracture during the low-impact fall.

3. How should you prepare this patient for transport?

Using as much padding as possible, secure the hip in the position found. Then secure the patient to a long backboard with ample padding to provide support for the injured leg. In some situations, you may be responsible for stabilizing the fracture site and preparing her for transport. In other cases, your role will be to keep her as comfortable as possible, maintain her body temperature to prevent shock, monitor her vital signs, and reassure her until additional EMS personnel and equipment arrive. Sometimes your role is to help prevent unnecessary movement of the patient, which prevents further pain or injury.

You are the EMR: CASE 4

1. What signs and symptoms of injuries does this patient exhibit?

In a situation like this, use all of the available information to make the best determination of the patient's injuries and to determine what treatment the patient needs. You can quickly get valuable information by evaluating the history of the incident. In this case, it appears that the roofer fell approximately 25 feet (8 m) from a roof onto a hard concrete sidewalk. A fall from this distance onto a hard surface has a high likelihood of producing a serious injury. A thorough patient examination will provide much information. This patient has abrasions and scrapes on his back indicating the possibility of internal injuries. He complains of pain on one part of his neck when you touch it. You note that one of his hands has a weaker grip than the other, which may indicate an injury to his spinal cord. Most important, you determine that he is not able to move his feet. These are all important signs and symptoms of a possible spinal cord injury. When performing an assessment on a patient who has experienced trauma, do not get tunnel vision when you find one injury. Continue your assessment to be sure you have completed a thorough patient examination to identify all the injuries the patient may have sustained, including life-threatening bleeding. Always carefully assess and monitor the ABCs. These indicators help you determine if there are additional injuries that might cause shortness of breath or shock.

2. How would you treat this patient?

Carefully assess and monitor the patient's ABCs, which will help you determine if there are internal injuries and the patient's overall condition. Because this patient has experienced a significant fall and is showing multiple signs and symptoms of a spinal injury, you need to stabilize the patient's neck and back to prevent movement that may cause additional injury. This patient will need to be moved using a spinal motion restriction device such as a backboard. However, there does not appear to be a need to move the patient before the arrival of additional EMS personnel and equipment. If the patient's neck is stabilized, there is no need to move him. Cover him to prevent shock. Continue to monitor the status of the patient's ABCs. Update responding EMS units and provide encouragement to the patient and to his coworkers. Sometimes an important role of the first responder is to prevent unnecessary movement and further injury to the patient because of the unwise actions of untrained people.

Prep Kit

Ready for Review

- Musculoskeletal injuries are caused by three types of MOI: direct force, indirect force, and twisting force.
- A fracture is a cracked or broken bone. Fractures can be closed (the bone is broken but there is no break in the skin) or open (the bone is broken and the overlying skin is lacerated).
- A dislocation is a disruption that tears the supporting ligaments of the joint.
- A sprain is a joint injury caused by excessive stretching of the supporting ligaments.
- The three steps in examining a patient with a limb injury include:
  - General assessment of the patient
  - Examination of the injured part
  - Evaluation of the circulation, sensation, and movement in the injured limb
- Regardless of their extent or severity, treat all limb injuries the same way in the field. For all open extremity wounds, first cover the entire wound with a dry, sterile dressing. Then apply firm but gentle pressure to control bleeding, if necessary. Then splint the injured limb.
- The three basic types of splints are rigid, soft, and traction.
- It takes two people to splint most limb injuries adequately: one to stabilize and support the extremity and one to apply the splint.
- Severe head and spinal cord injuries can result from many different types of trauma. These injuries are common causes of death and can lead to irreversible paralysis and permanent brain damage.
- Injuries of the head can be classified as open or closed. In a closed head injury, bleeding and swelling within the skull may increase pressure on the brain, leading to irreversible brain damage. An open injury of the head usually bleeds profusely.
- When a sign or symptom of a head injury is present, stabilize the patient's head and neck; maintain an open airway; support breathing; monitor circulation; check to see if CSF or blood is seeping; control bleeding with dry, sterile dressings; treat other serious injuries; and arrange for prompt transport.
- Airway obstruction is the primary danger in severe facial injuries.
- When facial injuries are present, stabilize the patient's head and neck; maintain an open airway; support breathing; monitor circulation; control bleeding with a dry, sterile dressing and apply direct pressure; treat other serious injuries; and arrange for prompt transport.
- When you suspect a spinal injury, do not move the patient during the examination. Further, do not allow the patient to move.
- When a sign or symptom of spinal injury is present, place the head and neck in a neutral in-line position; maintain an open airway; support breathing; monitor circulation; assess pulse, movement, and sensation; examine and treat other serious injuries; assist in establishing spinal motion restriction using an appropriate device; and arrange for prompt transport.
- The most common chest injuries are rib fractures, flail chest, and penetrating wounds.

Vital Vocabulary

abdominal breathing Breathing using only the diaphragm.

arm The upper portion of the upper extremity; from the shoulder to the elbow.

cerebrospinal fluid (CSF) A clear, watery, straw-colored fluid that fills the space between the brain and spinal cord and their protective coverings.

closed fracture A fracture in which the overlying skin has not been damaged.

closed head injury Injury where there is bleeding and/or swelling within the skull.

concussion A closed head injury that alters the way the brain functions; symptoms of a concussion include headache, loss of memory, and confusion. Also called a mild traumatic brain injury.

dislocation Disruption of a joint so that the bone ends are no longer in alignment.

flail chest A chest injury in which three or more ribs are broken in two or more places, resulting in the injured part of the chest moving in the opposite direction from the rest of the chest.

forearm The lower portion of the upper extremity; from the elbow to the wrist.

joint The point where two bones come in contact with each other.

leg The lower portion of the lower extremity; from the knee to the foot.

Prep Kit

mechanism of injury (MOI) The means by which a traumatic injury occurs.

open fracture Any fracture in which the overlying skin has been damaged.

osteoporosis Abnormal brittleness of the bones caused by loss of calcium; affected bones fracture easily.

paralysis Inability of an alert person to move voluntarily.

rigid splint Splint made from firm materials such as wood, aluminum, or plastic.

sling A bandage or material that helps to support the weight of an injured upper extremity.

soft splint A splint made from supple material that provides gentle support.

spinal motion restriction The general goal of maintaining the patient's spinal alignment throughout any treatment and movements that clinicians must perform.

sprain A joint injury in which the joint is partially or temporarily dislocated and some of the supporting ligaments are either stretched or torn.

thighbone The upper portion of the lower extremity; from the hip joint to the knee.

traction splint A splint that holds a lower extremity fracture in alignment by applying a constant, steady pull on the extremity.

trauma A wound or injury, either physical or psychological.

traumatic brain injury (TBI) A closed head injury that alters the way the brain functions; symptoms include headache, loss of memory, and confusion. A concussion is a mild traumatic brain injury.

vacuum splint A soft splint that becomes rigid when air is removed from the splint.

References

Baker CE, Martin P, Wilson MH, Ghajari M, Sharp DJ. The relationship between road traffic collision dynamics and traumatic brain injury pathology. *Brain Commun*. 202212;4(2):fcac033. doi:10.1093/braincomms/fcac033

Bliuc D, Tran T, Alarkawi D, et al. Patient self-assessment of walking ability and fracture risk in older Australian adults. *JAMA Netw Open*. 2024;7(1):e2352675. doi:10.1001/jamanetworkopen.2023.52675

Cho N, Kim S, Tran Z, et al. National trends and clinical outcomes following scooter injury in the United States: 2016–2020. *J Am Coll Surg*. 2024;238(3):254–260.

Migliorini F, Giorgino R, Hildebrand F, et al. Fragility fractures: risk factors and management in the elderly. *Medicina (Kaunas)*. 2021;57(10):1119.

Traumatic brain injury (TBI). National Institute of Neurological Disorders and Stroke website. https://www.ninds.nih.gov/health-information/disorders/traumatic-brain-injury-tbi. Reviewed October 15, 2024. Accessed November 15, 2024.

Assessment IN ACTION

You are dispatched to a single-family two-story home for a report of a fall from the roof. On arrival, you find a 32-year-old man who was stepping onto a ladder from the roof when the ladder moved away from the house, causing the patient to fall to the ground. The patient reports that he landed upright on both of his feet, probably because he was reaching for branches as he fell. The patient reports severe pain in the right lower leg and knee and is obviously frightened.

1. What kind of assessment should you perform on this patient?
   - **A.** Examine only the areas that are painful.
   - **B.** Examine only the upper extremities.
   - **C.** Perform a full-body assessment.
   - **D.** Complete a primary assessment only.
2. If a patient fell from the roof of a second story house and appeared to have multiple injuries, which of the following would be the most appropriate way to move the patient?
   - **A.** Perform a direct ground lift.
   - **B.** Have the patient slide onto the stretcher.
   - **C.** Log roll the patient onto a long backboard.
   - **D.** Perform a fireman's carry.
3. If you identify pain and deformity of the lower leg, what type of splint should you apply?
   - **A.** A sling
   - **B.** A rigid splint
   - **C.** A sling and swathe
   - **D.** A traction splint
4. Do you need to stabilize this patient's neck?
   - **A.** Yes
   - **B.** No
   - **C.** Only if he reports pain
   - **D.** Only if there is pain and bruising
5. You discover swelling, deformity, and an open wound on the patient's lower leg. How should you treat this wound?
   - **A.** Splint the leg.
   - **B.** Leave the wound exposed because it is associated with a possible fracture.
   - **C.** Cover the wound with a sterile dressing and then splint the leg.
   - **D.** Stop the bleeding with direct pressure, cover the wound with a sterile dressing, and splint the leg.
6. What is the general rule for splinting a fracture?
   - **A.** Stabilize the fracture site.
   - **B.** Stabilize the fracture site and the joint above it.
   - **C.** Stabilize the fracture site and the joint below it.
   - **D.** Stabilize the fracture site and the joints above and below it.
7. What is the general rule for splinting a joint?
   - **A.** Stabilize the joint only.
   - **B.** Stabilize the joint and the bone above it.
   - **C.** Stabilize the joint and the bone below it.
   - **D.** Stabilize the joint and the bones above and below it.
8. Why is it important to check and regularly recheck circulation, sensation, and movement in a patient with a limb injury?
9. Why is it important to consider the mechanism of injury when evaluating and treating patients who may have sustained a spinal injury?
10. Why do patients with severe penetrating chest injuries require rapid transport to an appropriate medical facility?

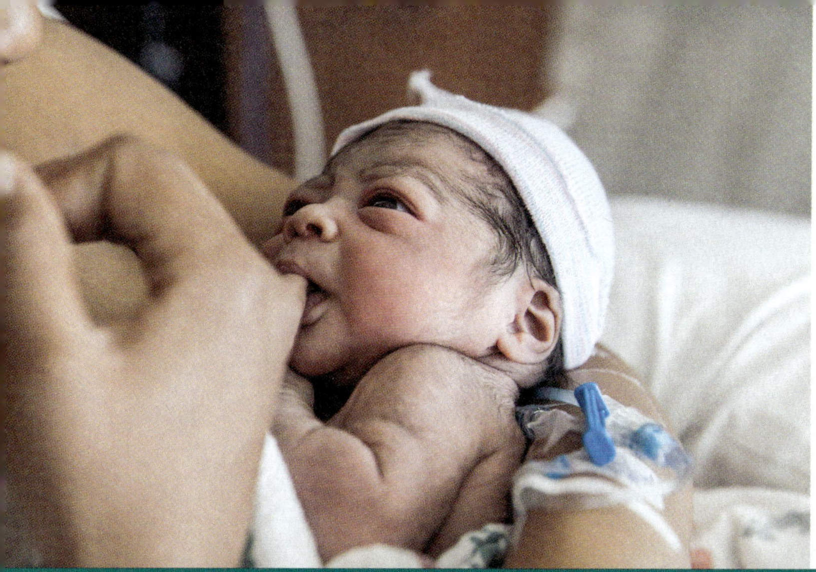

SECTION 6

Special Patient Populations

16 Childbirth

© Cavan Images-Offset/Shutterstock

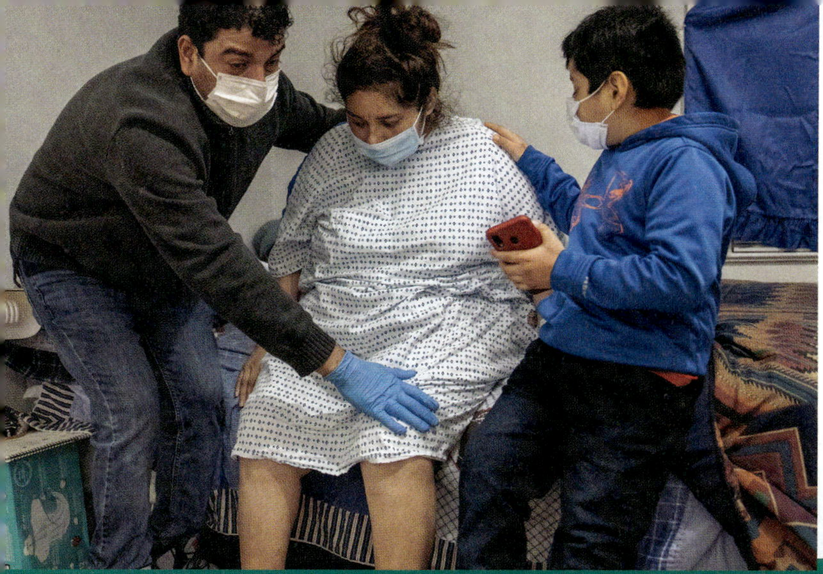

CHAPTER **16**

Childbirth

National EMS Education Standard Competencies

Special Patient Populations

Recognizes and manages life threats based on simple assessment findings for a patient with special needs while awaiting additional emergency response.

Obstetrics

- Normal delivery (pp 370–376)
- Vaginal bleeding in the pregnant patient (p 378)

Neonatal Care

- Newborn stabilization (pp 374–377)
- Neonatal resuscitation (pp 376–377)

Gynecology

- Shock associated with vaginal bleeding (p 378)

Trauma

Uses knowledge to recognize and manage life threats based on assessment findings for an acutely injured patient while awaiting additional emergency medical response.

Special Considerations in Trauma

- Pregnant patient (p 381)
- Pediatric patient (Section 5, *Trauma*)
- Geriatric patient (Section 5, *Trauma*)

Knowledge Objectives

1. Describe the anatomy and function of the female reproductive system. (p 370)
2. Explain the three stages of the labor process. (p 371)
3. Discuss how to determine whether there is time to transport the pregnant patient to the hospital for delivery. (pp 371–372)
4. Describe preparation for delivery of a newborn. (p 372)
5. Discuss the use of standard precautions in childbirth. (p 372)
6. List the equipment emergency medical responders (EMRs) should have for an emergency childbirth situation. (p 372)
7. Explain how to assist with delivery of a newborn. (pp 372–374)
8. Discuss the delivery of the placenta. (pp 374–376)
9. List the steps in resuscitating a newborn. (pp 376–377)
10. Describe the signs and symptoms and the treatment for the following complications of childbirth:
    - Ectopic pregnancy and shock (p 378)
    - Miscarriage and vaginal bleeding (p 378)
    - Premature birth (p 378)
    - Unbroken bag of waters (pp 378–380)
    - Prolapse of the umbilical cord (p 380)
    - Breech birth (p 380)
    - Stillborn delivery (pp 380–381)
    - Multiple births (p 381)
    - Excessive bleeding after delivery (p 381)
11. Explain how to care for a pregnant person who has been in a motor vehicle crash. (p 381)

Skills Objectives

1. Describe preparation for delivery of a newborn. (p 372)
2. Demonstrate the use of standard precautions in childbirth. (p 373; Skill Drill 16-1)
3. Demonstrate how to assist with delivery of a newborn. (pp 372–376)
4. Demonstrate delivery of the placenta. (pp 374–376)

© John Moore/Getty Images News/Getty Images

5. Demonstrate resuscitation of a newborn. (pp 376–377; Skill Drill 16-2)
6. Demonstrate treatment for the following complications of childbirth:
   - Ectopic pregnancy and shock (p 378)
   - Miscarriage and vaginal bleeding (p 378)
   - Premature birth (p 378)
   - Unbroken bag of waters (pp 378–380)
   - Prolapse of the umbilical cord (p 380)
   - Breech birth (p 380)
   - Stillborn delivery (pp 380–381)
   - Multiple births (p 381)
   - Excessive bleeding after delivery (p 381)

Introduction

As an emergency medical responder (EMR), you may assist in the birth of a child. A planned childbirth is itself an exciting, dramatic, and stressful event. An unplanned childbirth, where you are called to assist, can be even more dramatic and stressful. However, if you remember some easy steps, you can effectively assist in the birth process and offer comfort and support to both the mother and the newborn.

In general, pregnancy is not a surprise for the mother, who may be knowledgeable and well prepared for the birth process. However, there will be times when the timing of the childbirth catches everyone by surprise or a complication has developed, thus requiring a call for emergency medical services (EMS). As a first responder, you may not have the time or necessary assistance to transport the pregnant patient to the hospital. Therefore, you must be prepared to help your patient deliver the newborn in any location. In most cases, during the birth process, the newborn is being pushed out of the body; therefore, your part involves helping, guiding, and supporting the newborn. Following the birth, you will ensure that the newborn is breathing adequately and being kept warm.

Words of Wisdom

Childbirth is a normal and natural part of life. If you are concerned about your ability to handle such a situation, just remember that hundreds of thousands of deliveries occur in the world each day and result in healthy babies. In many countries, medical assistance at childbirth is the exception, not the rule.

In this chapter, you will learn about the three stages of the birth process. The two key indicators of an impending birth are the frequency of the **contractions** and the appearance of the newborn's head during a contraction, or **crowning**.

The Anatomy and Function of the Female Reproductive System

The major female reproductive organs are the ovaries, which produce eggs, and the **uterus (womb)**, which holds the fertilized egg as it develops during a pregnancy (the typical gestation period is 40 weeks). The egg released by the ovaries travels through the fallopian tubes to the uterus. The external opening of the female reproductive system is called the **birth canal**, which includes the lower part of the uterus and the **vagina**. The developing newborn (**fetus**) is surrounded by an amniotic sac for protection and floats in amniotic fluid. The **placenta**, or afterbirth, draws nutrients from the wall of the mother's uterus. These nutrients and oxygen are delivered to the fetus through the **umbilical cord**. **FIGURE 16-1** shows the anatomy of a pregnant person.

Assessing the Birth Situation

Should you help deliver the newborn on the scene or arrange for transport of the pregnant patient to the hospital? To make this decision, you need to understand that **labor** (the process of delivering a newborn) consists of three distinct stages.

YOU are the EMR — CASE 1

Just as you are completing your dinner, you and your partner are dispatched to a nearby office building for the report of a 27-year-old woman in labor. As you are responding, your dispatcher reports that the woman's "water has broken" and that her contractions are 4 minutes apart. The nearest EMS transport unit is 9 minutes away.

1. What information do you need to know before determining whether there is time to transport this woman to the hospital or whether you will need to assist her with the delivery?
2. What standard precautions do you need to take when assisting with the emergency delivery of a newborn?
3. What are the risks to a pregnant woman and fetus if they are involved in a motor vehicle crash?

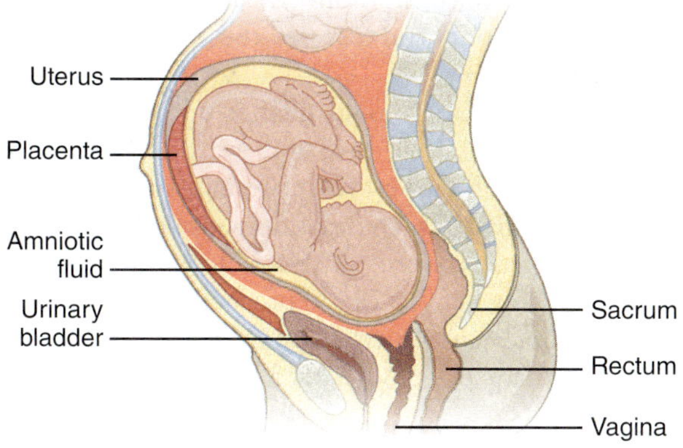

FIGURE 16-1 Anatomy of a pregnant person.
© Jones & Bartlett Learning

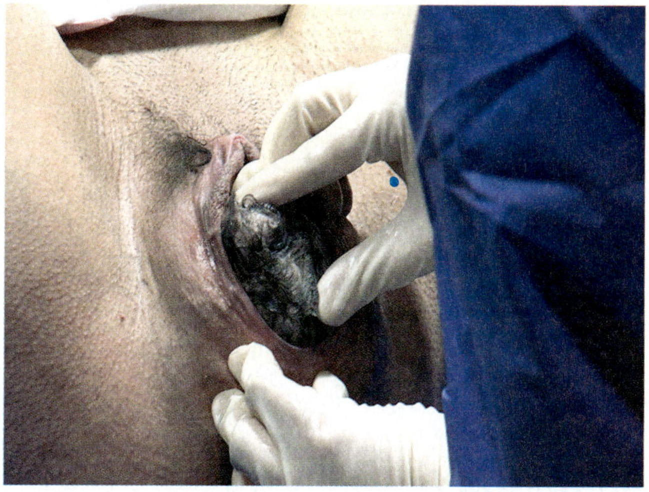

FIGURE 16-2 Crowning occurs when the newborn's head appears at the vaginal opening.
© University of Maryland Shock Trauma Center/MIEMSS

Stages of Labor

The first stage of labor is when the mother's body prepares for birth. This stage is characterized by the initial contractions, rupture of the **bag of waters** (the amniotic sac, which is the fluid in which the fetus floats), and discharge of the **bloody show** (a plug of mucus often mixed with blood). Check the patient's vaginal opening to confirm that crowning has not begun yet. Report your findings to the responding ambulance crew so that they can decide whether the patient is close to delivery or transport to the hospital is necessary.

The second stage involves the birth of the newborn. You will see the newborn's head crowning during contractions, at which time you must prepare to assist the patient with delivery (**FIGURE 16-2**). There is no time for transport now!

The third, and final, stage involves delivery of the placenta (afterbirth). You must assist in stabilizing the condition of the mother and newborn and delivering the placenta.

Is There Time to Reach the Hospital?

The following questions will help you to determine how close the pregnant patient is to delivery and whether there is time for transport to the hospital or whether you need to prepare for a delivery.

1. **Is this the patient's first pregnancy?** The length of labor for a first-time mother is usually longer than for a person who has already had a child. Patients experiencing their first labor will usually have more time to reach the hospital. It is also helpful to ask the patient the newborn's due date, although labor can start before this date.
2. **Has the patient experienced a bloody show?** As the newborn starts to descend toward the birth canal, the bloody show is expelled from the cervix and discharged from the vaginal opening. This usually occurs as the first stage of labor is about to begin.
3. **Has the bag of waters broken?** The bag of waters usually breaks toward the end of the first stage of labor and may give some idea of the progress of the birth process. In some patients, the bag of waters may not break until the birth is actually occurring (discussed later in the chapter).
4. **How frequent are the contractions?** If the contractions are more than 5 minutes apart, the patient can usually be transported to the hospital. Contractions less than 2 minutes apart usually indicate that delivery will occur soon and you need to prepare for delivery. If the contractions are 3 to 4 minutes apart, take the other factors listed here into account to make your decision.
5. **Does the patient feel an urge to move their bowels?** When the newborn's head is in the birth canal, it presses against the rectum and the pregnant patient may feel the urge to have a bowel movement. Do not allow the patient to go to the toilet. This urge is an indication that delivery is near.
6. **Is the newborn's head crowning?** Crowning indicates that the newborn will be born in the next few minutes and you need to be ready.
7. **Is transportation available?** Find out whether the ambulance is responding and how far it is to the hospital. Will bad weather, a natural disaster, or rush hour traffic prevent prompt arrival of transportation?

Timing Contraction Cycles

When you care for a patient in labor, time the contraction cycles from the beginning of one contraction to the beginning of the next (**FIGURE 16-3**). Do not time only the interval between contractions. If contractions are less than 3 minutes apart, delivery is close.

Detecting Crowning

To determine whether the newborn's head is crowning, you must observe the vaginal opening during a contraction. If you see the head crowning during the contraction, prepare for delivery (see Figure 16-2). There is no time for transport.

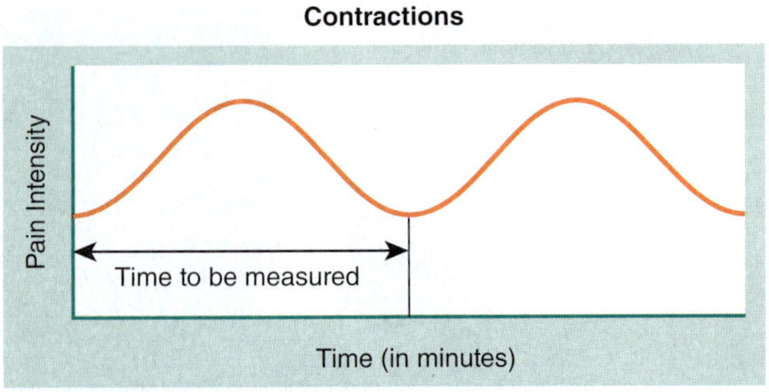

FIGURE 16-3 Time the contractions from the beginning of one to the beginning of the next.

© Jones & Bartlett Learning

Preparing for Delivery

As you prepare to assist the patient in the delivery, keep these two things in mind:

1. Calm the pregnant patient. Delivery is a natural process.
2. Calm yourself. You are there to help.

Because you are not in a hospital, you will not be able to maintain sterile conditions. However, be as clean as possible. Wash your hands thoroughly. If you do not have a sterile delivery kit, use the gloves from your jump kit (or even clean kitchen gloves, if they are available). Place the patient on a firm surface that is padded with blankets, folded sheets, or towels. Elevate the patient's hips 2 to 4 inches (5 to 10 cm) with pillows and blankets. Allow the patient to get in a comfortable position. This is often on their back with knees bent and feet flat on the surface beneath the patient.

Have plenty of clean towels ready to cover the newborn and to clean the mother after delivery has occurred. Childbirth involves blood and body fluids, so place towels or sheets on the floor around the delivery area to help soak up the fluids and to protect the mother and the newborn.

Standard Precautions and Childbirth

As the mother's contractions become more forceful, the newborn is gradually pushed down the birth canal. Because a person in childbirth will expel both blood and body fluids, take standard precautions during the delivery. Try to avoid getting blood or fluids on you. Use sterile gloves during any delivery whenever possible. Sterile gloves not only protect the mother and newborn from infection but also protect you from any bloodborne diseases the mother might have (**SKILL DRILL 16-1**).

Because body fluids could splatter on your face during the delivery process, wear face and eye protection to keep possible splatter out of your eyes, nose, and mouth. Wearing a surgical gown can help keep fluids off your body. As an EMR, you will not have all the protective equipment that is available in a hospital. Do what you can to prevent unnecessary exposure to body fluids and report all direct exposures of blood or fluids to the emergency physician or to your medical director.

Equipment

You should have a prepackaged obstetric (OB) delivery kit in your emergency care equipment (**FIGURE 16-4**). The delivery kit includes the following materials:

- Sterile gloves
- Umbilical cord clamp
- Sterile drapes and towels
- Sanitary pads
- Gauze pads (4 × 4 inch [10 × 10 cm])
- Towel or blanket for the newborn
- Bulb syringe
- Plastic placenta bag

In addition, you will need the following:

- Sheets or towels for the mother
- Suction (if available)
- Oxygen (if available and if you are trained to use it)
- Newborn-size face mask

If you do not have an OB delivery kit, look for appropriate substitute materials. You can find most of these items in your jump kit or in most homes. Even if you do not have any equipment, remember that you can still assist in delivering a newborn with only common sense and gloved hands.

Assisting With Delivery

As you prepare to assist with delivery, remember that there are two lives to be considered in this situation: the life of the mother and the life of the newborn. Do not neglect to perform a patient assessment on the mother. Determine whether the patient has any medical conditions. Obtain a baseline set of vital signs and repeat them at least every 15 minutes. Throughout the delivery process, continue to monitor the airway, breathing, and circulation.

YOU are the EMR **CASE 2**

Shortly after 0100 hours, you and your partner are dispatched to the home of a pregnant 32-year-old woman. When you arrive, you find her on the living room sofa. She is complaining of pain in her abdomen and says she is having contractions. She is sweating and generally uncomfortable.

1. What questions should you ask the patient about the contractions?
2. Why is it important to know whether this is her first pregnancy?
3. What stage of labor is she in?

SKILL DRILL 16-1

Putting on Sterile Gloves

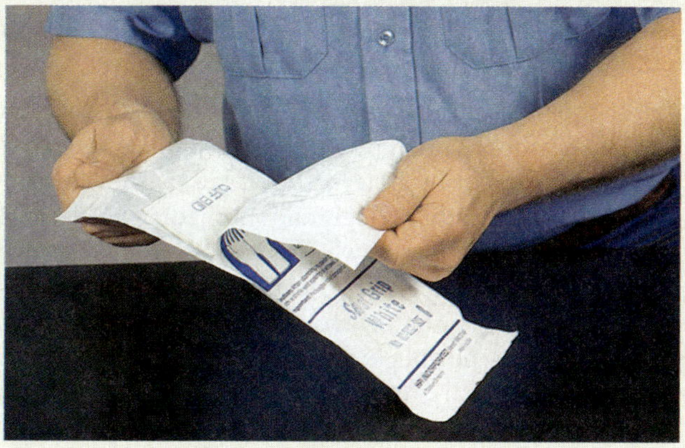

STEP 1 Carefully open the sterile glove package without touching the gloves.

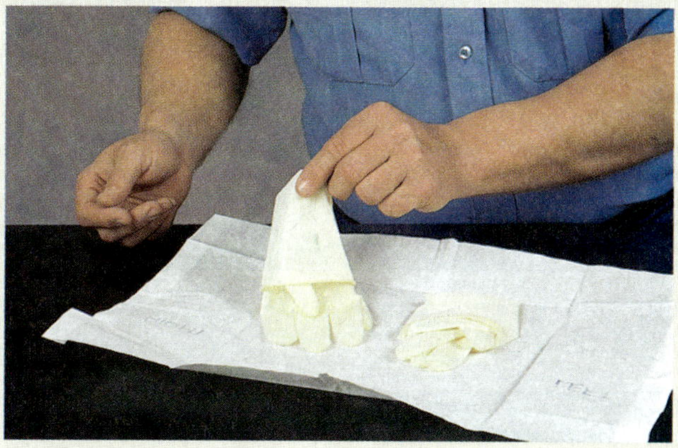

STEP 2 Pick up the first glove by grasping one edge.

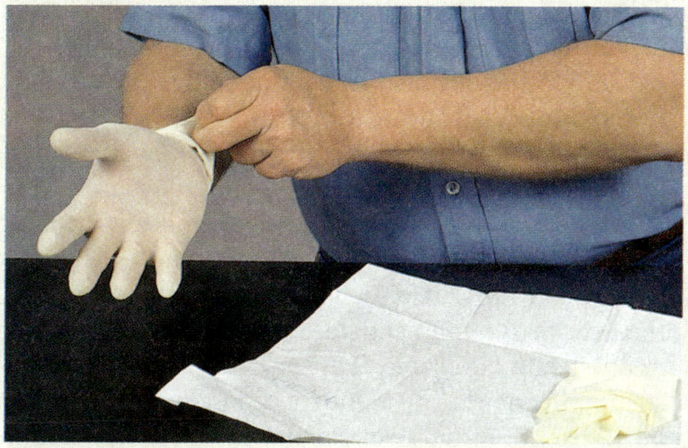

STEP 3 Pull on the first glove, being careful not to touch the outside of the glove.

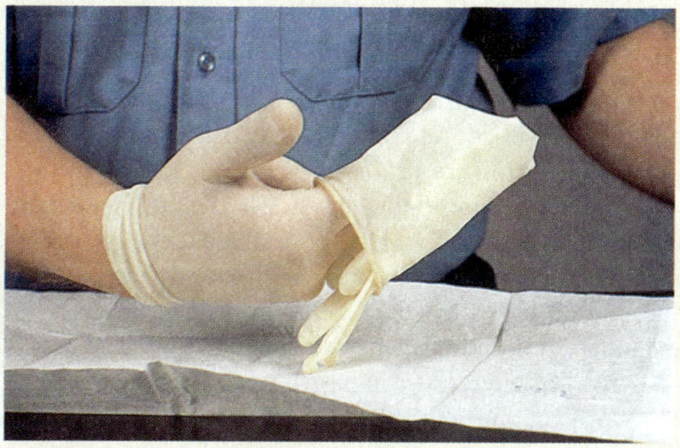

STEP 4 Grasp the second glove by sliding two fingers of your gloved hand inside the rolled edge.

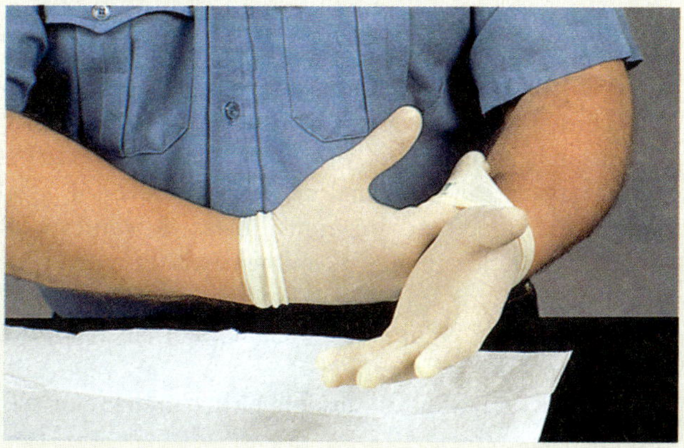

STEP 5 Put on the second glove.

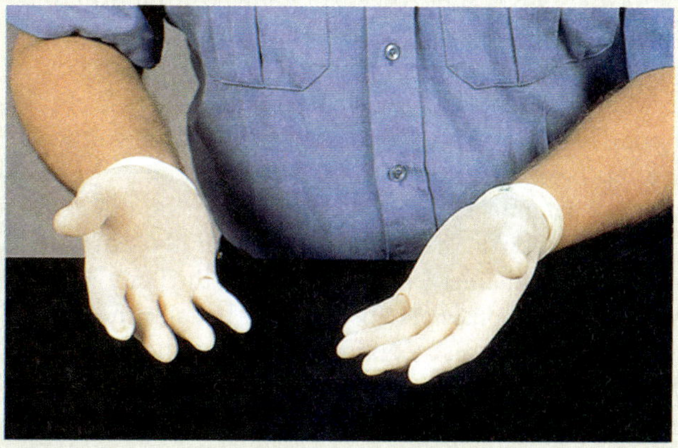

STEP 6 Keep the gloves as sterile as possible.

© Jones & Bartlett Learning. Courtesy of MIEMSS.

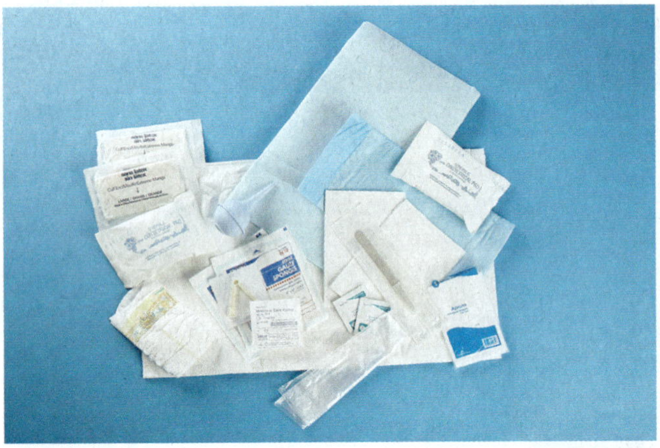

FIGURE 16-4 Commercial obstetric (OB) kit.

© Jones & Bartlett Learning

> **Words of Wisdom**
>
> Do not forget that pregnant patients can experience trauma or medical emergencies, too! It is important to perform a patient assessment to determine whether your patient has any additional medical conditions or has sustained a recent injury. It is easy to focus on the pregnancy and neglect other conditions.

Remember, your primary purpose is to assist in the delivery of the newborn. As mentioned, as delivery nears, the patient will feel pressure in the vaginal area, similar to the feeling of needing to move the bowels. This feeling is normal during the delivery process. Do not let the patient go to the bathroom and do not hold the patient's legs together.

Be as clean as possible during the entire delivery process. Take standard precautions. Do not touch the vaginal area except during the delivery. If you have a partner, have this person stay with you during the delivery.

The newborn's head should emerge slowly to prevent undue stress on the newborn and tearing of the vaginal tissues. As the head emerges, support the newborn's head and tell the mother to stop pushing. To help the patient stop pushing, advise taking quick, short breaths ("Blow as if blowing out a candle"). Some EMS systems advise their personnel to use the palm of the hand to provide slight counterpressure over the newborn's head to slow the birth process. Be sure to check with your medical director and follow your local protocols for the appropriate treatment in this situation.

Do not attempt to pull the newborn during the delivery. In a normal birth, the newborn will naturally turn to the side after the head emerges, and the rest of the body will be delivered spontaneously (**FIGURE 16-5**). Usually, the upper shoulder will deliver first. Continue to support the newborn's head and be ready to grasp the newborn in a clean towel. Remember, the newborn will be wet and slippery. As the torso and the legs are delivered, support the newborn with both hands. Grasp the newborn's feet as they are delivered. Keep the newborn's head at about the level of the mother's vagina. If the amniotic sac has not broken as the newborn's head starts to deliver, tear it with your fingers and push it away from the newborn's head and mouth.

As the head emerges, check to make sure the umbilical cord is not wrapped around the newborn's neck. If the cord is wrapped around the neck, attempt to slip the cord over the newborn's head. Never pull on the umbilical cord; it is extremely fragile. In a normal delivery, there is no need for you to cut the umbilical cord.

Caring for the Newborn

Note the time of the delivery so it can be properly reported on the newborn's birth certificate. As soon as you are holding the newborn in a clean towel, lay the newborn down between the mother's legs and immediately clear blood and mucus from the newborn's mouth and nose using a gauze pad or the cleanest object available. Many newborns will begin to breathe or cry without further assistance. If the baby does not begin to breathe spontaneously within a few seconds, **suction** the newborn's mouth and nose. Use a bulb syringe from the delivery kit if one is available (**FIGURE 16-6**). Suction the mouth first and then the nostrils. Be careful not to reach all the way to the back of the newborn's mouth. Discard the fluid into a towel, and repeat the procedure two to three times until the mouth and nostrils are clear. If a bulb syringe is not available, wipe the newborn's mouth and nose with a gauze pad. Drying and suctioning the newborn usually provides enough stimulation to induce breathing.

Place the newborn on the mother's abdomen if the mother and the newborn are breathing adequately. This step allows skin-to-skin contact and will help keep the newborn warm. Check again for blood or mucus in the newborn's mouth and nose. If present, wipe blood and mucus from the newborn's mouth and nose with sterile gauze or with the cleanest object available. If the newborn is still not breathing, suction the newborn's mouth and nose again. Rub the newborn's back or flick the soles of the newborn's feet to stimulate breathing (**FIGURE 16-7**). Use the towel to dry the newborn and then wrap the newborn in a blanket to keep the newborn warm. Place the newborn on the side with the head slightly lower than the trunk. This step will aid in the drainage of secretions from the airway.

Wait at least 60 seconds (long enough for the umbilical cord to stop pulsating), then clamp the cord with an umbilical cord clamp or tie it with gauze between the mother and the newborn. Remember, there is no need for you to cut the umbilical cord in a normal delivery. However, if you have sterile equipment and are trained to use it, you can cut the cord with sterile supplies. Keep the newborn warm and wait until more highly trained EMS personnel arrive. They will have the proper equipment to clamp and cut the umbilical cord in an approved manner.

In the rare event of multiple births, prepare for the second delivery.

Delivery of the Placenta

The placenta will deliver on its own, usually within 30 minutes of the newborn's delivery. Never pull on the umbilical cord to help deliver the placenta.

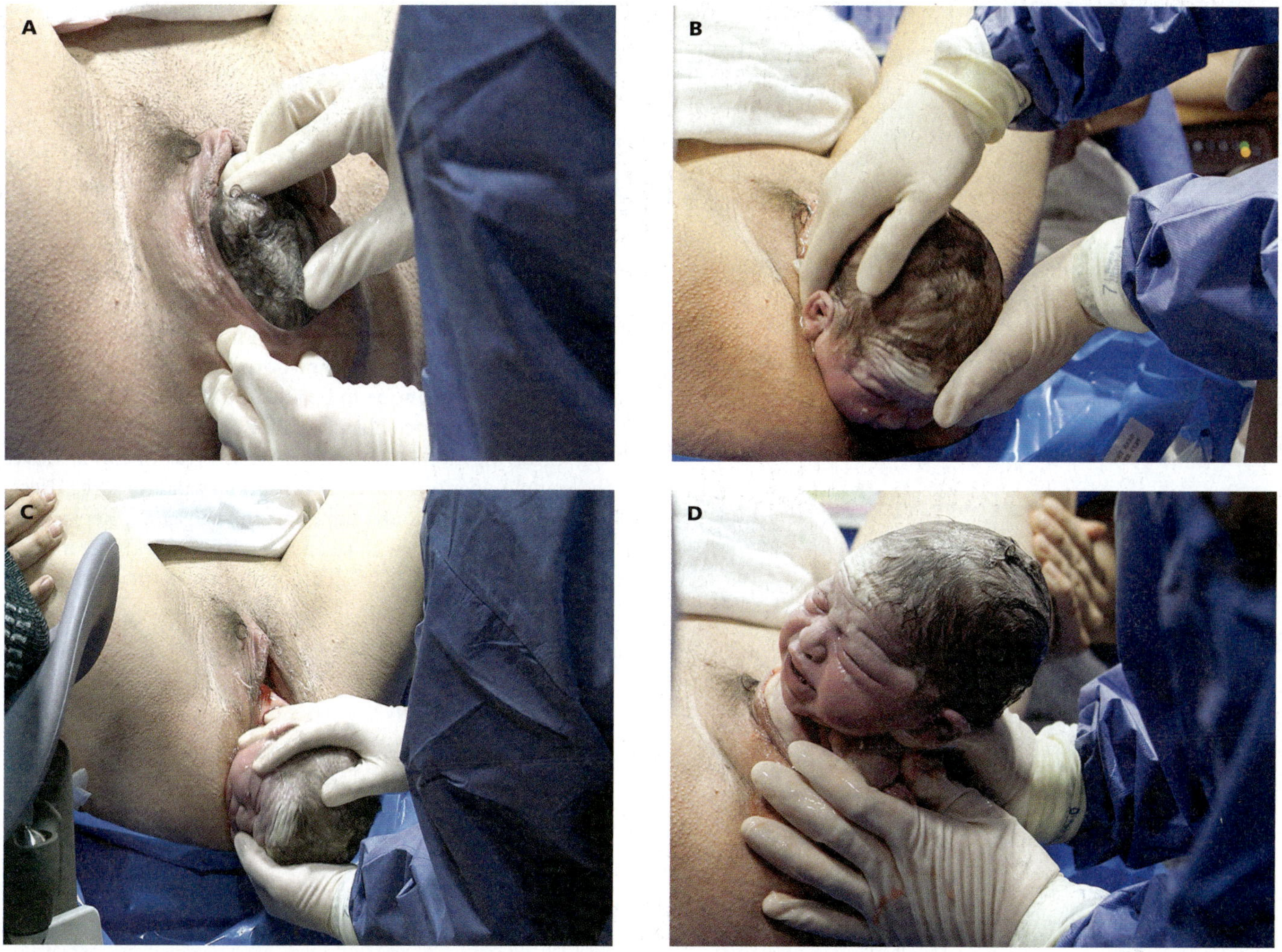

FIGURE 16-5 Phases of the second stage of labor. **A.** The head begins to deliver. **B.** Delivery of the head. **C.** Delivery of the upper shoulder. **D.** Delivery of the lower shoulder.

© University of Maryland Shock Trauma Center/MIEMSS

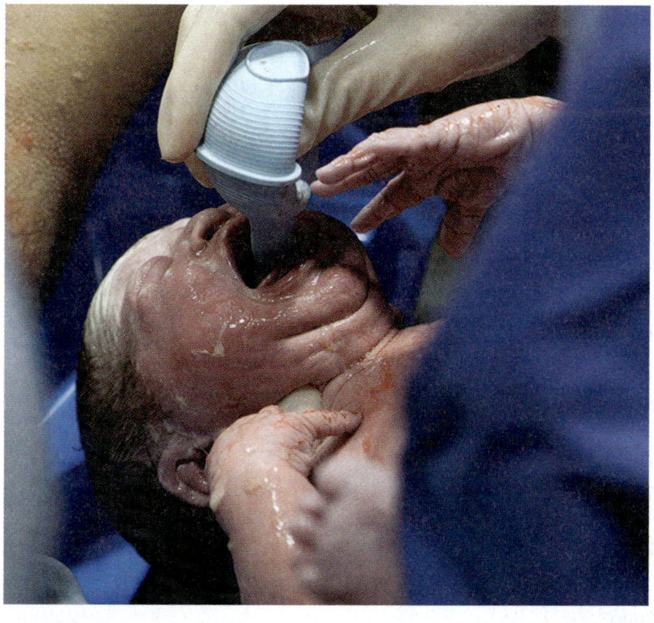

FIGURE 16-6 Suction the mouth and nose to clear the airway of mucus and amniotic fluid. Use a bulb syringe in a newborn's mouth first, then use the bulb syringe to suction the newborn's nose.

© University of Maryland Shock Trauma Center/MIEMSS

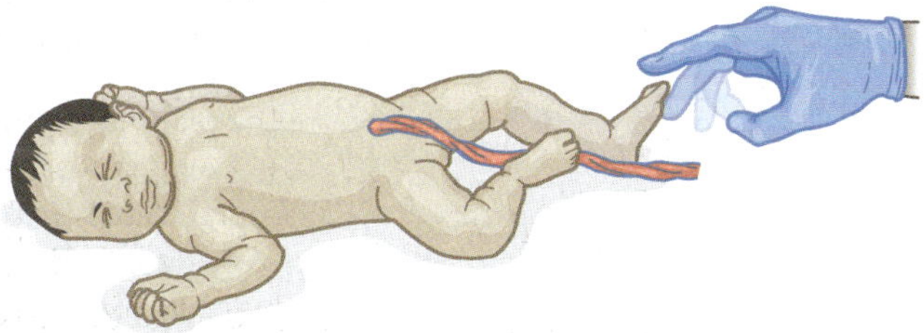

FIGURE 16-7 Gently flick your fingers against the soles of the feet to stimulate breathing in the newborn.

© Jones & Bartlett Learning

The safest and best method for the mother and the newborn is to leave the umbilical cord uncut and attached to the placenta and the newborn, at least until the transporting EMS unit arrives. After the placenta is delivered, place it in a plastic bag to be transported to the hospital with the mother and newborn so it can be examined by a physician. Try to keep the placenta at the same level as the newborn to help prevent any blood from the newborn flowing back out into the placenta. This step is especially important if you are unable to tie the umbilical cord (**FIGURE 16-8**). The mother

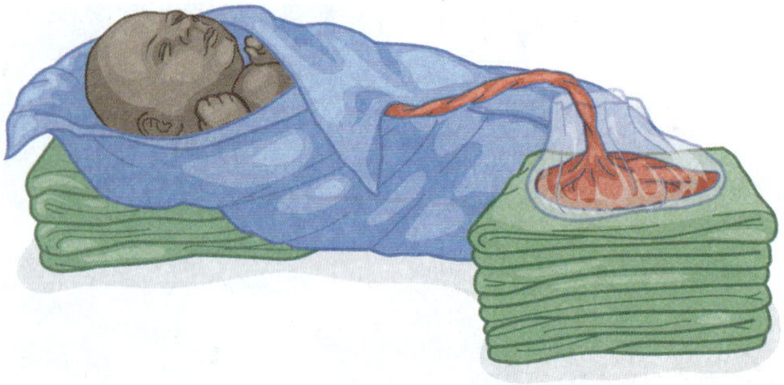

FIGURE 16-8 Following most normal deliveries, it is best for the EMR to keep the placenta, still attached at the cord, at the same level as the newborn during transport to the hospital.
© Jones & Bartlett Learning

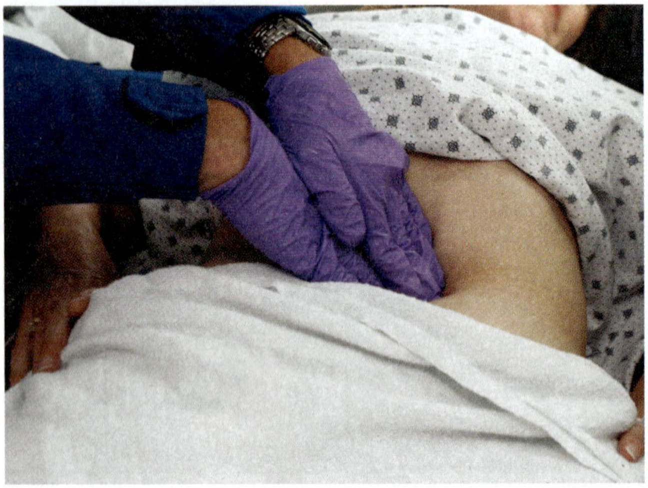

FIGURE 16-9 After delivery, massage the mother's abdomen in a firm, circular motion.
© Jones & Bartlett Learning

can be transported to the hospital before the placenta is delivered, if necessary.

Bleeding usually stops after the placenta is delivered. To help prevent postpartum hemorrhage, you can perform manual uterine massage. To massage the uterus, place one hand with fingers fully extended just above the mother's pubic bone. Use your other hand to press down into the abdomen and, using a circular motion, gently massage the uterus until it becomes firm. This process should take 3 to 5 minutes. As the uterus firms up, it should feel approximately the size of a softball or large grapefruit (**FIGURE 16-9**).

Aftercare of the Mother and Newborn

Continue to observe the mother and newborn carefully and keep them both warm. Cover the newborn's head and body to prevent the loss of body heat. Approximately every 3 to 5 minutes, recheck the uterus for firmness. Also recheck the vagina for any excessive bleeding. In a normal delivery, the mother will have approximately 10 to 16 fluid ounces, or 1 to 2 cups (300 to 500 mL), of blood loss. Continue to massage the uterus using a circular motion if it is not firm or if bleeding continues. Allowing the newborn to nurse at the mother's breast causes a hormone to be released that helps to contract the uterus and reduce bleeding after childbirth.

Clean the mother with clean, moist towels or cloths. Cover the vaginal opening with a clean sanitary pad or large dressing, but do not pack any materials in the vagina. Replace the used towels or sheets with clean ones, if possible. If the mother is thirsty, you can offer small amounts of water to drink.

Resuscitating the Newborn

Newborns who do not cry and breathe on their own within the first minute after birth require assistance breathing. Proceed with the steps listed in **SKILL DRILL 16-2**.

Special Populations

Assessment of the Newborn

The newborn should begin to cry right after birth. You should observe the following vital signs in a healthy, alert newborn:

- A respiratory rate of greater than 40 breaths per minute
- A pulse rate of greater than 100 beats per minute (Check the brachial pulse located at the inside of the infant's upper arm. Even for experienced health care clinicians, it is hard to accurately measure rapid heart rates.)

Throughout this process, try to dry the newborn and wrap the newborn in a clean, dry blanket to keep the newborn warm.

Special Populations

Preventing Hypothermia in the Newborn

Newborns must be kept warm. Dry the newborn and keep the body and head covered to prevent loss of body heat and hypothermia.

YOU are the EMR — **CASE 3**

You are dispatched to an apartment for a pregnant woman who is in labor. As you arrive on the scene, you find a 17-year-old who is 9 months pregnant. The teenager says she feels like she needs to move her bowels. As you examine the patient, you can see the top of the newborn's head.

1. What should be your first action?
2. What can you do to stimulate breathing in a newborn?

SKILL DRILL 16-2

Resuscitating a Newborn

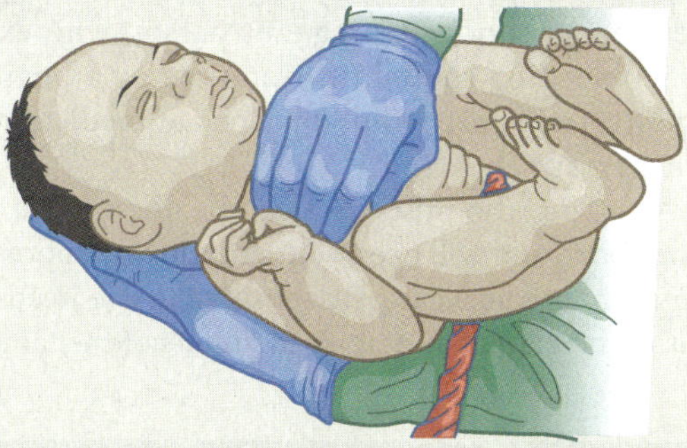

STEP 1 Tilt the newborn's head down and to the side to encourage drainage of mucus. Use a gauze pad to clear secretions from the newborn's mouth and nose. Suction the mouth and nose with a bulb syringe (if available).

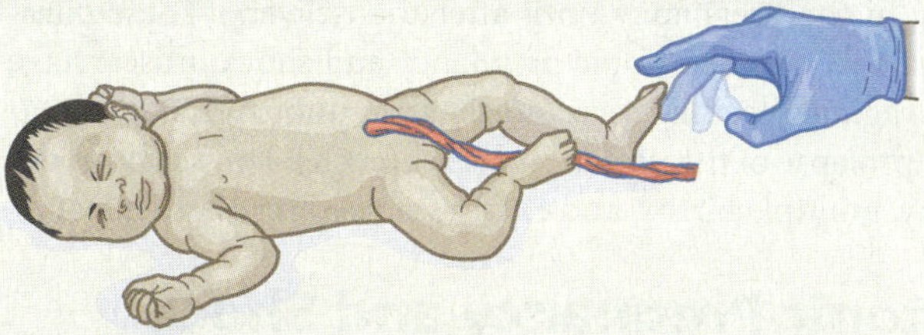

STEP 2 Dry, warm, and stimulate the newborn. Quickly dry the newborn with a clean towel. Use a second towel or blanket for warmth. This is usually enough stimulation for the newborn to begin breathing. If not, rub the back in a circular motion or gently flick your fingers against the soles of the newborn's feet. Do not handle the newborn roughly. A newborn responds best to simple, gentle techniques, but if the newborn is still not breathing, proceed to the next step.

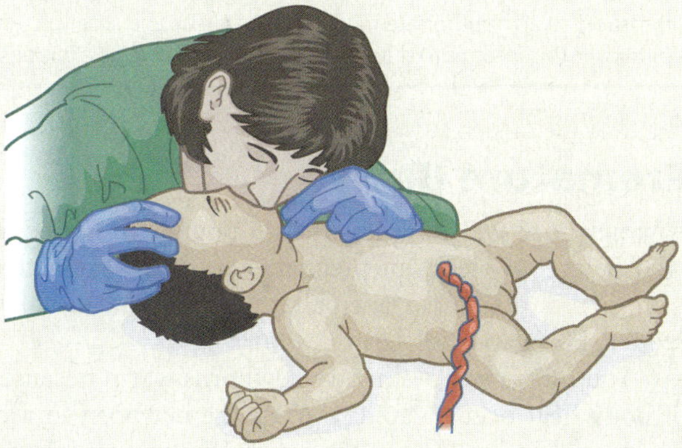

STEP 3 Begin mouth–to–mouth-and-nose or mouth-to-mask breathing by gently puffing twice into the newborn's mouth and nose with only enough force to cause the newborn's chest to rise. If the newborn begins to cry and breathe, support and assist respirations and recheck the airway to be sure it remains clear.

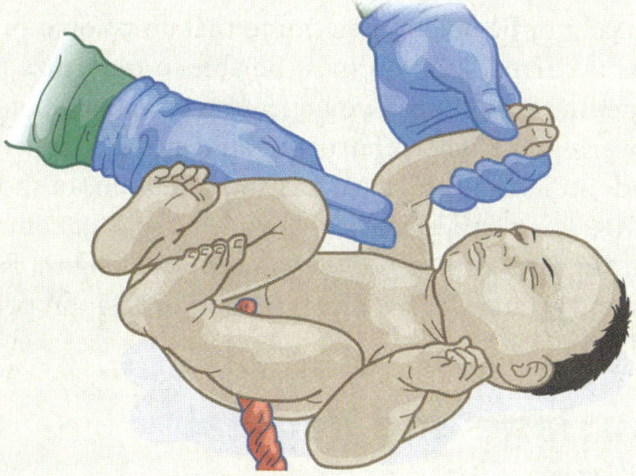

STEP 4 If the newborn is still not breathing, continue mouth–to–mouth-and-nose or mouth-to-mask breathing and check for a brachial pulse.

STEP 5 If you cannot feel a brachial pulse or if the heart rate is less than 60 beats per minute, begin chest compressions. See Chapter 8, *Professional Rescuer CPR*.

Continue cardiopulmonary resuscitation (CPR) until the newborn begins breathing adequately and has a strong pulse of over 60 beats per minute or until ambulance personnel take over. They should provide rapid transport to the hospital. Do not give up!

© Jones & Bartlett Learning

Complications of Pregnancy and Childbirth

Although most pregnancies and births are normal, be aware of possible complications that can occur any time between early in the pregnancy until after the delivery. These complications include ectopic pregnancy and shock, miscarriage and vaginal bleeding, premature birth, unbroken bag of waters, prolapse of the umbilical cord, breech birth, stillborn delivery, multiple births, and excessive bleeding after delivery.

Ectopic Pregnancy and Shock

Any female patient of childbearing age who presents with severe abdominal pain or signs and symptoms of shock (pale skin, dizziness, rapid pulse, decreased blood pressure, fainting) needs to be evaluated by a physician to determine whether a ruptured **ectopic pregnancy** has occurred. An ectopic pregnancy occurs when a fertilized egg becomes implanted in the fallopian tube rather than in the uterus. As the embryo starts to grow, it expands and causes the fallopian tube to rupture. This rupture causes sudden abdominal pain, internal bleeding, and shock.

You will not be able to determine that an ectopic pregnancy has occurred, but you must be able to recognize this life-threatening condition if you encounter a female patient of childbearing age who reports the sudden occurrence of severe abdominal pain and has signs and symptoms of shock. As an EMR, your treatment begins with a rapid patient assessment. Be sure to measure the patient's vital signs. Treat for shock and arrange for prompt transport to an appropriate medical facility.

Miscarriage and Vaginal Bleeding

A **miscarriage** (spontaneous abortion) is the delivery of an incomplete or underdeveloped fetus. A fetus before 20 weeks of pregnancy cannot survive outside the womb. If a miscarriage occurs, save the fetus and all the tissues that pass from the vagina. Control the patient's bleeding by placing a sanitary pad or other large dressing at the vaginal opening. Also treat for shock. Arrange for prompt transport to a hospital so that a physician can examine the patient and the fetal tissues and control any additional bleeding.

Vaginal bleeding in a pregnant patient is often the first sign of a miscarriage. It can also indicate a variety of other complications with the pregnancy. Any time a pregnant patient experiences vaginal bleeding, perform a patient assessment, obtain a good medical history, and obtain a set of vital signs to determine whether the patient is experiencing shock. A pregnant person who experiences vaginal bleeding should be examined by a physician. Arrange for transport to an appropriate medical facility for further treatment.

A patient who miscarries will be upset about the loss of the newborn and will need your emotional support as well as emergency medical care. Be sensitive to the needs and concerns of the patient and other members of the family.

> **Words of Wisdom**
>
> When you assess a pregnant patient, be sure to check the blood pressure. The normal systolic blood pressure for adults is 90 to 140 mm Hg. High blood pressure in pregnant patients can be a sign of a serious condition (preeclampsia) that leads to seizures and can be life threatening to the patient and fetus. If you obtain a high blood pressure reading in a pregnant patient in labor, arrange for prompt transport to an appropriate medical facility. Also, be sure to communicate this information to other emergency medical clinicians.

Premature Birth

Any newborn weighing less than 5 pounds (2 kg) or delivered before 36 weeks of pregnancy is called premature. A **premature newborn** is smaller, thinner, and usually has redder skin than a full-term newborn.

You must keep premature newborns warm because loss of body heat occurs rapidly. Wrap the newborn in a clean towel or sheet and cover the head. Wrapping a premature newborn in an additional length of aluminum foil can also help maintain body temperature. Arrange for prompt transport of mother and newborn to a medical facility.

Unbroken Bag of Waters

In rare instances, the bag of amniotic fluid that surrounds the newborn does not break. If the newborn is surrounded by the bag of waters as the head emerges, carefully break the bag and push it away from the nose and mouth so the

> **YOU are the EMR** — **CASE 4**
>
> At 0317 hours, you are dispatched to 927 Fallow Run for a report of a sick woman. You know the address is in a suburban part of town, but you wish you had more information about this call. As you arrive at the scene, you are met at the front door by an excited man wearing a robe over his nightclothes. He leads you to the bedroom and tells you that his wife woke him up just before he called 9-1-1 and reported severe pain in her abdomen. As you obtain a medical history from the 31-year-old patient, you learn that she has no medical conditions or allergies and takes no medications except for a vitamin pill. The last time she saw her physician was 3 months ago for strep throat.
>
> 1. What additional information do you need from this patient?
> 2. What type of care does this patient need?

Voices OF Experience

It was the morning of the 2004 Super Bowl. I was ending a 24-hour shift at the fire station and was looking forward to going home for a day of rest, relaxation, and football. We were finishing up the station duties when the dispatcher came on the radio and dispatched us for a 23-year-old woman who was reporting abdominal pain. As the address came across the radio, I could not help but think that it seemed oddly familiar. It took me a moment to process it; the address was mine. I was hit with a whirlwind of emotions and thought, "Is this really happening?" My wife and I had just found out that she was pregnant the previous week.

"There are a number of things that it could have been, but one thing was coming out on the top of my list: an ectopic pregnancy."

As we responded, I began running through the possible causes of her abdominal pain. There are a number of things that it could have been, but one thing was coming out on the top of my list: an ectopic pregnancy. We arrived to find my wife experiencing severe abdominal pain at 9/10 on a 0 to 10 scale. We placed her on oxygen, started an intravenous line, loaded her into the ambulance, and began the drive to the hospital. We were fortunate that day. After having a battery of tests, we found out the baby was fine; the reason for her pain was a kidney stone.

The next 8 months went by and she and the baby were doing well, until the 38th week. Suddenly, she began experiencing the signs and symptoms of preeclampsia; she started having some unusual swelling in her hands and lower legs and said she just was not feeling quite right. Her obstetrician ordered bed rest. Two weeks later, my wife woke me up in the middle of the night; her water had broken. Because it was her first pregnancy, we knew we did not have to rush to the hospital. We contacted our physician and patiently waited and timed her contractions. Suddenly, she started complaining of a headache and began having tremors in her arms.

I called 9-1-1, and within a few moments paramedics arrived. I explained that she had been diagnosed with preeclampsia 2 weeks earlier. They took her blood pressure and it was 190/110 mm Hg. We again loaded her into the ambulance for the drive to the hospital. I had never been so scared, but I knew I needed to be calm so that she did not become alarmed and risk making her situation worse. The last thing a patient with preeclampsia needs is extra stress. We were lucky for a second time when she delivered a healthy 6-pound 5-ounce (3-kg) baby boy.

As we progress through our training and then into our careers, we should always keep something in mind: you just never know who is going to benefit from the knowledge you gain and the lives that you will touch.

Richard Main, BS, NREMT-P
Lead EMT Instructor
National Center for Technical Instruction
Las Vegas, Nevada

Adapted from the personal Medical Identification Symbol of the American Medical Association.

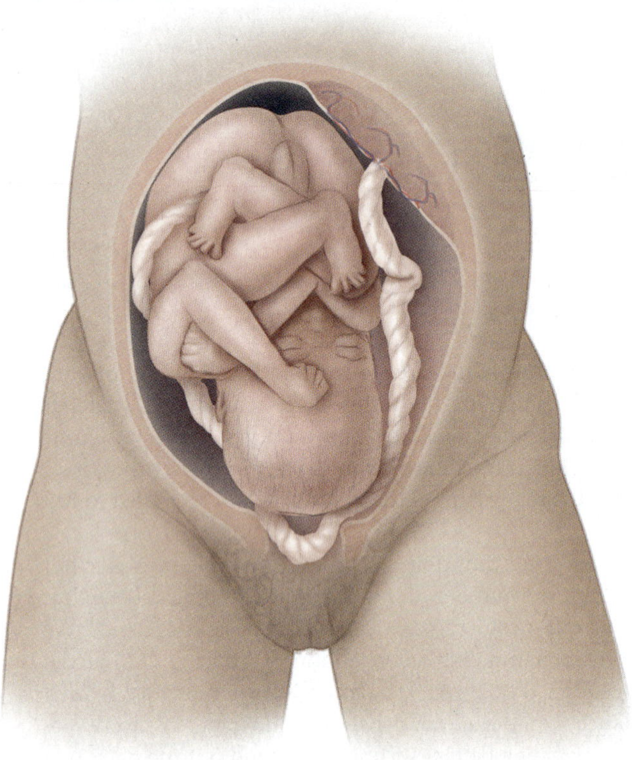

FIGURE 16-10 A prolapsed umbilical cord is a life-threatening situation for the fetus and must be treated at the hospital.
© Jones & Bartlett Learning

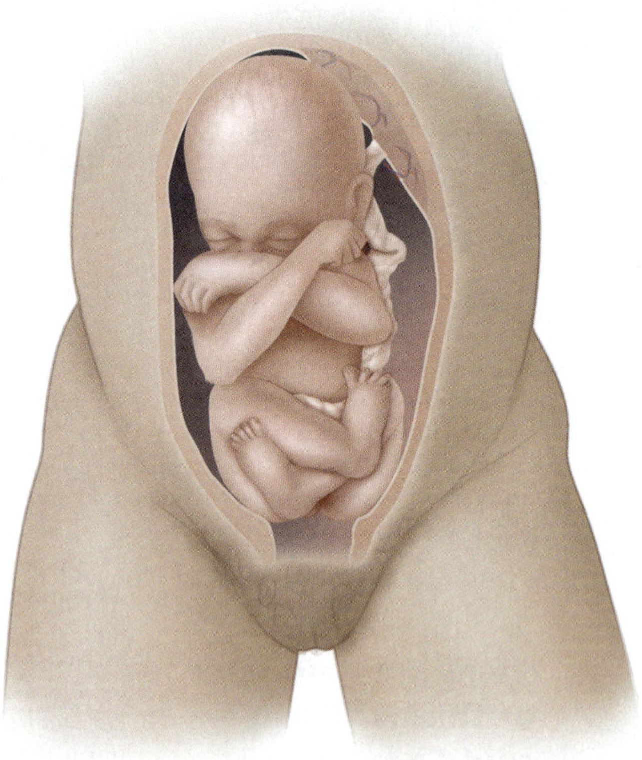

FIGURE 16-11 In a breech presentation, the buttocks are delivered first. Breech deliveries are usually slow, so you will often have time to transport the patient to the hospital.
© Jones & Bartlett Learning

newborn can breathe. Be careful not to injure the newborn in the process. Then suction the newborn's mouth, followed by the nose, to help the newborn begin to breathe.

Prolapse of the Umbilical Cord

On rare occasions, the umbilical cord appears from the vaginal opening before the fetus is delivered (**FIGURE 16-10**). This condition is called a **prolapsed umbilical cord**. The cord may be compressed between the newborn and the mother's pelvis during contractions, cutting off the newborn's blood supply. This condition is a serious emergency that requires immediate transport to a hospital.

Place the patient on their back and prop the hips and legs higher than the rest of the body with pillows, blankets, or articles of clothing. Keep the umbilical cord covered and moist, and do not try to push it back into the vagina. Administer oxygen to the patient if it is available and you are trained to use it. Arrange for rapid transport to the hospital.

Some EMS systems recommend placing the pregnant patient in a kneeling position (knee–chest position) to take the pressure off the umbilical cord. Check with your medical director regarding local procedures.

Breech Birth

In a breech birth, the newborn's buttocks, rather than the head, come down the birth canal first. This abnormal delivery can result in injury to the newborn and the mother (**FIGURE 16-11**).

If, instead of the normal crowning, you see a **breech presentation**, make every attempt to arrange for prompt transport to a medical facility. A breech birth slows the labor, so there will be more time for transport to the emergency department. If you are stranded and cannot transport the patient to the emergency department, you will have to assist with the breech birth.

Support the newborn's buttocks and legs as they are delivered; the head usually follows on its own. If the head does not deliver within 3 minutes, arrange for prompt transport to a hospital. Insert a gloved hand into the vagina and use your fingers to keep the newborn's airway open by forming a pocket over the newborn's nose and mouth.

In very rare cases, the arm or the leg is the first part of the newborn to appear in the birth canal. This circumstance, called limb presentation, is an extreme emergency that cannot be handled in the field. You must arrange for rapid transport to the hospital by ambulance.

> **Safety**
>
> When a newborn is in the breech position, do not attempt to pull the newborn out of the vagina!

Stillborn Delivery

Start and continue resuscitation on all newborns who are not breathing. However, sometimes a newborn dies in the uterus long before labor. The fetus will generally have an unpleasant odor and will not exhibit any signs of life. A lifeless fetus is referred to as a stillborn. In a situation like this, carefully wrap the stillborn newborn in a blanket and turn your attention to the mother to provide physical care and emotional support.

Multiple Births

In the event of multiple births (such as twins), another set of labor contractions will begin shortly after the delivery of the first newborn. A pregnant person generally knows of a multiple birth in advance. However, there are times when a multiple birth has not been previously diagnosed. Do not worry—just get ready to repeat the procedures you completed for delivering the first newborn.

Words of Wisdom

In the event of multiple births, there may be more than one placenta. If each fetus has its own placenta (such as with fraternal twins), the first placenta will usually deliver before the next newborn. If there is only one placenta (such as with identical twins), both newborns will deliver prior to the delivery of the placenta.

Excessive Bleeding After Delivery

In addition to the early bloody show that precedes birth, approximately 1 to 2 cups (300 to 500 mL) of blood loss occurs during normal childbirth. If the mother is bleeding severely, place one or more clean sanitary pads at the opening of the vagina, treat for shock, and arrange for rapid transport to the hospital by ambulance.

Remember to encourage the newborn to nurse at the mother's breast, because nursing contracts the uterus and can often help stop the bleeding. Massage the uterus with your hand, as described earlier in this chapter.

If the area between the mother's vagina and **anus** is torn and bleeding, treat it as you would an open wound. Apply direct pressure using sanitary pads or gauze dressings.

Trauma and Pregnant Patients

Pregnant patients may be subjected to various kinds of trauma, including motor vehicle crashes, falls, and assaults. A pregnant patient who has been involved in any type of trauma should be examined by a physician. The forces involved in even minor trauma may be enough to injure the mother or the unborn child, even though the fetus is usually well protected in the uterus.

Safety

Pregnant patients with no indication of trauma should be transported while lying on the left side to prevent putting pressure on the major abdominal organs and the inferior vena cava.

Promptly assess and arrange transport to the hospital of a pregnant patient who has been involved in a motor vehicle crash. If the patient exhibits signs or symptoms of shock, monitor the airway, breathing, and circulation. Arrange for administration of high-flow oxygen if available and if you are trained to use it. If the patient requires spinal motion restriction, tilt the long backboard approximately 30° (6 inches [15 cm]) to the left by placing pillows or folded blankets under the opposite side of the board. This position will relieve pressure on the uterus and the abdominal organs and will allow blood to return through the major veins in the abdomen.

In rare circumstances, a crash can be severe enough to kill the pregnant patient but not the fetus. High-quality CPR should be provided to the pregnant patient during transport to the closest medical facility.

Words of Wisdom

As part of your patient assessment, check to see whether the patient was wearing a seat belt. Pregnant patients are at lower risk for injury to the fetus and to themselves if they wear a seat belt.

YOU are the EMR SUMMARY

You are the EMR: CASE 1

1. What information do you need to know before determining whether there is time to transport this woman to the hospital or whether you will need to assist her with the delivery?

Consider the following seven factors to help you determine whether there is time to transport a pregnant patient to the hospital before the newborn is born:

- Is this the patient's first pregnancy?
- Has the patient experienced a bloody show?
- Has the bag of waters broken?
- How frequent are the contractions?
- Does the patient feel an urge to move the bowels?
- Is the infant's head crowning?
- Is transportation available?

2. What standard precautions do you need to take when assisting with the emergency delivery of a newborn?

During normal childbirth, the mother expels blood and body fluids. It is important to prevent yourself from coming in contact with blood and body fluids as much as possible. Use sterile gloves to protect you and to protect the

YOU are the EMR SUMMARY

patient. Protect your face and eyes from splatter by putting on a mask and eye protection, as well as a surgical gown if it is available. Be sure to thoroughly wash your hands or shower as soon as possible after you have completed the call.

3. What are the risks to a pregnant woman and fetus if they are involved in a motor vehicle crash?

Whenever a pregnant patient is involved in a motor vehicle crash, remember that there are two lives at risk: the life of the mother and the life of the unborn child. Any pregnant patient involved in a crash should be examined by a physician. Even a minor crash may injure the mother or fetus. Injuries may not be obvious right after the crash. As an EMR, you do not have the training or equipment to assess the seriousness of injuries to a pregnant patient and fetus. Treat the patient with special care and monitor carefully for signs and symptoms of injuries and shock. Transport the patient to an appropriate medical facility as soon as possible.

You are the EMR: CASE 2

1. What questions should you ask the patient about the contractions?

Ask the patient how long she has been having contractions and how frequently she is having contractions. The answers to these key questions will determine your next course of action. If the contractions are more than 5 minutes apart, you should be able to transport the woman to a nearby hospital. However, if the contractions are less than 2 minutes apart, she could be close to delivery. It is important for you to measure the contractions because many people either do not know how to measure the time between contractions or they do not accurately measure them in their excited state.

2. Why is it important to know whether this is her first pregnancy?

The time from the beginning of labor until the time of delivery is usually longer with the first child than with subsequent deliveries. Knowing whether the patient has had other children, along with the time between contractions, can help you make an informed decision about whether to transport or to prepare for an on-scene delivery.

3. What stage of labor is she in?

The woman is in the first stage of labor, in which her body is preparing for the birth. There are three stages of labor, beginning with the preparation of the mother's body for birth, which includes the breaking of the bag of waters, the bloody show, and contractions. The second stage is the actual birth, and the third stage is the delivery of the placenta.

You are the EMR: CASE 3

1. What should be your first action?

Prepare for the immediate birth of the newborn and prepare the area where the delivery is going to take place. If your medical gear includes a sterile delivery kit, use it. If not, use your EMR skills and improvise. Cover the area with clean towels and sheets. Use whatever personal protective equipment you may have because you will be exposed to blood and body fluids during the delivery.

2. What can you do to stimulate breathing in a newborn?

If the newborn is not breathing, suction the mouth and nose. You can also try rubbing the newborn's back or flicking the soles of the feet to stimulate breathing. If these techniques do not work, give two small mouth-to-mouth-and-nose rescue breaths. Dry the newborn as soon as possible and keep the newborn warm.

You are the EMR: CASE 4

1. What additional information do you need from this patient?

You need to determine what the patient had to eat last evening and ask her how she felt last evening. Ask the date of her last menstrual period to determine if there is any chance she is pregnant. Obtain a set of vital signs to see if she is in shock. Ask the patient if she has ever had pain like this before. Determine the severity of her pain using a 0 to 10 scale (10 being unspeakable pain).

2. What type of care does this patient need?

Sudden onset of severe abdominal pain in a young, healthy female patient often indicates a serious condition. Low blood pressure may indicate that she is in shock, but a normal blood pressure does not rule out a serious condition in its early stages. If the patient reports her menstrual period is late, suspect that she might be experiencing a ruptured ectopic pregnancy, which is a medical emergency. The only way to determine the cause of her pain is to arrange for her to be transported to an appropriate medical facility for evaluation by a physician.

Prep Kit

Ready for Review

- Childbirth is usually a happy event. As an EMR, your role is to assist in the delivery and offer comfort and support to the mother and newborn. In most cases, deliveries result in healthy babies.
- To estimate how soon a delivery will occur, assess the time between contractions and whether the newborn's head appears during a contraction (crowning). By using these two key indicators, you can determine whether to transport the pregnant patient to a medical facility or whether the birth will occur outside the hospital.
- Normal labor consists of three distinct stages:
  - The first stage is characterized by the following conditions: initial contractions occur, the bag of waters breaks, and the bloody show occurs, but the newborn's head does not appear.
  - The second stage involves the actual birth. You will see the newborn's head crowning during contractions, at which time you must prepare to assist the mother with delivery.
  - The third stage involves delivery of the placenta. You must assist in stabilizing the condition of the mother and newborn and delivering the placenta.
- Take standard precautions when assisting with delivery of a newborn.
- After the delivery, you have two patients to care for: the mother and the newborn.
- For infants who do not breathe on their own within the first minute after birth, you must proceed with the steps to resuscitate.
- Although most pregnancies and births are uneventful, be aware of possible complications, including ectopic pregnancy and shock, vaginal bleeding and miscarriage, premature birth, unbroken bag of waters, prolapse of the umbilical cord, breech birth, stillborn delivery, multiple births, and excessive bleeding after delivery.
- Promptly assess and arrange transport to the hospital for a pregnant patient who has been involved in a motor vehicle crash.

Vital Vocabulary

anus The distal or terminal ending of the gastrointestinal tract.

bag of waters The amniotic sac and fluid that surround the fetus before birth.

birth canal The vagina and the lower part of the uterus.

bloody show The plug of mucus that is discharged from the vagina when labor begins.

breech presentation A delivery in which the newborn's buttocks appear in the birth canal first, rather than the head.

contractions Muscular movements of the uterus that push the newborn out of the birth canal.

crowning Appearance of the newborn's head during a contraction as the newborn is pushed outward through the birth canal.

ectopic pregnancy A pregnancy that occurs outside the uterus, usually in a fallopian tube; usually terminates with the rupture of the fallopian tube.

fetus A developing newborn in the uterus or womb.

labor The process of delivering a newborn.

miscarriage Delivery of an incomplete or underdeveloped fetus before it is mature enough to survive outside the womb (approximately 20 weeks of pregnancy); also called spontaneous abortion.

placenta Life-support system of the fetus; also called the afterbirth.

premature newborn A newborn delivered before 36 weeks of gestation or who weighs less than 5 pounds (2 kg) at birth.

prolapsed umbilical cord A condition in which the umbilical cord appears before the newborn does; the newborn's head may compress the cord and cut off all circulation.

suction To aspirate (suck out) fluid by mechanical means.

umbilical cord Ropelike attachment between the mother and fetus; nourishment and waste products pass to and from the fetus and the mother through this cord.

uterus (womb) Muscular organ that holds and nourishes the developing fetus.

vagina The opening through which the newborn emerges.

Prep Kit

References

Chang AK. Pregnancy trauma. Medscape website. https://emedicine.medscape.com/article/796979-overview?-form=fpf. Updated July 15, 2024. Accessed November 4, 2024.

Committee on Practice Bulletins-Obstetrics. Practice bulletin No. 183: postpartum hemorrhage. *Obstet Gynecol*. 2017;130(4):e168–e186. doi:10.1097/AOG.0000000000002351

Osterman MJK, Hamilton BE, Martin JA, Driscoll AK, Valenzuela CP. Births: final data for 2022. *Natl Vital Stat Rep*. 2024 Apr;73(2):1–56.

Wyckoff MH, Singletary EM, Soar J, et al. 2021 International Consensus on Cardiopulmonary Resuscitation and Emergency Cardiovascular Care science with treatment recommendations: summary from the Basic Life Support; Advanced Life Support; Neonatal Life Support; Education, Implementation, and Teams; First Aid Task Forces; and the COVID-19 Working Group. *Resuscitation*. 2021;169:229–311.

Yamada NK, Szyld E, Strand ML, et al. 2023 American Heart Association and American Academy of Pediatrics focused update on neonatal resuscitation: an update to the American Heart Association Guidelines for Cardiopulmonary Resuscitation and Emergency Cardiovascular Care. *Pediatrics*. 2024;153(2):e2023065030. doi:10.1542/peds.2023-065030

Assessment IN ACTION

You and your partner are on standby at a high school football game when a man runs up to you screaming that his wife is "having a baby." The man tells you that his wife suddenly started having contractions and the next thing he knew, her water broke. He tells you his wife is 9 months pregnant with their first child and she is waiting in their vehicle. You grab your medical bag and head to the patient's vehicle.

1. Which of the following steps is NOT indicated in this case?
   - **A.** Gain information about the patient's pregnancy and medical history.
   - **B.** Put on gloves and prepare for birth.
   - **C.** Contact dispatch to request an EMS crew and a transport unit.
   - **D.** Massage the patient's abdomen to speed up the delivery process.
2. The patient is sitting in the back seat of the vehicle and is clearly in distress. She says her contractions are 2 minutes apart. What should you do?
   - **A.** Conduct a full patient assessment, including a secondary assessment.
   - **B.** Prepare to deliver the newborn.
   - **C.** Prepare for transport to the hospital.
   - **D.** Move the patient into a position of comfort.
3. Moments later, you see that the newborn's head is visible at the vaginal opening. What is this called?
   - **A.** Breech
   - **B.** Prolapse
   - **C.** Neonatal
   - **D.** Crowning
4. Because the head of the newborn is visible and you are in the field, what is the next most appropriate step?
   - **A.** Wait for emergency medical clinicians with a higher level of training.
   - **B.** Have a supply of clean towels ready.
   - **C.** Tell the woman to breathe slowly and push.
   - **D.** Tell the woman to stop pushing.
5. As soon as the head of the newborn is delivered, what should you do?
   - **A.** Look, listen, and feel for breathing.
   - **B.** Pull on the newborn's shoulders to get the rest of the body out.
   - **C.** Check the newborn's neck to be sure the umbilical cord is not wrapped around it.
   - **D.** Clamp the umbilical cord.
6. If the bag of waters has not broken once the newborn's head has delivered, what should you do?
   - **A.** Tear the bag with your fingers and push it away from the newborn's face.
   - **B.** Place your hand on the newborn's head to keep it from moving.
   - **C.** Be prepared to suction the newborn's mouth and nose with a bulb syringe.
   - **D.** Arrange for immediate transport.
7. Which of the following steps is NOT indicated if you have just delivered a healthy newborn?
   - **A.** Begin chest compressions.
   - **B.** Suction the airway if the newborn is having difficulty breathing.
   - **C.** Thoroughly dry the newborn.
   - **D.** Place the newborn on the mother's abdomen to allow skin-to-skin contact.
8. The newborn starts breathing and appears healthy. After wrapping the newborn in towels and placing the newborn on the mother's abdomen, what is your next step?
9. When should the umbilical cord be cut?
10. Why is a ruptured ectopic pregnancy a life-threatening emergency?

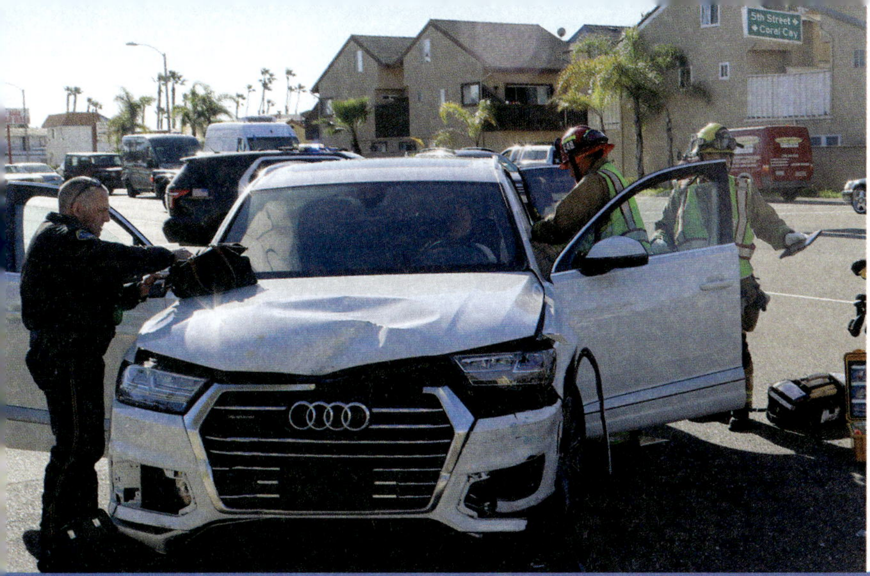

SECTION 7

EMS Operations

17 Transport Operations

18 Vehicle Extrication and Special Rescue

19 Incident Management

© mikeledray/Shutterstock

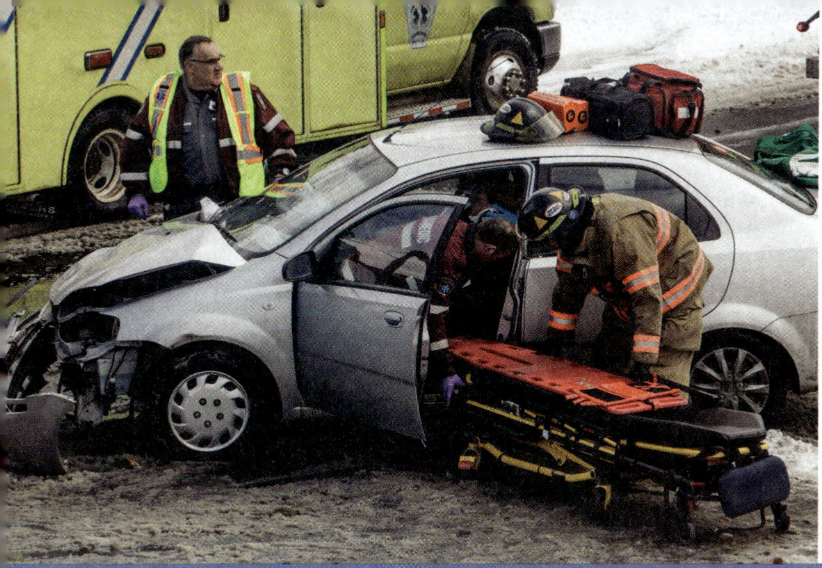

CHAPTER 17

Transport Operations

National EMS Education Standard Competencies

EMS Operations

Knowledge of operational roles and responsibilities to ensure patient, public, and personnel safety.

Emergency Response Vehicles

- Risks and responsibilities of emergency response and radio communications (pp 390–394)
- Risks and responsibilities of operating emergency vehicles (pp 390–394)

Air Medical

- Safe air medical operations (pp 390–394)
- Criteria for utilizing air medical response (pp 390–394)
- Medical risks/needs/advantages (pp 390–394)

Knowledge Objectives

1. Summarize the different phases of an emergency response. (pp 390–391)
2. Explain the importance of preparing for an emergency call. (p 390)
3. List the medical and nonmedical equipment needed to respond to a call. (p 390)
4. Explain the importance of reviewing dispatch information. (p 390)
5. Explain the safety precautions needed to ensure a safe emergency response. (pp 390–391)
6. Describe the actions emergency medical responders (EMRs) should take on arrival at an emergency scene. (p 391)
7. Describe the importance of transferring patient care to higher-level emergency medical services (EMS) personnel. (p 391)
8. Explain the postrun activities that follow the completion of an emergency response. (p 391)
9. Describe the guidelines for safe helicopter operations. (pp 391–394)
10. Describe the steps of setting up a helicopter landing zone. (p 392)
11. Describe the steps of loading patients into a helicopter. (p 394)

Skills Objectives

1. Demonstrate how to set up a helicopter landing zone. (p 392)
2. Demonstrate how to assist with loading a patient into a helicopter. (p 394)

© Benoit Daoust/Shutterstock

Introduction

To be an effective emergency medical responder (EMR), you need to prepare for an emergency medical services (EMS) call, review dispatch information, respond safely to the scene, perform a scene assessment, perform initial patient assessment and provide emergency care, update responding EMS units and transfer care to higher-level EMS personnel, and complete postrun activities. The first part of this chapter describes the phases of an EMS call and the tasks required to complete each of these phases safely. The second part of this chapter describes your role in helicopter medivac operations. It describes helicopter safety guidelines, how to set up a landing zone, and how to assist with loading patients into a helicopter.

Preparing for a Call

In your primary role as a law enforcement officer, firefighter, lifeguard, or security guard, you are also on call as an EMR. In preparing yourself for a call, you must understand your role as a member of the emergency medical system. Any vehicle used for emergency response, whether a fire department vehicle, a law enforcement vehicle, or your personal vehicle, must be ready to respond at all times. Follow a regular schedule to inspect and maintain all vehicles. Your department should provide a checklist to follow to ensure that everything is in working order, such as checking tire pressure, fluid levels, and fuel levels. Be prepared to respond promptly, using the most direct route available. Make sure you have the proper equipment to perform your job, including the medical equipment in your EMR life support kit, your personal safety equipment, and equipment to safeguard the incident scene. This equipment must be stocked and maintained on a regular basis according to the schedule specified by your agency. Suggested contents of the EMR life support kit are detailed in Chapter 1, *EMS Systems*.

Phases of an EMR Call

When you respond to an EMS call, make sure each task is carefully completed to ensure a safe and positive outcome to the incident.

Dispatch

The dispatch facility is a center that citizens can call to request emergency medical care. Most centers are part of a 9-1-1 system that is responsible for receiving emergency calls at a public safety answering point (PSAP) and then dispatching fire, police, and EMS. You should understand how the dispatch facility used by your department operates. Your job will be easier if the dispatcher obtains the proper information from the caller. Dispatchers should also be able to instruct callers on how to perform lifesaving techniques such as cardiopulmonary resuscitation until you arrive.

You may receive your dispatch information by telephone, radio, pager, computer terminal, or written printout. Regardless of the transmission method, the information should include the nature of the call, the name and location of the patient, the number of patients, and any special conditions at the scene. The dispatcher should also obtain a callback number in case you need more information from the caller. Without adequate dispatch information, you will not be able to respond properly.

Response to the Scene

Your first priority in responding to the scene is to get there quickly and safely. Consider traffic patterns and the time of day before you select the best route to the scene. Before you begin to respond, be sure you know how to get to the location of the call. Be certain that all personnel are properly seated and secured with approved seat belts. Keep all equipment secured so it does not injure someone in the event of a sudden stop or crash.

Use emergency lights and siren according to your state laws and according to the regulations of your agency. Evidence shows that patient outcome typically is not significantly improved by using lights and siren; thus, the increased risk of a vehicle crash caused by using lights and siren is often unwarranted. Always consider the risks versus benefits before engaging lights and siren. Also, remember that emergency lights and siren allow you to request the right of way; they do not guarantee it. You should be familiar with your local laws and regulations specific to responding in emergency mode.

Be especially careful at intersections and railroad crossings. Do not exceed the safe speed for the vehicle you are operating. Be aware that distractions such as radios, mobile devices, and global positioning systems (GPS) can contribute to vehicle crashes. Reduce your speed on unpaved roads, on wet or icy roads, and during periods of darkness or reduced visibility. Follow all safety procedures specified by your department. Above all else, drive defensively so you are not involved in a crash. Remember, your goal is to arrive on the scene safely.

YOU are the EMR **CASE 1**

At 2047 hours you are dispatched to 209 East Second Street for a report of a sick child with a high fever. You are informed that the child is located in Apartment 318. This address is approximately 7 minutes from your location.

1. Why is it important for you to understand the phases of an EMS call?
2. Why is it important to differentiate between East Second Street and West Second Street and to confirm the apartment number?
3. What steps do you need to take if you do not understand the location of the address given to you by your dispatcher?

Safety

Emergency lights and siren allow you to request the right of way but do not guarantee it. Drive defensively and safely.

Arrival at the Scene

When you arrive at the scene, remember to place your vehicle in a safe location to minimize the chance of injury and to avoid blocking the scene. Leave plenty of space for the ambulance and other arriving units. Consider how best to position your vehicle to effectively use your warning lights (**FIGURE 17-1**). Remember to perform a scene assessment as outlined in the patient assessment sequence. Look for safety hazards such as downed power lines, leaking fuel, broken glass, and fire, as well as potential biologic hazards. Control the flow of traffic to ensure the safety of responders, patients, and bystanders. Determine the number of patients and whether you need to call for additional resources. Be as efficient and organized as you can. Provide patient care using the knowledge and skills you have learned in this course. Call for additional resources if needed.

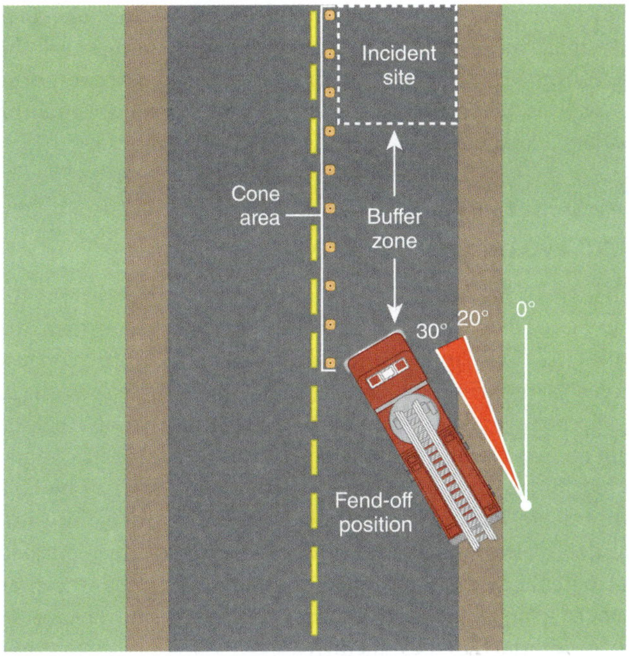

FIGURE 17-1 The "fend-off" position.
© Jones & Bartlett Learning

Perform Patient Assessment and Provide Emergency Care

Many of the activities you perform at the scene of an emergency are related to the assessment and treatment of patients. The knowledge and skills needed to perform patient assessment and provide treatment are detailed throughout this text. These skills are mentioned here only to give you an idea of where they fit within the phases of responding to an emergency call.

Safety

Always take standard precautions to prevent contamination by the patient's body fluids.

Transferring the Care of the Patient to Higher-Level EMS Personnel

As more highly trained EMS personnel arrive on the scene, you will have to transfer care of the patient to them. Update the responding EMS units by providing them with a brief report of the situation as you initially observed it, and tell them the results of your patient assessment and what care you have provided. Ask them if they have any questions for you. Finally, offer to assist other EMS personnel in caring for the patient.

Postrun Activities

You may think you are done with a call after you have cared for the patient and provided assistance to other EMS personnel; however, your job is not done until you have completed the paper or electronic patient care report. Documentation is important. In addition to completing the report, you must also clean your equipment and replace needed supplies. Only after you have completed these activities should you resume regular duties or notify your dispatcher or supervisor that you are ready for another call.

Helicopter Operations

Helicopters are used by EMS systems to reach patients, transport patients to medical facilities, and evacuate patients from otherwise inaccessible areas. If your EMS system uses a helicopter, obtain a copy of the ground operations procedures or schedule an orientation session with helicopter personnel so you will be prepared during an emergency. As an EMR, you

YOU are the EMR **CASE 2**

You arrive for work and find a new response vehicle in the garage. Your supervisor informs you that you will be using this vehicle during your shift. You have never seen this vehicle before and are not sure how everything works.

1. How can you verify that this vehicle is ready for response?
2. When should you tell the dispatch center that you are ready for response?

may be responsible for making the initial call for helicopter assistance or for setting up and preparing a landing site in the field. You need to know how to request a helicopter response as well as the criteria for calling a helicopter for trauma patients, medical patients, and wilderness response.

Determining the Need for Helicopter Transport

The use of helicopters to transport patients has several advantages. Helicopters can respond at speeds greater than 100 miles per hour (mph). They can travel above traffic congestion and into wilderness areas. They usually carry specialized equipment, and the personnel staffing them may include emergency medical technicians (EMTs), paramedics, registered nurses, and physicians. These personnel may be able to perform advanced life support (ALS) skills that are unavailable on ground ambulances. Helicopters are requested for patients with severe injuries or acute illnesses who may benefit from a higher level of care or more rapid transport to an appropriate medical facility.

However, helicopter transport has significant drawbacks. Helicopters should not be flown in bad weather, such as wind and freezing rain, and in conditions that reduce visibility, such as thunderstorms and blizzards. They are limited in the amount of weight they can carry, particularly in very hot temperatures and at high elevations. In some settings, sufficient space to establish a safe landing zone is not available.

The decision to request helicopter transport must also consider the door-to-door time. **Door-to-door time** is a measure of how long it takes from the time the patient is accessed to the time the patient reaches definitive care. Although a helicopter may be able to transport the patient from the scene to the hospital more quickly than a ground ambulance could, the extra time required for the helicopter to arrive on scene, or for the crew to land and deliver the patient to the emergency department, may make ground transport the overall faster option. In contrast, an obstruction, such as a traffic accident, could make the helicopter the faster choice even though the hospital is close to the emergency scene. Ultimately, the decision to use a helicopter is situational and must consider local protocols.

Helicopter Safety Guidelines

Helicopters can provide lifesaving transport for patients with serious injuries to an appropriate medical facility. However, helicopters are also dangerous to untrained personnel. The main rotor of the helicopter spins at more than 300 revolutions per minute (rpm) and may be just 4 feet (1 m) above the ground. The tail rotor spins at more than 3,000 rpm and may be invisible to an unwary person. Additionally, the rotors can generate a "wash," or blast of air, equivalent to winds of 60 to 80 mph. If you approach without caution, you may be severely injured by walking upright or by raising an arm above the head. It is important to understand safe helicopter operations.

Setting Up Landing Zones

When choosing a landing site, remember that pilots usually land and take off into the wind. The size of a **landing zone** will vary and depends on the size of the helicopter. Most civilian helicopters need a landing zone of at least 100 × 100 feet (30 × 30 m), or 10,000 square feet (approximately 900 m^2) (**FIGURE 17-2**). Military aircraft may need a larger area. The landing zone should be as flat as possible and free of debris that could become airborne in the 60-mph winds generated by the helicopter. Check carefully for any nearby electrical wires, which may be invisible to the pilot. If the site slopes or has any obstacles, notify the pilot.

Check with your helicopter service to see how you should secure and mark the perimeter of the site. Avoid using flags or other objects that can be blown away by the force of the helicopter rotor wash. Do not use fusees (red signal flares) because they create a fire hazard. Turn off unnecessary white lights and avoid flashing emergency lights because they interfere with the pilot's vision during landing and takeoff. Keep vehicles clear of the landing zone. Close the windows and doors of any nearby vehicles and remove

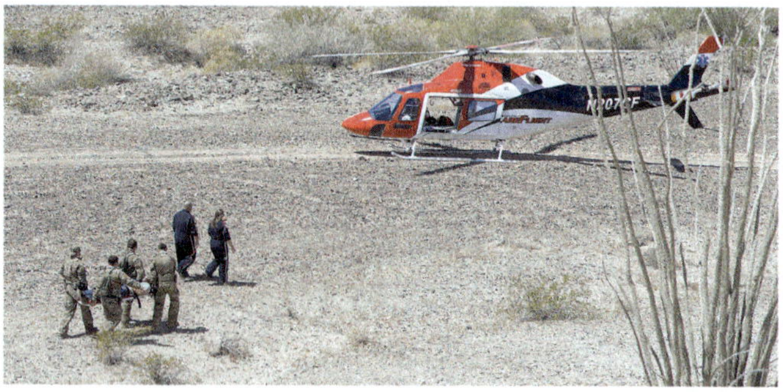

FIGURE 17-2 A landing zone must be large enough for a helicopter to safely land and take off.

© Randy Hoeft/Yuma Sun/AP Photo

YOU are the EMR **CASE 3**

You are dispatched to a motor vehicle crash at a busy intersection, which you recognize as the site of frequent crashes. When you arrive at the scene, you see two damaged vehicles in the middle of the intersection. Police officers have controlled traffic around the crash scene. All the occupants of the damaged vehicles appear to be standing near the crash scene.

1. How would you perform a scene assessment at this incident?
2. When should you request additional resources?

Voices of Experience

I had been an EMT for more than a year and worked for a local fire department in a mountain district outside of town. It was snowing and 6 inches (15 cm) of snow were already on the ground when we got a call for a 1-month-old infant with difficulty breathing. When I got to the house, the familiar red flashing lights marked the driveway and colored the falling snow.

Inside the home, the battalion chief looked relieved that I had arrived, but he was still very concerned. An infant girl, lying on her mother's lap, was having difficulty breathing. I administered high-flow oxygen and knew to sit the child upright. I auscultated her lungs and heard diffuse rhonchi. I gathered the SAMPLE [Signs and symptoms, Allergies, Medications, Pertinent past medical history, Last oral intake, Events leading up to the illness or injury] history from the mother and recognized a possible return of recent pneumonia.

> **"Always do what is in the best interest of your patient."**

I continually reassessed the patient. The oxygen seemed to help initially, and the infant's color and respiratory effort improved. The ALS ambulance had come up from town but was unable to make it up the steep 2-mile (3-km) hill to the house. We weighed the risks and benefits of bringing the paramedic up to us, but we still had to transport the patient down. We decided that the infant was doing better at this time and, because we were not supposed to transport patients, we would wait until the ambulance with four-wheel drive arrived. The ALS ambulance went back to town and the four-wheel drive ambulance was en route.

Minutes kept passing and the patient was getting tired; the improving trend started to reverse and the infant was back to her original presentation. Anxiously awaiting the paramedics, I made a deal with myself that if the child had any change in respiratory rate or rhythm, I would begin positive-pressure ventilation. I opened the pediatric kit and assembled the appropriate bag-mask device.

When the paramedics arrived, I was just about to begin ventilating. I gave a quick report and we dashed out to the ambulance. On the way to the hospital, we started to ventilate and administer bronchodilators with significant improvement.

The paramedic questioned why we did not take the patient down to the first ambulance. I explained that we made that decision because of the child's initial improvement and the issue of not being a transporting agency. He told me it is good to prioritize patient and crew safety, but "Always do what is in the best interest of your patient." Then, he looked me squarely in the eyes and said, "In EMS, you must always move forward toward higher levels of care. You cannot count on your interventions to fix the problem." Lesson learned and never forgotten!

Michael Dann, NREMT-P, BSN
Remote Medical International
Boulder, Colorado

Adapted from the personal Medical Identification Symbol of the American Medical Association.

any loose objects on the vehicles that could become airborne. Some helicopter services request that a charged hose line be available for fire emergencies.

> **Safety**
>
> 1. Be alert for electrical wires when identifying a landing zone for a helicopter.
> 2. Always approach helicopters from the front so the pilot can see you. Approaching a helicopter from the rear is dangerous because the tail rotor is nearly invisible when spinning.
> 3. Do not approach the helicopter until the pilot signals that it is safe to do so.
> 4. Helicopters are very noisy, and you may not be able to hear a shouted warning. Maintain eye contact with the pilot.
> 5. Keep low when you approach the helicopter to avoid the spinning rotor blades.
> 6. Follow the directions of the helicopter crew.

Loading Patients Into Helicopters

Certain safety precautions must be followed during the loading of a helicopter patient. Secure all loose clothing, sheets, and instruments such as stethoscopes. Use eye protection and a helmet, if available, to protect yourself from flying debris. Because helicopters can be very loud, also consider wearing hearing protection. Approach a helicopter from the front and only after the pilot or a crew member signals that it is safe (**FIGURE 17-3**).

The helicopter crew may need help carrying equipment to the patient. Follow their instructions. Give your patient care report to the crew, away from the helicopter's noise, and offer your assistance. It is more difficult to load a helicopter stretcher than an ambulance stretcher. Because loose sheets or blankets can blow off the stretcher, patients need to be packaged (prepared) properly and securely.

As an EMR, you can provide ground support and assistance during helicopter operations if you take proper safety precautions.

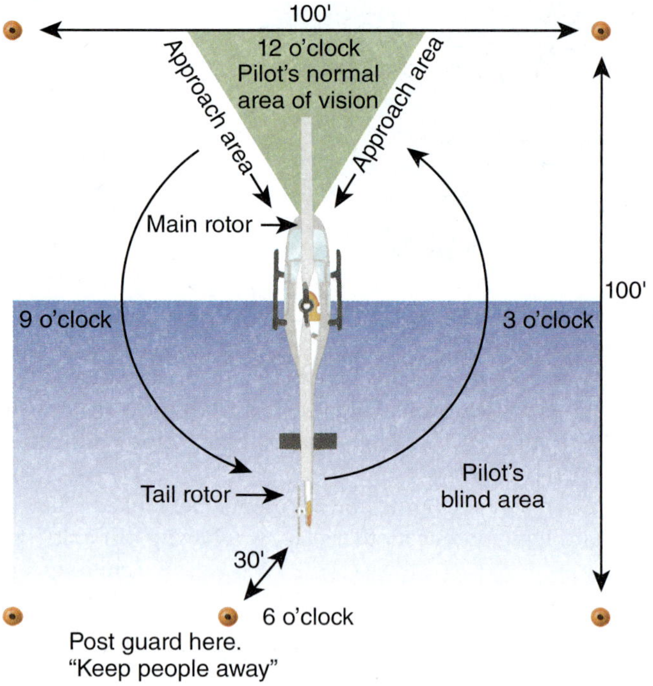

FIGURE 17-3 Approach helicopters from the front so the pilot can see you. The rear guard should be at least 30 feet (9.1 m) away from the tail rotor, which may not be visible when in motion. Blue indicates the pilot's blind area.

© Jones & Bartlett Learning

> **Safety**
>
> Keep the following guidelines in mind during helicopter operations:
>
> - DO NOT approach the helicopter landing zone unless necessary.
> - DO NOT approach a helicopter from the rear.
> - DO NOT run near a helicopter.
> - DO NOT raise your hand when approaching a helicopter.

YOU are the EMR — CASE 4

You are at the scene of a motorcycle crash. The EMS crew at the scene has decided to use a helicopter to transport the patient to the trauma center. You have been asked to help set up the landing zone.

1. What are some of the components of an ideal landing zone?
2. When would it be appropriate to use a helicopter for EMS transport?

YOU are the EMR SUMMARY

You are the EMR: CASE 1

1. Why is it important for you to understand the phases of an EMS call?

Understanding the phases of an EMS call helps you to understand the order in which these steps occur. It gives you a framework to follow as an emergency call progresses. It also helps you to understand your role during each phase of the call. By understanding your role at each step of this sequence, you will become a valuable member of the EMS team.

2. Why is it important to differentiate between East Second Street and West Second Street and to confirm the apartment number?

During dispatch, listen carefully to the address of the emergency call. Do not begin responding until you are sure you understand where you need to go. Responding to West Second Street when the patient is at East Second Street or arriving at the wrong apartment number may significantly delay your response and could compromise your safety.

3. What steps do you need to take if you do not understand the location of the address given to you by your dispatcher?

If you do not understand the location given by your dispatcher, you need to call the dispatcher back to clarify the patient's address. Alternatively, you can look it up in an address book or use a GPS. Do not begin responding until you know exactly where you are going.

You are the EMR: CASE 2

1. How can you verify that this vehicle is ready for response?

Your service may have a list of minimum equipment or materials required for response. Check the vehicle and use the equipment checklist to verify that all the necessary equipment is present and operational. These actions help you verify the vehicle is ready for response and show you where all the equipment is located. In addition to checking the equipment, make sure the vehicle is adequately fueled and fully operational. If for any reason the vehicle is not functioning properly, do not use it for response until the issues have been corrected.

2. When should you tell the dispatch center that you are ready for response?

Whenever your service introduces new equipment or a different vehicle with new operational features, do not make yourself available for response until you have been properly trained in the use of the new items. Although you might be able to "figure it out," this casual approach would put you and your patients at an additional safety risk. After you have been properly trained on the new features and equipment, make sure the unit is cleaned and properly stocked. After all of those tasks have been accomplished, you are then ready for response.

You are the EMR: CASE 3

1. How would you perform a scene assessment at this incident?

Always begin with scene safety. Dispatch information can provide clues regarding the situation and may indicate the need for additional resources. After you arrive at the scene, assess for any safety hazards; this includes potential biologic hazards. In this case, law enforcement officers have already controlled the traffic flow; therefore, the next step is to determine the number of patients and the potential nature of illness or mechanism of injury. Be sure to get a report from the law enforcement officers and to check the inside of each vehicle for additional patients. After you have completed these steps and acquired that information, determine whether any additional resources are needed.

2. When should you request additional resources?

After you have identified the need for additional resources, request them immediately. Do not wait to call for additional resources because you may find yourself in a situation that you are no longer able to handle by yourself. The delay could result in poor patient care. If it is determined that certain resources are no longer required, they can be easily recalled.

You are the EMR: CASE 4

1. What are some of the components of an ideal landing zone?

When you set up a landing zone, make sure the area is free of trees, electrical lines, and other obstructions. The area should be flat and free of debris. Most EMS helicopter services require a landing zone of at least 100 × 100 feet (30 × 30 m). Check with your local EMS helicopter services for specific landing zone requirements. If you notice any unavoidable hazards, make sure you communicate that information to the pilot.

2. When would it be appropriate to use a helicopter for EMS transport?

Helicopters are typically used in situations where the patient has sustained severe trauma or a major illness and will benefit from more rapid transport to an appropriate medical facility. With trauma patients, it is ideal to get the patient to a trauma center within 1 hour from the initial incident. Often, this can be easily accomplished through ground transport; however, depending on the distance from the medical facility and traffic congestion, it may be beneficial to use a helicopter to transport the patient to definitive care.

Prep Kit

Ready for Review

- In preparing yourself for a call, you must understand your role as a member of the emergency medical system and be prepared to respond promptly.
- As an emergency medical responder, you need the proper equipment on an emergency call, including the medical equipment in your life support kit, your personal safety equipment, and equipment to safeguard the incident scene.
- The phases of an emergency call include dispatch, response to the scene, arrival at the scene, initial patient assessment and emergency care, transfer of patient care to higher-level EMS personnel, and postrun activities.
- If you will be working with a medical helicopter, you need to know proper safety precautions and loading procedures for helicopter transport.
- By learning the simple but important skills involved in EMS operations, you can become an effective member of the EMS system in your community.

Vital Vocabulary

door-to-door time A measure of how long it takes from the time the patient is accessed to the time the patient reaches definitive care.

landing zone A designated area where a helicopter can safely land and take off. Most civilian helicopters need a landing zone of at least 100 × 100 feet (30 × 30 m), or 10,000 square feet (approximately 900 m^2).

References

Kupas DF. *Lights and Siren Use by Emergency Medical Services (EMS): Above All Do No Harm.* US Department of Transportation, National Highway Traffic Safety Administration, Office of Emergency Medical Services. https://www.ems.gov/assets/Lights_and_Sirens_Use_by_EMS_May_2017.pdf. Published May 2017. Accessed November 19, 2024.

Kupas DF, Zavadsky M, Burton B, et al. Joint statement on lights and siren vehicle operations on emergency medical services responses. *Prehosp Emerg Care.* 2022;26(3):459–461.

Assessment IN ACTION

You are dispatched to the Pleasant Elementary School at 125 School Street for a report of a 57-year-old man who is reporting chest pain and shortness of breath. Further information reveals that he is a janitor at the school. As you arrive on the scene, you are directed to the school boiler room. You find a man sitting in a chair. His skin is pale (compared with patient baseline), and he is sweating.

1. The dispatch center has all of the following responsibilities EXCEPT:
   - A. determining the resources and personnel needed to handle the emergency.
   - B. keeping the caller on the line until the incident is over.
   - C. notifying responders of the type and location of the emergency call.
   - D. receiving calls from people needing emergency medical assistance.
2. What phase of an emergency call is most risky for you as an EMR?
   - A. Arrival and scene assessment
   - B. Response to the scene
   - C. Transfer of patient care to higher-level EMS personnel
   - D. Each phase presents different hazards depending on the type of call. Any phase can be hazardous.
3. Hazardous conditions you might encounter at an emergency scene that would require you to request specially trained resources include all of the following EXCEPT:
   - A. weapons.
   - B. electrical hazards.
   - C. chemical fumes.
   - D. hemorrhaging.
4. All of the following information should be reported when transferring care of the patient to higher-level EMS personnel EXCEPT:
   - A. your partner's family problems.
   - B. your observations of the initial situation.
   - C. the care you provided.
   - D. the patient's vital signs.
5. Place the phases of an EMS call in the order in which they occur.
   1. Arrival at the scene
   2. Transfer of patient care to higher-level EMS personnel
   3. Response to the scene
   4. Initial patient assessment and emergency care
   5. Postrun activities
   6. Dispatch
   - A. 6, 3, 1, 4, 2, 5
   - B. 4, 6, 3, 1, 5, 2
   - C. 1, 6, 4, 5, 3, 2
   - D. 3, 1, 6, 2, 5, 4
6. The patient in this scenario is having chest pain. What are the pros and cons of using lights and siren during the response?
7. On the basis of the dispatch information, what type of equipment might be necessary when you arrive at the scene?
8. What other resources might be necessary when treating this patient?
9. What are your responsibilities when higher-trained EMS clinicians arrive?
10. When should you make yourself available for another call?

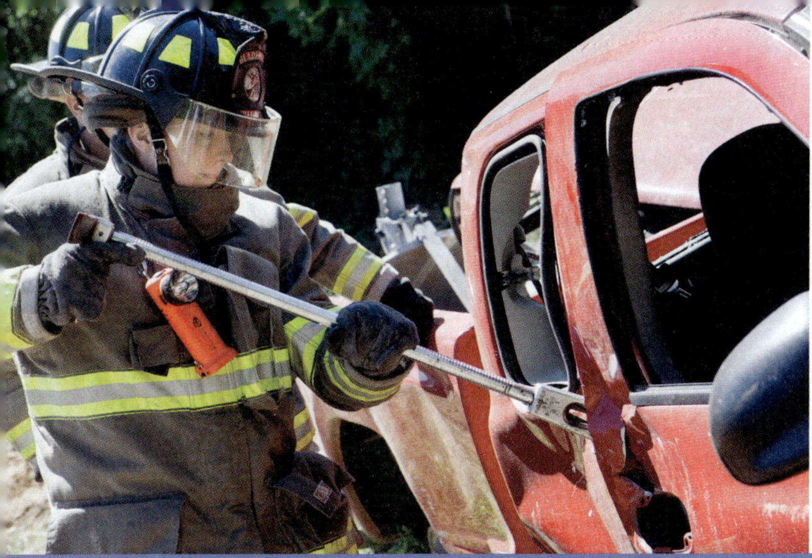

CHAPTER 18

Vehicle Extrication and Special Rescue

National EMS Education Standard Competencies

EMS Operations

Knowledge of operational roles and responsibilities to ensure patient, public, and personnel safety.

Rescue Operations

- Safety principles of rescue operations (pp 400–415)

Knowledge Objectives

1. Discuss the role of emergency medical responders (EMRs) during extrication. (p 400)
2. Identify the seven steps in the extrication process. (p 400)
3. List the various methods of gaining access to a patient. (p 400)
4. Describe the simple extrication procedures that an EMR can perform. (pp 400–408)
5. Identify the complex extrication procedures that require specifically trained personnel. (pp 400–408)
6. Discuss the role of EMRs in special rescue situations, including the following:
   - Water rescue (pp 408–409)
   - Diving-related emergencies (pp 409–411)
   - Ice rescue (p 411)
   - Confined space rescue (p 412)
   - Farm rescue (pp 412–415)
   - Bus rescue (p 415)

Skills Objectives

1. Demonstrate how to provide airway management to a patient who is trapped in a vehicle. (p 407; Skill Drill 18-1)
2. Demonstrate the role of EMRs in special rescue situations. (pp 400–408; pp 409–412; pp 412–415)
3. Demonstrate the steps EMRs can take in assisting with a water rescue. (pp 408–412)
4. Demonstrate the initial treatment of a patient in the water. (pp 409–410; Skill Drill 18-2)
5. Demonstrate the initial treatment of a patient experiencing a diving-related emergency. (pp 409–411)
6. Demonstrate the steps EMRs can take in assisting with an ice rescue. (p 411)
7. Demonstrate the steps EMRs can take in assisting with a confined space rescue. (p 412)
8. Demonstrate the steps EMRs can take in assisting with farm rescue incidents. (pp 412–415)
9. Demonstrate the steps EMRs can take in assisting with bus crashes. (p 415)

© Michael Cavazos/The News-Journal/AP Photo

Introduction

The first part of this chapter covers the steps you can take as an emergency medical responder (EMR) to perform simple extrication procedures and to assist other rescuers with patient extrication. The extrication process consists of seven steps, beginning with your arrival on the scene and ending with the removal of the patient from a position of **entrapment**. As an EMR, you may not be directly involved in all seven of the extrication steps, but you should be aware of the entire process. You cannot provide effective assistance unless you fully understand what must be done and how each step is accomplished. By learning these steps, you can provide valuable care for the patient until other rescuers arrive. After the arrival of additional rescuers, your role may change to assisting them in administering further care.

The second part of this chapter covers special rescue situations. These challenging situations can be life threatening to both the rescuer and the patient. Special rescue situations include water rescue, diving emergencies, ice rescue, confined space rescue, farm emergencies, and bus crashes. This chapter provides you with the guidelines for handling these situations. In each situation, your first objective is to maintain your personal safety. Do not perform any rescue procedures that could endanger either yourself or the patient.

Extrication

This section describes simple techniques you can use to access, treat, and remove patients who are trapped inside crashed vehicles. As an EMR, it is essential for you to think quickly and to use the principles and guidelines that are presented here. You will also need several hours of practical exercises to become skilled in the process of **extrication**.

Your EMR course should include a demonstration of the entire extrication operation. Become familiar with extrication equipment, its use, and the hazards involved in the extrication process. You should know what equipment is available in your community and how to summon this equipment. Rescue personnel usually use extrication techniques for motor vehicle crashes, but many of these same principles are applicable in other situations. Resourcefulness, common sense, and knowledge gained through training are key attributes of the EMR and underlie every act of patient care.

The safety of all rescuers and patients is an important consideration during the extrication process. Ideally, you should wear protective equipment similar to that worn by a firefighter: full bunker gear consisting of a coat, pants, boots, helmet with face shield, and gloves. Minimally, you should wear a helmet with a face shield or goggles and gloves.

A situation in which a patient is trapped in a motor vehicle can be complex enough to tax the skills and resources of even the most highly trained and well-equipped emergency medical services (EMS) system. To ensure the best patient care, many different agencies may need to cooperate: law enforcement, the fire department, EMS, and sometimes the utility company and a wrecker operator. It requires coordination and practice to achieve the cooperation and mutual understanding that is needed for a safe, smooth extrication effort.

As you read this section, keep in mind these basic guidelines:

- Know the limitations of your training, equipment, and skills.
- Identify any hazards (power lines, gasoline, or other hazardous materials).
- Control those hazards for which you are trained and equipped.
- Gain access to the patients.
- Provide patient care and stabilization.
- Move the patients only if absolutely necessary.

As an EMR, you have two primary extrication goals: (1) to obtain safe access to the patients and (2) to ensure patient stabilization. To achieve these goals, your role in the extrication process can be divided into the steps that are discussed next. Think safety first to avoid injury. An injured rescuer becomes an additional patient.

As the first trained rescuer on the scene, the actions you take can make the difference between an organized and a disorganized rescue effort, perhaps even the difference between life and death! You set the stage, and you have an essential role in the extrication process.

Words of Wisdom

The steps in the vehicle extrication process include the following:

1. Conduct a scene assessment or an overview of the incident and its surroundings.
2. Stabilize the scene, control any hazards, and stabilize the vehicle.
3. Gain access to the patients.
4. Provide initial emergency care.
5. Help disentangle the patients.
6. Help prepare the patients for removal.
7. Help remove the patients.

Step 1: Conduct a Scene Assessment

As soon as you are dispatched to the incident, begin to plan for what you are likely to find on arrival. For instance, you may know that a certain type of crash frequently occurs at a particular intersection or along a specific stretch of highway. Do not, however, become complacent about responding to the "same old thing." Use your knowledge, but be flexible.

If the dispatch information is complete, you will know the types of any vehicles involved (for example, two cars, a single vehicle and tree, or a truck and a motorcycle) and whether there are any injured or trapped people, burning vehicles, or hazardous materials present.

As you approach the scene and before you exit your vehicle, perform a scene assessment, which includes a visual overview of the entire incident and its surroundings (**FIGURE 18-1**). Remember, you must locate the patients before you can treat them! Rapidly determine the extent of

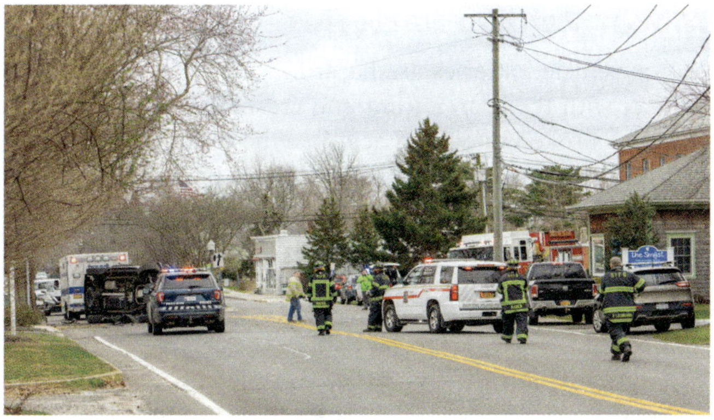

FIGURE 18-1 As you approach an incident, look over the entire scene.
© Gavin Zeigler/Alamy Stock Photo

the incident, estimate the number of patients, and try to locate any hazards that may be present. Then call for whatever additional resources you may need to manage the incident.

Step 2: Stabilize the Scene and Control Hazards

It is especially important to keep a sharp lookout for hazards that can result in injury, disability, or death to a patient, yourself, other emergency personnel, or bystanders. Some of the most common hazards found at motor vehicle crash scenes include infectious diseases, traffic, bystanders, spilled fuel or other hazardous material, automotive batteries, downed electrical wires, unstable vehicles, and vehicle fires (**FIGURE 18-2**).

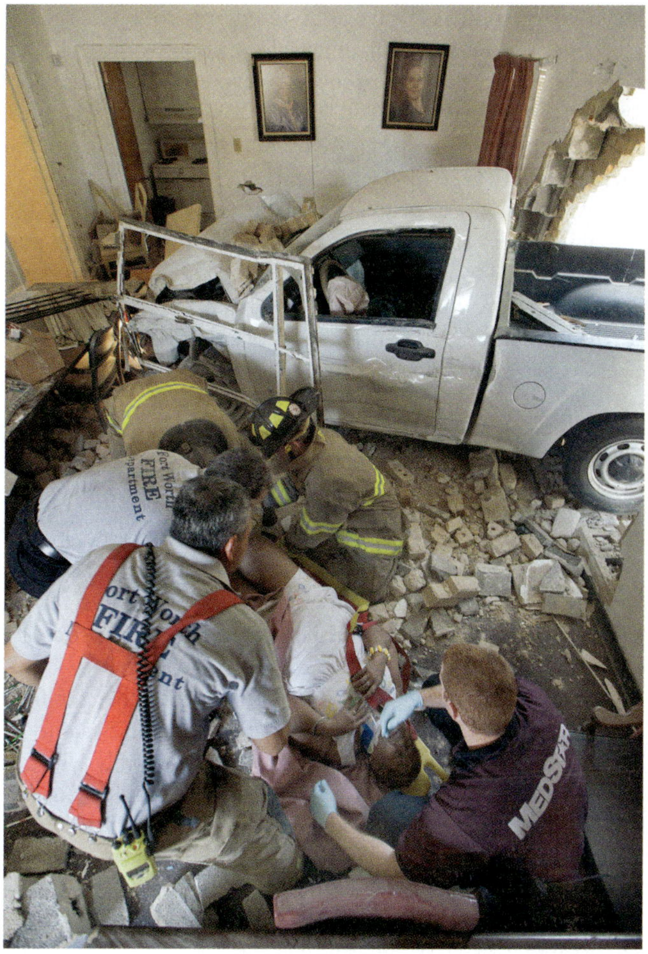

FIGURE 18-2 A single incident scene may contain many hazards.
© Glen E. Ellman

Personal Exposure

Many patients involved in motor vehicle crashes will have soft-tissue injuries and active bleeding from open wounds or from their mouth or nose. Take standard precautions at all motor vehicle crash scenes, including gloves and eye protection. If sharp glass or metal is present, you should wear heavy-duty leather gloves over your latex or vinyl gloves; otherwise, vinyl or latex gloves should offer sufficient protection.

Traffic Hazards

First, park your vehicle and other emergency vehicles so that they protect the scene and warn oncoming traffic to avoid the crash site. In most situations, park your vehicle in a location that does not obstruct open traffic lanes, but do not hesitate to use your vehicle to block traffic to protect yourself, your patients, and other rescuers. If you are first on scene, you should position your vehicle 100 feet (30 m) before the scene. If other emergency personnel are already on the scene, park your vehicle 100 feet (30 m) past the scene. Maintaining this distance not only creates a buffer zone from oncoming traffic, it also leaves space for other responding vehicles (for example, fire truck, ambulance) to park near the actual crash.

Consider the design of your vehicle's warning lights and park so you can use them to their best advantage. Do not

YOU are the EMR — CASE 1

At 2330 hours on a rainy night, you are dispatched for a report of a vehicle crash approximately 3 miles (5 km) from your location. As you are responding, your dispatcher tells you that this has been reported as a single-vehicle crash. As you approach the scene, you note that the vehicle has struck a power pole and that the pole has been sheared off close to the ground. Closer examination reveals that there are downed power lines. One power line is resting on the hood of the car. From a distance, you see one patient in the driver's seat. She appears to be dazed and slightly confused.

1. What initial actions do you need to take to stabilize the scene and ensure scene safety?
2. What other resources are needed for an incident like this?
3. What actions can you take once the scene is safe?

leave your trunk lid open after removing your emergency equipment because the lid may block your warning lights. Remember to wear an approved safety vest and other personal protective equipment. Traffic cones, safety triangles, and portable warning signs are used by some departments to increase safety at roadway incidents.

Another way to protect the scene is to ignite **fusees** (or warning flares) as soon as possible. Place the fusees up and down the road to warn oncoming traffic and give other drivers time to slow down safely. After you have taken these protective measures, survey the scene for other hazards. Always keep fusees away from flammable liquids.

Bystanders

Keep bystanders away from the crash scene to minimize the danger to themselves and patients. It is not usually enough to ask everyone to stay away. Give specific directions such as "Move back to the other side of the road" or "Move back onto the sidewalk." Sometimes you can pick one or two bystanders and ask them to assist you in keeping others away from the scene.

If available, either a rope or police or fire barrier tape is effective for establishing an off-limits area. Bystanders respond appropriately to such barriers and usually will not cross them after they are set up. While it may not seem appropriate to you for bystanders to record your delivery of patient care, you are operating in the public space, and thus public recording is allowed and likely to occur. Keep in mind when operating on an emergency scene: someone is always recording.

Spilled Fuel

Gasoline or diesel fuel spills are common during motor vehicle crashes. Expect to find a fuel spill if a motor vehicle has been hit near the rear, is on its side, or is upside down. If a fuel spill is present (or if the vehicle is in a position that suggests a fuel spill could occur), call the fire department to minimize the fire hazard and to clean up any spilled fuel.

If the patient is trapped in a motor vehicle that is leaking fuel and the fire department has not arrived, consider covering the fuel with dirt. Some rescuers carry cat litter with them for this purpose. Covering the fuel reduces the amount of vapor coming from the spill, which, in turn, reduces the danger of fire. Fuel vapors tend to stay close to the ground and will travel with the wind. In addition to fuel, other potentially hazardous fluids may leak from a wrecked vehicle, including motor oil, transmission fluid, power steering fluid, and antifreeze. Rescuers should keep in mind that any fuel absorbed in dirt or litter remains a fire hazard, including for personnel involved in scene cleanup, and must be handled and documented properly.

> **Safety**
>
> Keep all sources of ignition, such as cigarettes and flares, well away from a fuel spill.

Motor Vehicle Batteries

Motor vehicle batteries are hazardous, and you must avoid contact with them. In a front-end crash, the battery may already be broken open and acid may be leaking. Reduce the possibility of an electrical short circuit by turning off the vehicle's ignition. Do not attempt to disconnect the battery unless you have received special training in the proper way to do this and have the necessary tools. You could be injured by a short circuit, explosion, or contact with battery acid. Remember that hybrid vehicles and electric vehicles may have several batteries, or batteries that extend through the base of the vehicle. These batteries operate at much higher voltage than regular automotive batteries and present a greater risk of electric shock. Approach hybrid and electric vehicles cautiously.

Electric Vehicles

Electric vehicles (EVs) present a unique and dangerous challenge for rescuers. While they are less likely to catch on fire than their internal combustion engine or hybrid counterparts, when they do catch on fire, they present particularly intense heat and additional risks relating to high-voltage cables and hazardous materials. In addition, no extinguishing agents currently available are fully effective on these fires, and reignition is a threat for hours or even days after the initial event. The lithium-ion batteries often used in EVs, along with other safety features designed to assist drivers, further increase the risk to responders.

When responding to fires that involve EVs, EMRs should be careful not to assume the EV is not running simply because no engine noises can be heard. These vehicles often do not produce perceptible noises, especially on a noisy scene. If an EV is running, responders need to know how and where to shut off the high-voltage system, or wait for the proper person to do so. Finally, EMRs should know that EVs use more high-strength steel to lower vehicle weight. These materials can make it more difficult to access trapped occupants. After the vehicle is turned off, the keys should be stored away from the vehicle to help prevent it from turning back on.

Downed Electrical Wires

Downed electrical wires may be caused by high winds, ice buildup, a vehicle crashing into a utility pole, a fallen tree, or a building fire. Sometimes, downed electrical wires explode in arcs of spectacular flashes and sparks; other times, they simply lie across the vehicle, fully charged with electricity and capable of causing injury or death.

> **Safety**
>
> Treat all downed wires as if they are charged (live) until you receive specific clearance from the electric company. Even if the lights are out along the street where the wires are down, never assume that the wires are deenergized. Be especially alert for downed wires after a storm that has blown down trees and tree limbs.

Locate the wires but avoid contact. If a vehicle has a downed wire across it and passengers are trapped inside, immediately instruct the passengers to stay inside the vehicle. Then summon the utility company and fire department. Move bystanders back in all directions to at least the distance between two power poles.

Do not forget that electrical hazards can come from other sources as well, including traffic light control boxes and underground power feeds. Be sure to check everywhere, including under the vehicles, for electrical hazards. However, do not attempt to manage electrical hazards yourself at vehicle crash scenes.

Words of Wisdom

Remember these guidelines when you encounter a motor vehicle that is in contact with electrical wires:

- If the wire is draped over the vehicle, instruct trapped persons to remain inside the vehicle. Any attempt to remove either the wire or the passengers may result in serious injury or death to yourself as well as the passengers.
- Keep all bystanders away from the vehicle.
- Call for immediate assistance from the utility company.
- Call the fire department for assistance.
- Call for the police department to help secure the scene by directing traffic away from the downed power lines.

Vehicle Stability

Assume that every vehicle involved in a crash is unstable, unless you have confirmed that it has been stabilized. A vehicle that is positioned on a hill, on its side, upside down, or teetering over the edge of an embankment or bridge is obviously unstable (**FIGURE 18-3**). However, no matter how stable the vehicle appears to be, it may suddenly roll away or topple over. Be sure to check and ensure the stability of every vehicle before you attempt to enter it or treat the passengers inside.

Safety

Even vehicles that are positioned upright on all four wheels should be stabilized. This includes making sure the vehicle is in park with the engine off and the emergency brake engaged.

Vehicle on Its Wheels. If the vehicle is upright and on its wheels, you can ensure stability by **chocking** the front or back of each wheel with hubcaps or pieces of wood (**FIGURE 18-4**). If you can gain access to the inside of the vehicle, place the transmission in park, be sure the ignition has been turned off, and set the parking brake to prevent the vehicle from moving. You can also deflate the tires by safely cutting or pulling the valve stems (**FIGURE 18-5**).

Safety

If wooden blocks or commercial chocks are not available for chocking the wheels, improvise by using materials found at the scene.

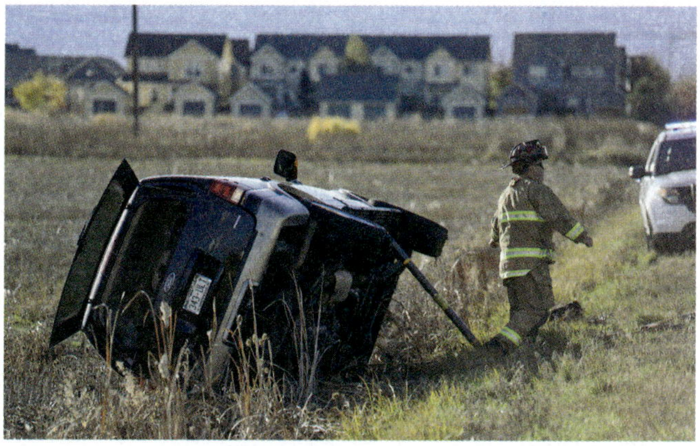

FIGURE 18-3 A vehicle positioned on its roof or side is obviously unstable.

© MediaNews Group/Boulder Daily Camera/Getty Images

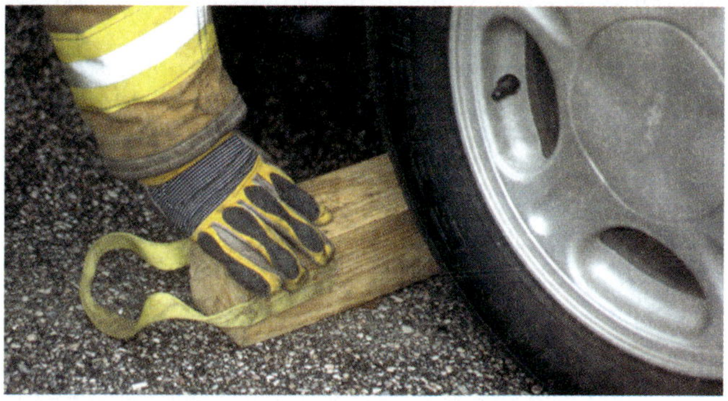

FIGURE 18-4 Chock the wheels.

© Jones & Bartlett Learning

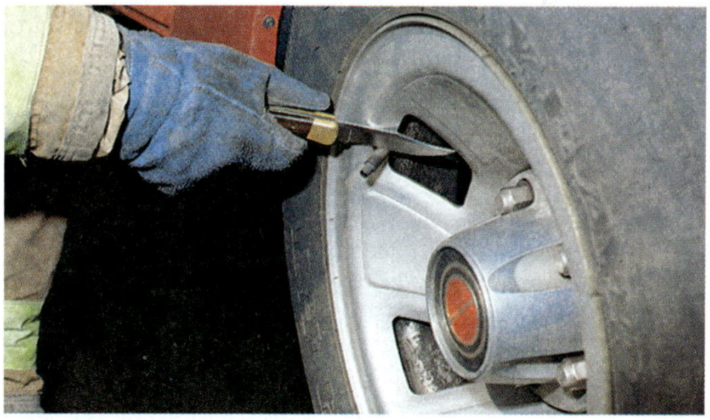

FIGURE 18-5 Deflating the tires can help stabilize the vehicle.

© Jones & Bartlett Learning

Vehicle on Its Side or Upside Down. A vehicle that is positioned on its side is extremely unstable. Fortunately, this position is unusual. Stabilizing a vehicle on its side is beyond the range of skills and equipment for many EMRs and should be handled by a specifically trained rescue crew or the fire department. Many fire departments and rescue crews carry **wooden cribbing**, step chocks, or special jacks to manage this situation. If you must enter a vehicle that is on its side to respond to a life-threatening situation, do not climb on the vehicle. Carefully break the rear window glass and enter through the back of the vehicle. Bend over or crouch down to stay close to the ground. This will help prevent upsetting the vehicle's center of gravity. Your purpose is to keep the vehicle in the position found. Any movement could cause the vehicle to shift. Gaining access to a patient is further discussed later in this chapter.

An upside-down vehicle is relatively stable, but cribbing is still necessary to prevent rocking of the vehicle with entry into and egress from the vehicle.

Consider other potential hazards in this situation. Flammable fuel and other fluids may have been spilled and must be handled by the fire department. Also consider burn hazards. A catalytic converter, which may be exposed when a vehicle is on its side or upside down, is extremely hot.

Vehicle Fires

Even though fires happen infrequently at motor vehicle crash sites, they are a cause of great concern among EMS personnel. There are two types of fires related to motor vehicle crashes: impact fires and postimpact fires.

Impact fires occur when the fuel tank ruptures during the crash. The vehicle is usually rapidly engulfed in flames, and it soon becomes impossible to approach it for a rescue attempt. Passengers rescued from this type of fire are usually saved by bystanders and witnesses to the crash who act immediately to remove them.

Postimpact fires are often caused by electrical short circuits. You can help to prevent them by turning off the ignition, as discussed previously. These fires usually do not develop into major fires if prompt action is taken. Should a fire occur, first turn off the ignition. Then attempt to extinguish the fire with a portable fire extinguisher. Remove the passengers from the vehicle as soon as possible. Hybrid or electric vehicles may contain multiple batteries that can overheat and ignite. Fires can occur for several hours following a crash.

If you arrive at a crash scene and find a motor vehicle on fire with people trapped inside, remember the following procedures:

- Use a dry chemical fire extinguisher if available (**FIGURE 18-6**). Most dry chemical fire extinguishers can be used on ordinary combustibles, flammable liquids, or electrical fires. Be sure you know how to use the extinguisher in your vehicle.
- Immediately have someone else gather fire extinguishers from other vehicles at the scene. Do not wait until your extinguisher runs out.
- Use your extinguisher to keep flames out of the passenger compartment. Aim for the base of the fire and ensure that you are not pushing the fire toward the passenger compartment.
- Do not be overly worried about discharging the extinguisher onto the passengers; the dry chemical powder is nontoxic. However, the dry chemical can be corrosive, so you should watch for respiratory conditions.
- Remove the patients as quickly as possible, but take care because they may have sustained injuries.
- Move everyone at least 50 feet (15 m) away from any vehicle that is on fire.
- Stay away from the front and rear ends of a burning vehicle. Modern bumpers contain air-filled cylinders that can explode forcefully when exposed to fire. Tires will also heat up during a vehicle fire and the increase in pressure can cause them to explode.
- If no one is in a burning vehicle, it is often better to move to a safe distance away from the vehicle and not attempt to extinguish the fire unless you are trained and have adequate resources.

Safety

Be alert for vehicles that are powered by alternative fuels, which present special electrical and fire hazards. These include propane-powered vehicles, compressed natural gas–powered vehicles, battery-powered vehicles, and hybrid vehicles.

Safety

Do not mistake hot water vapor from a damaged radiator for smoke from an engine compartment fire. If the smoke disappears rapidly (10 to 15 feet [3 to 5 m] away from the vehicle), it is probably steam and not smoke.

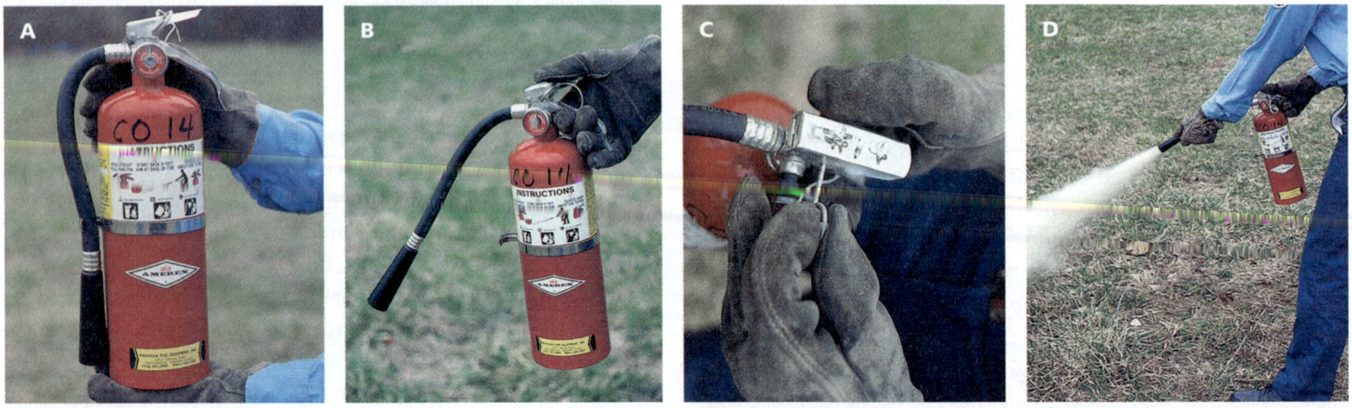

FIGURE 18-6 Use of a dry chemical fire extinguisher. **A.** Check the pressure gauge. **B.** Release the hose. **C.** Pull the locking pin. **D.** Discharge at the base of the fire.

© Jones & Bartlett Learning. Courtesy of MIEMSS.

Step 3: Gain Access to the Patients

The third step in the extrication process is to gain access to the patients. You cannot begin to examine and treat the patients until you have gained access to them. This section discusses the two methods you can use to achieve access. First, try to gain access through the doors. If this does not work, try to gain access through a window.

Access Through Doors

Most patients involved in a motor vehicle crash can be reached simply by stabilizing the vehicle and then opening a door or window. Try all the doors first, even if they appear to be badly damaged. It is an embarrassing waste of time and energy to open a jammed door with heavy rescue equipment when another door can be opened easily and without any equipment. Attempt to open the least damaged door first. If it is locked and the patient is alert, ask the patient if they can unlock the door or lower the window (**FIGURE 18-7**).

Access Through Windows

If you believe that any passenger's condition is serious enough to require immediate care (for example, if the passengers do not appear to be breathing) and you cannot enter through a door, you should break a window.

Do not try to break and enter through the windshield because it is made of plastic-laminated glass (**FIGURE 18-8**) and must be cut. The side and rear windows are usually made of **tempered glass** in older vehicles and will break easily into small pieces when hit with a spring-loaded center punch or fire axe. Because these windows do not pose a safety threat when broken correctly, they should be your primary access route. In newer vehicles, front side windows are composed of **plastic-laminated glass**. Rear windows in the majority of vehicles are still made of tempered glass, making it an option for access.

Words of Wisdom

The Federal Motor Vehicle Safety Standard 226 (FMVSS 226) went into effect in September 2018, with the aim of reducing the potential for ejections or partial ejections through side windows during rollover or side-impact crashes. This standard requires all vehicles weighing 4,536 pounds (2,057 kg) or less to have laminated glass side windows. Since punches will not shatter laminated glass, these windows must be cut to enable access to patients. You can usually identify the type of glass by looking for an identification label on a bottom corner of the window (**FIGURE 18-9**).

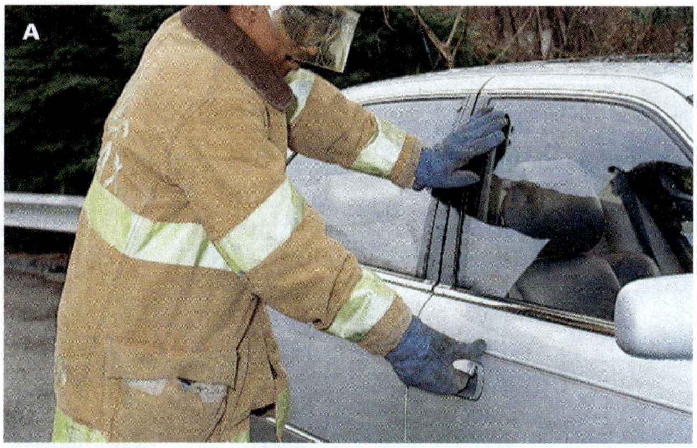

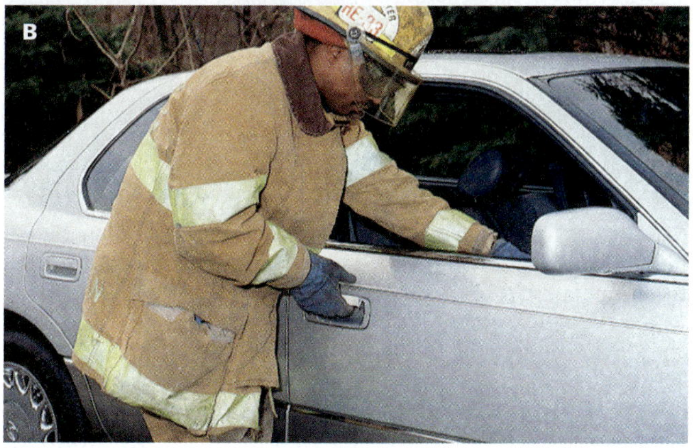

FIGURE 18-7 Access the vehicle through the doors, if possible. **A.** Try all exterior door handles first. **B.** If the door cannot be opened from the outside, once the window is lowered or broken, try the inside and outside handles at the same time.

© Jones & Bartlett Learning. Courtesy of MIEMSS.

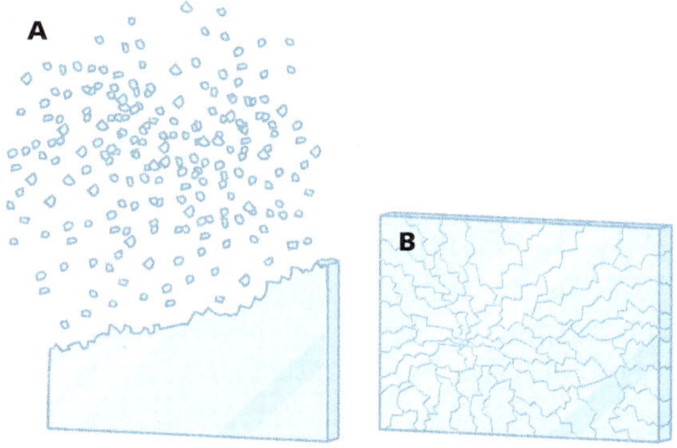

FIGURE 18-8 **A.** Tempered glass shatters when impacted with high force. **B.** Laminated glass may crack when impacted, but the embedded plastic layer holds the pieces in place.

© Jones & Bartlett Learning

YOU are the EMR — CASE 2

As you are returning to your station following a routine call, you notice tire skid marks on the road. You reduce your speed and discover a broken guardrail. You and your crew stop to investigate further. You find a sport utility vehicle (SUV) that has skidded from the roadway, catapulted through the guardrail, and traveled approximately 20 feet (6 m) down an embankment. The wrecked SUV is resting on the passenger side of the vehicle. A bystander says she thinks three passengers are inside.

1. What concerns you most about this scene?
2. What are the important aspects of the scene assessment for this particular scene?

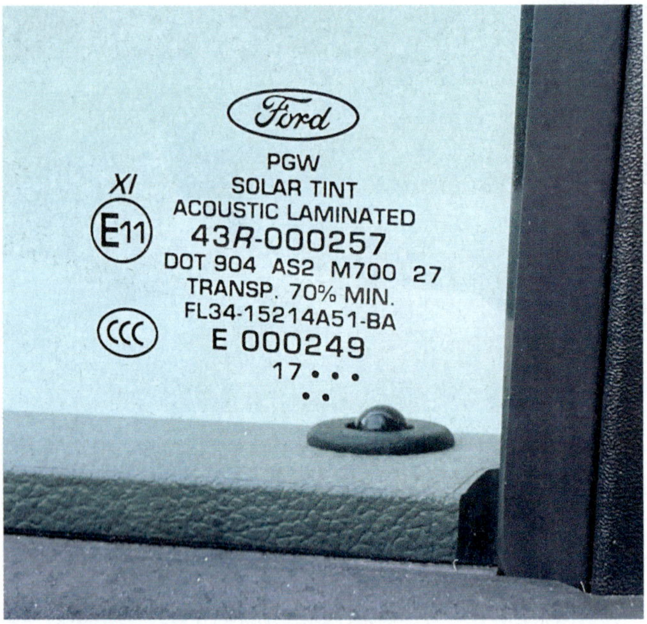

FIGURE 18-9 Laminated glass cannot be shattered with a punch; it must be cut. To determine the type of glass in a vehicle window, read the identification label in the bottom corner.

© Jones & Bartlett Learning

A spring-loaded center punch (available from many hardware stores) should be carried in your EMR jump kit (**FIGURE 18-10**). It can be used rapidly and takes up little room in the kit and is nearly always successful in breaking tempered glass in the side and rear windows on the first try.

If you must break a window to open a door or gain access, try to break one that is the farthest from the patient. However, if the patient's condition warrants your immediate entry, do not hesitate to break the closest side or rear window, even if the glass will fall onto a patient. If possible, have the patient cover their face when you are breaking glass, which may help to prevent injuries from glass shards.

Tempered pieces of glass do not usually pose a danger to people trapped in vehicles. Advise EMS personnel if a passenger is covered with broken glass so they can notify the hospital emergency department. If there is glass on a passenger, pick off the glass; do not brush it off.

> **Words of Wisdom**
>
> Remember: Try before you pry!

After breaking the window, use your gloved hands to pull out the remaining glass from the window frame so it does not fall onto any passengers or injure any rescuers.

If you are using something other than a spring-loaded center punch to break the window, always aim for a lower corner. That way, the window frame will help prevent the tool (such as a tire iron, fire axe, or large screwdriver) from sailing into the vehicle and hitting the person inside.

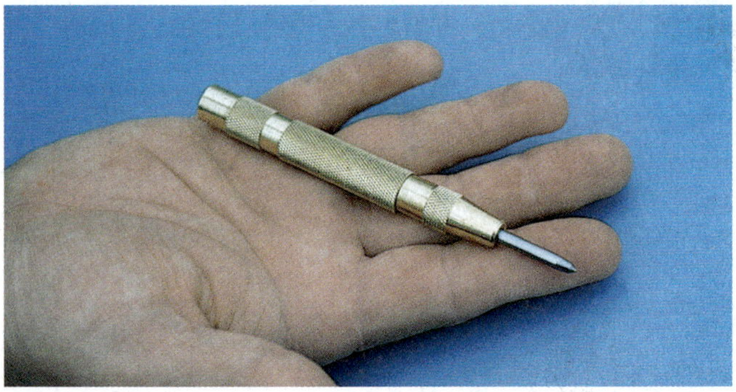

FIGURE 18-10 Spring-loaded center punch for breaking tempered glass.

© Jones & Bartlett Learning. Courtesy of MIEMSS.

> **Safety**
>
> Always warn trapped vehicle passengers that you are going to break the glass.

After you have broken the glass and removed the remaining pieces of glass from the frame, try to unlock the door again. Release the locking mechanism, and then use both the inside and outside door handles at the same time. This will often enable you to force a jammed locking mechanism, even in a door that appears to be badly damaged.

Using the simple techniques described and illustrated in this section, you should be able to gain access to nearly all patients involved in a motor vehicle crash, even those who are trapped in an upside-down vehicle.

When you gain access to a crashed vehicle, be alert for airbags that have not deployed. Airbags are mounted in the steering wheel on the driver's side and in the dashboard on the passenger's side. In newer vehicles, supplemental airbags may also be mounted on the sides of the vehicle or around the rear seats. If the airbags did not deploy during the crash, they represent a hazard to rescuers because they may unexpectedly deploy and cause injuries. Even though battery cables have been severed, the lines can still hold a charge and the airbags can still deploy. To limit your risk of injury from an airbag, your goal should be to assist passengers in exiting the vehicle or to remove the passengers as safely and quickly as possible. If you must enter the vehicle, try to maintain at least 10 inches (25 cm) between yourself and an undeployed airbag, which may require using the backseat to access passengers in the front seats. The risk of damaging an unexploded airbag increases when using extrication tools.

If you cannot gain access to the vehicle, you must do what you can to assist the patient. This means stabilizing the vehicle and protecting the scene until the proper equipment arrives.

Step 4: Provide Initial Emergency Care

After you gain access to the passengers, immediately begin emergency medical care. Conduct a primary assessment on every patient. After you determine the status of each patient,

SKILL DRILL 18-1

Airway Management in a Vehicle

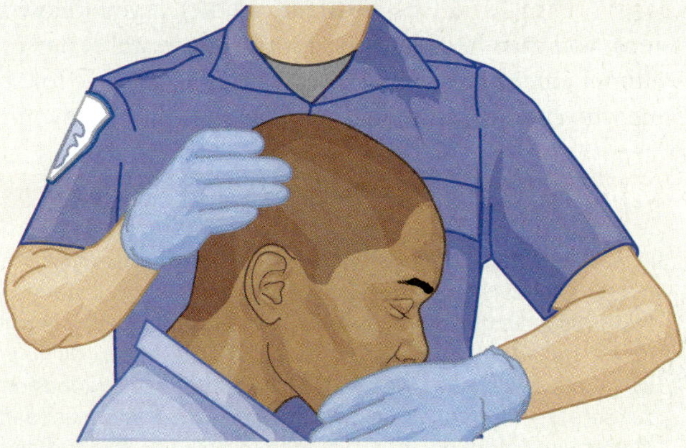

STEP 1 Place one hand under the patient's chin and your other hand on the back of the patient's head.

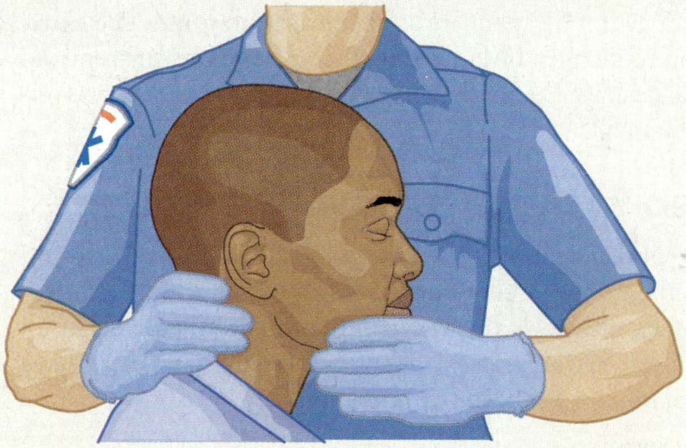

STEP 2 Raise the patient's head to a neutral position to open the airway.

© Jones & Bartlett Learning

you should monitor the ABCs (airway, breathing, and circulation), control bleeding, treat for shock, manually stabilize the cervical spine, and provide emotional support. Stay calm, and do not forget to maintain the patient's body temperature by covering the patient with a blanket. If you have time, you can conduct a secondary assessment (physical exam).

Leave the patients in the vehicle unless it is on fire or the patients are otherwise in immediate danger. If the patient is not maintaining their airway or breathing sufficiently, which you may discover during your primary assessment, you will need to rapidly extricate your patient.

SKILL DRILL 18-1 shows how to perform initial airway management when the patient is in a vehicle.

> **Words of Wisdom**
>
> Remember, passengers may be thrown around inside the vehicle during a collision. You must ensure there are no other victims in the vehicle, which includes checking the trunk.

Step 5: Help With Patient Disentanglement

Extrication operates on the principle of "removing the vehicle from around the patient." This process usually requires tools and specialized equipment, such as air chisels, manual or powered hydraulic rams and cutters, and airbags. In some serious extrication situations, disentanglement can take up to 30 minutes and requires advanced training (**FIGURE 18-11**). In some situations, you can make the patient more comfortable and give yourself more room to work by carefully moving the front seat back or by raising the adjustable steering wheel.

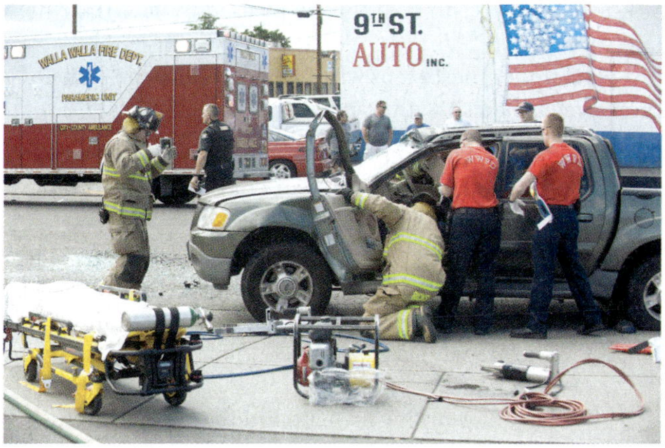

FIGURE 18-11 Serious entrapment situations require teamwork.

© Michael Lopez/Walla Walla Union-Bulletin/AP Photo

Some rescue crews use the concept of the **Golden Hour**, sometimes called the Golden Period, when managing serious trauma situations. The concept of the Golden Hour is that because serious trauma patients have the highest risk of death in the first hour after an incident; efforts should be made to get the patient to the hospital within that first hour. While there is limited evidence that the patient will suddenly deteriorate after 60 minutes, you should work diligently to free the patient from their entrapment so they may be transported to the hospital as soon as possible.

Step 6: Help Prepare the Patient for Removal

As disentanglement proceeds, help prepare the patient for removal from the vehicle by applying dressings, bandages, and splints, as needed, and maintaining manual stabilization of the head and cervical spine. If you are trained in the procedures and equipment for spinal motion restriction, you may be able to assist in this effort. See Chapter 3, *Lifting and Moving Patients*.

It is important to realize that the access route to the patient may not be adequate as an extrication route. The extrication route must be large enough to permit the safe removal of the packaged patient, whereas the access route may be relatively small.

Step 7: Help Remove the Patient

Once packaged, the patient is removed from the vehicle and placed onto the stretcher of the transporting ambulance. Remember, although you may not be directly involved in all seven extrication steps, your actions and assistance can have a vital impact on the entire operation.

Review of the Extrication Process

Your familiarity with the phases of the extrication effort may enable you to assist the rescue and extrication crews. Take the time to find out about the rescue and extrication resources in your community. Ask the crews how you can assist them; they will probably be pleased to have your help and support.

Remember these steps when you arrive on the scene of a motor vehicle crash with trapped passengers:

- Call for additional resources and extrication help.
- Specify the number and types of vehicles involved.
- Do not stand idly by while waiting for help. You should:
  - Identify and contain safety hazards.
  - Park your vehicle so that its headlights and warning lights can be used to protect and light the scene.
  - Clear a working area around the site of the crash before you or rescue personnel attempt to stabilize the vehicle or vehicles.
  - Use your head! Think and use the tools you already have.
  - Remember to try opening the doors first, rather than breaking windows.
  - After you gain access to the patient, assess and monitor their condition.
  - Above all, remain calm.

Water and Ice Rescue

You may encounter situations in which a person needs to be rescued from the water. The person may be fatigued, may have sustained an underwater diving injury, may have gotten caught in a strong current, or may have fallen through the ice in the winter. This text does not intend to teach the skills of a certified lifeguard; however, the following information does describe some simple techniques you can use to perform a water or ice rescue without endangering your own safety.

Water Rescue

When you see a person struggling in the water, your first impulse may be to jump in to assist. However, that action may not result in a successful rescue and can endanger your own life. If you are faced with a water rescue situation, remember to **reach, throw, row, go** (**FIGURE 18-12**). If you follow these steps, you may be able to perform a successful water rescue without entering the water. It may even be possible for someone who cannot swim to rescue a person who is drowning.

> **Safety**
>
> In many communities, a flash flood is a common occurrence. Flash floods occur as the result of sudden and continuing rainstorms that overwhelm the ability of streams and storm sewer systems to handle the runoff. Flash floods may cause water to quickly flow over roadways in low-lying areas. Most rescues during floods occur because motorists drive into low-lying areas that are flooded. Almost one-half of deaths resulting from flash floods in the United States occur in vehicles. Be cautious about driving through standing water, and be aware of the dangers posed by floodwaters that cover roadways. According to the Federal Emergency Management Agency, a foot of water will float many vehicles. These floodwaters can contain strong currents and can be deadly. Do not venture into floodwaters without proper training and equipment.

Reach

Use any readily available object to reach the distressed person in the water. If the person is close to shore, a branch, pole, oar, or paddle may be long enough. If you are at a swimming pool, there may be a specifically designed pole available for this purpose.

Throw

If you cannot reach the person, throw something that can float or that the victim can grab. At a swimming pool, dock, or supervised beach, a **flotation device** (such as a ring buoy) may be available. Some public safety departments carry a specifically constructed **rescue throw bag** that contains a rope that can be thrown to a distressed person in the water. If your department carries a throw rope, you need instruction and practice in its use. If no buoy or throw bag is available, improvise. Throw a rope, plastic milk jug, or a sealed polystyrene plastic (Styrofoam) cooler. Even a spare tire can support several people in the water.

> **Words of Wisdom**
>
> If you use something like a plastic milk jug or picnic jug to throw to a person in the water, fill the container with approximately 1 inch (3 cm) of water to add weight before you seal it and throw it to the person.

Row

If you cannot reach the person by throwing something that floats, you may be able to row out to the drowning person if a small boat or canoe is available. Consider this option only if you know how to operate or propel the craft properly. Protect yourself by wearing an approved personal flotation device.

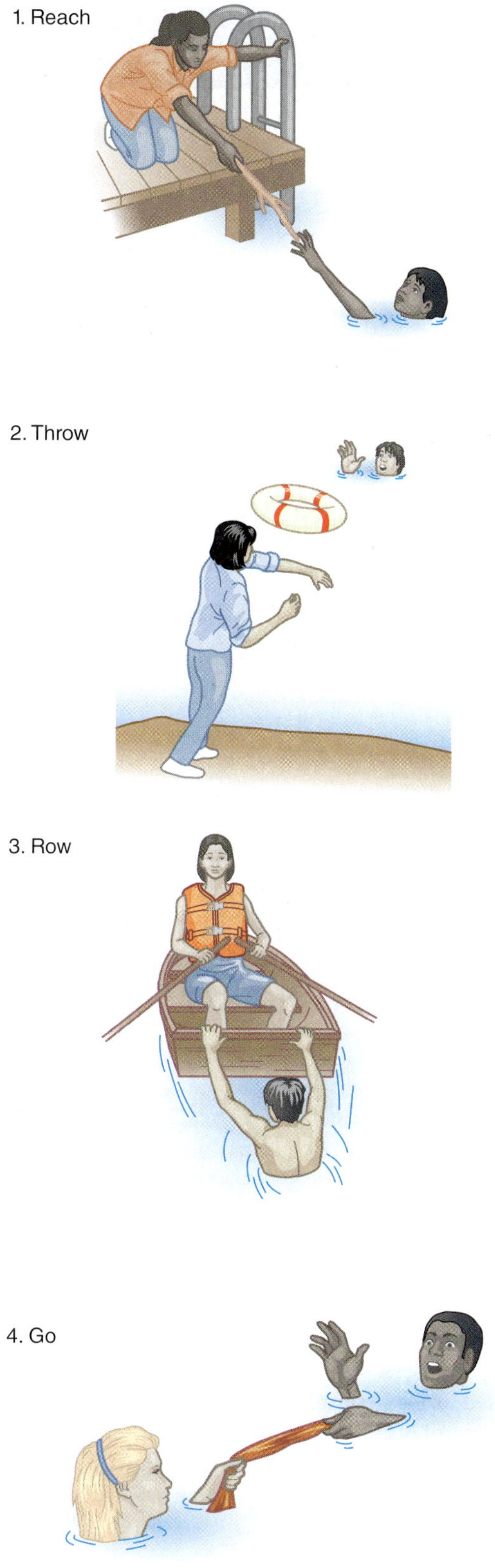

FIGURE 18-12 The rules for water rescue.
© Jones & Bartlett Learning

Go

As a last resort, you may have to go into the water to save the person. Enter the water only if you are a capable swimmer trained in lifesaving techniques. Remove heavy clothing before entering the water. Take a flotation device with you if one is available.

Safety

A current in a stream or a strong current (**riptide**) at ocean beaches can pull both the distressed person and the rescuer rapidly away from shore. In an area below a dam, rapids, or a waterfall, deadly currents may be present. Never attempt to enter the water if you are not trained for these conditions. If you do, it is likely that both you and the distressed person will need to be rescued.

Initial Treatment of a Person in the Water

If you are involved in a water rescue situation, your primary concerns for the patient are to open an airway, establish breathing and circulation, and stabilize the head and neck in case of spinal cord injuries. Turn a patient faceup who is facedown in the water (**SKILL DRILL 18-2**).

Use the jaw-thrust maneuver to open the airway. Do not hyperextend the neck because of the high risk of associated spinal cord injuries. Look, listen, and feel for signs of breathing. If the patient is not breathing, start rescue breathing while the patient is still in the water (**FIGURE 18-13**). Ventilation will be much easier if you can stand on the bottom of the body of water.

If the patient has experienced cardiac arrest, quickly stabilize the head and neck and remove the patient from the water. Place the patient on a hard surface before you begin cardiopulmonary resuscitation (CPR). See Chapter 8, *Professional Rescuer CPR*.

Assume the presence of a spinal cord injury if an alert patient in the water reports numbness or tingling in the arms or legs, is unable to move the extremities, or reports neck pain. Support the patient by floating a backboard in the water under the patient (**FIGURE 18-14**). Strap the patient to the backboard, stabilize the head and neck, and remove the patient from the water. Many jurisdictions require swimming pools to have a backboard at poolside. If a rigid device is unavailable and the patient must be removed from the water before EMS personnel arrive, multiple people can lift and support the patient using their hands (**FIGURE 18-15**).

Words of Wisdom

If a backboard is unavailable, you can use a chaise lounge, door, or piece of plywood to provide rigid support under the patient. One rescuer should give the commands to lift, move, and set down the patient.

Diving Emergencies

As an EMR, you may be called to care for people who have experienced an emergency while diving. Most recreational divers use a self-contained underwater breathing apparatus (scuba). Scuba gear consists of an air tank, a regulator, a mouthpiece, and a face mask. Commercial divers use either scuba gear or equipment that supplies air through a hose.

Most underwater diving emergencies occur in coastal regions or in areas with large lakes. Diving mishaps can cause

SKILL DRILL 18-2

Turning a Patient in the Water

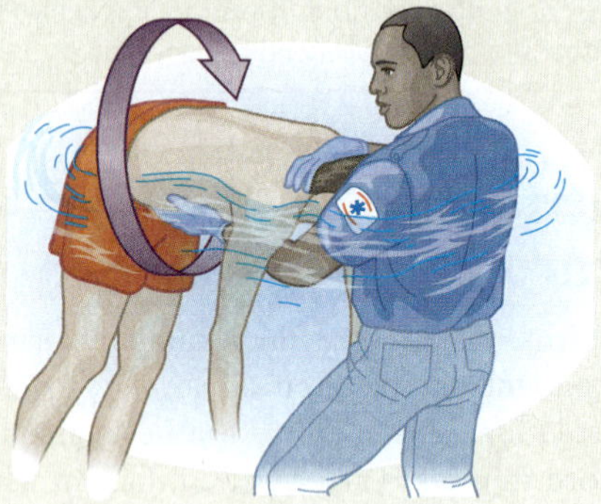

STEP 1 Support the back and head with one hand. Place your other hand on the front of the patient to keep the head and neck stabilized.

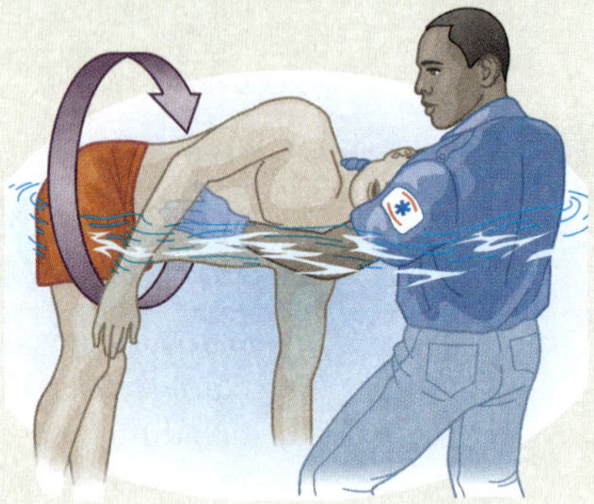

STEP 2 Keep the head in the neutral position and carefully turn the patient as a unit.

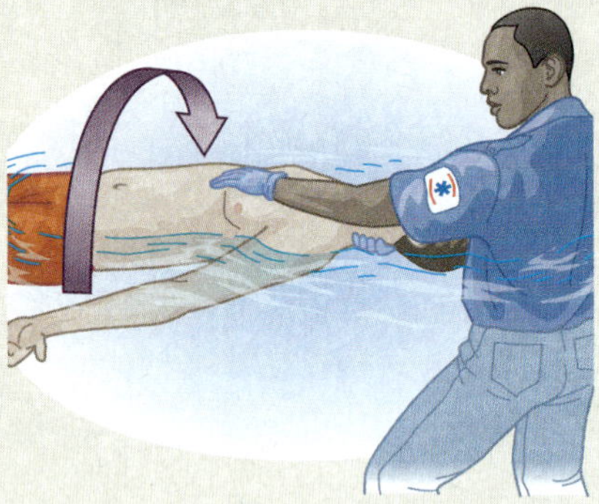

STEP 3 Stabilize the patient's head and neck.

© Jones & Bartlett Learning

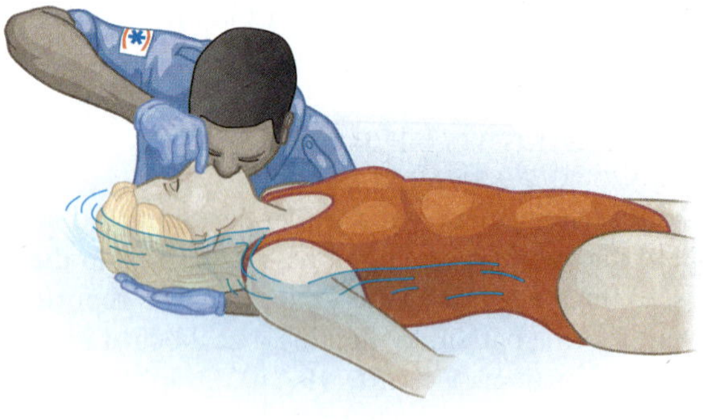

FIGURE 18-13 Begin rescue breathing in the water.

© Jones & Bartlett Learning

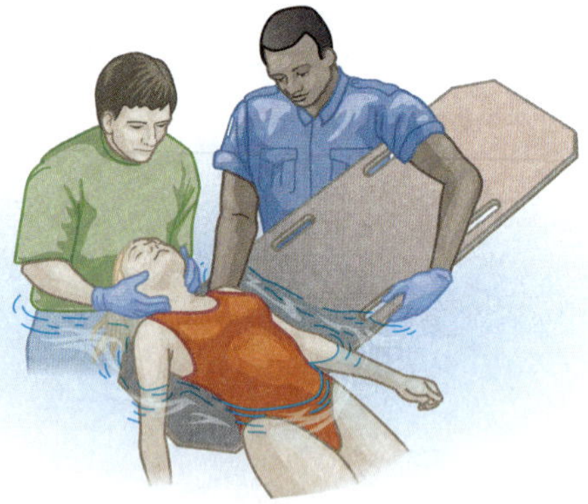

FIGURE 18-14 Apply the backboard while the patient is still in the water.

© Jones & Bartlett Learning

trauma, near drowning, or specialized injuries. In situations involving trauma or drowning, remove the patient from the water and treat the patient using information and skills you have already learned.

Two specialized conditions that are associated with diving are **air embolism** and **decompression sickness (the bends)**. Usually, you will not be able to differentiate between these two conditions. Both are caused by air bubbles being released in the body as a result of the changes in pressure while diving. If an air bubble affects the brain or spinal cord, the signs and symptoms may be similar to those of a stroke, including dizziness, difficulty speaking, difficulty seeing, and a decreased level of consciousness. The patient may have difficulty in maintaining an open airway. If the air bubble causes a collapsed lung, the signs and symptoms will include chest pain, shortness of breath, and pink or bloody froth coming

YOU are the EMR — CASE 3

You respond to the scene of a vehicle that has rolled over. The dispatcher informs you that the vehicle landed on its roof and two passengers are trapped inside. When you arrive at the scene, you find a minivan on its roof. As you approach the vehicle, you determine that the scene is safe and the vehicle is stable. You notice two patients in the vehicle; both appear unresponsive.

1. What could you do to assist in the extrication of these patients before rescue arrives?
2. What are the steps for using a spring-loaded center punch?

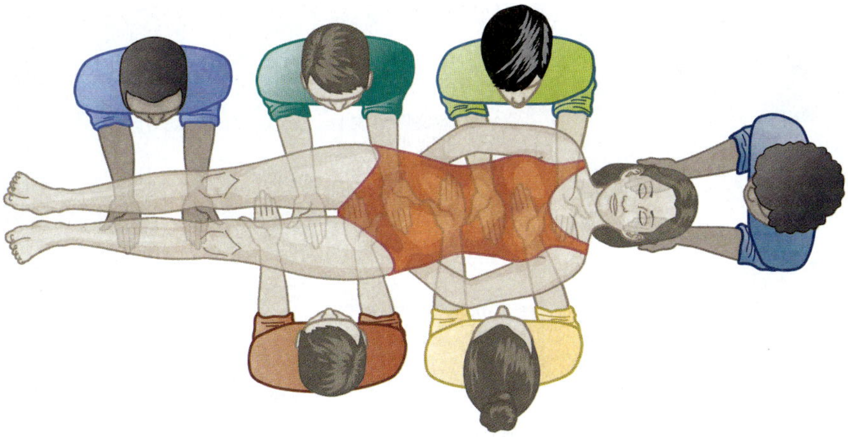

FIGURE 18-15 In emergency situations, a patient can be removed from the water using multiple people.
© Jones & Bartlett Learning

from the mouth or nose. If the air bubble obstructs blood flow to the abdomen, the patient will experience severe abdominal pain and may be bent over. If the air bubble involves a joint, there will be severe pain in that joint.

To treat a patient with a suspected air embolism or decompression sickness, maintain the patient's ABCs and a normal body temperature. Oxygen should be administered as soon as it is available. Administer oxygen only if you have received the proper training and have the approval of your medical director. Some physicians recommend placing the patient on the left side with the head of the patient slightly lowered. This may help to prevent further damage if there is an air bubble in the central nervous system. A patient who has experienced a diving-related emergency may need to be transported to a hospital that is equipped with a hyperbaric (recompression) chamber. If you live in an area where diving is common, you should receive specialized training and be familiar with the local protocols of your EMS system.

Ice Rescue

Ice rescue is extremely hazardous because ice is changeable and should always be considered unsafe. Think safety first; do not exceed the limits of your training and do not put yourself at undue risk. You cannot save anyone if you fall through the ice yourself. As soon as you arrive at the scene of an ice rescue, visually mark the location where the person was last seen. This will enable other rescuers to concentrate their efforts on a limited area. Know who is responsible for ice rescue in your community and call this team as soon as possible.

The basic rules of ice rescue are the same as water rescue: reach, throw, row, go. Reach for the person using anything that will extend your natural stretch, such as a ladder, a pike pole, a tree branch, or a backboard. Next, throw a flotation device, throw rope, or anything that floats to pull in the person. Third, row or propel a small boat to the person if you can break through the ice, or use a toboggan to get across the ice. Using a toboggan will spread your weight over a wider area and reduce your chances of falling through the ice. Be sure that you have a rope and that the boat or toboggan is secured to the shore as well. Finally, if you must go, secure yourself to shore with a rope around your waist, lie on your stomach, and proceed across the ice. Spreading your weight over a wider area reduces your chances of falling through the ice (**FIGURE 18-16**). Maintain good communication with other rescuers.

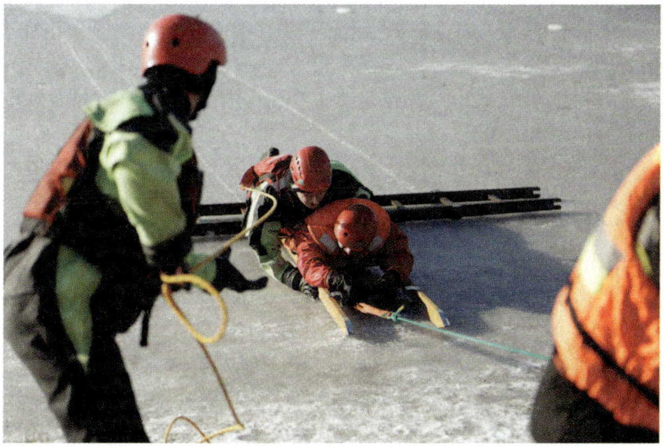

FIGURE 18-16 Ice rescue. The ladder distributes the rescuer's weight over a larger area, making it less likely that the rescuer will also fall into the water.
© praszkiewicz/Shutterstock

A motor vehicle on the ice presents a risky situation. Instruct the vehicle's occupants to avoid unnecessary movement. If the vehicle has not gone through the ice, instruct the occupants to open the vehicle's doors. This may help to slow the sinking of the vehicle if the ice breaks. If the doors cannot be opened, instruct the occupants to open the windows so they have a better escape route. If you must approach the vehicle, remember that the added weight of rescuers can cause movement of the vehicle. Do not place your head inside the vehicle because if it sinks, you may be unable to get out.

During ice rescues, both the people on the ice or in the water and the rescuers are at risk for hypothermia. Keep all rescuers as warm as possible by ensuring everyone is wearing clothing suitable for the climate. Rescue personnel who are not directly involved in the rescue operation should remain

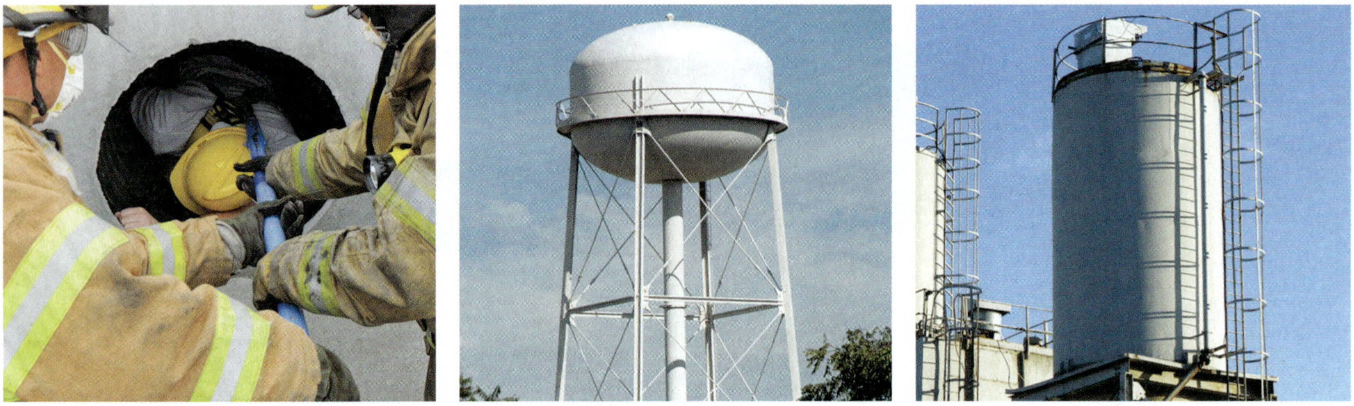

FIGURE 18-17 Confined spaces may have insufficient oxygen to support life without the use of a self-contained breathing apparatus.
A: © Jones & Bartlett Learning; B: © Harris Shiffman/Shutterstock; C: © Joe Gough/Shutterstock.

in a warm vehicle until they are needed. Remove wet clothing from rescued people, and dry them off and warm them as soon as possible after they are removed from the water. If the patient has no pulse, start CPR and continue until the patient has been transported to a hospital. See Chapter 13, *Environmental Emergencies*, for more information on treating hypothermia.

Confined Space Rescue

Confined spaces are structures designed to keep something in or out. Confined spaces may be below ground, ground level, or elevated structures. Below-ground confined spaces include manholes, utility vaults or storage tanks, old mines, cisterns, and wells. Ground-level confined spaces include industrial tanks and farm storage silos. Elevated confined spaces include water towers and storage tanks.

Rescue situations involving confined spaces have two deadly hazards. The first hazard is respiratory. The confined space may have insufficient oxygen to support life, or it may be filled with a poisonous gas (**FIGURE 18-17**). Never enter a confined space without the proper respiratory protection or else you risk becoming a patient yourself.

The second hazard in a confined space is the danger of collapse. In a mine, for example, rescuers may need to shore up (support) the confined space before they can safely enter. Confined space rescue requires a specifically trained team. As soon as you determine there is a confined space situation, call for additional assistance and do not enter the space until help arrives.

If a worker in a confined space begins to feel sick because of a lack of oxygen or the presence of a poisonous gas, coworkers may assume the worker is having a heart attack. Therefore, the call you receive may be for a "sick person." When you arrive on the scene, take time to assess the scene carefully. If a patient is in a confined space, do not enter unless you are part of a team trained in confined space rescue and have adequate respiratory equipment for you and your team to work in this deadly environment. Otherwise, wait for properly equipped and specifically trained personnel to access, treat, and remove the patient.

Safety

Many would-be rescuers have lost their lives during confined space incidents. Do not enter a confined space without proper breathing apparatus and special training.

Farm Rescue

Farms are located throughout most parts of the country. They range from a few acres of land with limited machinery and a small number of animals to large complexes that contain many acres of land, heavy-duty machinery, and thousands of large animals. Farm emergencies pose a wide variety of challenges for rescuers, including possible delays in reaching the patient. Because many farmers work by themselves, the discovery and reporting of an emergency may not occur immediately. Once notification of an incident is received, there may be a lengthy response in getting to a farm if it is located in a remote area. After rescuers arrive at a farm, it may be hard to pinpoint the exact location of the emergency. Poorly maintained roads, nonexistent roads, and muddy soil may require you to leave your vehicle some distance from the patient.

YOU are the EMR **CASE 4**

You are dispatched to an emergency at a farm. On arrival at the scene, you are told a man was working outside when he heard an explosion inside the silo. He reports three people were inside the silo at the time of the explosion. You notice smoke coming from the silo.

1. What additional resources will you potentially need at this scene?
2. What are the potential hazards associated with farm rescue incidents?

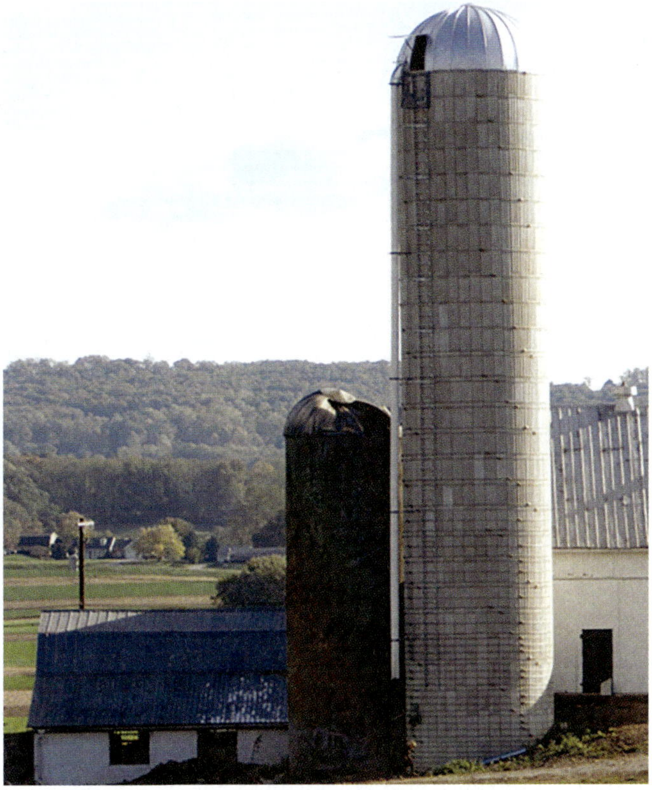

FIGURE 18-18 Farm silos represent high-angle hazards, confined space hazards, and explosive hazards.
© Nancy Hixson/Shutterstock

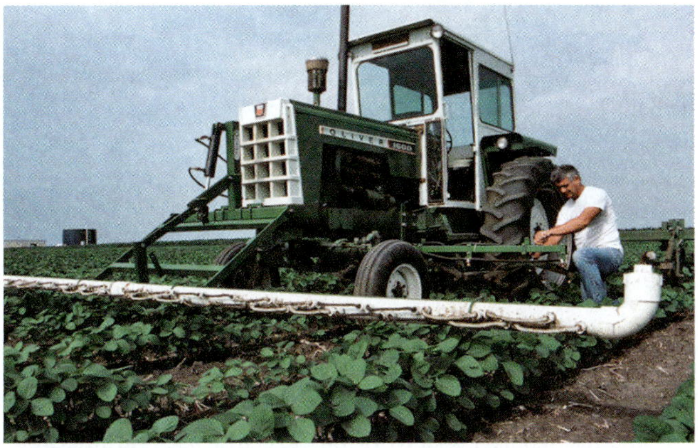

FIGURE 18-19 Farm machinery is involved in many farm rescue situations.
Courtesy of Lynn Betts/NRCS.

TABLE 18-1 The Seven Steps of Extrication

1. Conduct a scene assessment or an overview of the incident and its surroundings, and call for sufficient help.
2. Stabilize the scene, control any hazards, and stabilize the vehicle.
3. Gain access to the patients, if possible.
4. Provide initial emergency care.
5. Help disentangle the patients.
6. Help prepare the patients for removal.
7. Help remove the patients.

© Jones & Bartlett Learning

Farms contain a wide variety of hazards. Animals can seriously injure farmers and pose a serious risk to rescuers. Be alert for the dangers posed by animals. Also, farms contain a wide range of chemicals that can be hazardous. These include pesticides, herbicides (weed-killing chemicals), and fertilizers such as anhydrous ammonia. Any of these chemicals, if improperly handled, can create a dangerous situation for farmers and rescuers. Incidents involving hazardous materials are not always on highways. In addition, farms use many electric-powered machines. Be alert for the shock hazard posed by the presence of electrical lines and electrical devices on any part of a farm. Additional information regarding pesticides can be found in Chapter 11, *Poisoning and Substance Use*.

Some injuries involve tall barns or silos and often require rescuers who are trained in high-angle rescue techniques (**FIGURE 18-18**). Some farm silos are sealed and are designed to operate in an oxygen-deficient atmosphere. Always treat a silo as a hazardous confined space. Under certain conditions, gases given off by the contents of a silo can explode. Some farms also contain below-grade manure storage pits. These pits may be filled with poisonous gases or be deficient in oxygen. Do not enter any confined space or enclosed below-grade structure without proper self-contained breathing apparatus and proper training.

Farms also contain a wide variety of machinery. Machinery is used in every step of growing crops and raising animals. Accidents with farm machinery often involve rollovers of farm tractors, entrapment in machinery, or severing of body tissue by sharp objects (**FIGURE 18-19**). Tractor rollovers are more common with older tractors, which do not have roll bars or reinforced cabs. Rollovers most commonly occur on steep slopes and often result in the operator being pinned beneath the tractor. Entrapments can occur with many types of crop-harvesting equipment or mechanized animal feeding systems. Power take-off equipment, which converts power from a tractor's engine to supplementary equipment through a spinning shaft, can catch clothing and can quickly entrap a person. Rescuers should understand that such equipment may continue to spin due to mechanical failure or inertia even after the tractor is turned off.

As an EMR, your role in farm rescues consists of stabilizing the scene and providing initial medical care for the patient. Follow the seven steps of extrication (**TABLE 18-1**). Perform a careful scene assessment to determine the scope of the incident. Shut off any electric power and turn off any machinery that is still running, if possible. Call for adequate assistance from fire, rescue, and EMS organizations. In some communities, rescue personnel use farm implement mechanics for assistance with complex farm rescues. Helicopter transport of the patient may be beneficial. Remember, it is better to call for help and not need it than it is to delay adequate help from arriving at the scene.

Stabilize any hazards that you can while keeping yourself and the patient safe. Realize that you do not have the training

Voices OF Experience

The call came in as a possible back injury. It seemed to be a routine call on an average day at a large manufacturing facility where I was working part time as a paramedic in the medical clinic. Routine, that is, until I found out that the patient was three stories high on a remote part of the roof with limited access. The report came from a coworker stating that an electrician had fallen approximately 15 feet (5 m) from a scaffold, striking a large pipe on the way to the roof.

En route to the scene, I met the plant safety officer. He told me that there was some confusion as to the exact location of the injured person and he was not sure which access would get us there. Because of the unknowns of the call and the access problems, we decided to call our local fire/rescue department; they are well trained in unusual patient evacuations. Meanwhile, I was on the radio with the coworker, trying to find out the status of the patient.

> **"With everyone's help the patient was placed on oxygen, his fracture splinted, and a full spinal package completed."**

Fortunately, at this facility we have security personnel who are cross-trained as EMRs. The next report received was from a security/EMR staff member who had just arrived at the scene. He was able to tell us which access point to use and gave me a report stating that the patient was lying supine with a reduced level of consciousness. At this time, he was only responding to verbal stimulation. He had an open airway with no obvious bleeding. The secondary assessment showed a possible fracture to the left lower leg with stable vital signs.

I arrived at the scene along with two other security/EMR personnel. They had the long backboard, spinal packaging equipment, and a Stokes litter. My rapid trauma assessment found the patient just as the first EMR had reported. By now fire and rescue personnel had arrived and began to set up to lower the patient off the side of the structure. With everyone's help the patient was placed on oxygen, his fracture splinted, and a full spinal package completed. The patient was placed in the Stokes litter and successfully lowered as the EMS unit waited. He was transported to a local trauma center where he was treated and had a complete recovery from his injuries.

This was a great example, showing that having well-trained EMRs available with a good incident command system in place and local mutual aid response can lead to the best possible outcome for the patient.

Russ L. Miller, WEMT-Paramedic
Instructor/Coordinator
Past EMS Program Director, Cleveland State Community College
Director, Wilderness Safety Consultants
Delano, Tennessee

Adapted from the personal Medical Identification Symbol of the American Medical Association.

and equipment to stabilize all rescue scenes. If possible, gain access to the patient. Provide initial emergency care to the patient: establish responsiveness, support the patient's ABCs, control bleeding, and maintain the patient's body temperature. It is important to talk with the patient and provide emotional support. As other rescuers arrive on the scene, help them to disentangle the patient, prepare the patient for removal, and remove the patient.

Your actions at a farm rescue incident can make a lifesaving difference to the patient. Farm rescues can be challenging, but they require you to follow the same steps of patient care and extrication that you would use for other types of emergencies. Above all, remember your safety and the safety of the patient.

Bus Rescue

Buses operate in most communities. School buses transport students to school and to school-sponsored events. Cities operate fleets of municipal buses over established routes. Charter buses transport people of all ages to special events and on vacation trips. Specifically equipped buses transport people with limited mobility. Interstate buses transport people all over the country.

Because of the large numbers of people being transported by buses, significant potential exists for bus crashes to occur in any community. Bus crashes range from minor incidents with no injuries to mass-casualty incidents; therefore, you need to understand some guidelines for providing care to patients involved in bus crashes. A mass-casualty incident refers to any accident or situation involving more patients than you can handle with the initial resources available.

If you are an EMR at a bus crash, perform a scene assessment or an overview of the scene and call for adequate police, fire, and EMS resources. Establish an incident command system if there are multiple casualties. Set up a one-way traffic pattern for responding vehicles to avoid congestion and gridlock at the emergency scene. For example, you might direct all responding emergency vehicles to approach the scene from the east and depart the scene traveling toward the west. If multiple patients must be removed from a bus, pass equipment into the bus through one door or window and remove the patients through a second door or window. This will improve the efficiency of the extrication process. If many patients are involved, triage them using your agency's designated triage system or the triage system that is used in your department. This system is used for sorting and treating patients in mass-casualty situations. The START triage system is explained in Chapter 19, *Incident Management*.

You are not expected to handle the command functions at a bus crash involving multiple casualties. However, you may be the only trained person on the scene for the first several minutes of an incident. Knowing some of the basic elements of handling this type of incident will help to improve the efficiency and effectiveness of the care given to the patients (**FIGURE 18-20**).

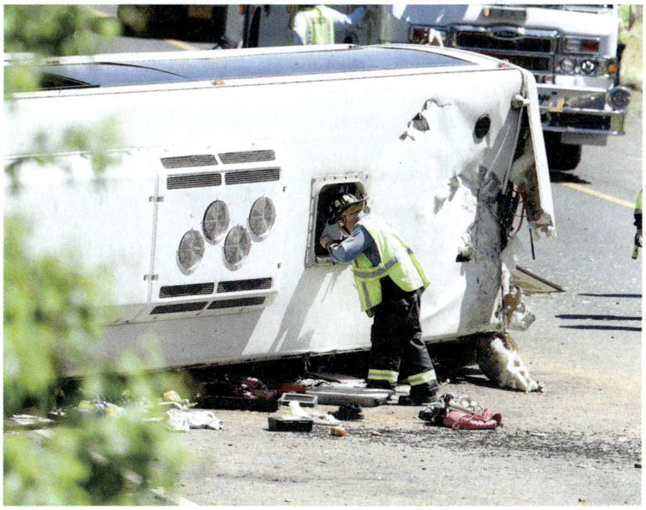

FIGURE 18-20 A bus crash requires an effective incident command system.

© Matt Button/ZUMA Press, Inc./Alamy Stock Photo

YOU are the EMR — SUMMARY

You are the EMR: CASE 1

1. What initial actions do you need to take to stabilize the scene and ensure scene safety?

Your first actions on the scene of an emergency incident should be to keep yourself and other rescuers safe and to ensure the safety of patients and bystanders at the scene. In this case, your active overview of the scene has determined that there are downed power lines, which create a deadly hazard for rescuers and for the patient. EMRs are not equipped or trained to determine if these lines are energized with electricity. Therefore, you must assume they are a life threat to the patient and to rescuers. One of your first actions after determining that there are power lines down is to notify dispatch that you need an emergency response from the electric utility to disconnect the power to these wires. In addition, remember that downed lines present a hazard to motorists and bystanders entering the area. This is especially true under conditions of dark and inclement weather. Because your patient appears to be dazed and slightly confused, it is especially important to talk with her from a safe location and instruct her to stay in her car until it has been confirmed that the downed wires are safe. Take steps to ensure that there is adequate

YOU are the EMR SUMMARY

traffic control to prevent drivers from entering the hazard area and that adequate resources have been requested to handle the situation.

2. What other resources are needed for an incident like this?

This incident represents a somewhat complex situation that requires additional resources. The additional resources needed include the following: the electric utility company, emergency responders with transport capabilities, adequate law enforcement resources to handle traffic control, fire department to address fire hazards, and a rescue company if extrication services will be needed to remove the patient from the vehicle. Even though it is not possible to begin patient care and extrication until the electric wires have been rendered safe, it is important to get all needed resources en route to the scene as soon as possible. You can always cancel the resource if they are not needed. Remember that as a first responder you will often be the eyes and ears of your dispatcher. They will not always know what is needed until you give them an assessment of the conditions on the scene.

3. What actions can you take once the scene is safe?

Once the power has been rendered safe by the electric utility company and the traffic flow has been controlled, it is safe for you to begin the steps needed to further stabilize the scene and to begin to care for the patient and to extricate her, if necessary. In this situation, the following steps might be involved:

1. Control any additional hazards.
2. Stabilize the vehicle to keep it from moving.
3. Gain access to the patient, if possible. Try the doors first; if access is not possible through a door, consider breaking and entering through a window to remove the patient.
4. Provide initial emergency care, including controlling external hemorrhaging, establishing spinal motion restriction, and maintaining body temperature.
5. Help disentangle the patient.
6. Help prepare the patient for removal.
7. Help remove the patient.

For each rescue situation you will need to determine which steps you can undertake safely and how much you can do, but in general these same principles apply to help determine what actions you can take once the scene is safe.

You are the EMR: CASE 2

1. What concerns you most about this scene?

Unlike when you are officially dispatched to an emergency, you have discovered an unreported incident and do not have any information about it from your dispatcher. Your first step is to park your vehicle in a safe place where it protects the scene as much as possible from oncoming traffic. If other responders are with you, coordinate your activities with them. Based on your overview of this scene and information from the bystander, you have enough information to call dispatch and report that you are out of service at the scene of a vehicle crash. You will probably need law enforcement personnel for traffic control, EMS units to provide care and transportation for three patients, an extrication crew to remove the patients from the SUV, and additional personnel to help transport the patients up the embankment. Because there is an increased chance of flammable fluids escaping from the overturned SUV, you should also request fire suppression units, although in most jurisdictions they are included in the response to all motor vehicle crashes with reports of injury. At some point, a tow truck (wrecker) operator will be needed to retrieve and remove the damaged vehicle. To provide the best possible care for these patients, request additional resources as soon as possible and get them en route to your location. After a more thorough overview of the scene, you may determine that some of those units will not be needed, at which time you can notify your dispatcher to cancel their response. The additional units can return to service before they arrive on the scene.

2. What are the important aspects of the scene assessment for this particular scene?

Your first priority is to immediately identify any threat to your safety, other responders, and bystanders. In this case, realize that most overturned vehicles are unstable. As an EMR, you may not have the resources necessary to stabilize this vehicle before the arrival of additional resources. Sometimes you can help alert patients to extricate themselves. At other times you may be able to use improvised resources to stabilize the vehicle. However, do not forget that the best course of action may be to wait for further assistance before attempting to enter an unstable, overturned vehicle, which would make the situation worse and endanger your own safety and potentially that of the patients. As mentioned previously, survey the scene and any patients for the mechanism of injury and determine the need for additional resources. Determine the possible number of patients, and verify the appropriate EMS response. In addition, remember to treat every patient as potentially infectious and take standard precautions to prevent any exposure to blood or body fluids.

You are the EMR: CASE 3

1. What could you do to assist in the extrication of these patients before rescue arrives?

Because these two patients are unresponsive, consider them to be in critical condition. You have determined that the scene is safe and that the vehicle is stable; therefore, attempt to gain access to the patients. Attempt to open

YOU are the EMR SUMMARY

the doors. Entrance through open windows is also an option. If the doors cannot be opened and the windows are closed, consider breaking a window with a spring-loaded center punch. Use caution when performing this task. The breaking of glass can cause injury to you and the patients. You should break the window that is farthest away from the patients.

2. What are the steps for using a spring-loaded center punch?

1. Wear heavy-duty leather gloves and eye protection, if available.
2. Place the spring-loaded center punch at the lower corner of the window.
3. Press on the center punch to break the window.
4. With gloved hands, remove the broken glass to the outside of the vehicle.
5. Enter the vehicle through the window.

You are the EMR: CASE 4

1. What additional resources will you potentially need at this scene?

Someone reported an explosion, and smoke is coming from the silo; therefore, fire suppression apparatus and personnel will be needed at the scene. Farms use a wide variety of chemicals in their operations, so be alert for the presence of pesticides, herbicides, and fertilizers, which may indicate the need for a hazardous materials (hazmat) team. This incident involves an enclosed silo, which means that you are dealing with a confined space rescue. Because no one should enter a confined space without proper training and self-contained breathing apparatus, a properly trained rescue crew is needed. You also need to be alert for electrical hazards, the need for ladders to access the silo, and the presence of dangerous equipment. Electric power needs to be disabled before rescue personnel begin operations. As with any emergency, request sufficient EMS units for patient care and transportation. If the farm is located a long distance from an appropriate medical facility, you may need to request helicopter transport. While the rescue efforts progress, continue to monitor the operation for any additional resources that are needed.

2. What are the potential hazards associated with farm rescue incidents?

Farms are a major source of hazards for emergency workers. During your scene assessment, consider the presence of chemicals such as pesticides, herbicides, and fertilizers, which are commonly used on farms. Farmers also use heavy equipment with specialized functions. Unless you are trained to handle farm equipment or have received specialized rescue training, keep a safe distance from the equipment until trained help arrives and the power to this equipment has been disabled. Farm equipment entrapments may require specialized expertise and tools from a farm implement dealer. You should know your local protocol for accessing these resources. In addition to their specialized functions, farm equipment is extremely heavy. Additional care needs to be taken when stabilizing these pieces of machinery before rescue attempts are made. Finally, whenever operating around a farm scene, be alert for animals that may be close to you.

Prep Kit

Ready for Review

- As an EMR, you may not be directly involved in all seven of the extrication steps, but you should be aware of the entire process.
- Water rescue, ice rescue, underwater diving emergencies, confined space rescue, farm rescue, and bus crashes are situations that require extensive skills and special training. It is important to help the patient, but not at the expense of your own safety.
- In water and ice rescue situations, there are four simple steps you can take to help the person without endangering yourself: reach out to the person with an object, throw a flotation device to the person, row to the person in a boat, or go to the person if you are adequately trained to do so (reach, throw, row, go).
- You may not be able to distinguish between the two major medical emergencies created by underwater diving incidents (air embolism and decompression sickness), but you can provide basic care and summon appropriate assistance.
- In confined space rescue, your primary goals are to call for additional assistance and prevent other people, including yourself, from becoming patients.
- Farm emergencies and bus crashes are complex rescue situations; however, if you follow simple steps, you can often stabilize these situations and provide initial aid to patients.

Prep Kit

Vital Vocabulary

air embolism A bubble of air obstructing a blood vessel.

chocking A piece of wood or metal that is placed in front of or behind a wheel to prevent vehicle movement.

decompression sickness (the bends) A condition seen in divers in which gas, especially nitrogen, forms bubbles in blood vessels, obstructing them.

entrapment A situation in which a person is caught (trapped) within a vehicle, room, or container with no way out or has a limb or other body part trapped.

extrication Removal from a difficult situation or position; removal of a patient from a wrecked vehicle or other place of entrapment.

flotation device A life ring, life buoy, or other floating device used in water rescue.

fusees Warning devices or flares that burn with a red color; usually used in scene protection at motor vehicle crash sites.

Golden Hour A concept of emergency patient care that attempts to place a trauma patient into definitive medical care in the shortest time to achieve the best possible outcome; also called the Golden Period.

plastic-laminated glass Safety glass that cracks but does not shatter when impacted; the embedded plastic layer holds the pieces in place.

reach, throw, row, go A sequence of four actions that should be taken in water rescue situations.

rescue throw bag A water rescue device consisting of a small cloth bag and a waterproof rope used for rescuing people from the water.

riptide Unusually strong surface currents flowing outward from a seashore that can present a hazard to swimmers.

tempered glass Safety glass that breaks into small pieces when hit with a sharp, pointed object.

wooden cribbing Wooden boards used for vehicle stabilization or bracing.

References

First responders are getting new help with EV challenges. Government Technology website. https://www.govtech.com/public-safety/first-responders-are-getting-new-help-with-ev-challenges. Published February 13, 2024. Accessed November 19, 2024.

Heightman AJ. New laminated side windows will pose access problems for unprepared first-arriving EMS and fire units. *JEMS* website. https://www.jems.com/equipment-gear/new-laminated-side-windows-will-pose-access-problems-for-unprepared-first-arriving-ems-fire-units/. Published August 9, 2021. Accessed November 19, 2024.

National Highway Traffic Safety Administration. *National Emergency Medical Services Education Standards.* https://www.ems.gov/assets/EMS_Education-Standards_2021_FNL.pdf. EMS.gov website. Published 2021. Accessed November 19, 2024.

National Oceanic and Atmospheric Administration, US Department of Commerce. Floods: the awesome power. National Weather Service website. https://www.weather.gov/media/bis/Floods.pdf. Published March 2005. Accessed November 19, 2024.

National Oceanic and Atmospheric Administration, US Department of Commerce. Turn around, don't drown. National Weather Service website. https://www.weather.gov/tsa/hydro_tadd. Accessed November 19, 2024.

Selman J, Spickett J, Jansz J, Mullins B. An investigation into the rate and mechanism of incident of work-related confined space fatalities. *Saf Sci.* 2018:109;333–343.

Assessment IN ACTION

You are dispatched to the intersection of Shelbourne Falls Road and State Route 324 for a motor vehicle crash. On arrival, you find a small pickup truck that has struck a utility pole. The power line is resting on the roof of the truck. Two occupants are in the vehicle. Both appear to be alert and oriented. There appears to be smoke coming from a nearby utility pole. (Questions 1–3 relate to this scenario.)

1. What is your first step in this situation?

- **A.** Perform a scene assessment.
- **B.** Call for additional assistance.
- **C.** Assess the patient's ABCs.
- **D.** Begin removing the patients from the vehicle.

2. What additional resources would probably NOT be needed at this scene?

- **A.** Electric company
- **B.** Hazmat team
- **C.** Fire department
- **D.** Additional ambulance

3. What is the greatest hazard at this scene?

- **A.** Battery acid
- **B.** Transmission fluid
- **C.** Fuel leakage
- **D.** Live power line

You and your family are at the local swimming pool enjoying a break from the summer heat when you notice two boys playing near the shallow end of the pool. A few minutes later, you hear a boy screaming, "Scott fell into the pool and hit his head on the bottom step! Help!" As you approach the side of the pool, you see a young boy floating facedown in the pool. (Questions 4–10 relate to this scenario.)

4. What is your first priority in the treatment of this patient?

- **A.** Remove the patient from the water.
- **B.** Establish an airway.
- **C.** Turn the patient over.
- **D.** Begin chest compressions.

5. Performing rescue breathing on the patient while still in the water is easiest if:

- **A.** the patient is smaller than you.
- **B.** you can stand on the bottom.
- **C.** you are an expert swimmer.
- **D.** you are using a flotation device.

6. What maneuver should you use to open the patient's airway?

- **A.** Head tilt–chin lift
- **B.** Head tilt–jaw thrust
- **C.** Jaw thrust
- **D.** Head tilt–neck lift

7. What are the steps for turning the patient so that he is facing up?

8. After the patient is out of the water, how would you assess this patient?

9. If this patient is in cardiac arrest, what special precautions do you need to take when using an automated external defibrillator (AED)?

10. If a backboard is not available for use with this patient, what are possible substitutions?

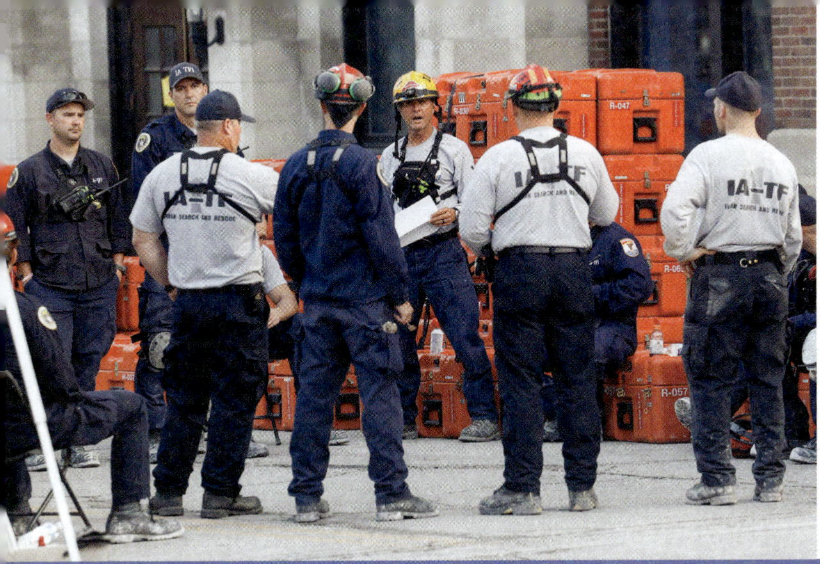

CHAPTER 19

Incident Management

National EMS Education Standard Competencies

EMS Operations

Knowledge of operational roles and responsibilities to ensure patient, public, and personnel safety.

Incident Management

- Establish and work within the incident management system. (pp 421–437)

Multiple-Casualty Incidents*

- Operational goals (pp 424–430)
- Field triage (pp 422–424; pp 426–430)

Hazardous Materials Awareness

- Risks and responsibilities of operating on the scene of a hazardous materials incident (pp 431–437)

Mass-Casualty Incidents Due to Terrorism and Disaster

- Risks and responsibilities of operating on the scene of a natural or human-made disaster (pp 431–436)

Knowledge Objectives

1. State the responsibilities of emergency medical responders (EMRs) in incidents where hazardous materials are present. (pp 424–431)
2. Describe the actions EMRs should take in hazardous materials (hazmat) incidents before the arrival of specifically trained personnel. (pp 431–437)
3. Discuss the different areas of a hazmat scene. (p 422)
4. Define a mass-casualty incident. (p 424)
5. Describe the role of EMRs in a mass-casualty incident. (pp 424–431)
6. Explain the steps in the START triage system. (pp 426–430)
7. Describe the purpose of the National Incident Management System. (p 430)
8. Define terrorism and weapons of mass destruction. (p 431)
9. Describe potential terrorist targets and risks. (p 431)
10. Explain the risks posed by explosives and incendiary devices. (pp 431–437)
11. Explain the risks posed by the following chemical agents:
    - Pulmonary agents (p 432)
    - Metabolic agents (p 432)
    - Insecticides (p 434)
    - Nerve agents (p 434)
    - Blister agents (p 434)
12. Explain the risks posed by biologic agents. (p 435)
13. Explain the risks posed by radiologic agents. (p 435)
14. Describe the role of EMRs in a terrorist event. (p 436)

Skills Objectives

1. Demonstrate the actions EMRs should take in hazmat incidents before the arrival of specifically trained personnel. (pp 422–425)
2. Demonstrate triage of a mass-casualty incident using the START triage system. (pp 426–431)

*This text uses the term mass-casualty incident.

© Nikos Frazier/Quad City Times/ AP Photo

Introduction

This chapter covers hazardous materials (hazmat) incidents, mass-casualty incidents (MCIs), the National Incident Management System (NIMS), and terrorism awareness. You should be able to identify the signs of a hazmat incident and prevent injury to yourself and to others in the first minutes of the incident. Because you may be called to assist with an MCI, you should understand the purpose of an incident management system and the NIMS framework. Your knowledge of basic triage and your ability to use the START triage system are also important.

The last section of this chapter is designed to increase your awareness of terrorism. In addition to defining terrorism, you will learn the types of structures and facilities terrorists might target and how terrorists might use explosive, incendiary, chemical, biologic, and radiologic agents to cause mass destruction. You will also learn the importance of safety, preparedness, and the use of the incident command system (ICS).

Hazmat Incidents

A **hazardous material** is any substance that is toxic, poisonous, radioactive, flammable, or explosive and can cause injury or death with exposure. During a **hazmat incident**, your top priority is to protect yourself and bystanders from exposure and contamination.

A very important step when handling any hazmat incident is to identify the substances involved. Federal law requires all vehicles containing certain quantities of hazardous materials to display a hazmat placard, which is a large diamond-shaped indicator placed on all sides of transport vehicles that carry hazardous materials. When you see a hazmat placard, you know that a potential problem could exist. You will have to find the proper response to the problem before beginning patient treatment (**FIGURE 19-1**). The placard should also have a four-digit identification number, which can be used to identify the substance and to obtain emergency information.

The *Emergency Response Guidebook*, published by the US Department of Transportation, lists the most common hazardous materials, their four-digit identification numbers, and the proper emergency actions to take to control the scene. It also describes the emergency medical care of patients who become ill or injured after exposure to these substances (**FIGURE 19-2**). This guidebook is updated every 3 to 4 years. You should carry an up-to-date copy of this guidebook in your vehicle or have electronic access to it at all times. You can download a free copy of the guidebook at the Pipeline and Hazardous Materials Safety Administration website, and an app is available as a free download for both Android and iOS platforms.

Unless you have received specialized training in handling hazardous materials and can take the necessary precautions to protect yourself, you should keep away from the contaminated area, or hot zone. As soon as you recognize that a hazmat incident exists, notify your dispatcher so other responders will be aware of the situation.

> **Safety**
>
> If you believe that a crash may involve hazardous materials, stop uphill and upwind at a distance from the crash. Then determine whether the vehicle is marked with a placard. A pair of binoculars, which can be stored in your vehicle or the jump kit, is helpful for identifying these markings from a safe distance. The placard indicates the class of material being transported.
>
> Also note the presence of leaking fluids. The presence of odors or fumes may be the first indication of hazardous materials located in buildings. If you believe that a hazardous material is present, call for assistance from the agency that handles hazardous materials in your community. Remain far away from any suspected hazmat incident so you do not become an additional casualty.

Once the trained hazmat rescuers have been properly protected, these rescuers need to identify the source of the hazardous materials and remove anyone who has been exposed to the hazard. Sometimes hazmat teams can stop the escape of the hazardous material by shutting off a leak or by absorbing spilled chemicals. Once people have been removed from the contaminated area, they need to be decontaminated by trained personnel, assessed for any injuries, given necessary emergency medical care, and transported to a hospital.

Few specific antidotes or treatments exist for most hazmat injuries. Consequently, the emergency treatment you can provide to patients who have been exposed to hazardous materials is usually aimed at supportive care. Because most fatalities and serious injuries sustained in hazmat incidents result from breathing problems, you must constantly reevaluate the patient's vital signs, including breathing status, so that a patient whose condition worsens can be moved to a higher triage level.

> **Words of Wisdom**
>
> Anyone who is working at the scene of a hazmat emergency should understand the terminology used to differentiate separate parts of the hazmat scene:
>
> - **Hot zone**. The contaminated area where people may be exposed to sharp metal edges, broken glass, toxic substances, lethal rays, or ignition or explosion of hazardous materials.
> - **Warm zone**. The controlled area where personnel and equipment **decontamination** and hot zone support take place.
> - **Cold zone**. The controlled safe area that contains the command post and other support functions needed in the incident.
>
> Only specifically trained and equipped personnel should be in the hot zone and the warm zone.

> **Safety**
>
> Your top priority in a possible hazmat incident is to protect yourself and any bystanders from exposure and contamination. Contaminated patients can contaminate unprotected rescuers!

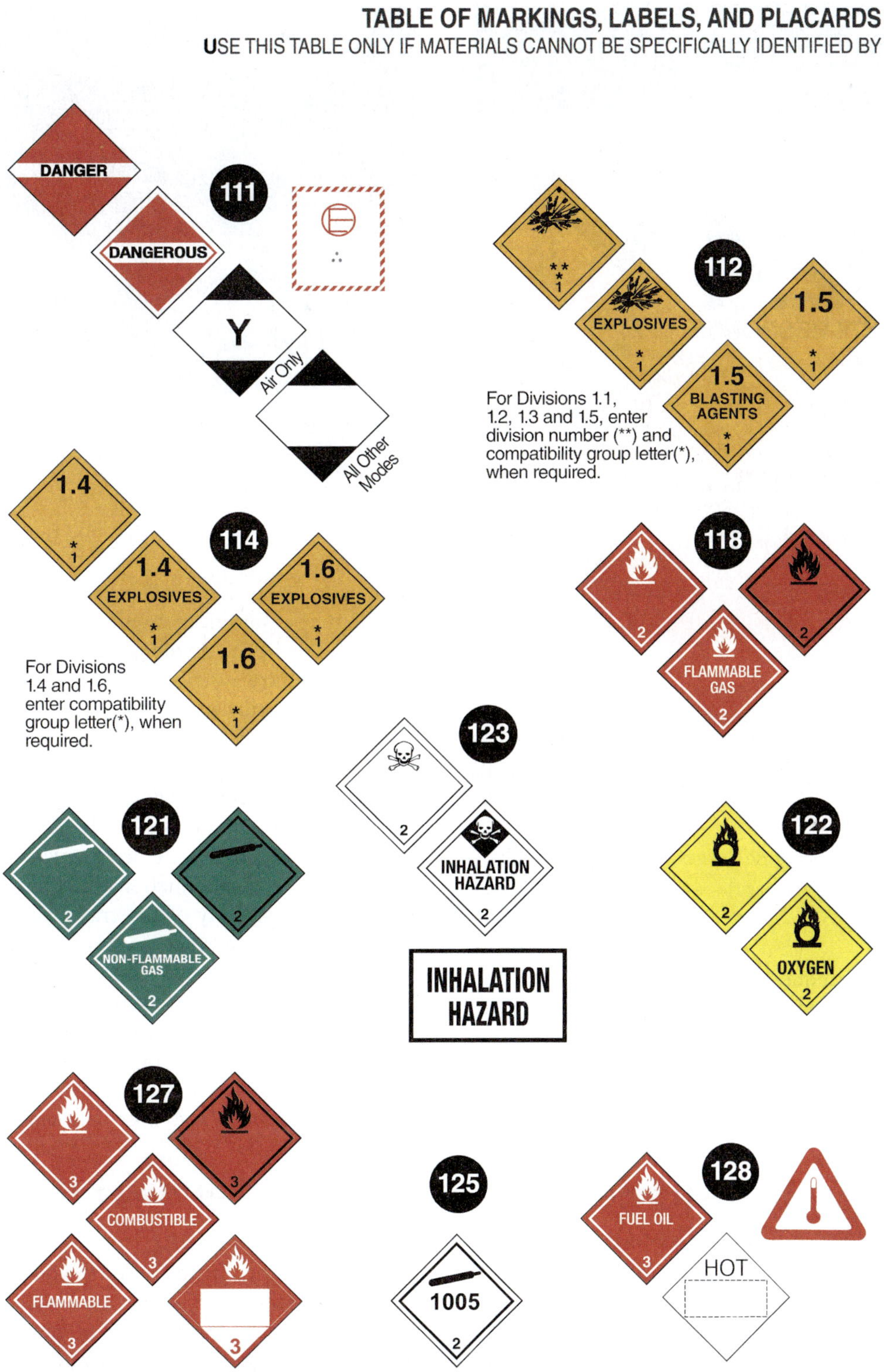

FIGURE 19-1 The US Department of Transportation uses labels, placards, and markings (such as those found in the *Emergency Response Guidebook*) to give a general idea of the hazardous materials inside a particular container or cargo tank. Look for these placards when you arrive on an emergency scene. They are required when hazardous materials are present. Be aware that shipments with small quantities of hazardous materials may not be required to be labeled with placards.

Courtesy of the US Department of Transportation.

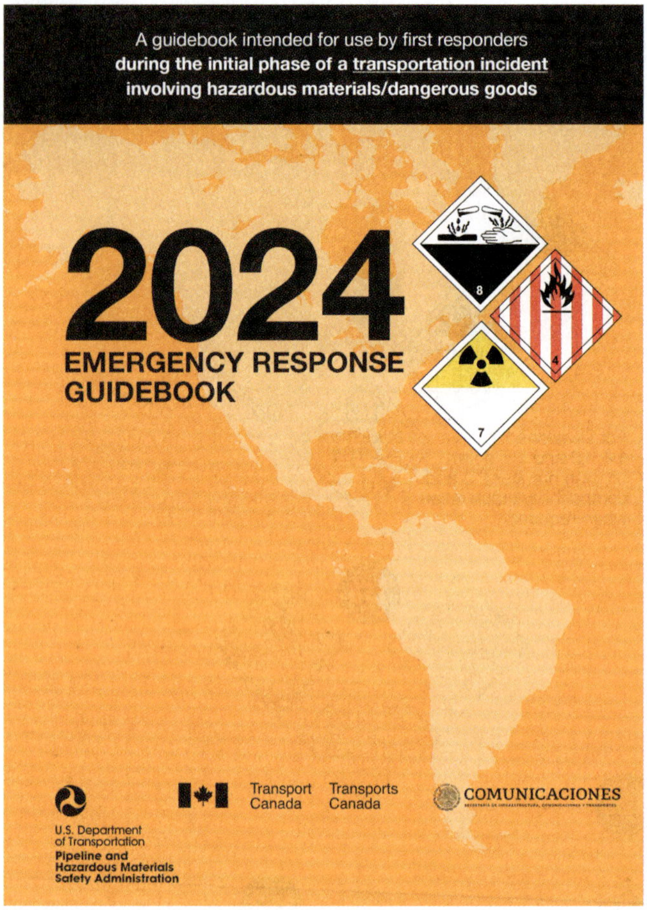

FIGURE 19-2 *Emergency Response Guidebook.*
Courtesy of the US Department of Transportation.

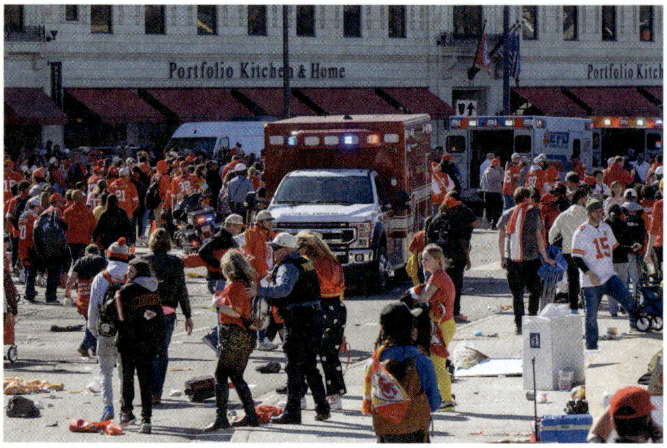

FIGURE 19-3 A mass shooting occurred during the Kansas City Chiefs' Super Bowl victory celebration in 2024.
© Reed Hoffmann/AP Photo

Because of the unique aspects of responding to and working at a hazmat incident, as an emergency medical responder (EMR), you should receive specific additional training in hazardous waste operations and emergency response (often referred to as HAZWOPER) to the emergency medical response level.

Mass-Casualty Incidents

As an EMR, you may face situations in which there is more than one sick or injured person. These situations may range from a serious motor vehicle crash with three or four injured people to a building explosion with dozens of injured people. A **mass-casualty incident (MCI)** is an emergency in which there are more patients than there are resources (ambulances), either on scene or en route, ready to treat and transport patients. In these situations, how do you determine which patient to treat first?

You must first be able to recognize the situation as an MCI. An MCI typically refers to any call that involves three or more patients, any situation that places such a great demand on available equipment or personnel that the system would require a **mutual aid** response (an agreement between neighboring emergency medical services [EMS] systems to respond when local resources are insufficient to handle the response), or any incident that has the potential to create one of the previously mentioned situations. These incidents require a very different method of operation from routine emergency medical calls. During some MCIs, you may be on the scene 15 to 20 minutes before additional assistance arrives, and it may be 45 to 60 minutes before enough rescue resources are available.

No easy formula exists for deciding when to shift from normal operations into the techniques of the MCI. Simulations provide realistic situations, but there are many variables, including the severity of the crash, access routes, available resources, response times, levels of emergency training, and overall experience of the EMS system.

Your goal should be to provide the greatest medical benefit for the greatest number of people and to match patients' medical needs with appropriate treatment and transport. To accomplish this goal, you must identify those patients most in need of treatment and those who can wait.

The Visual Survey: The Eye Sees It All

As you are on the way to the scene, you should mentally prepare yourself for what you may find (**FIGURE 19-3**). Perhaps you have responded to other accidents at the same location. You should ask yourself the following questions: Where will additional assistance come from? How long will it take for them to arrive?

When you arrive at the scene of a major incident, focus on staying as calm as possible. Make a visual assessment of the entire accident scene. This visual survey, as part of the scene size-up, gives you an initial impression of the overall situation, including the potential number of patients and, possibly, the severity of their injuries. The visual survey enables you to estimate how much and what kind of assistance you will need to handle the situation.

Your Initial Radio Report: Creating a Verbal Image

The initial radio report is often the most important radio message of a major emergency because it sets the emotional and operational stage for everything that follows. As you prepare for that first vital report, use clear language, be concise, be calm, and do not shout into the equipment. Give the communications center a concise verbal picture of the scene.

The key points to communicate are as follows:

1. Location of the incident
2. Type of incident
3. Any hazards
4. Approximate number of patients
5. Types of assistance required

Be as specific with your requests as possible. A good rule of thumb in mass-casualty situations is to request one ambulance for every five patients. For example, for 35 patients, request seven ambulances; for 23 patients, request five ambulances; and so forth. Be aware however, that this ratio will vary from one jurisdiction to another and also based on the number of casualties. Know your local protocols for the number of ambulances to be requested as a function of the number of injured victims. After taking several deep breaths (to give yourself time to absorb what you have seen and to try to calm your voice), you might give the following radio report for a crash involving a city bus: "This is a major crash involving a truck and a city bus on Highway 233, approximately 2 miles west of Route 510. There are approximately 35 victims. There are multiple people trapped. Repeat: This is a major crash. I am requesting the fire department, rescue squad, seven ambulances, and medevac helicopters at this time. Dispatch additional police units to assist." Note that air medical operations may be required, particularly in rural areas. For a discussion of working with helicopters, see Chapter 17, *Transport Operations.*

Follow the protocols of your department when calling for additional resources:

1. Determine the perimeters for emergency vehicles only and exclude all other vehicles.
2. Establish a one-way route for emergency traffic to approach the scene and a separate one-way route for emergency traffic to exit the scene. This will prevent roads from becoming blocked for incoming units.
3. Allow adequate room for emergency vehicles that need to be close to the scene.
4. Keep vehicles and personnel at a designated staging area nearby if they are not needed at the scene.

Words of Wisdom

Studies have shown that the failure to provide adequate traffic control at an emergency scene is a common and often fatal error in MCIs. Immediately after radioing for additional assistance, you should establish a traffic control plan. Establishing a one-way traffic pattern will help to avoid confusion and congestion at the incident site. This process should take only a few minutes.

Traffic Incident Management

Many EMS calls involve traffic hazards. When incidents occur on highways, it is important to protect the incident scene to prevent further injury to responders, patients, and other motorists. Achieving this objective requires planning and coordination between EMS, law enforcement, fire services, and highway departments. **Traffic incident management (TIM)** is a system that specifies where to place vehicles and warning devices to achieve a safe scene while highway incidents are being resolved. TIM involves the following concepts (**FIGURE 19-4**):

- **Advanced warning area.** This area gives motorists ample warning of an incident ahead and is usually marked with a pink diamond warning sign on a flashing signboard or a portable sign.
- **Transition area.** This area is marked by flares or cones to move the traffic away from the incident.
- **Buffer space.** This area starts to slow traffic and funnel it away from the incident.
- **Protection vehicle.** This vehicle is positioned directly upstream from the incident to block and direct traffic.
- **Work space.** This is the area of the emergency incident. It needs to remain open and safe from any traffic hazards to allow emergency crews to work safely with as little disruption of traffic as possible.
- **Termination area.** This area is immediately downstream from the incident and allows motorists to resume normal traffic flow.

YOU are the EMR — CASE 1

In the middle of the night, you are dispatched for a report of a vehicle crash. A delivery truck lost control during a heavy rainstorm and hit a large oak tree. As you arrive at the scene, you find a package delivery truck that hit a tree on a residential road that runs through your community. There is still a light rain falling. Dispatch reports that because of the heavy volume of calls during the storm, the nearest EMS unit has an estimated arrival time of 8 to 9 minutes.

1. What initial actions should you take at this scene?
2. What initial actions should you take if this incident turns out to be an MCI?

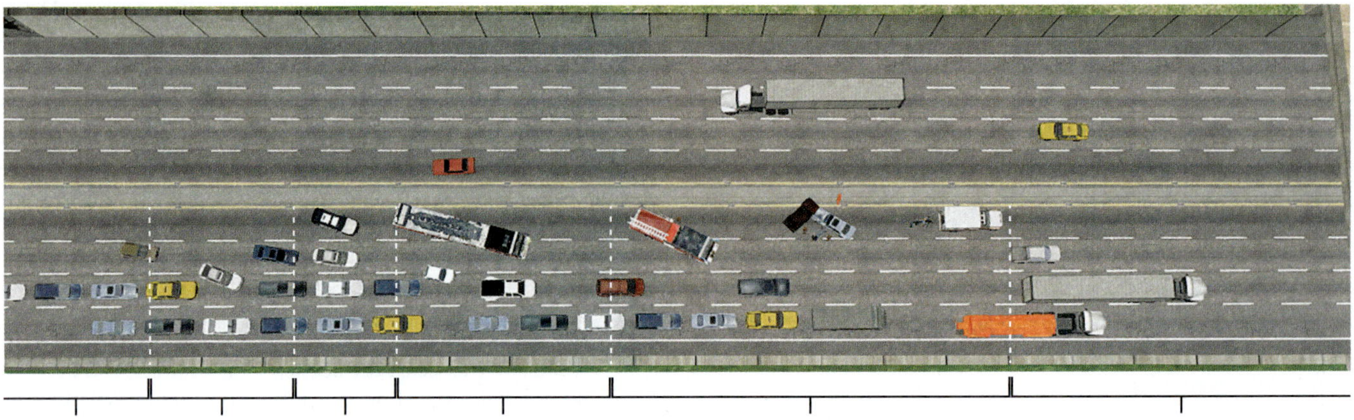

FIGURE 19-4 Example of a traffic incident management system.
Courtesy of FAAC, Inc. Based on original figure by Emergency Responder Safety Institute.

You need to learn your role in the TIM system that is used in your community.

Casualty Sorting: Creating Order Out of Chaos

The sorting of patients into groups according to their need for medical treatment is called **triage**. Triage is a French word that has come to mean **casualty sorting** in the emergency medical care field. The purpose of casualty sorting is to determine the order in which patients should be treated based on the severity of their injuries so that the most good can be done for the greatest number of people.

Ideally, your casualty-sorting system should be simple and fast, based on the skills and knowledge you already have. Do not worry about making a specific diagnosis before categorizing patients; a casualty-sorting system is meant to provide the basis for a system of rapid, lifesaving actions. A casualty-sorting system focuses your activities in the middle of a chaotic and confusing environment. You must identify and separate patients rapidly, according to the severity of their injuries and their need for treatment.

Avoid spending undue time treating the first or second patient you see. Remember, your job is to get to each patient as quickly as possible, conduct a primary assessment, and assign patients to broad triage categories based on their need for treatment.

You should not stop during this assessment, except to correct airway and severe bleeding problems quickly. Your job is to sort (triage) the patients. Other rescuers will provide follow-up treatment.

Different communities use many variations of triage systems, and you will need to learn the specific role that you have in your community's triage plan. Many EMS systems rely on the **START triage** system because it is simple and easy to remember and implement. START stands for Simple Triage And Rapid Treatment. This system lets EMRs triage each patient in 60 seconds or less based on three primary observations: breathing, circulation, and mental status.

The START triage system is designed to help rescuers find the most seriously injured patients. While determining injury severity, they may take the time required to open a blocked airway and manage severe bleeding. As more rescue personnel arrive, patients can be triaged again for further evaluation, treatment, stabilization, and transport.

Street Smarts

The experience of responding to an MCI can be extremely stressful for all responders. Certain roles, such as triage officer, are especially stressful. When you are triaging patients, use your triage protocols to guide you through this process. You are expected to do your best, but keep in mind that there is no perfect way to handle an overwhelming incident. After an MCI, it may be helpful for you to talk with your peers, a mentor, a supervisor, or a counselor. Many departments offer an employee assistance program to help employees cope with a wide variety of stressful situations. Taking care of your own mental well-being should be a priority throughout your career. See Chapter 12, *Behavioral Emergencies*, for a discussion of peer support and critical incident stress debriefing.

Triage Tagging: Telling Others What You Have Found

Patients are tagged so that other rescuers arriving at the scene can easily recognize their triage level. Patients are tagged using colored surveyor's tape or colored paper tags, depending on the method selected by your local EMS system (**FIGURE 19-5**).

The START triage system consists of four categories of triage, each with its own color code:

- **Priority 1 (red tag).** Immediate care: injuries are life threatening. These patients cannot be stabilized at the scene and need to be transported to an appropriate medical facility as soon as possible. An example of a red tag patient might be a patient who has sustained severe chest trauma, is breathing at a

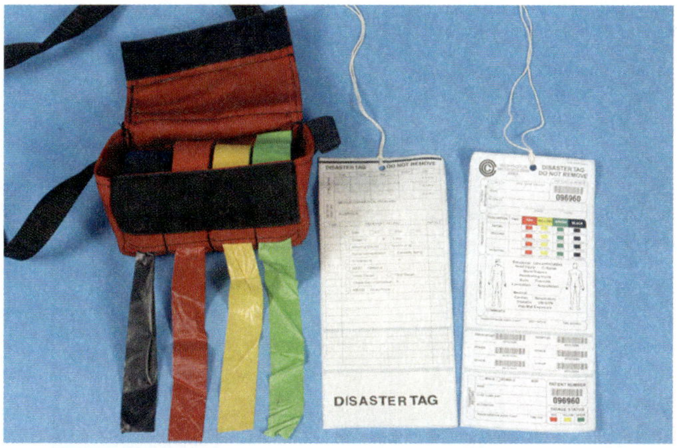

FIGURE 19-5 A. Triage tape. **B.** Triage tag (back). **C.** Triage tag (front).
© Jones & Bartlett Learning. Courtesy of MIEMSS.

rate of greater than 30 times per minute, and is pale and sweaty.

- **Priority 2 (yellow tag).** Urgent care: care can be delayed up to 1 hour. These patients have sustained serious injuries, but they can survive a delay of up to 1 hour in getting to an appropriate medical facility. An example of a yellow tag patient might be a person who is in pain from a deformity to the femur but is responsive to your verbal commands and is not showing signs and symptoms of shock.
- **Priority 3 (green tag).** Delayed care, minor care, or hold (walking wounded): care can be delayed up to 3 hours. These patients are the ones who are able to walk to a designated area away from the immediate area of the incident. They may have isolated upper extremity injuries, cuts, and bruises, but they are responsive and are not showing signs and symptoms of shock.
- **Priority 4 (black tag).** Patient is dead; no care is required. These patients have sustained injuries that are obviously incompatible with life, or they have no pulse or respirations. Note that some branches of the military use both a black triage color (deceased) and a blue triage color (unlikely to survive transport).

You need to learn the triage system that is used by your department.

The First Step in START: Get Up and Walk

The first step in START is to ask everyone who can get up and walk to move away from the immediate rescue scene to a designated safe area. If patients can get up and walk, they rarely have life-threatening injuries. These patients are the walking wounded and are designated as Priority 3 (green tag/delayed care). A patient who reports pain when attempting to walk or move should not be forced to move.

With these patients separated in a safe location, you can now concentrate on the patients who are left in the rescue scene.

The Second Step in START Triage: Begin Where You Stand

Begin the second step of the START triage system by moving from where you stand. Move in an orderly and systematic manner through the remaining patients, stopping at each patient to provide a quick assessment and tagging. The stop at each patient should never take more than 1 minute.

Your job is to find and tag the Priority 1 patients: those who require immediate attention. Examine these patients, treat life-threatening airway and breathing conditions, tag the patients with a red tag, and move on.

How to Evaluate Patients Using Breathing, Circulation, and Mental Status

The START triage system is based on the three observations: breathing, circulation, and mental status. Each patient must be evaluated quickly, in a systematic manner, starting with breathing (**FIGURE 19-6**).

Breathing: It All Starts Here. If the patient is breathing, you need to determine the breathing rate. Patients with breathing rates of greater than 30 breaths per minute are tagged Priority 1 (red tag/immediate). These patients are showing one of the primary signs of shock and need immediate medical care as soon as it is available.

If the patient is breathing at a rate of less than 30 breaths per minute, move on to the circulation and mental status observations to complete your 60-second survey.

If the patient is not breathing, quickly clear the mouth of any foreign matter. Use the head tilt–chin lift maneuver to open the airway. In a mass-casualty situation, you may not have time to stabilize every injured patient's spine properly. Open the airway, position the patient to maintain the airway, and, if the patient breathes, tag the patient Priority 1. Patients who need help maintaining an open airway are Priority 1. If you are in doubt as to the patient's ability to breathe, tag the patient as Priority 1. If the patient is not breathing and does not start to breathe with simple airway maneuvers, tag the patient Priority 4 (black tag; deceased).

Circulation: Is Oxygen Getting Around? The second part of the triage test is the patient's circulation. The best field method for checking circulation (to see if the heart is circulating blood adequately) is to check the patient's carotid pulse. The carotid pulse is close to the heart. It is large and easily felt in the neck. To check the carotid pulse, place your index and middle fingers on the larynx and slide your fingers into the groove between the larynx and the muscles at the side of the neck. You must keep your fingers there for 5 to 10 seconds to find and measure the pulse rate. If the carotid pulse is weak or irregular, tag the patient Priority 1. If the carotid pulse is strong, or a radial pulse is present, move on to the mental status observation, the third step of the triage system.

Treat patients with a weak carotid pulse for shock by laying the patient supine. Then try to stop any severe bleeding.

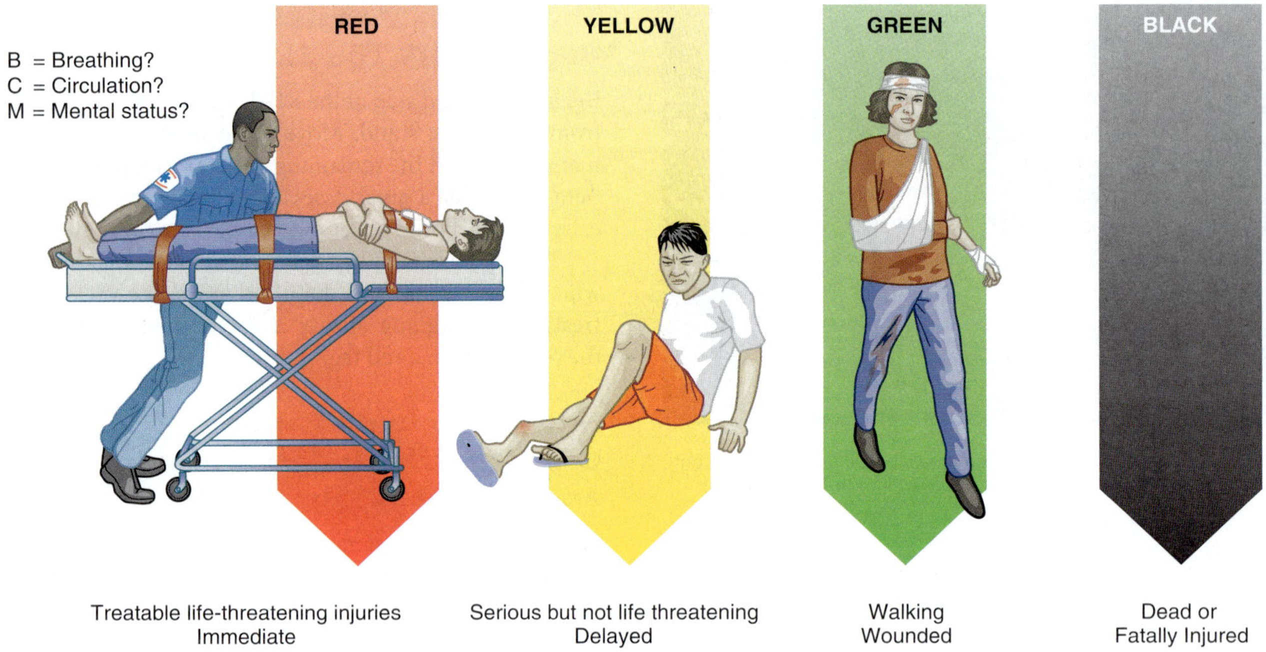

FIGURE 19-6 Use the START triage system to sort patients into appropriate groups for treatment.
© Jones & Bartlett Learning

Do not spend time controlling the bleeding yourself unless you can quickly apply a tourniquet to the bleeding area. Get the patient to assist with controlling the bleeding or ask one of the walking wounded, Priority 3 (green tag) patients, to help. These patients are often eager to assist with emergency treatment. If the pulse is absent, tag the patient as Priority 4 (black tag).

Mental Status: Open Your Eyes. The final part of the triage test is the mental status of the patient. This observation is performed on patients who have adequate breathing and adequate circulation. First, determine whether the patient responds to verbal stimuli. Ask the patient to follow a simple command, such as "Open your eyes," "Close your eyes," or "Squeeze my hand." Patients who can follow these simple commands and have adequate breathing and adequate circulation are tagged Priority 2 (yellow tag). According to the AVPU scale (Awake and alert, responsive to Verbal stimuli, responsive to Pain, Unresponsive), such patients are considered to be alert and responsive to verbal stimuli. A patient who cannot follow this type of simple command is unresponsive to verbal stimuli, according to the AVPU scale. Tag these patients as Priority 1 (red tag).

START Is Just the Beginning. In every situation involving the sorting of casualties, your goal is to find, stabilize, and move Priority 1 patients first. The START triage system is designed to help you find the most seriously injured patients. As more rescue personnel arrive at the scene, the patients will be triaged again for further evaluation, treatment, stabilization, and transport. As more EMS personnel arrive, you should turn over the responsibilities of triage to a person with more training. Each MCI should have a person designated as the triage officer.

Remember, injured patients do not always remain in the same condition. The process of shock may continue, and some conditions will become more serious as time goes by. As time and resources permit, go back and reassess the condition of Priority 2 and Priority 3 patients to detect changes in their conditions that may require upgrading the patients to Priority 1 attention (**FIGURE 19-7**).

Street Smarts

Patients with life-threatening internal injuries may be quiet. Do not assume that patients who do not vocalize their pain or distress are stable or uninjured.

Working at an MCI

You may or may not be the first person to arrive at the scene of an MCI. If other rescuers are already at the scene when you arrive, be sure to report to the incident commander before going to work. Because many activities are going on at the same time, the incident commander will assign you to an area where your help and skills can best be used. The incident commander, based on training and local protocols, is in charge of the rescue operation. An effective ICS depends on integrated, agreed-on protocols and procedures involving fire department, law enforcement, and EMS personnel.

If you are the first on the scene, you will have to make the initial overview, clearly and accurately report the situation to your dispatcher, and conduct the initial START triage.

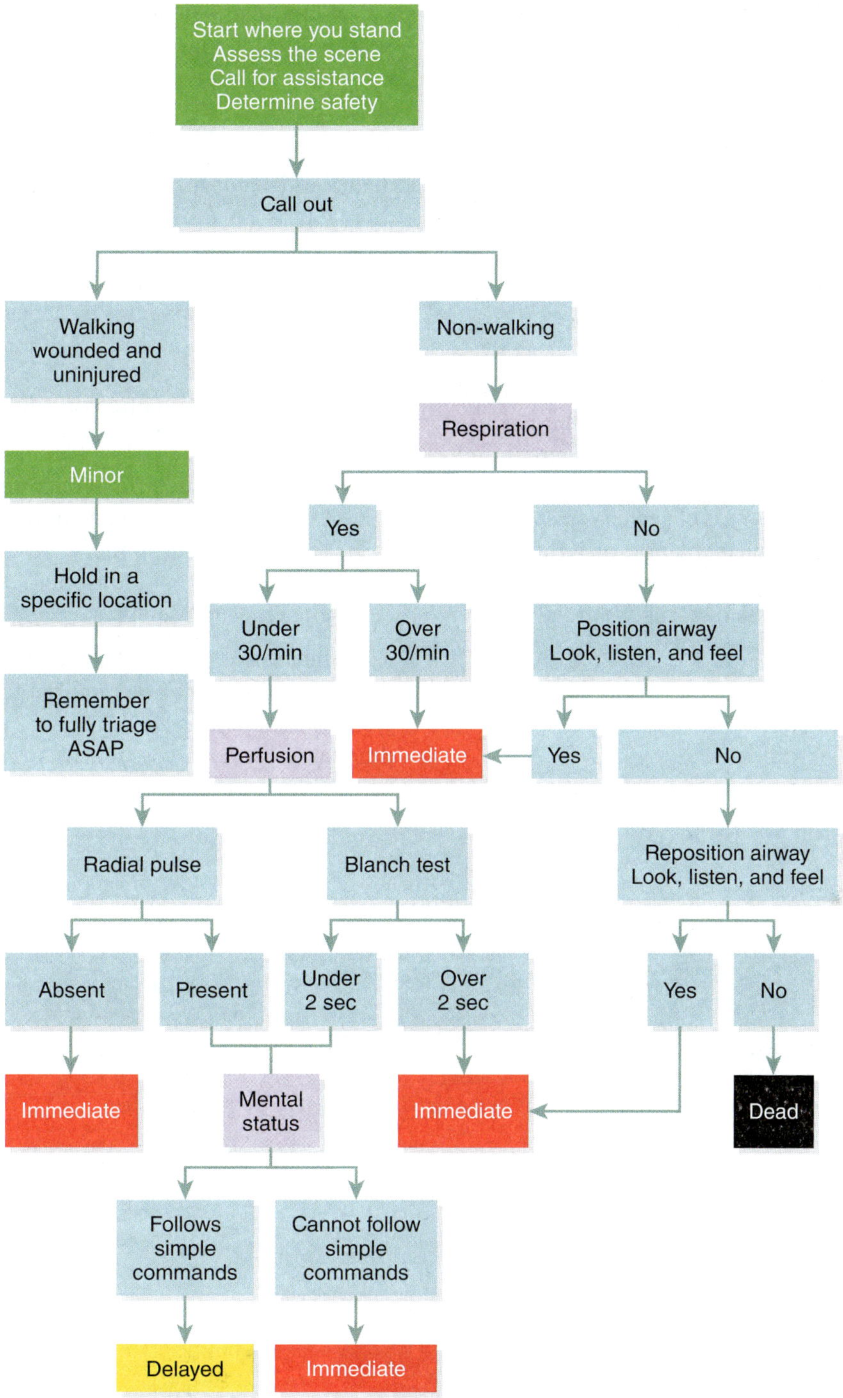

FIGURE 19-7 START algorithm.

Courtesy of Los Angeles Fire Department: Disaster Preparedness Section.

In addition, you most likely will be called on to participate in many other ways during MCIs.

As more highly trained rescue and EMS personnel arrive at the scene, accurately report your findings to the person in charge by using a format similar to that used in the initial arrival report. Note the following information:

- Approximate number of patients
- Number of patients you have triaged into each of the four levels
- Additional assistance required
- Other important information

After you have reported this information, you may be assigned to provide emergency medical care to patients, to help move patients, or to assist with ambulance or helicopter transport. You may also be asked to assist with traffic control or setting up a landing zone, or to help provide fire protection, depending on your training.

Treatment

At an MCI, remember you are trying to do the most good for the most patients. Do not get sidetracked by spending too much time treating the first patient you encounter.

National Incident Management System

The **National Incident Management System (NIMS)** has been developed by the US Department of Homeland Security to provide a comprehensive, consistent, and unified approach to handling emergency incidents. NIMS is designed to effectively and efficiently handle the immediate response to, mitigation of, and long-term recovery from natural and human-made incidents of all sizes, from small to massive. NIMS is designed to address all types of agencies responding to these disasters. Effective implementation of NIMS helps local government agencies work with regional, state, and federal agencies during all phases of a major emergency incident. It is flexible yet contains the following standardized components (**FIGURE 19-8**):

- Resource Management
- Command and Coordination
- Communications and Information Management

Additional information on NIMS is available at the Federal Emergency Management Agency website.

Incident Command System

The **incident command system (ICS)** is part of the Command and Coordination component of NIMS. EMS, and thus you as an EMR, will function within this portion of NIMS. The ICS is designed to provide an effective and efficient approach to managing and coordinating incidents. It provides a flexible, standardized incident management structure. You should understand the function of the ICS and your role within it.

The major benefits of the ICS are as follows (**FIGURE 19-9**):

1. A clearly defined chain of command
2. The use of common terminology
3. The safety of responders
4. The achievement of response objectives
5. The efficient use of resources

The federal government requires many agencies to use the ICS, and you may be required to become trained in this system. Different levels of training are offered through traditional and online courses. It is recommended that EMRs be certified in the following courses: ICS-100: Introduction

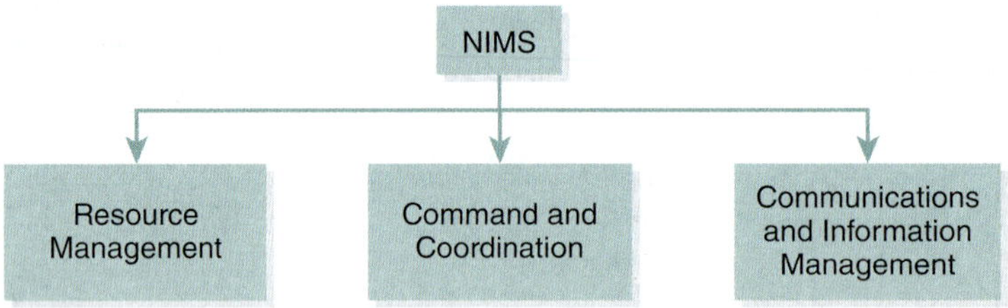

FIGURE 19-8 Components of the National Incident Management System (NIMS).

© Jones & Bartlett Learning

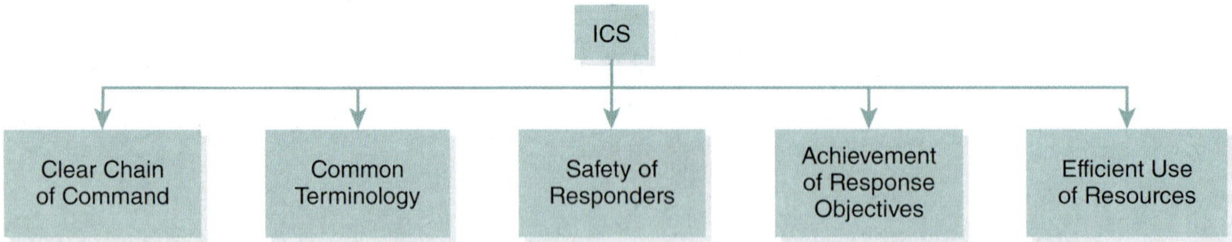

FIGURE 19-9 Major benefits of the incident command system (ICS).

© Jones & Bartlett Learning

YOU are the EMR **CASE 2**

You respond to a motor vehicle collision involving three vehicles. You arrive at the scene after EMS and are assigned to assist with triage. All patients who could walk were triaged as green prior to your arrival. As you approach your first patient, you kneel beside her and assess her breathing. You note she has a respiratory rate of 24 breaths per minute and the respirations are nonlabored. She has a weak carotid pulse, and no peripheral pulses are felt in her wrists.

1. In what triage category does this patient belong?
2. What is the appropriate treatment for this patient?

to ICS and ICS-200: Basic ICS for Initial Response. Take advantage of training in incident management. It will help you understand and work within the incident management system. FEMA offers online training through its website (https://training.fema.gov/emiweb/is/icsresource/trainingmaterials/).

Terrorism Awareness

Terrorism is the systematic use of violence by a group to intimidate a population or government to achieve a political goal. Terrorism receives considerable public attention and is a high-profile crime. Domestic terrorism is caused by a country's own citizens. For example, the bombing of an abortion clinic by an American citizen is considered an act of domestic terrorism. International terrorism is caused by people from another country. The attacks on the World Trade Center and the Pentagon on September 11, 2001, were international terrorist acts.

A terrorist attack may involve limited property damage with no injuries or it may involve the deaths of many people. The success of terrorist activities is measured by the intimidation produced, not just by the value of the property lost or the number of lives lost. Terrorists might use a wide variety of methods to incite terror, including guns, explosives, fire, chemicals, viruses, bacteria, and radiation.

Many agents used by terrorists are the same agents that produce hazards for EMRs in everyday accidents and emergencies. A building collapse caused by a natural gas explosion and a building collapse caused by a terrorist attack are both collapsed buildings. They share many of the same hazards and require many of the same safety precautions for rescuers. The accidental release of a chemical causes a hazmat emergency; an intentional release of the same chemical by terrorists becomes a terrorist event. Still, the safety precautions required for rescuers at both events are similar. A radiation leak from a nuclear power plant releases the same type of radiation that would be released by a terrorist. The safety principles remain the same in all types of scenarios: assess the scene for risks to yourself, your crew, and others, and maintain situational awareness at all times.

Safety

When responding to a known or suspected terrorist event, EMRs must remain vigilant for the possibility of secondary devices that are intentionally directed at first responders. Be aware of places where a secondary device could be hidden, including abandoned vehicles, trash dumpsters, debris piles, newspaper boxes, mailboxes, and storm sewers. This vigilance should extend to areas outside the immediate zone of the attack.

Weapons of Mass Destruction

A **weapon of mass destruction (WMD)** is any agent designed to bring about mass death, casualties, and/or massive damage to property and infrastructure (such as bridges, tunnels, airports, electrical power plants, and seaports). These instruments of death and destruction include explosive, chemical, biologic, and nuclear weapons. To date, the preferred WMD for terrorists has been explosive devices. Terrorist groups have favored tactics that use truck or car bombs or pedestrian suicide bombers. Many previous terrorist attempts to use either chemical or biologic weapons to their full capacity have been unsuccessful. Nonetheless, as an EMR, you should understand the destructive potential of these weapons.

Potential Targets and Risks

To understand the threat that terrorists pose to people and places, you need to consider the places that terrorists might identify as targets for terrorist activities. Remember, terrorists strive to incite fear to achieve a political or ideologic goal, and their motives do not limit their choice of targets. Bridges, tunnels, pipelines, and harbors constitute infrastructure targets. The Washington Monument and the Statue of Liberty are examples of symbolic targets. Housing developments and automobile dealerships have been targeted by ecoterrorists. Computer networks and data systems might be targets for cyberterrorists. Farms and agricultural installations might be targets for terrorists trying to destroy or taint the nation's food sources. Civilian targets such as schools, government buildings, places of worship, and shopping centers represent high-visibility targets for terrorists (**FIGURE 19-10**). Taken collectively, a wide variety of places, representing most components of society, might be considered as targets. In an open society in which people are largely free to move around as they wish, a person committed to performing a terrorist act can access most of the components of the infrastructure and turn any one of them into a target.

Despite measures to heighten security, a terrorist event can occur at any time. You should always be alert for hazards: those associated with a terrorist event as well as those connected to any other emergency. In any discussion of the

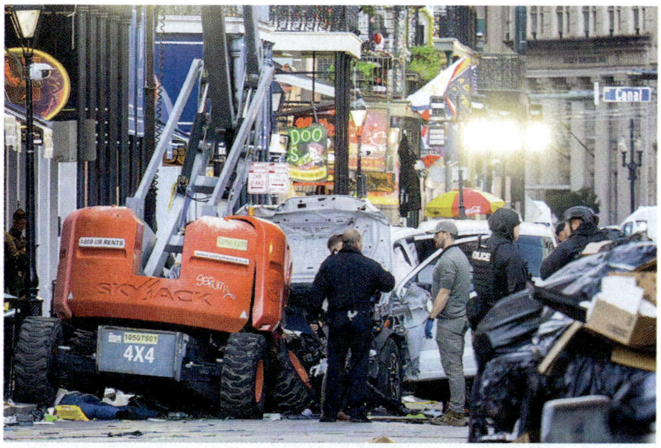

FIGURE 19-10 Terrorists may attack civilians by targeting schools, churches, stores, and other public areas. On New Year's Day in 2025, a terrorist drove a pickup truck onto a crowded sidewalk on Bourbon Street in New Orleans, resulting in 15 deaths (including his own) and more than 50 injuries.

© MATTHEW HINTON/AFP/Getty Images

risks of terrorist attacks, it is important to consider that the number of terrorism-related events is relatively low when compared with other types of events. Although you should be prepared for terrorist events, most of the emergency calls you answer will relate to heart disease, cancer, car crashes, isolated acts of violence, and other common causes.

Agents and Devices

A wide variety of agents and devices can be used to incite terror, including explosive devices, incendiary devices, chemical agents, biologic agents, and radiologic agents. You need to understand how these devices are used and what safety precautions you need to take to ensure scene safety for yourself, other rescuers, and bystanders.

Explosives and Incendiary Devices

Explosives are used to produce a concussion that destroys property and inflicts injury and death. Some explosive devices, also known as **incendiary devices**, are designed to start fires. Incendiary devices can be as simple as a homemade firebomb or as complex as a highly technical device that may have been stolen from the military (**FIGURE 19-11**). An explosive device can be hand carried or transported in a heavy truck. Often the first indication that an explosive or incendiary device is present is the explosion or fire that results from the deployment of the device. In some parts of the world, suicide terrorists carry explosive devices on their person and set them off to kill themselves and others.

WMD Safety Considerations

In times of increased concern about terrorist activity, travelers and the general public are urged to be alert for bags or luggage left unattended. Be aware of suspicious vehicles and report them to the proper law enforcement officials. If you are called to respond to an explosion, be alert for safety hazards that may have been created by the explosion or by a terrorist. Do not enter any area that may be unsafe until properly trained personnel are able to assess the risks. Be alert for the possibility of a second explosive device that is timed to explode when rescuers are on the scene. Use the same safety skills you developed for other types of emergency situations to keep yourself safe.

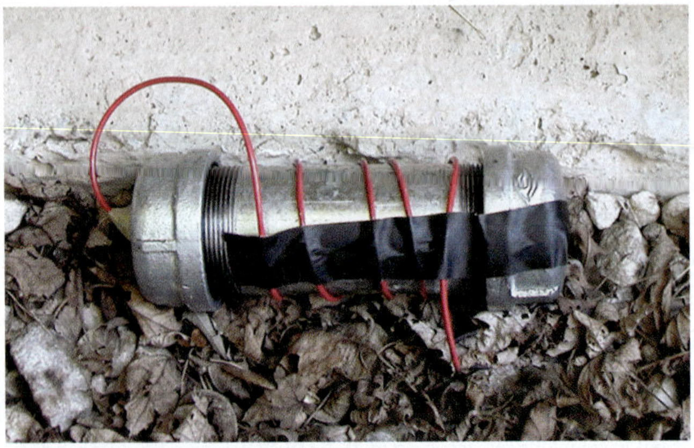

FIGURE 19-11 A pipe bomb is a simple explosive device.
Courtesy of Captain David Jackson, Saginaw Township Fire Department.

When dealing with a WMD scene, it is safe to assume you will not be able to enter where the event has occurred; nor do you want to. The best location for staging is upwind and uphill from the incident. Wait for assistance from those who are trained in assessing and managing WMD scenes.

Chemical Agents

Many different types of chemicals can be used as terrorist weapons. Chemicals used in industrial processes can be used to intentionally inflict harm on people. For example, chlorine is a gas that is used in many industrial processes and in water purification, but it was also used as a poisonous gas in World War I. Many of the **chemical agents** that could be used by terrorists are the same chemicals that create hazmat incidents when accidentally released.

Chemical agents are liquids or gases that are used to kill or injure and can be divided into the following categories:

- Pulmonary (choking) agents
- Metabolic agents
- Insecticides
- Nerve agents
- Blister agents

Pulmonary Agents. **Pulmonary agents** are gases that cause immediate harm and injury. Their primary route of entry into the body is through the airway into the lungs. Once these chemicals are inhaled, they damage lung tissue, which causes fluid to escape into the lungs and results in pulmonary edema. Pulmonary agents cause intense coughing, gasping, shortness of breath, and difficulty breathing. Two common pulmonary agents are chlorine and phosgene. Phosgene gas is produced by burning Freon, which is found in most domestic air conditioners. The odor of this gas is similar to that of freshly mowed grass. The symptoms of phosgene gas exposure may be delayed for several hours after inhalation of the gas.

Although pulmonary agents could be weapons of choice for terrorists, these chemicals are also present in a variety of domestic and industrial settings and might also be encountered following an accidental release. The safety precautions for phosgene release are to keep a safe distance away until properly trained hazmat personnel can handle the situation.

Metabolic Agents. **Metabolic agents** affect the body's ability to use oxygen at the cellular level. The most common metabolic agents are cyanides. Cyanides are produced in large quantities and are used in gold and silver mining, photography, and plastics processing. Cyanide is also produced by the combustion of plastics and textiles, so there is the potential for cyanide poisoning in any house fire. Contact with cyanides produces shortness of breath, flushed skin, rapid heartbeat, seizures, coma, and cardiac arrest. The safety precautions for cyanide release are to keep a safe distance away until properly trained hazmat personnel can handle the situation.

Voices OF Experience

I had just finished my regular 8-hour paramedic shift in Lorain, Ohio. It was 2400 hours, and I was about halfway through my 20-minute drive home, when I heard a distant thud to the south, toward Elyria. When I looked in the direction of the sound, I thought I saw a glow reflecting off the clouds in the distance. The EMS agency I worked for covered both Lorain and Elyria, so I took the next right turn and headed toward the glow.

There had been an explosion at the Aztec chemical plant, which was inconveniently located in the middle of a city of approximately 50,000 residents. This occurred in the days before everyone had cell phones, and I didn't want to interfere with priority traffic by talking on the radio. One of the most important rules to remember as an emergency medical responder, and one of the most easily forgotten in the excitement of the moment is: Don't make things worse!

> **"When the time comes, you must do what you have been trained to do."**

As I drove toward the scene, I looked for flags or smoke to check the wind direction. I was in luck; I was upwind. When I got into town, I could hear from the radio traffic that both fire and medical incident command were up and running. When there was a lull in radio traffic, I called dispatch and was directed to report to dispatch at the central station.

When I arrived at dispatch, I was told to wait for an assignment with several other off-duty personnel who were already there. After about an hour, we were sent to various schools where evacuation shelters were being set up by the Red Cross. Although the fire department had not been able to identify the chemicals released, there were reports of respiratory distress.

My partner and I took a squad and reported to one of the designated schools. What we saw on our arrival was amazing. Volunteers from the Red Cross were calmly and efficiently setting up. They had already designated areas for decontamination, canteen, families, and intake. They had set up coolers, water, chairs, and cots, and they were bringing in food—and the explosion had occurred less than 2 hours before. Most of the volunteers were older adults, and they operated in a calm, friendly, and professional manner.

We were asked to set up a medical station to evaluate people who weren't feeling well. The chemical released was eventually reported to be a mild respiratory irritant. The explosion was caused by a worker, who was the only one to die in the blast. By morning, everyone was allowed to go back home.

It doesn't matter what caused a mass-casualty incident—accident, terrorism, or criminal violence—many of the principles of responding remain the same. Emergency medical responders must respond quickly, but more importantly, they must respond wisely, calmly, and efficiently. The greatest service you can perform at a disorganized scene is to create order out of chaos, calm out of calamity. To do so, you must consciously work to control your emotions as well as your physiologic response to stress. Slow down, breathe slowly and deeply, and lower your voice. Tunnel vision is your worst enemy. Force yourself to look around, in all directions and dimensions, and use all of your senses. These skills do not come naturally. To be good in a crisis you must train and retrain, and when the time comes, you must do what you have been trained to do.

Guy H. Haskell, PhD, NREMT-P
Firefighter, Benton Township Volunteer Fire Department, Unionville, Indiana
Paramedic, Brown Township Fire and Rescue, Mooresville, Indiana
Director, Emergency Medical and Safety Services Consultants, Bloomington, Indiana

Adapted from the personal Medical Identification Symbol of the American Medical Association.

Insecticides. Insecticides are a class of poisonous chemicals that are inhaled or absorbed through the skin. Many insecticides belong to a class of chemicals called organophosphates. Absorption of these chemicals produces the following symptoms: salivation, sweating, lacrimation (excessive tearing), urination, diarrhea, gastric upset, emesis (vomiting), and miosis (pupil constriction). The acronym for these symptoms is the word SLUDGEM:

- **S** Salivation, sweating
- **L** Lacrimation (excessive tearing of the eyes)
- **U** Urination
- **D** Defecation, drooling, diarrhea
- **G** Gastrointestinal upset and cramps
- **E** Emesis (vomiting)
- **M** Muscle twitching/miosis (pinpoint pupils)

Because insecticides are readily available, they could be used as agents by terrorists. It is important to realize that far more emergency responders have experienced accidental contact with insecticides in routine calls than during terrorist-related events. If you encounter an incident involving an insecticide, keep bystanders far enough away to prevent additional contact with the chemical. If you encounter an emergency involving multiple people with SLUDGEM symptoms, assume you are dealing with poisoning from this type of chemical and call for assistance from a trained hazmat team. Do not make contact with contaminated patients until they have been through decontamination by trained personnel to prevent the spread of contamination.

Nerve Agents. Nerve agents are among the deadliest chemicals developed. These chemicals can kill large numbers of people with small quantities and cause cardiac arrest within seconds to minutes of exposure. Discovered by scientists in search of a superior pesticide, nerve agents are much stronger organophosphates than those found in insecticides. Nerve agents, like insecticides, block an essential enzyme in the nervous system and cause SLUDGEM-like symptoms. Four of the most commonly mentioned nerve agents are sarin, soman, tabun, and V agent (VX).

In an emergency situation, your primary responsibility is to keep yourself, other rescuers, and bystanders from becoming contaminated. A well-trained hazmat team in special protective equipment is needed to remove and decontaminate people exposed to these agents. The DuoDote kit is a nerve agent antidote kit (NAAK) that contains two drugs in a single auto-injector that counteract the effects of nerve agents.

Blister Agents. When blister agents come in contact with the skin, they produce burnlike blisters. If the vapors of these agents are inhaled, they cause burns of the respiratory system. Blister agents produce pain, skin irritation, eye irritation, severe shortness of breath, and severe coughing. Blister agents include sulfur mustard and Lewisite. As with other chemical agents, blister agents pose a threat to rescuers. Only well-trained and properly dressed rescuers with a self-contained breathing apparatus (SCBA) should approach a scene that might contain these agents. **TABLE 19-1** lists characteristics of some chemical agents.

This brief summary about chemical agents will not make you an expert; rather, it is intended to provide you with enough information to help you realize the chemicals that might be used by terrorists, while deadly, are in the same classes as many of the chemicals encountered by hazmat

TABLE 19-1 Characteristics of Chemical Agents

Type	Name (Military Designation)	Odor	Lethality	Onset of Symptoms	Primary Route of Exposure
Pulmonary agents	Chlorine (Cl) Phosgene (CG)	Bleach (Cl) Cut grass (CG)	Causes irritation, choking (Cl) Severe pulmonary edema (CG)	Immediate (Cl) Delayed (CG)	Vapor hazard
Metabolic agents	Hydrogen cyanide (AC) Cyanogen chloride (CK)	Almonds (AC) Irritating (CK)	Highly lethal chemical gases; can kill within minutes; effects are reversible with antidotes	Immediate	Vapor hazard
Nerve agents	Tabun (GA) Sarin (GB) Soman (GD) V agent (VX)	Fruity or none	Most lethal chemical agents; can kill within minutes; effects are reversible with antidotes	Immediate	Both vapor and contact (GA, GD) Vapor hazard (GB) Contact hazard (VX)
Blister agents	Mustard (H) Lewisite (L) Phosgene oxime (CX)	Garlic (H) Geranium (L)	Causes large blisters to form on victims; may severely damage upper airway if vapors are inhaled; severe, intense pain and gray skin discoloration	Delayed (H) Immediate (L, CX)	Primarily contact, with some vapor hazard

© Jones & Bartlett Learning

teams. Any time there are multiple people experiencing unexplained symptoms, you should suspect a common agent as the cause. Your primary role is to recognize that a problem exists and to avoid contaminating yourself, other rescuers, and bystanders. Stay upwind from any potential source and call for assistance from a properly trained hazmat team.

Biologic Agents

Biologic agents are naturally occurring substances that produce diseases. They may be bacteria, such as anthrax or the plague, or viruses, such as smallpox or hemorrhagic fever. Many biologic agents caused epidemics of disease in the past. Some of these agents, such as smallpox, have been wiped out; the last natural case of smallpox was seen in 1977. However, the smallpox organism has been maintained in laboratories and could be used intentionally to infect people. Although biologic agents are hard to disperse to large numbers of people, there is some concern that they could be used as a deadly weapon by terrorists.

Safety

Remember, hazardous chemical releases and terrorist events often result in large numbers of patients who are experiencing the same symptoms at the same time. For example, the report of multiple patients reporting difficulty breathing in the subway at rush hour, when no hint of smoke is evident, is cause for suspicion. You must resist the urge to rush into scenes when there are multiple victims from an unknown cause.

If terrorists intentionally dispersed a biologic agent, the organism would have to come in contact with people in sufficient quantities to produce an illness. These diseases have an **incubation period**, which is the time between exposure to a disease organism to the time the person begins to show symptoms of the disease. This means that if people were exposed to an infectious organism today, it might be several days before they would show signs of the disease. The first awareness of a biologic terrorist incident would probably come from hospital emergency departments and public health departments. Your role in biologic incidents is to report unusual patterns of illness and keep up to date on current information from your medical director and public health department.

Safety considerations for EMRs include being alert for unusual patterns of diseases with flulike symptoms. You should make every effort to review current information about disease trends from your medical director and public health department. Practice appropriate standard precautions for the signs and symptoms exhibited by every patient. If you have any indications that a call might involve a biologic agent, call for specifically trained assistance and wait in a safe location.

You need to be aware of multiple potential risks of exposure to biologic agents. For example, if the agent is in the form of a powder, such as in the October 2001 attacks involving anthrax-laced letters mailed through the US Postal Service, the incident must be handled by hazmat specialists. Patients who have come into direct contact with the agent need to be decontaminated before any EMS contact or treatment is initiated.

Safety

Remember to take standard precautions any time there is a chance that an infectious disease organism might be present. Because many biologic materials are transmitted by air or indirect contact, standard precautions include wearing gloves, a gown, and a HEPA (high-efficiency particulate air) mask.

Radiologic Agents

Ionizing radiation is a kind of energy that is formed by the decay of a naturally occurring or human-made radioactive source. **Radiation** is used in hospitals, research facilities, and nuclear power plants, and it is also used for military weapons. Exposure to excess amounts of radiation can cause delayed illnesses, such as an increase in the rate of certain cancers. Exposure to large amounts of radiation can cause people to become violently ill within a few hours of exposure and may cause death within hours or days. **TABLE 19-2** lists some signs and symptoms of radiation sickness.

Radiation is a hidden hazard that is similar to electricity. You cannot see, feel, or detect radiation with any of your normal body senses. Special instruments are needed to detect and measure the amount of radiation that is present (**FIGURE 19-12**).

Some concern exists that terrorists could detonate an explosive device containing a small amount of radioactive

YOU are the EMR **CASE 3**

You are called to assist an EMS team at the scene of a fire at a plastics factory. When you arrive, you are informed that a smoky fire inside the building has almost been extinguished by the fire department. As you approach the scene, you are directed by the incident commander to assist with the treatment of three patients in a treatment area. The patients all report shortness of breath and have flushed skin and a rapid heart rate. The patients tell you they were working in the plastics factory when some of the materials caught fire, and they breathed in some smoke while escaping from the fire.

1. On the basis of the patients' signs and symptoms and the history surrounding the incident, what type of agent do you think is involved?
2. How would you ensure you are in a safe location?

TABLE 19-2 Common Signs of Acute Radiation Sickness

Low exposure	Nausea, vomiting, diarrhea
Moderate exposure	Superficial burns, hair loss, depletion of the immune system (death of white blood cells), cancer
Severe exposure	Partial- and full-thickness burns, cancer, death

© Jones & Bartlett Learning

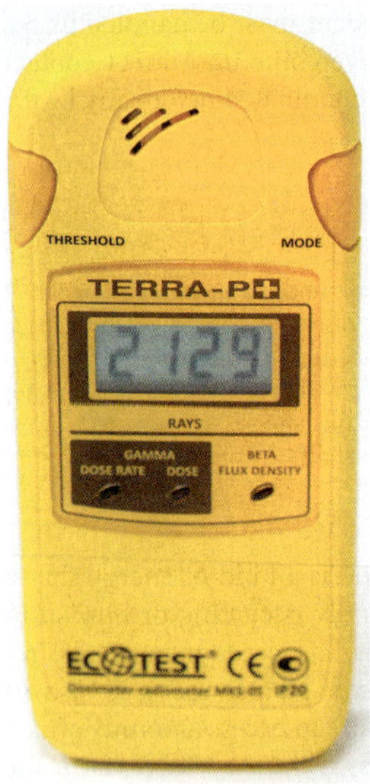

FIGURE 19-12 A personal dosimeter measures the amount of radioactive exposure received by an individual.
© rootstock/Shutterstock

material (known as a **dirty bomb**). Such an explosion would spread radioactive material over the area of the explosion and thereby contaminate anyone in the vicinity. In a situation like this, rescuers would have no means of determining whether radioactivity was present unless special monitors were used to check for radiation. Unless there was a warning issued about such an event, rescuers might not know about the presence of radiation.

As an EMR, you need to be alert to warnings about incidents involving radiation. If the presence of radiation is suspected, you should stay away from a blast or suspicious site until specifically trained teams check for the presence of radiation with special monitoring devices. Know what agencies in your community are equipped to handle such an event.

Words of Wisdom

One way to remember the classes of substances that could be used by terrorists is with the acronym B-NICE:

B Biologic
N Nuclear
I Incendiary devices
C Chemicals
E Explosives

Your Response to Terrorist Events

The threat of terrorist activity is frightening to most people. It is important that all emergency responders have some awareness and knowledge of the various tactics and agents terrorists might use. Emergency response personnel need to develop an all-hazards approach for managing these emergencies. Keep in mind that agents used by terrorists could be the same agents that you are already trained to deal with: explosions, fires, toxic chemicals, hazardous materials, infectious diseases, and radiation. Although you may feel apprehensive about responding to a terrorist event, remember the same safety rules apply in all emergencies: good scene safety and diligent use of standard precautions.

To prepare for a terrorist event, master the skills that enable you to be a good EMR. Be prepared and know the limits of your training. Many types of terrorist events require you to stay a certain distance away to avoid contaminating additional people. Teams with special training are required to manage incidents involving special hazards. Be alert for secondary devices placed by a terrorist and set to detonate after emergency responders arrive at the scene.

Terrorist events can affect large numbers of people. Establish an ICS as soon as possible (**FIGURE 19-13**). Know your role in working within the ICS. Treat these incidents as mass-casualty situations. Establish good working relationships with appropriate local, state, and federal agencies.

EMRs have a vital role in working at terrorist events. You can do the most good by following your training and not exceeding your skill level. Always be alert for your safety, the safety of other rescuers, and the safety of patients. Remember, you cannot be an effective rescuer if you become a victim yourself.

YOU are the EMR **CASE 4**

You are responding to an explosion in the downtown area. As you approach the scene, you see a cloud of smoke coming from a building. While you wait for the hazmat team at a safe distance, you see people walking out of the building toward your vehicle. The people are coughing, have blisters on their skin, and look like they are having difficulty breathing.

1. What agent is most likely causing these signs and symptoms?
2. What other resources will potentially be needed at this scene?

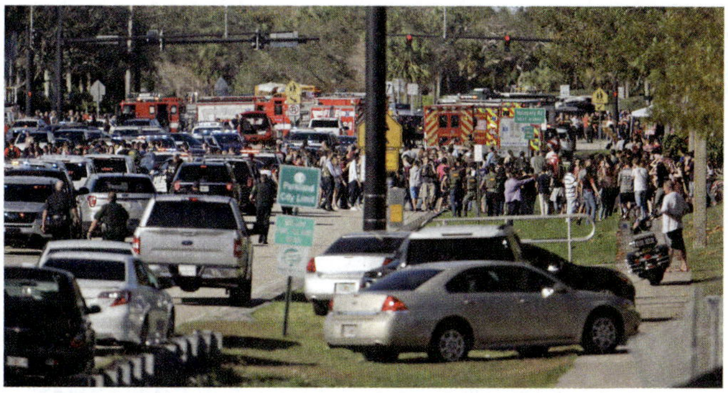

FIGURE 19-13 An incident command system needs to be set up for large-scale terrorist and mass-casualty events.
© Amy Beth Bennett/*Sun Sentinel*/Tribune News Service via Getty Images

Words of Wisdom

Terrorism is no longer something that happens "somewhere else," as the attacks on the World Trade Center, the Pentagon, and the Walmart in El Paso, Texas, proved. As an EMR, be aware of the possibility of a terrorist event. Realize that a major incident may be dispatched as a routine call. Your skill in assessing scene safety could be vital in saving lives. Be especially alert for clues that point toward special hazards, and take advantage of training offered in your local community.

YOU are the EMR SUMMARY

You are the EMR: CASE 1

1. What initial actions should you take at this scene?

Your role in an incident that may involve hazardous materials is to look for and identify, from a safe distance, any hazardous materials involved while protecting yourself and keeping yourself and others away from the hazardous materials. The actual mitigation of a hazmat incident needs to be accomplished by a specifically trained hazmat team.

2. What initial actions should you take if this incident turns out to be an MCI?

Your role as an EMR in an MCI is as follows:

- Determine the approximate number of patients.
- Determine the number of patients that you have triaged.
- Report any additional assistance required.
- Report any other important information.

You are the EMR: CASE 2

1. In what triage category does this patient belong?

The patient's respirations are 24, which is within acceptable limits, and by itself is not a reason for concern. This patient did not walk to the green triage area, so you can suspect she has some type of injury that kept her from joining this group. As you assess her circulatory status you note a weak carotid pulse and no palpable radial pulse in the wrist. These findings place this patient in the immediate category. This patient should receive a red tag and be immediately taken to the treatment area and prepared for transport. At this point an assessment of the patient's mental status would not serve to change her triage assessment from the red category. Take spinal precautions into consideration when attempting to move this patient.

2. What is the appropriate treatment for this patient?

There appears to be a decrease in the patient's circulation; therefore, you should begin immediate treatment for shock. After taking spinal precautions into consideration, lay the patient supine. Attempt to identify and correct any sources of external bleeding. Cover the patient with a blanket to maintain body temperature. Transport as soon as possible.

You are the EMR: CASE 3

1. On the basis of the patients' signs and symptoms and the history surrounding the incident, what type of agent do you think is involved?

The burning or combustion of materials involving plastics has the potential to release numerous toxins. The most likely type of agent affecting these patients is a pulmonary agent that they have inhaled. A wide variety of chemicals are present in plastics and can be released during a fire. It is impossible to identify specific toxins without sophisticated testing. You need to treat the symptoms the patients are experiencing. Also, you need to confirm with the hazmat team that you are in a location that is removed from toxic fumes and that you will not be contaminated by the patients.

2. How would you ensure you are in a safe location?

You need to check with the hazmat team. One of the responsibilities of the hazmat team is to designate areas or zones at an incident involving hazardous materials. Hot zones are designated for the area immediately involved with the hazardous material. Warm zones are outside the immediate hazardous area but still pose a risk to people who are not properly protected. This is typically an area where patients exposed to the agent are decontaminated.

YOU are the EMR SUMMARY

After decontamination, patients are sent to the cold zone. Cold zones are safe areas for non-hazmat personnel to operate without fear of exposure to the agent. Although safety considerations still need to be exercised, this is a safe area for the triage and treatment of patients.

You are the EMR: CASE 4

1. What agent is most likely causing these signs and symptoms?

Many agents can cause respiratory distress; however, agents that cause blistering of the skin and trouble breathing are not that common. These patients are likely experiencing an exposure to a blistering agent, such as mustard gas or Lewisite. These agents produce burnlike blisters and can cause burns of the respiratory system, resulting in respiratory distress.

2. What other resources will potentially be needed at this scene?

Hazmat services will be your primary resource at this scene. However, there are other resources that may be necessary. The fire department typically works in conjunction with the hazmat team and EMS. Police may be needed to help control the scene and to assist in area evacuation. In addition, your local health department and the Red Cross may be needed as well.

Prep Kit

Ready for Review

- Because you may be the first trained person on the scene of an incident involving hazardous materials, you must be able to identify the signs of a potential hazmat incident and respond appropriately.
- During a hazmat incident, your top priority is to recognize that a hazard is present and protect yourself and bystanders from exposure and contamination from the hazardous material.
- You should understand the role of an EMR during the first few minutes of an MCI.
- The START triage system is a simple triage system that you can use at MCIs. It serves to sort patients into groups so that the most serious patients are treated and transported first.
- The National Incident Management System (NIMS) is designed to provide a unified approach to emergency incidents of any size that involve multiple agencies anywhere in the United States. All emergency responders need to have some understanding of this system.
- Terrorist attacks, although rare, are a concern for emergency responders. The goal of terrorists is to intimidate a population or government. Terrorists may use a wide variety of methods to incite terror, including the use of explosives, fire, chemicals, viruses, bacteria, and radiation.
- Chemical agents are human-made substances that can have devastating effects on living organisms. Types consist of pulmonary, metabolic, insecticide, nerve, and blister agents.
- Biologic agents are organisms that cause disease. They are generally found in nature and can be weaponized to maximize the number of people exposed to the germ.
- Radiologic weapons can create a massive amount of destruction. This type of weapon includes radiologic dispersal devices, also known as dirty bombs.
- EMRs need to consider their safety, the safety of other rescuers, and the safety of bystanders whenever responding to a terrorist-related event. Your responsibility as an EMR in many of these situations is to identify potential threats, ensure safety, and call for specifically trained personnel to deal with these threats.

Vital Vocabulary

biologic agents Naturally occurring substances that cause disease. Terrorists may use bacteria, viruses, or toxins to intentionally cause epidemics of disease.

blister agents Chemicals that cause the skin to blister.

casualty sorting The sorting of patients to determine the order in which patients should be treated and transported.

chemical agents Compounds that can be used by terrorists to inflict harm.

cold zone The controlled area that contains the command post and other support functions needed in the incident.

decontamination The process of reducing or preventing the spread of contaminants at a hazardous materials event.

Prep Kit

dirty bomb An explosive device using conventional explosives that is designed to spread radioactive material over a wide area.

explosives Substances that release energy in a sudden and uncontrolled manner when detonated.

hazardous material Any substance that is toxic, poisonous, radioactive, flammable, or explosive and can cause injury or death with exposure.

hazmat incident An emergency involving a hazardous material (often abbreviated hazmat as an adjective).

hot zone A contaminated area.

incendiary devices Substances or weapons designed to start a fire.

incident command system (ICS) A system of people, procedures, and equipment designed to improve emergency response operations at situations of all types and complexities.

incubation period The time between exposure to a disease organism and the time the person begins to show symptoms of the disease.

insecticides Chemicals that are formulated to kill insects but that can intentionally or accidentally cause injury or death to humans when inhaled or absorbed through the skin.

mass-casualty incident (MCI) An accident or situation involving more patients than the responding agency can handle with the initial resources available.

metabolic agents Substances that are intended to produce injury or death by disrupting the body's ability to use oxygen and chemical reactions at the cellular level.

mutual aid An agreement between neighboring EMS systems to respond when local resources are insufficient to handle the response.

National Incident Management System (NIMS) A system developed by the US Department of Homeland Security for managing an emergency incident, which may require the response of many different agencies; designed to provide a comprehensive, efficient, and effective management approach from initial response through recovery.

nerve agents Deadly toxic substances that attack the central nervous system.

pulmonary agents Substances that produce respiratory distress or illness.

radiation The electromagnetic energy that is released from a radioactive material or a dirty bomb.

START triage A patient sorting process based on three primary observations: breathing, circulation, and mental status. START stands for Simple Triage And Rapid Treatment.

terrorism A systematic use of violence to intimidate or to achieve a political goal.

traffic incident management (TIM) A system that specifies where to place vehicles and warning devices to achieve a safe scene while highway incidents are being resolved.

triage The sorting of patients into groups according to the severity of their injuries; used to determine priorities for medical treatment and transport.

warm zone The controlled area where personnel and equipment decontamination and hot zone support take place.

weapon of mass destruction (WMD) Any agent designed to bring about mass death, casualties, and/or massive damage to property and infrastructure (bridges, tunnels, airports, electrical power plants, and seaports).

References

Chemical Hazards Emergency Medical Management. START adult triage algorithm: text version. US Department of Health and Human Services. https://chemm.hhs.gov/startalgotext.htm. Updated December 26, 2024. Accessed January 27, 2025.

Department of Homeland Security. *National Incident Management System*. Federal Emergency Management Agency website. https://www.fema.gov/emergency-managers/nims. Updated March 21, 2024. Accessed January 27, 2025.

National EMS Management Association. *Operational Templates and Guidance for EMS Mass Incident Deployment*. Emmitsburg, MD: US Fire Administration; 2012. https://www.usfa.fema.gov/downloads/pdf/publications/templates_guidance_ems_mass_incident_deployment.pdf. Accessed January 27, 2025.

NFPA 3000, Standard for an Active Shooter/Hostile Event Response Program. National Fire Protection Administration website. https://www.nfpa.org/product/nfpa-3000-standard/p3000code#. Published 2024. Accessed January 27, 2025.

US Department of Transportation. *2024 Emergency Response Guidebook*. Pipelines and Hazardous Materials Safety Administration website. https://www.phmsa.dot.gov/sites/phmsa.dot.gov/files/2024-04/ERG2024-Eng-Web-a.pdf. Published 2024. Accessed January 27, 2025.

Assessment IN ACTION

You are dispatched for a report of several students who are short of breath and coughing at a local high school. As you arrive at the school, you find several students in the parking lot who are experiencing difficulty breathing.

1. Which of the following should NOT be one of your first actions?
   - A. Park upwind of the school.
   - B. Call for additional assistance.
   - C. Enter the school building to investigate.
   - D. Transmit an initial report to the dispatcher.
2. What type of assistance is probably not needed right away?
   - A. Fire department support
   - B. Hazmat team
   - C. Law enforcement personnel
   - D. Highway department
3. What type of substance should you suspect might be involved in this incident?
   - A. Blister agent
   - B. Pulmonary agent
   - C. Insecticide
   - D. Chemical agent
4. What is the first step in the START triage system?
   - A. Begin tagging patients.
   - B. Walk among the injured patients.
   - C. Instruct patients who can walk to move to a specified area.
   - D. Ask patients individually if they can walk to a different area.
5. Match each of the following colors with the appropriate level of triage in the START system.
   - A. Green
   - B. Black
   - C. Red
   - D. Yellow

   _______ Immediate care/life threatening
   _______ Urgent care/can be delayed up to 1 hour
   _______ Patient is dead; no care required
   _______ Care can be delayed up to 3 hours
6. What are the key points to communicate to the dispatcher when you are at the scene of an MCI?
7. What are your primary goals when assessing patients in an MCI?
8. What types of treatment do you want to avoid in an MCI?
9. Do you need consent to begin treatment of these patients?
10. What are the possibilities for additional people to become symptomatic at the scene?

Appendix: Medical Terminology

As an emergency medical responder (EMR), it is important that you have some knowledge of medical terminology. The medical terms you will most often use as an EMR are identified throughout the text. This appendix explains some rules for breaking down medical terms and introduces additional terms that you may encounter.

Understanding key terms, symbols, and abbreviations is important for effective communication and documentation. Once you understand medical jargon, you will be able to communicate more effectively with other members of the emergency medical services (EMS), health care, and public safety teams.

Anatomy of a Medical Term

Medical terms are made of distinct parts that perform specific functions. Each term may include one or more of the following parts:

- **Word root:** the foundation of the word
- **Prefix:** a word part that occurs before the word root
- **Suffix:** a word part that occurs after the word root
- **Combining vowels:** vowels that join one or more word roots to other components of a term

The meaning of each part and the manner in which the parts come together determine the word's meaning. Changing or deleting any of those parts can significantly change the meaning.

Word Roots

The main part or stem of a word is called a word root, sometimes referred to as a *root word.* A word root conveys the essential meaning of the word and frequently indicates a body part. Most terms have at least one word root, and some have more than one word root. A frequently used medical term is cardiopulmonary resuscitation. *Cardiopulmonary* breaks down as follows: *cardi* is a word root meaning "heart," and *pulmon* is a word root meaning "lungs." By performing *cardiopulmonary* resuscitation (CPR), you introduce air into the *lungs* and circulate blood by compressing the *heart* to resuscitate the patient.

Note that some word roots may also be used as prefixes or suffixes for other terms.

Examples of some word roots are shown in **TABLE A-1**.

Prefixes

A prefix is the part of a term that appears at the beginning of a word. It generally describes location and intensity. Prefixes are frequently found in everyday language (for example, *au*topilot, *sub*marine, *tri*cycle), as well as in medical and scientific terminology. Not all medical terms have prefixes.

A prefix gives the word root a specific meaning. When a medical word contains a prefix, the meaning of the word is altered. For example, *pnea* is the word root for breathing. Adding the prefix *a-* (without), *brady-* (slow), or *tachy-* (rapid) to this word root creates three very different terms:

- a/pnea (without breathing)
- brady/pnea (slow breathing)
- tachy/pnea (rapid breathing)

Some common prefixes are shown in **TABLE A-2**.

Suffixes

Suffixes are placed at the end of words and usually indicate a procedure, condition, disease, or part of speech. A commonly used suffix is *-itis*, which means "inflammation." When this suffix is paired with the word root *arthro-*, meaning "joint," the resulting word is *arthritis*, an inflammation of the joints.

Some common suffixes are listed in **TABLE A-3**.

TABLE A-1 Common Word Roots in EMS

Root	Meaning	Example	Definition of Example
cardi	heart	tachycardia	fast heart rate
hepat	liver	hepatomegaly	enlargement of the liver
nephr	kidney	nephropathy	disease of the kidney
neur	nerves	neurologist	physician who specializes in diseases of the nervous system
psych	mind	psychology	study of the mind
thorac	chest	thoracic	pertaining to the chest or thorax

© Jones & Bartlett Learning

TABLE A-2 Common Prefixes in EMS

Prefix	Meaning	Example	Definition of Example
hyper-	over, excessive, high	hyperventilation	fast ventilations
hypo-	under, below normal	hypoperfusion	below-normal blood flow to vital organs
tachy-	rapid, fast	tachycardia	fast heart rate
brady-	slow	bradypnea	slow breathing
pre-	before	prenatal	occurring before birth
post-	after, behind	postsurgical	occurring after surgery

© Jones & Bartlett Learning

TABLE A-3 Common Suffixes in EMS

Suffix	Meaning	Example	Definition of Example
-al	pertaining to	syncopal	pertaining to syncope
-algia	pertaining to pain	arthralgia	joint pain
-ectomy	surgical removal of	appendectomy	surgical removal of the appendix
-ic	pertaining to	diaphoretic	pertaining to diaphoresis
-itis	inflammation of	epiglottitis	inflammation of the epiglottis
-logy	study of	cardiology	the study of the heart
-logist	specialist	pulmonologist	specialist in diseases of the lung
-megaly	enlargement	cardiomegaly	enlargement of the heart
-meter	measuring instrument	sphygmomanometer	instrument to measure blood pressure
-oma	tumor (usually referring to cancer)	lymphoma	cancer of the lymphatic system
-pathy	disease	nephropathy	diseases of the kidneys

© Jones & Bartlett Learning

Combining Vowels

A combining vowel is the part of a term that connects a word root to a suffix or other word root. In most cases, the combining vowel is an *o*; however, it may also be an *i* or an *e*. A combining vowel is usually used when joining a suffix that begins with a consonant or when joining another word root. For example, take the term *gastroenterology*, the study of diseases of the stomach and small intestines:

- gastr/o + enter/o + logy
- stomach + small intestines + the study of

In this term, *gastr* and *enter* are both word roots, *-logy* is the suffix, and *o* is the combining vowel (used twice). The combining vowel helps ease the pronunciation of the term. Without the vowel, the term would be rather difficult to pronounce: *gastrenterlogy.*

A combining vowel shown with the word root is called a combining form. Here are a few of the most common combining forms you will see:

- cardi/o (heart)
- gastr/o (stomach)
- hepat/o (liver)
- arthr/o (joint)
- oste/o (bone)
- pulmon/o (lungs)

Putting the Parts Together

You can use your knowledge of word parts to decipher the meaning of a full term. The following summarizes the rules covered thus far:

1. The prefix, if included in a term, is always at the beginning of the term.
2. The suffix, if included in a term, is always at the end.
3. A combining vowel may be used between word parts to aid in pronunciation.

When trying to define a term, begin with the suffix and work backward. If the term also contains a prefix, define the suffix, followed by the prefix, and then the word root. Here are some examples:

- nephropathy
  nephr/o/pathy
  -pathy (suffix meaning "disease")
  o (combining form)
  nephr (word root meaning "kidney")
  nephropathy = disease of the kidney
- dysuria
  dys/ur/ia
  -ia (suffix meaning "condition of")
  dys- (prefix meaning "difficult, painful, or abnormal")
  ur (word root meaning "urine")
  dysuria = painful urination (pain when urinating) or difficulty urinating
- hyperemesis
  hyper/emesis
  hyper- (prefix meaning "excessive")
  emesis (word root meaning "vomiting")
  hyperemesis = excessive vomiting
- analgesic
  an/alges/ic
  -ic (suffix meaning "pertaining to")
  an- (prefix meaning "without" or "absence of")
  alges (word root meaning "pain")
  analgesic = pertaining to no pain

Plural Endings

To change a term from a singular to plural form, certain rules apply. Often, you simply add an *s* to the word (*lung* becomes *lungs*). However, for some medical terms, making the plural

Words of Wisdom

How the parts of a term are combined determines its meaning. Accurate spelling, especially when some words are pronounced almost the same way, is essential in medical terminology. For example, the suffix *-phasia* means speaking, whereas *-phagia* means eating or swallowing. The prefix *dys-* means difficult or painful. Combining those two parts, *dysphasia* means difficulty speaking, whereas *dysphagia* means difficulty eating or swallowing. These are very different terms, and the two words, although spelled differently, sound almost identical. Likewise, the terms *ilium* and *ileum* are pronounced exactly the same but refer to different anatomic parts. The ilium is the largest bone of the pelvis, and the ileum is the last part of the small intestine. Knowing anatomy and the context of how these words are used will help you correctly determine (and spell) the term in a given situation.

form is more complicated. You may encounter the following rules when converting terms from singular to plural:

1. The singular ending *a* changes to *ae* when plural.
   - Example: *vertebra* becomes *vertebrae*.
2. The singular ending *is* changes to *es* when plural.
   - Example: *diagnosis* becomes *diagnoses*.
3. The singular ending *ex* or *ix* changes to *ices*.
   - Example: *apex* becomes *apices*.
4. The singular ending *on* or *um* changes to *a*.
   - Examples: *ganglion* becomes *ganglia*; *ovum* becomes *ova*.
5. The singular ending *us* changes to *i*.
   - Example: *bronchus* becomes *bronchi*.

Special Word Parts

As already described, prefixes appear at the beginning of a word, before the word root. Prefixes used to indicate numbers, colors, and directions are described in the following sections. Look at the prefixes, meanings, and examples. Can you think of other terms using the same prefix with another root? Do you see how it changes the meaning?

Numbers

Several prefixes are used to indicate if a term involves a number such as one-half, one, or two or more parts or sides. Common prefixes for numbers are listed in **TABLE A-4**.

Colors

Several word roots are used to describe color. The most common include those listed in **TABLE A-5**.

Position and Direction

Prefixes can also be used to describe a position, direction, or location. The most common include those listed in **TABLE A-6**.

Movement

The following terms relate to movement (**FIGURE A-1**):

- **Flexion:** the bending of a joint
- **Extension:** the straightening of a joint
- **Adduction:** motion toward the midline
- **Abduction:** motion away from the midline

TABLE A-4 Common Number Prefixes

Prefix	Meaning	Example	Definition of Example
uni-	one	unilateral	one side
dipl-	two; double	diplopia	double vision
null-	none	nullipara	never given birth
primi-	first	primigravida	pregnant for the first time
multi-	many	multiparous	giving birth to more than one offspring at a time
bi-	two	bilateral	pertaining to both sides
tri-	three	trigeminy	irregular heartbeat of two normal beats followed by one premature beat
quad-	four	quadriplegic	paralysis of all four extremities
tetra-	four	tetralogy of Fallot	a congenital defect involving four anatomic abnormalities of the heart
semi-	half; partial	semiconscious	partially conscious
hemi-	half; one-sided	hemiplegia	paralysis on one side of the body
ambi-	both	ambidextrous	able to use either hand equally well
pan-	all, entire	pandemic	an epidemic over a wide area

© Jones & Bartlett Learning

TABLE A-5 Word Roots That Describe Color

Root	Meaning	Example	Definition of Example
cyan/o	blue	cyanosis	blue discoloration of the skin
leuk/o	white	leukocyte	white blood cells that fight infection
erythr/o	red	erythrocyte	red blood cells that contain hemoglobin to carry oxygen
cirrh/o	yellow-orange	cirrhosis	inflammation of the liver causing yellow-orange pigmentation of the liver
melan/o	black	melena	black, tarry stool typically caused by upper gastrointestinal bleeding

© Jones & Bartlett Learning

Words of Wisdom

Some of the words used to describe a patient's skin presentation, such as pallor and cyanosis, originate from Greek or Latin terms indicating specific colors. For example, *jaundice* is derived from the Latin term *galbinus*, meaning "greenish yellow." *Pallor* is derived from the Latin term *pallidus*, meaning "without color" and in many contexts has come to indicate "whiteness." In medicine, these terms have clinical importance in conveying a pathologic process, not a specific color. Pallor may indeed present as whiteness in the skin of a person with a light complexion, but it may appear as grayness in the skin of a person with a darker complexion. In either case, the clinical importance is that the person appears to be experiencing poor perfusion. When assessing a patient's skin color, you must understand how a pathologic process may present in that particular person, with consideration of their baseline skin tone. In patients with dark skin, you may need to assess areas such as the oral mucosa, conjunctiva, nail beds, or palms.

TABLE A-6 Prefixes That Describe Position

Prefix	Meaning	Example	Definition of Example
To/From			
ab-	away from	abduction	away from the point of reference
ad-	to, toward	adduction	toward the center
Above/Below/Around			
de-	down, from, away	decay	to waste away
circum-	around, about	circumferential burn	a burn around an entire area (arm, chest, abdomen, etc.)
peri-	around	pericardium	the sac around the heart
trans-	across, through, beyond	transvaginal	across or through the vagina
epi-	above, upon, on	epigastric	above or over the stomach
supra-	above, over	suprasternal notch	top of the sternum
retro-	behind	retroperitoneal	the area behind the peritoneum
sub-	under, beneath	subcutaneous	beneath the skin
infra-	below, under	infraclavicular	below the clavicle
para-	near, beside, beyond, apart from	parasternal	beside the sternum
contra-	against, opposite	contraindicated	something that is not indicated
Outside/Inside			
ecto-	out, outside	ectopic pregnancy	pregnancy in which the embryo attaches outside the uterus
endo-	within	endoscopy	examining inside someone's body (with an endoscope)
extra-	outside, in addition	extraneous	outside the organism and not belonging to it
intra-	inside, within	intrauterine	within the uterus
ipsi-	same	ipsilateral	on or affecting the same side

© Jones & Bartlett Learning

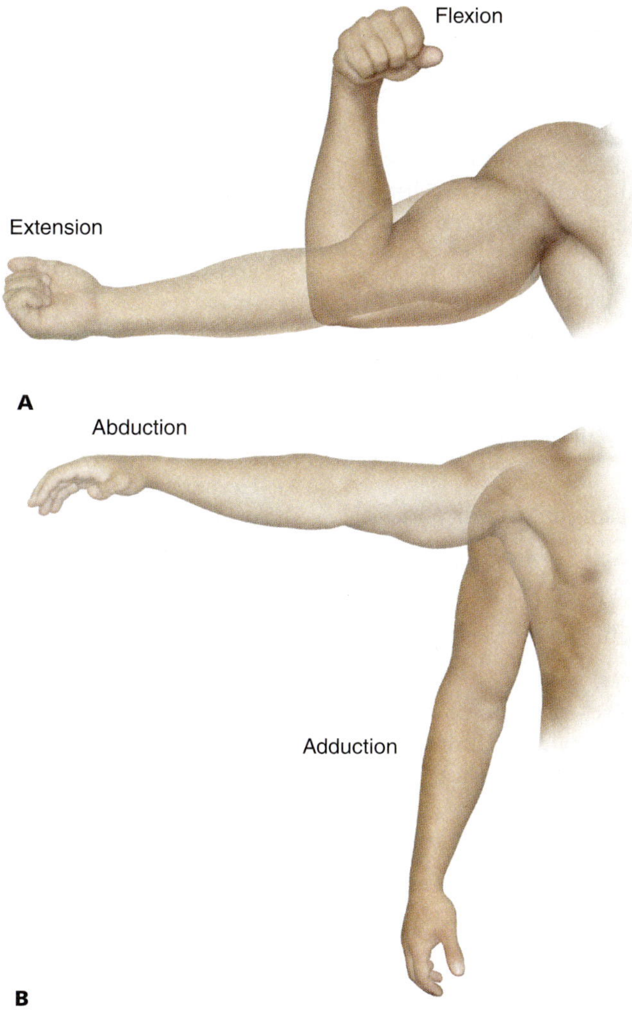

FIGURE A-1 **A.** Flexion and extension at the elbow. **B.** Adduction and abduction at the shoulder.
© Jones & Bartlett Learning

Glossary

abandonment Failure of the emergency medical responder to continue emergency medical treatment until relieved by someone with the same or a higher level of training.

abdomen The body cavity between the thorax and the pelvis that contains the major organs of digestion and excretion.

abdominal aortic aneurysm (AAA) A condition in which the layers of the aorta in the abdomen weaken. This causes blood to leak between the layers of the artery, causing it to bulge and sometimes rupture.

abdominal breathing Breathing using only the diaphragm.

abrasion Loss or damage of skin as a result of a body part being rubbed or scraped across a rough or hard surface.

acid A chemical substance with a pH level of less than 7.0 that can cause severe burns.

acute abdomen The sudden onset of abdominal pain caused by disease or trauma that irritates the lining of the abdominal cavity and requires immediate medical or surgical treatment.

acute respiratory distress syndrome (ARDS) A condition in which severe lung injury produces swelling and fluid buildup in the alveoli, possibly leading to respiratory failure.

advanced emergency medical technician (AEMT) A person who is qualified to perform basic life support skills and limited advanced life support skills.

advance directive A legal document that indicates what a person wants done if they are unable to make their own medical decisions. Advance directives include living wills, durable powers of attorney for health care, and do not resuscitate orders.

advanced life support (ALS) The use of specialized equipment (such as cardiac monitors and defibrillators) and specialized techniques (such as intravenous fluid administration, drug infusion, and endotracheal intubation) to stabilize a patient's condition.

air embolism A bubble of air obstructing a blood vessel.

airway The passages from the openings of the mouth and nose to the air sacs in the lungs through which air enters and leaves the lungs.

airway obstruction Partial (mild) or complete (severe) obstruction of the respiratory passages resulting from blockage by food, small objects, or vomitus.

altered mental status A sudden or gradual decrease in the person's level of responsiveness; measured using the AVPU scale.

alveolar ventilation The exchange of oxygen and carbon dioxide that occurs in the alveoli.

alveoli The air sacs of the lungs where the exchange of oxygen and carbon dioxide takes place.

Alzheimer disease The most common subtype of dementia, characterized by confusion, memory failure, disorientation, speech disturbances, and inability to carry out purposeful movements.

amphetamines Stimulants that produce a general mood elevation, improve task performance, suppress appetite, or prevent sleepiness.

anaphylactic shock A type of shock caused by an extreme allergic reaction to certain foods, medications, or insect bites and stings.

angina pectoris Chest pain with squeezing or tightness in the chest caused by an inadequate flow of blood to the heart muscle.

anterior The front surface of the body.

antivenin A serum that counteracts the effect of venom from an animal or insect.

anus The distal or terminal ending of the gastrointestinal tract.

appropriate medical facility A hospital or medical clinic with adequate medical resources to provide continuing care to sick or injured patients who have been transported after field treatment by emergency medical responders.

arm The upper portion of the upper extremity; from the shoulder to the elbow.

arm-to-arm drag An emergency move that consists of the rescuer grasping the patient's arms from behind; used to remove a patient from a hazardous environment.

arterial bleeding Serious bleeding from an artery in which blood frequently pulses or spurts from an open wound.

aspiration Breathing in foreign matter such as food, drink, or vomitus into the airway or lungs.

aspirator A suction device.

assessment-based care A system of patient evaluation in which the chief complaint of the patient and other signs and symptoms are gathered. The care given is based on this information rather than on a formal diagnosis.

asthma A disease in which the airway becomes narrowed and inflamed, resulting in episodes of shortness of breath because of air being trapped in the small air sacs of the lungs.

atherosclerosis A disease characterized by thickening and destruction of the arterial walls and caused by fatty deposits within them; the arteries lose the ability to dilate and carry blood.

atria The two upper chambers of the heart.

auscultation Listening to sounds with a stethoscope.

automated external defibrillator (AED) A portable, battery-powered device that recognizes ventricular fibrillation (and ventricular tachycardia) and advises when a countershock is indicated. The device delivers an electric shock to patients with ventricular fibrillation.

AVPU scale A scale to measure a patient's level of consciousness. The letters stand for Alert, Verbal, Pain, and Unresponsive.

avulsion An injury in which a piece of skin is torn completely loose or is left hanging as a flap.

backboard A straight board used for splinting, extricating, and transporting patients with suspected spinal injuries.

bag-mask device A patient ventilation device that consists of a bag, one-way valves, and a face mask.

bag of waters The amniotic sac and fluid that surround the fetus before birth.

bariatric Relating to or specializing in the prevention and treatment of obesity.

base A chemical with a pH level of greater than 7.0. Bases are also called caustics or alkalis.

base station A powerful two-way radio that is permanently mounted in a communications center.

basic life support (BLS) Emergency lifesaving procedures performed without advanced emergency procedures to stabilize the condition of patients who have experienced sudden illness or injury.

bath salts The common name for certain types of synthetic stimulant-type drugs.

behavioral emergency A situation in which the patient exhibits abnormal behavior that is unacceptable or cannot be tolerated by the patient or by family, friends, or the community.

biologic agents Naturally occurring substances that cause disease. Terrorists may use bacteria, viruses, or toxins to intentionally cause epidemics of disease.

birth canal The vagina and the lower part of the uterus.

blanket drag An emergency move in which a rescuer encloses a patient in a blanket and drags the patient to safety.

blister agents Chemicals that cause the skin to blister.

blood pressure The pressure of the circulating blood against the walls of the arteries.

bloody show The plug of mucus that is discharged from the vagina when labor begins.

bounding pulse A very strong pulse (similar to the pulse that follows physical exertion such as running or lifting heavy objects).

brachial pulse The pulse located on the arm between the elbow and shoulder; used for checking the pulse in infants.

breech presentation A delivery in which the newborn's buttocks appear in the birth canal first, rather than the head.

bronchi The two main branches of the trachea that lead into the right and left lungs. Within the lungs, they branch into smaller airways.

bronchiolitis Inflammation of the small airways (bronchioles) in the lungs.

bronchitis Inflammation of the airways (bronchi) in the lungs.

bruise Injury caused by a blunt object striking the body and crushing the tissue beneath the skin; also called a contusion.

capillaries The smallest blood vessels that connect small arteries and small veins. Capillary walls serve as the membrane to exchange oxygen and carbon dioxide.

capillary bleeding Bleeding from the capillaries in which blood oozes from the open wound.

capillary refill The ability of the circulatory system to restore blood to the capillary blood vessels after it has been squeezed out by the examiner.

carbon dioxide The gas formed as a waste product of metabolism and excreted through the respiratory system during exhalation.

carbon monoxide A colorless, odorless, tasteless, poisonous gas formed by incomplete combustion, such as in a fire.

cardiac arrest Cessation of breathing and a heartbeat.

cardiogenic shock A type of shock resulting from inadequate functioning of the heart.

cardiopulmonary resuscitation (CPR) The combination of chest compressions and rescue breathing used to establish adequate ventilation and circulation in a pulseless, nonbreathing patient.

carotid artery The principal arteries of the neck; they supply blood to the face, head, and brain.

carotid pulse The pulse that can be felt on each side of the neck where the carotid artery is close to the skin.

cartilage A tough, elastic form of connective tissue that covers the ends of most bones to form joints; also found in some specific areas such as the nose and the ears.

casualty sorting The sorting of patients to determine the order in which patients should be treated and transported.

cellular respiration The use of oxygen by the cells to carry out their specific activities; also called cellular metabolism.

central nervous system (CNS) The brain and spinal cord.

cerebrospinal fluid (CSF) A clear, watery, straw-colored fluid that fills the space between the brain and spinal cord and their protective coverings.

certification The process by which a person, institution, or program is evaluated and recognized as meeting certain standards to ensure safe and ethical patient care.

cervical collar A neck brace that partially stabilizes the neck following injury.

cervical spine That section of the spinal column consisting of the seven vertebrae located in the neck.

channel An assigned frequency or frequencies that are used to carry voice and/or data communications.

chemical agents Compounds that can be used by terrorists to inflict harm.

chemical burns Burns that occur when any toxic substance comes in contact with the skin. Most chemical burns are caused by strong acids or alkalis.

chest compressions A means of applying artificial circulation by applying rhythmic pressure and relaxation on the lower half of the sternum.

chief complaint The patient's response to questions such as "What happened?" or "What's wrong?"

child A person between the age of 1 year and the onset of puberty (age 12 to 14 years).

chocking A piece of wood or metal that is placed in front of or behind a wheel to prevent vehicle movement.

chronic obstructive pulmonary disease (COPD) A slow process of destruction of the airways, alveoli, and pulmonary blood vessels caused by chronic bronchial obstruction (emphysema).

circulatory system The heart and blood vessels, which together are responsible for the continuous flow of blood throughout the body.

clavicle The collarbone.

closed fracture A fracture in which the overlying skin has not been damaged.

closed head injury Injury where there is bleeding and/or swelling within the skull.

closed wound Injury in which soft-tissue damage occurs beneath the skin but there is no break in the surface of the skin.

clothes drag An emergency move used to remove a patient from a hazardous environment; performed by grasping the patient's clothes and moving the patient headfirst from the unsafe area.

cocaine A powerful stimulant that induces an extreme state of euphoria. Legitimately, it is a potent local anesthetic. On the street, it is commonly known as coke. Crack cocaine, crack, or rock is a solid, smokable form of cocaine.

coccyx The tailbone; the small bone at the base of the spinal column.

cold zone The controlled area that contains the command post and other support functions needed in the incident.

coma A state of unresponsiveness from which the patient cannot be aroused.

communication The transmission of information to another person.

computer-aided dispatch (CAD) A communications system that assists 9-1-1 dispatchers to prioritize and record calls, coordinate information that is incoming from multiple streams, and effectively dispatch appropriate responder personnel.

concussion A closed head injury that alters the way the brain functions; symptoms of a concussion include headache, loss of memory, and confusion. Also called a mild traumatic brain injury.

consent Permission to provide care.

continuum of care The concept of consistent patient care across the entire health care team from first patient contact to patient discharge.

contractions Muscular movements of the uterus that push the newborn out of the birth canal.

cradle-in-arms carry A one-rescuer patient movement technique used primarily for children; the patient is cradled in the hollow formed by the rescuer's arms and chest.

cravat A swathe of cloth made by folding a triangular bandage; applied around the injured body part to stabilize the injury or secure other dressing/bandaging materials over a wound.

crew resource management (CRM) A set of procedures for use in environments where human error can have disastrous consequences. It empowers people within a team to communicate effectively with one another with a goal of improving team situational awareness, patient and crew safety, and overall communication.

critical incident stress debriefing (CISD) A system of psychological support designed to reduce stress on emergency personnel after a major stress-producing incident.

critical incident stress management (CISM) A process that confronts the responses to critical incidents and defuses them, directing the emergency services personnel toward physical and emotional equilibrium.

croup Inflammation and narrowing of the air passages in young children, causing a barking cough, hoarseness, and a harsh, high-pitched breathing sound.

crowning Appearance of the newborn's head during a contraction as the newborn is pushed outward through the birth canal.

cultural competence The ability to effectively interact with others regardless of their social, cultural, and linguistic background.

cultural humility The attribute of being curious about others and keeping an open mind when interacting with people from an unfamiliar culture.

cyanosis Blue discoloration of the skin or mucous membranes resulting from poor oxygenation of the circulating blood.

decision-making capacity Ability to understand and process information and make a choice regarding appropriate medical care.

decompression sickness (the bends) A condition seen in divers in which gas, especially nitrogen, forms bubbles in blood vessels, obstructing them.

decontamination The process of reducing or preventing the spread of contaminants at a hazardous materials event.

defibrillation The process of delivering an electric shock through a person's chest wall and heart to establish normal heart contraction rhythms.

delirium tremens (DTs) A severe, often fatal, complication of alcohol withdrawal that most commonly occurs 3 to 4 days after withdrawal (though it can occur as late as 10 days after withdrawal). It is characterized by restlessness, fever, sweating, confusion, disorientation, agitation, hallucinations, and convulsions.

dementia A progressive, irreversible decline in mental functioning marked by memory impairment and decrease in reasoning, judgment, comprehension, and ability to communicate verbally.

dependent lividity Blood settling to the lowest point of the body after death, causing discoloration of the skin.

depression A psychiatric disorder marked by persistent feelings of sadness, hopelessness, and decreased interest in daily activities. The person may have persistent thoughts of suicide.

diabetes A disease in which the body is unable to use glucose normally because of a deficiency or total lack of insulin.

diaphragm A muscular dome that separates the chest from the abdominal cavity. Contraction of the diaphragm and the chest wall muscles brings air into the lungs; relaxation expels air from the lungs.

diastolic pressure The measurement of pressure exerted against the walls of the arteries while the left ventricle of the heart is at rest.

digestive system The gastrointestinal tract (stomach and intestines), mouth, salivary glands, pharynx, esophagus, liver, gallbladder, pancreas, rectum, and anus, which together are responsible for the absorption of food and the elimination of solid waste from the body.

digital messaging Technology that includes email, text messages, and social media, which are increasingly used by EMRs to send and receive various types of information.

dirty bomb An explosive device using conventional explosives that is designed to spread radioactive material over a wide area.

dislocation Disruption of a joint so that the bone ends are no longer in alignment.

distal Describing structures that are farther from the trunk (or torso) or nearer to the free end of an extremity. Opposite of proximal.

documentation A recorded description, whether handwritten or electronic, of the emergency situation and the patient care provided.

do not resuscitate (DNR) order A written request giving permission to medical personnel not to attempt resuscitation in the event of cardiac arrest.

door-to-door time A measure of how long it takes from the time the patient is accessed to the time the patient reaches definitive care.

dressing Any of various materials placed directly on a wound to control bleeding and prevent further contamination.

drowning The process of experiencing respiratory impairment from submersion or immersion in liquid.

durable power of attorney for health care A legal document that allows a patient to designate another person to make medical decisions on their behalf if they are unable to make their own treatment decisions.

duty to act An emergency medical responder's legal responsibility to respond quickly to an emergency scene and provide medical care (within the limits of training and available equipment).

dyspnea Shortness of breath or difficulty breathing.

ectopic pregnancy A pregnancy that occurs outside the uterus, usually in a fallopian tube; usually terminates with the rupture of the fallopian tube.

elder abuse An action taken by a family member or caregiver that results in the physical, emotional, financial, or sexual harm to a person older than 65 years; also includes neglect.

electrical burns Burns caused by an electrical current that enters the body at one point (producing an entrance wound), travels through the body tissues and organs, and exits the body (producing an exit wound).

emergency medical responder (EMR) A person who is qualified to provide basic lifesaving interventions until a more highly trained clinician arrives on the scene.

emergency medical technician (EMT) A person who is qualified to provide basic life support and certain other noninvasive prehospital medical procedures.

emergency response communications center A fire, police, or emergency medical services agency; a 9-1-1 center; or a seven-digit telephone number used by one or all of the emergency agencies to receive and dispatch requests for emergency care; also called a public safety answering point.

emotional shock A state of shock caused by a sudden illness, an accident, or the death of a loved one; technically referred to as psychogenic shock.

empathy The ability to share another person's feelings or ideas.

emphysema Damage to the small air sacs (alveoli) in the lungs, which decreases the amount of working lung capacity, resulting in shortness of breath.

entrance wound The point where an object such as a bullet enters the body.

entrapment A situation in which a person is caught (trapped) within a vehicle, room, or container with no way out or has a limb or other body part trapped.

epidemic An infectious disease or condition that affects many people at the same time in the same geographic area.

epiglottis The valve located at the upper end of the voice box that prevents food from entering the larynx.

epiglottitis Severe inflammation and swelling of the epiglottis; a life-threatening situation.

epilepsy A disease manifested by seizures, caused by an abnormal focus of electrical activity in the brain.

esophagus The tube through which food passes. It starts at the throat and ends at the stomach.

exhalation The act of breathing out.

exit wound The point where an object such as a bullet passes out of the body.

explosives Substances that release energy in a sudden and uncontrolled manner when detonated.

expressed consent Authorization to provide care or transport that is given explicitly, whether verbally or nonverbally.

external respiration The exchange of gases between the lungs and blood.

extremities The arms and legs.

extrication Removal from a difficult situation or position; removal of a patient from a wrecked vehicle or other place of entrapment.

face mask A clear plastic mask used for oxygen administration that covers the mouth and nose.

femoral pulse The pulse taken at the groin.

femur The thighbone; the longest and one of the strongest bones in the body.

fetus A developing newborn in the uterus or womb.

fibula The smaller of the two bones that form the lower leg, located on the lateral side.

firefighter drag A method of moving a patient without lifting or carrying; used when the patient is heavier than the rescuer. The rescuer places the patient's tied hands around their neck and drags the patient by crawling on the hands and knees.

flail chest A chest injury in which three or more ribs are broken in two or more places, resulting in the injured part of the chest moving in the opposite direction from the rest of the chest.

floating ribs The 11th and 12th ribs; they do not connect to the sternum.

flotation device A life ring, life buoy, or other floating device used in water rescue.

flowmeter A device on oxygen cylinders used to control and measure the flow of oxygen.

forearm The lower portion of the upper extremity; from the elbow to the wrist.

fractures Breaks in a bone.

frostbite Partial or complete freezing of the skin and deeper tissues caused by exposure to the cold.

full-thickness burns Burns that extend through the skin and into the underlying tissues; the most serious class of burns.

fusees Warning devices or flares that burn with a red color; usually used in scene protection at motor vehicle crash sites.

gag reflex A strong involuntary effort to vomit caused by something being placed or caught in the throat.

gastric distention Inflation of the stomach caused when excessive pressures are used during artificial ventilation and air is directed into the stomach rather than the lungs.

generalized seizures Seizures characterized by contractions of all the body's muscle groups that may last for 1 to 2 minutes; formerly known as grand mal seizures.

genitourinary system The organs of reproduction, together with the organs involved in the production and excretion of urine.

Golden Hour A concept of emergency patient care that attempts to place a trauma patient into definitive medical care in the shortest time to achieve the best possible outcome; also called the Golden Period.

Good Samaritan laws Laws that encourage citizens to voluntarily help an injured or suddenly ill person by minimizing the liability for any errors or omissions in providing good faith emergency care.

gunshot wound A puncture wound caused by a bullet or shotgun pellets.

hallucinogens Chemicals that cause a person to see visions or hear sounds that are not real.

hazardous material Any substance that is toxic, poisonous, radioactive, flammable, or explosive and can cause injury or death with exposure.

hazmat incident An emergency involving a hazardous material (often abbreviated hazmat as an adjective).

head tilt–chin lift maneuver A method of opening the airway by tilting the patient's head backward and lifting the chin forward, bringing the entire lower jaw with it.

heart failure Heart disease characterized by breathlessness, fluid retention in the lungs, and generalized swelling of the body.

heat cramps Painful muscle spasms that usually occur after vigorous exercise in hot weather and are generally relieved by rest and drinking water.

heat exhaustion A form of shock that occurs from significant fluid loss and too many electrolytes through very heavy sweating after exposure to heat.

heatstroke A condition of rapidly rising internal body temperature that occurs when the body's mechanisms for releasing heat are overwhelmed. Can result in death if left untreated.

Heimlich maneuver A method of relieving an upper airway obstruction by delivering a series of manual thrusts to the abdomen.

hemorrhage Excessive bleeding.

hemostatic agents Chemical compounds that slow or stop bleeding by assisting with clot formation.

hives An allergic skin disorder marked by patches of swelling, redness, and intense itching.

hospice A health care program that brings together a variety of caregivers to provide physical, emotional, spiritual, social, and economic care for patients who have terminal illnesses and a short life expectancy.

hot zone A contaminated area.

human trafficking The illegal exploitation of a person through force, fraud, or coercion.

humerus The upper arm bone.

hyperglycemia A condition of high blood sugar that occurs when the body has too much glucose and not enough insulin.

hypertension High blood pressure.

hypoglycemia A condition of low blood sugar that occurs in a person with diabetes who has taken too much insulin or has not eaten enough food.

hypotension Low blood pressure.

hypothermia A condition in which the internal (or core) body temperature falls below 95°F (35°C) after prolonged exposure to cool or freezing temperatures.

impaled object An object such as a knife, splinter of wood, or glass that penetrates the skin and remains in the body.

implied consent Authorization to provide care or transport that is assumed because the individual is unresponsive, underage, or so badly injured or ill that they cannot respond.

incendiary devices Substances or weapons designed to start a fire.

incident command system (ICS) A system of people, procedures, and equipment designed to improve emergency response operations at situations of all types and complexities.

incision A type of laceration that is made with a sharp object such as a knife.

incubation period The time between exposure to a disease organism and the time the person begins to show symptoms of the disease.

infant A person younger than 1 year.

inferior Nearer to the feet than the head.

informed consent Authorization to provide care or transport that is given by a patient who has decision-making capacity after the potential risks, benefits, and alternatives to treatment have been explained.

inhalation The act of breathing in.

insecticides Chemicals that are formulated to kill insects but that can intentionally or accidentally cause injury or death to humans when inhaled or absorbed through the skin.

insulin A hormone produced by the pancreas that enables glucose in the blood to be used by the cells of the body; supplementary insulin is used in the treatment and control of diabetes mellitus.

internal respiration The exchange of gases between the blood and tissue cells.

intravenous (IV) fluids Fluids other than blood or blood products infused into the vascular system to maintain an adequate circulatory blood volume.

jaw-thrust maneuver A method of opening the airway by bringing the patient's jaw forward without extending the neck.

joint The point where two bones come in contact with each other.

labor The process of delivering a newborn.

laceration An open wound caused by a sharp object or by blunt force; can have ragged or sharp edges.

landing zone A designated area where a helicopter can safely land and take off. Most civilian helicopters need a landing zone of at least 100 × 100 feet (30 × 30 m).

laryngospasm A spasm of the muscles of the larynx or vocal cords resulting in an inability to breathe.

larynx A structure composed of cartilage in the neck that guards the entrance to the windpipe and functions as the organ of voice; also called the voice box.

lateral Away from the midline of the body.

leg The lower portion of the lower extremity; from the knee to the foot.

ligaments Fibrous bands that connect bones to bones and support and strengthen joints.

living will A legal document that states the types of medical care a person wants, or wants withheld, if they are unable to make their own treatment decisions. Living wills may include do not resuscitate orders.

log rolling A technique used to move a patient onto a long backboard; four rescuers work together to ensure spinal alignment while turning the patient onto a side.

lower extremity The body part consisting of the thigh, leg, ankle, and foot.

lumbar spine The lower part of the back formed by the lowest five nonfused vertebrae.

lungs The organs that supply the body with oxygen and eliminate carbon dioxide from the blood.

mandible The lower jaw.

manual suction device A hand-powered device used for clearing the upper airway of mucus, blood, or vomitus.

mask-to-stoma breathing A means of providing rescue breathing to patients who, because of surgical removal of the larynx, have a stoma.

mass-casualty incident (MCI) An accident or situation involving more patients than the responding agency can handle with the initial resources available.

mechanical suction device A battery-powered pump or an oxygen-powered aspirator used for clearing the upper airway of mucus, blood, or vomitus.

mechanism of injury (MOI) The means by which a traumatic injury occurs.

medial Closer to the midline of the body.

medication cross-check A team-based communication method to verify that the proper medication is being given by the correct route of administration to the correct patient.

metabolic agents Substances that are intended to produce injury or death by disrupting the body's ability to use oxygen and chemical reactions at the cellular level.

metered-dose inhaler (MDI) A miniature spray container used to direct medications through the mouth and into the lungs.

midline An imaginary vertical line drawn from the head to toe that divides the body into equal left and right sides.

minute ventilation The amount of air pulled into the lungs and removed from the lungs in 1 minute.

miscarriage Delivery of an incomplete or underdeveloped fetus before it is mature enough to survive outside the womb (approximately 20 weeks of pregnancy); also called spontaneous abortion.

mobile data terminal (MDT) A computer terminal mounted in a vehicle that sends and receives data through a radio communications system.

mobile radio A two-way radio that is permanently mounted in an emergency vehicle that draws electricity from the electrical system of the vehicle.

mottling Patchy skin discoloration caused by too little or too much circulation.

mouth-to-mask ventilation device A piece of equipment that consists of a mask, a one-way valve, and a mouthpiece. Rescue breathing is performed by breathing into the mouthpiece after placing the mask over the patient's mouth and nose.

multisystem trauma An injury that affects more than one body system.

musculoskeletal system The bones and voluntary muscles of the body.

mutual aid An agreement between neighboring EMS systems to respond when local resources are insufficient to handle the response.

nasal airway An airway adjunct that is inserted into the nostril of a patient who is unable to maintain a natural airway; also called a nasopharyngeal airway.

nasal cannula A clear plastic tube, used to deliver oxygen, that fits onto the patient's nose.

nasopharynx The posterior part of the nose.

National Incident Management System (NIMS) A system developed by the US Department of Homeland Security for managing an emergency incident, which may require the response of many different agencies; designed to provide a comprehensive, efficient, and effective management approach from initial response through recovery.

negligence Deviation from the accepted standard of care resulting in further injury to the patient.

nerve agents Deadly toxic substances that attack the central nervous system.

nerves Fiber tracts or pathways that carry messages from the spinal cord and brain to all body parts and back; sensory, motor, or a combination of both.

nervous system The brain, spinal cord, and nerves.

neurogenic shock A type of shock in which injury to the spinal cord allows the vessels to expand, causing blood to pool below the level of the injury. The brain, heart, lungs, and other vital organs are deprived of blood.

nitroglycerin A medication used to treat angina pectoris; increases blood flow and oxygen supply to alleviate the pain of angina pectoris.

occlusive dressing An airtight dressing or bandage for a wound.

one-person walking assist A method in which one rescuer supports the patient from a side while walking; used if the patient is able to bear their own weight.

one-rescuer CPR Cardiopulmonary resuscitation performed by one rescuer.

on-scene peer support Stress counselors at the scene of stressful incidents who help emergency personnel deal with stress.

open fracture Any fracture in which the overlying skin has been damaged.

open wound Injury that breaks open the skin or mucous membrane.

opioids Medications that relieve pain, including prescription drugs such as morphine, oxycodone, and hydrocodone and illicit drugs such as heroin, which is produced from the morphine in poppy plants.

oral airway An airway adjunct that is inserted into the mouth to keep the tongue from blocking the upper airway; also called an oropharyngeal airway.

oropharynx The posterior part of the mouth.

osteoporosis Abnormal brittleness of the bones caused by loss of calcium; affected bones fracture easily.

oxygen A colorless, odorless gas that is essential for life.

oxygenation The process of loading oxygen molecules onto hemoglobin molecules in the bloodstream.

pack-strap carry A one-person carry in which the rescuer backs into the patient and positions the patients such that their armpits are over the rescuer's shoulders and the arms hang over the rescuer's chest; the rescuer holds the patient's wrists with one hand and carries the patient, with one hand free.

paging systems Communications systems used to send voice or text messages over a radio system to specially designed radio receivers.

palpation Examination by touch.

pandemic An infectious disease or condition that affects many people at the same time in the many geographic areas of the world; a global disease outbreak.

paralysis Inability of an alert person to move voluntarily.

paramedic A person trained and certified to provide advanced life support.

partial-thickness burns Burns in which the outer layers of skin are burned; these burns are characterized by blister formation.

patent Open, clear of obstruction.

pathogens Microorganisms that are capable of causing disease.

pediatric assessment triangle (PAT) An assessment tool that measures the severity of a child's illness or injury by evaluating the child's appearance, work of breathing, and circulation to the skin.

pelvis The closed bony ring, consisting of the sacrum and the pelvic bones, that connects the trunk to the lower extremities.

pharmacology The study of the effects of drugs and chemicals on people and animals.

pharynx The throat.

placenta Life-support system of the fetus; also called the afterbirth.

plasma The clear, yellowish fluid of the blood that carries blood cells, transports nutrients, and removes cellular waste materials.

plastic-laminated glass Safety glass that cracks but does not shatter when impacted; the embedded plastic layer holds the pieces in place.

platelets Microscopic disk-shaped elements in the blood that are essential to the formation of a blood clot, the mechanism that stops bleeding.

pneumonia An infection that causes inflammation of the air sacs within the lungs.

pocket mask A mechanical breathing device used to administer mouth-to-mask rescue breathing.

poison Any substance that may cause injury or death if relatively small amounts are ingested, inhaled, absorbed, applied to, or injected into the body.

portable radio A handheld, battery-operated, two-way radio.

portable stretcher A lightweight, nonwheeled device for transporting a patient; used in small spaces where the wheeled ambulance stretcher cannot be used.

posterior The back surface of the body.

posterior tibial pulse The pulse that can be felt on the inner aspect of the ankle, just behind the ankle bone.

posttraumatic stress disorder (PTSD) A mental health or behavioral condition triggered by experiencing or witnessing a terrifying event.

preincident stress education Training about stress and stress reactions conducted for public safety personnel before they are exposed to stressful situations.

premature newborn A newborn delivered before 36 weeks of gestation or who weighs less than 5 pounds (2 kg) at birth.

pressure point An anatomic location where a blood vessel lies near a bone; pressure can be applied to this point to help control bleeding.

primary assessment The first actions taken to form an impression of the patient's condition; to determine the patient's responsiveness and introduce yourself to the patient; to check the patient's airway, breathing, and circulation; and to acknowledge the patient's chief complaint. Sometimes called the initial patient assessment.

prolapsed umbilical cord A condition in which the umbilical cord appears before the newborn does; the newborn's head may compress the cord and cut off all circulation.

proximal Closer to the trunk (or torso). Opposite of distal.

psychogenic shock A type of shock caused by a temporary reduction in blood supply to the brain; commonly referred to as fainting.

psychotic behavior Mental disturbance characterized by abnormal thought processes and/or the loss of contact with reality.

public safety answering point (PSAP) A fire, police, or emergency medical services agency; a 9-1-1 center; or a seven-digit telephone number used by one or all of the emergency agencies to receive and dispatch requests for emergency care; also called an emergency response communications center.

pulmonary agents Substances that produce respiratory distress or illness.

pulse The wave of pressure created by the heart as it contracts and forces blood out into the major arteries.

pulse oximeter A machine that consists of a monitor and a sensing probe that measures the oxygen saturation in the capillary beds.

pulse oximetry An assessment tool that measures oxygen saturation in the capillary beds.

puncture A wound resulting from a bullet, knife, ice pick, splinter, or any other pointed object.

pupils The circular openings in the middle of the eye.

quality assurance A reactive process that involves monitoring compliance against a standard to identify problems that have already occurred.

quality improvement A proactive process that involves making changes to a system to improve performance.

rabies An acute viral infection of the central nervous system transmitted by the bite of an infected animal.

radial pulse The pulse located on the inside of the wrist on the thumb side.

radiation The electromagnetic energy that is released from a radioactive material or a dirty bomb.

radius The bone on the thumb side of the forearm.

reach, throw, row, go A sequence of four actions that should be taken in water rescue situations.

recovery position A side-lying position that helps an unresponsive patient maintain an open airway.

redirection A means of focusing the patient's attention on the immediate situation or crisis.

repeater A radio system that automatically retransmits a radio signal on a different frequency.

rescue breathing An artificial means of breathing for a patient.

rescue throw bag A water rescue device consisting of a small cloth bag and a waterproof rope used for rescuing people from the water.

respiration The exchange of oxygen and carbon dioxide in the alveoli as well as the tissues of the body; classified as external, internal, or cellular.

respiratory arrest Sudden stoppage of breathing.

respiratory burns Burns to the respiratory system that result from inhaling superheated air.

respiratory distress A condition marked by difficulty breathing and an abnormal respiratory rate or effort; can range from mild to severe and can progress to respiratory failure.

respiratory failure A condition in which oxygen levels are too low to meet the body's needs and ventilation is impaired, leading to high carbon dioxide levels; accompanied by serious signs and symptoms and must be corrected quickly.

respiratory rate The speed at which a person is breathing (measured in breaths per minute).

respiratory system All body structures that contribute to normal breathing.

restatement The act of rephrasing a person's statement to demonstrate that the person is being heard and understood.

ribs The paired arches of bone, 12 on either side, that extend from the thoracic vertebrae toward the anterior midline of the trunk.

rigid splint Splint made from firm materials such as wood, aluminum, or plastic.

riptide Unusually strong surface currents flowing outward from a seashore that can present a hazard to swimmers.

road rash An abrasion caused by sliding on pavement. Usually seen after motorcycle or bicycle accidents.

rule of nines A means of calculating the amount of body surface burned; for adults, the body is divided into sections, each of which constitutes approximately 9% or 18% of the total body surface area; these percentages vary slightly for children.

sacrum One of three bones (the others being the two pelvic bones) that makes up the pelvic ring; forms the base of the spine.

saline Salt water.

SAMPLE history A patient's medical history. The letters stand for Signs and Symptoms, Allergies, Medications, Pertinent past medical history, Last oral intake, Events associated with or leading up to the illness or injury.

scene assessment A step within the patient assessment process that includes a visual survey, or an overview of the incident and its surroundings, and a quick assessment of the scene and the surroundings to provide information about scene safety and the mechanism of injury or nature of illness before you enter and begin patient care.

scoop stretcher A firm device used to carry a patient; can be split into halves and applied to the patient from both sides.

secondary assessment The step in the patient assessment sequence in which you carefully examine the patient from head to toe and measure vital signs.

seizure A neurologic episode that causes uncoordinated muscular activity, resulting from a surge of electrical activity in the brain.

self-contained breathing apparatus (SCBA) A complete unit for delivery of air to a rescuer who enters a contaminated area; contains a mask, regulator, and air supply.

senile dementia A general term for dementia that occurs in older people.

sepsis A severe complication of infection that occurs when chemicals are released into the bloodstream and trigger an inflammatory response throughout the body.

septic shock A type of shock in which the blood pressure drops dramatically as a result of severe infection; often results in death.

shock A state of collapse of the cardiovascular system; the state of inadequate delivery of blood to the organs of the body.

shoulder girdles The three bones of the upper extremity; each shoulder supports the clavicle, the scapula, and the humerus.

sign A condition observed in a patient, such as bleeding or the temperature of a patient's skin.

situational awareness Knowledge and understanding of one's surroundings and the ability to recognize potential risks to the safety of the patient or EMS team.

situational crisis A state of emotional upset or turmoil caused by a sudden and disruptive event.

skull The bones of the head, collectively; the protective structure for the brain.

sling A bandage or material that helps to support the weight of an injured upper extremity.

soft splint A splint made from supple material that provides gentle support.

spinal motion restriction The general goal of maintaining the patient's spinal alignment throughout any treatment and movements that clinicians must perform.

splint A means of stabilizing an injured body part by using a rigid or soft support.

spontaneous nosebleed A nosebleed with no apparent cause.

sprain A joint injury in which the joint is partially or temporarily dislocated and some of the supporting ligaments are either stretched or torn.

stair chair A small portable device used for transporting a patient in a sitting position.

standard of care The actions expected of a clinician in accordance with their level of education and experience.

standard precautions An infection control concept that treats all body fluids as potentially infectious.

standing orders Written documents, signed by the EMS system's medical director, that outline specific directions, permissions, and sometimes prohibitions regarding patient care; also called protocols.

START triage A patient sorting process based on three primary observations: breathing, circulation, and mental status. START stands for Simple Triage And Rapid Treatment.

sternum The breastbone.

stoma A surgical opening in the neck that connects the windpipe (trachea) to the skin.

stridor A harsh, high-pitched respiratory sound, generally heard during inhalation, that is caused by partial blockage or narrowing of the upper airway.

stroke A brain attack caused by a blood clot or a broken blood vessel in the brain. Strokes can result in trouble speaking, inability to move parts of the body, confusion, or unresponsiveness.

submersion injury An injury resulting from being beneath the surface of water or another liquid.

suction To aspirate (suck out) fluid by mechanical means.

suctioning Aspirating (sucking out) fluid in the mouth or airway by mechanical means.

suicide The intentional causing of one's own death. It is especially common among older and chronically ill people.

superficial burns Burns in which only the outermost layers of skin are injured.

superior Closer to the head or above a body part.

symptom A condition the patient tells you, such as "I feel dizzy."

systolic pressure The measurement of blood pressure exerted against the walls of the arteries during contraction of the heart.

telemetry A process in which electronic signals are transmitted and received by radio or telephone; commonly used for sending electrocardiogram tracings.

tempered glass Safety glass that breaks into small pieces when hit with a sharp, pointed object.

tendons Tough, ropelike cords of fibrous tissue that attach muscle to bone.

terrorism A systematic use of violence to intimidate or to achieve a political goal.

thermal burns Burns caused by heat; the most common type of burn.

thighbone The upper portion of the lower extremity; from the hip joint to the knee.

thoracic spine The 12 vertebrae that attach to the 12 ribs; the upper part of the back.

thready pulse A barely palpable pulse.

tibia The shinbone; the larger of the two bones of the lower leg.

topographic anatomy The superficial landmarks on the body that serve as location guides to the structures that lie beneath them.

toxic Poisonous.

trachea The windpipe.

traction splint A splint that holds a lower extremity fracture in alignment by applying a constant, steady pull on the extremity.

traffic incident management (TIM) A system that specifies where to place vehicles and warning devices to achieve a safe scene while highway incidents are being resolved.

trauma In the context of emergency response, a physical wound or injury; in other contexts, trauma may also refer to events producing psychological distress.

traumatic brain injury (TBI) A closed head injury that alters the way the brain functions; symptoms include headache, loss of memory, and confusion. A concussion is a mild traumatic brain injury.

triage The sorting of patients into groups according to the severity of their injuries; used to determine priorities for medical treatment and transport.

trunked communications system A computer-controlled radio system that allows the sharing of a few radio frequencies among a large group of users.

two-person chair carry A method of carrying a patient in which two rescuers use a chair to support the weight of the patient.

two-person extremity carry A method of carrying a patient out of tight quarters in which two rescuers use the patient's extremities, one reaching under the patient's arms and holding the wrists and the other backing between the patient's legs and holding the legs, to carry the patient; requires no equipment.

two-person seat carry A method of carrying a patient in which two rescuers link arms behind the patient's back and under the patient's knees; requires no equipment.

two-person walking assist A method in which two rescuers support the patient's full weight from each side while walking; used when a patient cannot bear their own weight.

two-rescuer CPR Cardiopulmonary resuscitation performed by two rescuers.

ulna The bone on the little-finger side of the forearm.

umbilical cord Ropelike attachment between the mother and fetus; nourishment and waste products pass to and from the fetus and the mother through this cord.

upper extremity The body part consisting of the arm, forearm, wrist, and hand.

uterus (womb) Muscular organ that holds and nourishes the developing fetus.

vacuum splint A soft splint that becomes rigid when air is removed from the splint.

vagina The opening through which the newborn emerges.

venous bleeding External bleeding from a vein, characterized by steady flow; the bleeding may be profuse and life threatening.

ventilation The physical act of moving air into and out of the lungs; also called pulmonary ventilation.

ventricles The two lower chambers of the heart.

ventricular fibrillation An uncoordinated muscular quivering of the heart; the most common abnormal rhythm causing cardiac arrest; often referred to as V-fib.

vertebrae The 33 bones of the spinal column: 7 cervical, 12 thoracic, 5 lumbar, 5 sacral, and 4 coccygeal vertebrae.

vital signs Measurements or critical parameters used to assess the patient's immediate health condition, including pulse, capillary refill, skin condition, temperature, respirations, and blood pressure.

warm zone The controlled area where personnel and equipment decontamination and hot zone support take place.

weapon of mass destruction (WMD) Any agent designed to bring about mass death, casualties, and/or massive damage to property and infrastructure (bridges, tunnels, airports, electrical power plants, and seaports).

wooden cribbing Wooden boards used for vehicle stabilization or bracing.

xiphoid process The flexible cartilage at the lower tip of the sternum.

Index

Note: Page number followed by *f* and *t* denote figures and tables, respectively.

A

abandonment, 70–71, 170
abdomen
  acute, 229
  assessment, 195
abdominal breathing, 357
abdominal pain, 228–230, 229*f*
abdominal thrusts, 137
abdominal wounds. *See specific wounds*
abduction at shoulder, 443, 445*f*
abortion, spontaneous, 378
abrasion, 310, 310*f*
absorbed poisons, 242, 248
abuse. *See also specific entries*
  cycles of, 265
acceptance, as stage of grieving process, 23
acid, 244
activated charcoal, 244, 244*f*
actual consent, 69
acute respiratory distress syndrome (ARDS), 224
Adam's apple, 156, 186
additional resources, scene assessment, 183
adduction at shoulder, 443, 445*f*
adequate breathing, signs of, 127
adolescents, 106
advance directives, 70
advanced emergency medical technicians (AEMTs), 6
advanced life support (ALS), 6, 42, 223, 302
advanced medical devices, 233–234, 233*f*
advanced medical needs, patients with, 233
AEDs. *See* automated external defibrillators
AEMTs. *See* advanced emergency medical technicians
aerobic exercise, 24
agents and devices, terrorism. *See specific agents and devices*
air embolism, 410
air splint, 340, 341, 342*f*
  to leg, 350
airbags, 406, 407
airborne pathogens, 25, 27, 27–28*f*
  standard precautions for, 29–30
airway adjuncts
  nasal airway, 125–126, 126*f*
  oral airway, 124–125, 124*f*
airway, breathing, and circulation (ABCs), 116, 184. *See also* airway; breathing; circulation
  treatment for shock, 301–302
airway management, 115–117
  airway, 120–126
    airway adjuncts, 124–126, 124*f*, 126*f*
    blocked, 121–122, 121*f*
    finger sweeps, 122
    fluids, foreign bodies, or dentures, 122
    maintaining, 124
    opening, 126
    recovery position, 124, 124*f*
    responsiveness, 120, 120*f*
    review, 133, 135–136
    suctioning, 122–123, 124*f*
  breathing
    adequate, signs of, 127
    bag-mask device, 131–134, 132*f*, 135*f*
    checking, 126–129, 127*f*
    correcting, 129–133
    inadequate, signs of, 127, 129
    mouth-to-barrier rescue, 130–132, 131*f*
    mouth-to-mask rescue, 130, 130*f*
    mouth-to-mouth rescue, 131
    rescue on children and infants, 135–136
    review, 133, 135–136
  foreign body airway obstruction
    in adult, 137–139, 138–139*f*
    causes of, 136, 137*f*
    in child, 139, 139–140*f*
    in infant, 139–141, 140–141*f*
    types of, 136–137
  oxygen administration. *See* oxygen administration
  pulse oximetry, 144–145, 144*f*
  respiratory system, anatomy and function of, 117–118, 118–119*f*
  special considerations
    airway management in vehicle, 145–146
    dental appliances, 145
    gastric distention, 145
    stomas, rescue breathing for, 145, 145*f*
  in vehicle, 407
alcohol, 21, 23
  internal bleeding and, 303
  misuse, 250
alkali. *See* base
ALS. *See* advanced life support
altered level of consciousness, 216
altered mental status, 215–216
alveolar ventilation, 117
alveoli, 99, 117, 119*f*
Alzheimer disease, 272
ambulance stretchers, wheeled. *See* wheeled ambulance stretchers
ambulance transport, 9, 9*f*
ammonia, 245, 246*f*
amniotic fluid, 370, 371*f*. *See also* bag of waters
amphetamine misuse, 251
amputations, 311–312, 311–312*f*
analgesic, 442
anaphylactic shock, 247, 300
  treatment for, 303
anger, 261–262
  as stage of grieving process, 23
angina pectoris, 218–219, 218*f*
animal
  bites and stings, 246–248, 247*f*
  hazards, 34
ankle, 334
  and foot injuries, 350, 351
  pulse, 348, 350*f*
anterior, meaning of, 98
antivenin, 248
anus, 381
appropriate medical facility, 6
arm-to-arm drag, 42, 43*f*
armed patient, 268
arrival at scene
  emergency medical responder call, 391, 391*f*
  functions of radio communications, 82, 82*f*
arterial bleeding, 304
arteries, 298
artificial ventilation, 118
aspiration/aspirator, 123, 193
aspirin, 219
assessment-based care model, 178
assessment. See individual entries for history taking, primary assessment, scene assessment, secondary assessment, and reassessment
asthma, 222–223, 223*f*, 233*f*
atherosclerosis, 218
atrium, 100, 152, 153*f*, 298, 298*f*
attitude/conduct, 12, 12*f*
auscultation, 199–200, 199*f*, 200*t*
automated external defibrillators (AEDs), 166–169, 168*f*, 285
avoidance, posttraumatic stress disorder and, 270
AVPU scale, 185, 201, 216
avulsions, 311–312, 311–312*f*

B

B-NICE acronym, 436
back
  assessment, 195
  wounds, 317, 317*f*
backboard, 192
bag-mask device, 125, 131–134, 132*f*, 135*f*
bag of waters, 371
  unbroken, 378, 380
ball-and-socket joints, 103, 103*f*
bandaging, 313–314, 313*f*
  extremity wound, 318, 319*f*
  impaled object, 316*f*
bargaining, as stage of grieving process, 23
bariatric stretchers, 49
base, 244
base station, 80
basic life support (BLS), 5, 42
bath salts, 251
battery-powered suction device, 123, 123*f*
Battle sign, 354, 355*f*

behavioral emergencies, 260–261
  coping with work-related stress
    critical incident stress debriefing, 273
    peer support, 273–274
  crisis management. *See* crisis management
  medical and legal considerations, 272–273
  mental health considerations
    dementia, 272
    depression, 272
  patient assessment in, 260, 260*f*
  situational crisis
    anger, 261–262
    defined, 261
    denial, 261
    high-anxiety or emotional shock, 261
    remorse or grief, 262
below-grade rescue, 34
below-ground confined spaces, 412
bile, 104
biologic agents, 435
birth canal, 104, 370
birth situation assessment
  stages of labor, 371, 371*f*
  time to reach hospital, 371
  timing contraction cycles, 371, 372*f*
bites and stings, 245–248, 247*f*, 320
  animal, 246
  environmental emergencies, 287
  insect, 246–247, 247*f*
bladder, 104
blanket drag, 42, 43*f*
blanket roll, 59–60
bleeding. *See also specific entries*
  direct pressure, 304–305, 305*f*
  from ear, 355, 356*f*
  elevation, 305
  excessive bleeding after delivery, 381
  external blood loss, controlling, 304–309, 304*f*
  internal blood loss, 304
  patient assessment for, 297, 297*f*
  pressure points, 306–307, 307*f*, 308*f*
  standard precautions and control, 309, 309–310*f*
  tourniquet application, 305–309, 305*f*, 307–309*f*
  vaginal bleeding in pregnant patient, 378
blister agents, 434–435, 434*t*
blocked cardiac artery, 219, 219*f*
blood, components of, 101, 298, 299*f*
blood pressure, 199–200, 299–300
  auscultation, checking by, 199–200, 199*f*, 200*t*
  cuff, 198–199, 199*f*
  normal, 198
  palpation, checking by, 198–199, 199*f*
bloodborne pathogens, 27, 231
  standard precautions for, 27, 27–28*f*
bloody show, 371
BLS. *See* basic life support
body language
  communication by, 262–263, 263*f*
  as nonverbal communication, 85
body mechanics, 41, 41*f*
body systems, 98. *See also specific systems*
body temperature, 302
bone marrow, 334
bounding pulse, 197
brachial arteries, 152, 192, 333
brachial artery pressure point, 306–307, 307*f*
brachial pulse, 154, 157–158, 158*f*, 187, 187*f*, 197, 199
brain, 103–104, 353
  attack. *See* stroke
  damage, 126, 154
  death, 117
  injury to, unequal pupils and, 200, 201*f*
breath odors assessment, 195
breathing. *See* airway management
breech birth, 380, 380*f*
broken ribs, 164
bronchi, 117
bronchioles, 99
bronchitis, chronic, 222
bruises (contusions), 310, 312
burn sheet, 322, 322*f*
burns
  cause or type of, 321–324
  chemical, 323, 323*f*
  depth, 320–321, 320–321*f*
  electrical, 323–324, 323–324*f*
  extent of, 321, 321*f*
  respiratory, 322
  thermal, 322, 322*f*
bus rescue, 415, 415*f*
bystanders, 402

C

caffeine, 21–22
cancer, 230
capillaries, 99, 117, 298
  bleeding, 304, 304*f*
capillary refill, 197–198, 198*f*
  on splinted injured leg, 351, 351*f*
carbon dioxide, 99, 99*f*
carbon monoxide poisoning, 245
cardiac arrest, 154, 218, 220, 222, 230
  and hypothermia, 284–285
  signs and symptoms of, 220
cardiac chain of survival, 155, 155*f*
cardiac compressions
  on adult, 156–157
  on child, 158
  on infant, 157–158, 158*f*
cardiac event, 155
cardiac muscles, 103, 335, 335*f*
cardiac pacemaker, 233–234
cardiac patients and clothes drag, 42
cardiogenic shock, 299
cardiopulmonary resuscitation (CPR), 42, 42*f*, 116, 151–152, 220, 284, 285, 441
  adult CPR
    one-rescuer adult CPR, 158–159, 160*f*
    switching positions during, 162
    two-rescuer adult CPR, 159–160, 161*f*
  child CPR, 163–164, 164*f*
  complications of
    broken ribs, 164
    gastric distention, 165
    hyperventilation, 166
    regurgitation, 165
  components of, 154–155
  compression-only, 157
  creating sufficient space for, 166, 166*f*
  early defibrillation by EMRs, 166–169, 168*f*
  effective, signs of, 164
  infant CPR
    one-rescuer infant CPR, 162–163, 162–163*f*
    two-rescuer infant CPR, 163, 163*f*
  legal implications of, 170
  starting, 155–156
  stopping, 156
  training, 170
carotid artery, 101, 101*f*, 152, 197
carotid pulse, 152, 186, 186*f*, 197
cartilage, 102
casualty sorting, 426–428, 427*f*, 428*f*
CAT tourniquet, 305*f*
caustic. *See* base
central nervous system (CNS), 103–104, 251
cerebrospinal fluid (CSF), 353, 354*f*
certification, 14, 69
cervical collar, 53, 53–54*f*
cervical spine, 102, 333, 334*f*
  stabilizing, 358
cervical vertebrae, 102*f*
chemical agents
  blister agents, 434–435, 434*t*
  characteristics of, 434*t*
  insecticides, 434
  metabolic agents, 432
  nerve agents, 434
  pulmonary agents, 432
chemical burn, 323, 323*f*
chest (thorax), 334
  assessment, 194
  compressions, 152
  flail chest, 360–361, 361*f*
    treatment of, 360–361
  pain, 155
  penetrating chest wounds, 361–362, 361–362*f*
    treatment of, 361–362
  rib fractures, 360
    treatment of, 360
chest-thrust maneuver, 138, 138*f*
chest wounds, 317, 317*f*
  penetrating, 361–362, 361–362*f*
chief complaint, 188
  investigation, 188–189, 188*f*
  reassessment, 203
child abuse, 265–266, 265*f*
childbirth
  assisting with delivery, 372
    newborn, caring for, 374, 375*f*
    placenta, delivery of, 374–376, 376*f*
  birth situation assessment
    stages of labor, 371, 371*f*
    time to reach hospital, 371
    timing contraction cycles, 371, 372*f*
  complications of, 378
    breech birth, 380, 380*f*
    ectopic pregnancy and shock, 378
    excessive bleeding after delivery, 381
    miscarriage and vaginal bleeding, 378
    multiple births, 381
    premature birth, 378
    prolapsed umbilical cord, 380, 380*f*
    stillborn delivery, 380–381
    unbroken bag of waters, 378, 380
  equipment, 372, 374*f*
  level of responsiveness assessment, 185
  mother and newborn, aftercare of, 376
  resuscitating newborn, 376–377

standard precautions and, 372, 373
trauma and pregnant patients, 381
children, 158
airway obstruction in, 139, 139–140*f*
car seats and, 57, 57*f*
cardiac compression, 158
cardiopulmonary resuscitation
one-rescuer and two-rescuer child CPR, 163–164, 164*f*
oral airway insertion, 126
rescue breathing on, 135
respiratory systems, 99
traumatic shock in, 303–304
weight-based dosing in, 232
chlorine gas, 245, 246, 432
chocking, 403, 403*f*
chronic obstructive pulmonary disease (COPD), 222, 224
Cincinnati Prehospital Stroke Scale, 224, 225*t*
circulation, 427–428
assessment, 186–187, 186–187*f*
to skin, 202
circulatory system, 100–101, 100–101*f*, 298–299, 298*f*
anatomy and function of, 152–154, 153–154*f*
CISD. *See* critical incident stress debriefing
CISM. *See* critical incident stress management
clavicle, 194
cleaning, equipment, 34
closed abdominal wounds, 317–318
closed-ended questions, 86
closed fracture, 336, 336*f*
closed head injury, 354, 354*f*
closed wounds, 310
clot-busting drugs, 225
clothes drag, 42, 42*f*
CNS. *See* central nervous system
cocaine, 251, 254
coccygeal vertebrae, 102*f*
coccyx, 102, 333, 334*f*
codeine, 251
cold, exposure to
frostbite, 282–283, 283*f*
hypothermia, 284–285, 284*t*
cold water drowning, 287
cold zone, 422
collapse, danger of, 412
collarbone (clavicle), 333
colors (description), 443, 444*t*
coma, 248
combining vowels, 441, 442
communicable diseases, infectious diseases vs., 25
communication. *See* data and communication systems
compression-only CPR, 157
computer-based (electronic) records, 92, 92*f*
concepts. *See* medical, legal, and ethical issues
concussion, 355
confidentiality, 73
confined space
hazards, 413*f*
rescue, 34, 412, 412*f*
consent, 69
for minors, 69, 69*f*
of patients with mental illness, 69–70
constricted pupils, 200, 200*f*
continuum of care, 4
contraction cycles, 370, 371, 372*f*
control external hemorrhage, 302
COPD. *See* chronic obstructive pulmonary disease
Coronavirus disease 2019 (COVID-19), 25, 130, 230
precautions for, 29
CPR. *See* cardiopulmonary resuscitation
cradle-in-arms carry, 44, 45*f*
cravat, 313, 313*f*
crew resource management (CRM), 25
crib death. *See* sudden infant death syndrome
crime scene operations, 73–74, 74*f*
crime/violence, 33
crisis management
armed patient, 268–269
child abuse, 265–266, 265*f*
communicating with patient, 262–263, 262–263*f*
communication skills, 263–264
empathy, 263
redirection, 263
restatement, 263
crowd control, 264
cycles of abuse, 265
death and dying, 271, 271*f*
domestic violence, 264–265
elder abuse, 266, 266*f*
emergency medical responder, role of, 262
emotional crises
attempted suicide, 268–269, 269*t*
posttraumatic stress disorder, 269–270
sexual assault, 270–271
violence against EMRs, 268
prevention, 263
violent patients, 266, 266*f*
critical incident stress debriefing (CISD), 24, 273
critical incident stress management (CISM), 24
CRM. *See* crew resource management
croup, 223
crowds, 33
control, 264
crowning, 370, 371, 371*f*
CSF. *See* cerebrospinal fluid
cultural competence, 85
cultural humility, 85
cultural norms, respecting, 85–86
cuts, 311
cyanides, 432
cyanosis, 187

D

data and communications systems
data systems, 81, 81*f*
radio communications, functions of
arrival at scene, 82
channel, 80
dispatch, 81
postrun activities, 83, 83*t*
response to scene, 81–82, 82*f*
transfer of patient care to other EMS personnel, 82–83
update responding EMS units, 82
voice systems
radio systems, 80, 80*f*
telephone systems, 81
DCAP-BTLS mnemonic, 191
dead spots, communications, 80
death and dying, 23, 271, 271*f*
decapitation, 71, 156
decompression sickness (bends), 410
decontamination, 422
defibrillation, 6, 166–169, 168*f*
automated external, 166–169
delirium tremens (DTs), 250
delivery. *See* childbirth
dementia, 272
denial, 261
as stage of grieving process, 23
dental appliances, 145
dentures, check for, 122
dependent lividity, 71, 156
depression, 272
as stage of grieving process, 23
dermis, 105, 105*f*
developmental disabilities, 264
diabetes, 226
diabetic coma, 228
hyperglycemic emergency, 226–228, 228*t*
hypoglycemic emergencies, 226, 226*f*
signs and symptoms of, 226
diabetic coma, 228
diaphragm, 99, 100*f*
diastolic pressure, 198, 199
diesel fuel spills, 402
diet, 21, 21*f*
digestive system, 104, 104*f*
digital messaging, 81
dilated pupils, 200, 200*f*
direct (or online) medical control, 14
direct contact, 25
direct force, 335
direct ground lift, 46–47
direct pressure, 304–305, 305*f*
dirty bomb, 436
disease transmission, 25–28, 27–28*f*
disentanglement, help with patient, 407, 407*f*
disinfection, equipment, 34
dislocations, 336–337. *See also specific dislocations*
dispatch, 5, 5*f*, 31
emergency medical responder call, 390
functions of radio communications, 81
information, reviewing, 180–181, 180*f*
disposable respirator, 28*f*
distal, meaning of, 98
diving emergencies, 409–411
DNR order. *See* do not resuscitate (DNR) order
do not resuscitate (DNR) order, 70
documentation, 74, 80, 92, 92*f*
domestic terrorism, 431
domestic violence, 264–265
door-to-door time, 392
doors, access through, 405
dosimeter, 435–436, 436*f*
DOTS mnemonic, 191
downed electrical wires, 402–403
dressing, 304–305, 312–313, 312*f*
drowning, environmental emergencies, 287
drugs
misuse, 250–254
poisoning death rates, 243*f*
dry chemical fire extinguisher, 404, 404*f*
DTs. *See* delirium tremens
DuoDote kit, 249, 434
durable power of attorney for health care, 70
Duragesic. *See* fentanyl

duty to act, 68, 68*f*
dysphagia, 443
dysphasia, 443
dyspnea, 222–223
dysuria, 442

E

early adulthood, 106
ectopic pregnancy, 378
elbow injuries, 344, 344*f*
elder abuse, 266, 266*f*
electric vehicles (EVs), 402
electrical burn, 323–324, 323–324*f*
electrical hazards, 33, 403
electronic records, 92, 92*f*
elevation, 305
emergency lights, 390
emergency medical responder (EMR)
  defibrillation by, 166–169, 168*f*
  roles and responsibilities of, 12, 12*f*, 262
  training, 9, 9*f*
    assistance of other EMS clinicians, 10
    goals of, 10, 10*f*, 11*t*
    life support kit, 10, 10*f*, 11*t*
    how to improvise, 10
    what not to do, 10
  violence against, 268
    prevention, 268
emergency medical service (EMS) systems, 4*f*, 20
  certification, 14
  history of, 7–8, 8*f*
  public health, roles in, 6–7
  quality management, 14
emergency medical technicians (EMTs), 4, 5
emergency movement of patients, 42
  ambulatory patients, walking assists for
    one-person walking assist, 47, 48*f*
    two-person walking assist, 47–48, 48*f*
  emergency drags
    arm-to-arm drag 42, 43*f*
    blanket drag, 42, 43*f*
    clothes drag, 42, 42*f*
    firefighter drag, 43, 43*f*
    from vehicle, 43–44, 44*f*
  equipment
    portable stretchers, 49
    stair chairs, 49, 50*f*
    wheeled ambulance stretchers, 49, 49*f*
  nonambulatory patients, carries for
    cradle-in-arms carry, 44, 45*f*
    direct ground lift, 46–47
    pack-strap carry, 45–46, 46*f*
    transferring patient from bed to stretcher, 47, 48*f*
    two-person chair carry, 44–45, 45*f*
    two-person extremity carry, 44, 44*f*
    two-person seat carry, 44, 45*f*
  spinal motion restriction devices
    long backboards, 50, 50*f*
    scoop stretchers, 52, 52*f*
    short backboard devices, 53–54, 54*f*
emergency response communications center, 4
Emergency Response Guidebook, 422, 423*f*, 424*f*
emotional crises
  attempted suicide, 268–269, 269*t*
  posttraumatic stress disorder, 269–270
emotional shock, 261
empathy, 263
EMR. *See* emergency medical responder
EMR-administered medications, 233
EMS. *See* emergency medical service (EMS) systems
EMT tourniquet, 305*f*
EMTs. *See* emergency medical technicians
entrance wound, 311
entrapment, 400
environmental conditions, 34
environmental emergencies
  bites and stings, 287
  drowning and submersion, 287
  exposure to cold
    frostbite, 83*f*, 282–283
    hypothermia, 284–285
  exposure to heat
    heat cramps, 281
    heat exhaustion, 281
    heatstroke, 281–282, 282*f*, 282*t*
  lightning injuries, 287
  patient assessment for, 280, 280*f*
epidemics, 230, 231*t*
epidermis, 105, 105*f*
epiglottis, 99, 117
epiglottitis, 223–224
epilepsy, 216
epinephrineauto-injector (EpiPen), 247, 248, 303
Epsom salt, 251
esophagus, 117
ethical responsibilities and competence, 68–69
exhalation, 118, 119*f*, 194
exit wound, 311
explosives, 432, 432*f*
  hazards, 413*f*
expressed consent, 69
exsanguinating bleeding, airway, breathing, circulation (XABCs), 332
extension at elbow, 443, 445*f*
external bleeding, 300, 302–306, 304*f*, 308, 310
  control of, 304–309, 304*f*
extremities, 44. *See also specific entries*
  assessment, 195
  injuries, signs and symptoms, 337
  wounds, 318, 319*f*
extrication
  disentanglement, help with patient, 407, 407*f*
  gaining access to patients
    through doors, 405, 405*f*
    through windows, 405–406, 405–406*f*
  initial emergency care, 406–407
  patient removal, 407–408
  scene assessment, 400–401, 401*f*
eye contact, 84–85
eyes
  assessment, 193
  chemical burns to, 323, 323*f*
  injuries, 316, 316*f*

F

face
  assessment, 194
  injuries, 356
  masks, 143
  wounds, 314, 314*f*
face-to-face conversations, 84
facial expressions, 87
fainting, 300, 308
farm machinery, 413, 413*f*
farm rescue, 412–415, 413*f*, 413*t*
farm silos, 413, 413*f*
febrile seizures, 231
female reproductive system, 104, 370, 371*f*
femoral artery, 101, 101*f*, 152
  pressure point, 306–307, 307*f*, 308*f*
femoral fractures, 348
femoral pulse, 154
femur, 334
fentanyl (Duragesic), 251
fetus, 370
fibula, 334
finger injuries, 344–345, 346*f*
finger sweeps, 122
firefighter drag, 43, 43*f*
firefighters, 5, 5*f*, 282
flail chest, 194, 360–361, 361*f*
flexible suction catheter, 123, 124*f*
flexion at elbow, 443, 445*f*
floating ribs, 102, 334, 334*f*
flotation device, 408
flowmeter, 142, 142*f*
flu shots, 31
foam blocks, 53, 58, 61*f*
folded cardboard splints, 341, 341*f*
foot, 334
forearminjuries, 333–334
foreign body. *See* airway management
four-person log roll, 56
fractures, 194, 336, 336*f*. *See also specific fractures*
frostbite, 282–283, 283*f*
frostnip, 283
full-thickness burns (third-degree burns), 320, 321*f*
fused joints, 103
fusees, 392, 402

G

GA. *See* tabun
gag reflex, 125
gases, exchange of, 119*f*
gasoline, 244, 402
gastric distention, 145, 165
gastroenterology, 442
GB. *See* sarin
GD. *See* soman
general impression, 184
generalized seizures, 216
genital wounds, 318
genitourinary system, 104
gloves
  removing, 29
  sterile, 373
go (water rescue), 409, 409*f*
Golden Hour (or Period), 407
Good Samaritan laws, 73
grand mal seizures. *See* generalized seizures
grief, 262
grieving process, 23, 262
groin (femoral) artery, 101, 101*f*, 152
ground-level confined spaces, 412
gunshot wound, 311, 318, 320, 320*f*

H

hallucinogens, 253
hand, 333
  gestures, 88
  injuries, 344–345, 346*f*

handwashing, 31
handoff report, 204, 204*f*
hands-only CPR, 157
hazardous materials (hazmat), 400, 422
  placards to identify, 246*f*
  scene assessment, 33
hazards
  high-angle, 413*f*
  scene assessment, 181
  stabilization of. *See* stabilization of scene and hazards
  of supplemental oxygen, 144
head, 333
  assessment, 193
  bandage, 312, 312*f*
  injuries, 354*f*
    mechanisms of injury, 353–354, 354*f*
    signs and symptoms of, 354–355, 355*f*
    treatment of, 355, 356*f*
    types of, 354, 354*f*
head tilt–chin lift maneuver, 121, 121*f*
head/spine injuries, suspected
  backboards, 53
  car seats and children, 57, 57*f*
  cervical collar, 53, 53–54*f*
  log rolling, 54–57
  short backboard devices, 53–54, 54*f*
  stabilizing the patient's head, 58–61, 61*f*
  straps and strapping techniques, 57–58, 58*f*
Health Insurance Portability and Accountability Act of 1996, 73
heart, 100, 100*f*, 152, 153*f*
  conditions
    angina pectoris, 218–219, 218*f*
    heart attack, 219–220, 219*f*
    heart failure, 221, 221*f*, 299
heat, exposure to
  heat cramps, 281
  heat exhaustion, 281
  heatstroke, 281–282, 282*f*, 282*t*
Heimlich maneuver, 137
helicopter transport, 391–394
  determining need for, 392
  loading patients, 394, 394*f*
  setting up landing zones, 392–394, 392*f*
hemodialysis, 230
hemorrhage, 302
hemostatic agents, 306
HEPA. *See* high-efficiency particulate air respirator
hepatitis B, 27
heroin, 251, 253, 254
high anxiety, 261
high-efficiency particulate air (HEPA) respirator, 27, 27*f*
  steps for donning, 27, 27–28*f*
hinge joints, 103, 103*f*
hip
  dislocation, 347
  fractures, 347
  injuries, 347, 347*f*
history taking
  chief complaint investigation, 188–189, 188*f*
  SAMPLE history, 189–190, 189*t*
hives, 247
hospice, 232
hospital emergency care, 6*f*, 8
hot zone, 422
human body, 97
  body systems, 98
    circulatory system, 100–101, 100–101*f*
    digestive system, 104, 104*f*
    genitourinary system, 104
    joints, 103, 103*f*
    muscular system, 103
    nervous system, 103–104, 104*f*
    pelvis, 102
    respiratory system, 99–100, 99–100*f*
    rib cage, 102, 102*f*
    shoulder girdles, 102
    skeletal system, 101–103, 102*f*
    skin, 105, 105*f*
    skull, 101
    spine, 101–102
    upper extremity, 102
  stages of life, growth and development, 105–108
    vital signs, 106–108, 106*t*, 108*t*
  topographic anatomy, 98, 98*f*
human immunodeficiency virus (HIV), 27
humerus bone, 102, 333
hydration, 21–22, 21*f*
hydrocodone (Vicodin), 251
hyperemesis, 442
hyperglycemia. *See* diabetic coma
hypertension, 90, 198
hyperventilation, 166
hypoglycemia, 226
hypotension, 198
hypothermia, 284–285, 284*t*, 300

I

ice rescue, 34, 411–412, 411*f*
ICS. *See* incident command system
ileum, 443
ilium, 443
immunizations, 31
impact fires, 404
impaled object, 310
  dressing and bandaging, 317, 318*f*
  in eye, 316
implantable defibrillator, 233, 234
implied consent, 69
improvised splints, 342, 342*f*, 346*f*
inadequate breathing, signs of, 127, 129
incendiary devices, 432, 432*f*
incident command system (ICS), 430–431, 430*f*
incident management
  hazmat incidents, 422–424, 423–424*f*
  mass-casualty incidents, 424
    casualty sorting, 426–428, 427*f*, 428*f*
    initial radio report, 425
    traffic incident management, 425–426
    visual survey, 424, 424*f*
    working at, 428–431, 430*f*
  terrorism awareness. *See* terrorism
incision, laceration, 311
incubation period, 435
indirect (or off-line) medical control, 14
indirect force, 335
industrial chemicals, 248
infants, 106, 157
  airway obstruction in, 139–141, 140–141*f*
  brachial pulse, check for, 187, 187*f*
  cardiac compression, 157–158, 158*f*
  cardiopulmonary resuscitation
    one-rescuer infant CPR, 162–163, 162–163*f*
    two-rescuer infant CPR, 163, 163*f*
  level of responsiveness assessment, 185
  rescue breathing on, 135–136
  respiratory system, 99, 120
infectious diseases, 25–31, 230, 401
  disease transmission methods, 25–28, 27–28*f*
  immunizations, 31
  personal protective equipment, 29*f*, 30–31
  standard precautions, 28, 29*f*
inferior, meaning of, 98
informed consent, 69
ingested poisons, 242, 243
  activated charcoal, 244, 244*f*
  signs and symptoms, 243
  treatment for, 243–244
inhalants, 253–254
inhalation, 118, 119*f*, 194
inhaled poisons, 242
  carbon monoxide, 245
  irritants, 245–246, 246*f*
  treatment for, 246
initial emergency care, 406–407
initial patient assessment. *See* primary assessment
initial treatment of person in water, 409, 410–411*f*
injected poisons, 242
  insect bites and stings, 246–247, 247*f*
  snakebites, 248
injuries. *See also specific injuries*
  to muscles and bones, patient assessment of, 332–333, 332*f*
insect bites and stings, 246–247, 247*f*
insecticides, 248, 249, 434
instant glucose, 226*f*
insulin, 104, 226
intentional self-poisoning, 254
internal bleeding and blood loss, shock by, 303, 308
international terrorism, 431
interoperability, 80
intranasal administration, naloxone, 251, 253, 253*f*
intravenous (IV) fluids, 302
intrusive memories, posttraumatic stress disorder and, 270
involuntary muscle. *See* smooth muscle
irritants, 245–246, 246*f*

J

jaundice, 187
jaw-thrust maneuver, 121–122, 121*f*, 409
jawbone, 333
joints, 103, 103*f*, 334. *See also specific joints*

K

Kendrick Extrication Device (KED), 54, 54*f*
kidneys, 104
  dialysis, 230, 230*f*
knee
  injuries, 348, 350, 350*f*
  joint, 348, 350, 350*f*
kneecap (patella), 334

L

labor, stages of, 371, 371*f*
laceration, 311, 311*f*
landing zones, setting up, 392–394, 392*f*
language, 85
large-scale terrorists, 437*f*
laryngospasm, 285
larynx, 99
lateral, meaning of, 98
laundry detergent pods and children, 244
law enforcement personnel, 5, 5*f*
leg, 196, 334
  injuries, 350
legal concepts. *See* medical, legal, and ethical issues
legal implications of cardiopulmonary resuscitation, 170
level of responsiveness
  primary assessment, 184, 185*f*
  secondary assessment, 201
Lewisite, 434
life, stages of, 105–108
  vital signs, 106–108, 106*t*, 108*t*
life-threatening internal injuries, 428
life threats
  defined, 184
  rapidly assess the ABCs to, 185–186
lifting and moving patients
  body mechanics, 41, 41*f*
  emergency movement of patients. *See* emergency movement of patients
  general principles, 40
  recovery position, 40–41, 40*f*
  suspected head or spine injuries, treatment of
    backboards, 53
    cervical collar, 53, 53–54*f*
    log rolling, 54–57
    short backboard devices, 53–54, 54*f*
    straps and strapping techniques, 57–58, 58*f*
ligaments, 102, 103
lightning injuries, 287
limb injury
  circulation, sensation, and movement, 338–340
  examination of, 337–338, 337–338*f*
  general patient assessment, 337
limb presentation, 380
liver, 104, 104*f*
living will, 70
loading patients, into helicopters, 394, 394*f*
log rolling, 54–57
long backboards, 50, 50*f*
lower extremities, 102–103, 196, 334
LSD. *See* lysergic acid diethylamide
lumbar spine, 102, 333, 334*f*
lumbar vertebrae, 102*f*
lungs, 117
lysergic acid diethylamide (LSD), 253

M

male reproductive system, 104
mammalian diving reflex, 287
mandible, 117
manual suction device, 123, 123*f*
mass-casualty incidents, 34, 415, 424, 437*f*
  defined, 424
  initial radio report, 425
  traffic incident management, 425–426
  visual survey, 424, 424*f*
  working at, 428–431, 430*f*
MDI. *See* metered-dose inhaler
MDT. *See* mobile data terminal
mechanical suction devices, 123, 123–124*f*
mechanism of breathing, 100*f*
mechanism of injury (MOI), 182, 182*f*
  head injuries, 353–354, 354*f*
  musculoskeletal injuries, 335–336, 335*f*
  spinal injuries, 356–357, 357*f*
medial, meaning of, 98
medical and legal considerations, 272–273
medical conditions, 261
    altered mental status, 215–216
    seizures, 216–218
medical identification, 192, 192*f*
medical, legal, and ethical issues
  advance directives, 70
  consent
    for minors, 69, 69*f*
    of patients with mental illness, 69–70
  crime scene operations, 73–74, 74*f*
  documentation, 74
  duty to act, 68, 68*f*
  ethical responsibilities and competence, 68–69
  Good Samaritan laws, 73
  HIPAA, 73
  legal concepts, 70
    abandonment, 70–71
    confidentiality, 73
    negligence, 71–73
    patient dead at the scene, 71, 71*f*
  refusal of care, 70
  reportable events, 73
  scope of practice, 68
  standard of care, 68
medical orders for life-sustaining treatment (MOLST), 70
medical oversight, 14
medical power of attorney, 70
medical terminology, 90, 90*t*, 441–445
MedicAlert, 192
medication administration, rights of, 219
medication cross-check, 232
medication properties, 232
medication safety principles, 232
meditation, 24
meningitis, 27
mental illness, 69–70
mental status, 428, 428*f*. *See also* altered mental status
mescaline, 253
metabolic agents, 432
metered-dose inhaler (MDI), 144
methicillin-resistant *Staphylococcus aureus* (MRSA), 25
middle adulthood, 106
midline, meaning of, 98
mild airway obstruction, 137
mind-altering substances, 261
minors, consent for, 69, 69*f*
minute ventilation, 117
miscarriage, 378
mobile data terminal (MDT), 81, 81*f*
mobile phones, 81
mobile radio, 80
molded plastic/aluminum splints, 341
MOLST. *See* medical orders for life-sustaining treatment
morphine, 251
motor vehicle batteries, 402
motor vehicle crashes
  animals in, 34
  hazards after, 33
  responding to, 31–32
  sharp objects in, 34
motorcycle, 357–360
mottling, 202
mouth assessment, 193
mouth-to-barrier rescue breathing, 130–132, 131*f*
mouth-to-mask rescue breathing, 130, 130*f*
mouth-to-mask ventilation device, 130, 130*f*
mouth-to-mouth rescue breathing, 131
mouth-to-stoma breathing, 145
movement terms, 445*f*
moving patients. *See* lifting and moving patients
MRSA. *See* methicillin-resistant *Staphylococcus aureus*
multiple births, 381
multisystem trauma, 324
musculoskeletal injuries
  limb injury
    circulation, sensation, and movement, 338–340
    examination of, 337–338, 338*f*
    general patient assessment, 337
  mechanism of injury, 335–336, 335*f*
  standard precautions and, 337
  treatment of. *See* splinting
  types of
    dislocations, 336–337
    fractures, 336, 336*f*
    sprains and strains, 337
mutual aid, 424
myocardial infarction. *See* heart attack

N

naloxone (Narcan), 251, 253
Narcan. *See* naloxone
nasal airway, 125–126, 126*f*
nasal cannula, 142–143, 142–143*f*
nasopharyngeal airway. *See* nasal airway
nasopharynx, 117
National Academy of Sciences, 7
National Highway Traffic Safety Administration (NHTSA), 8, 8*f*
National Incident Management System (NIMS), 430, 430*f*
National Research Council, 7
National Suicide Prevention Lifeline, 269
nature of illness (NOI), 182, 182*f*
neck
  artery, 101, 101*f*, 152
  assessment, 194
  breathers, 145
  wounds, 316–317, 316*f*
neglect, child abuse, 266
negligence, 71–73
nephropathy, 442
nerve agents, 249–250, 434
nerves, 103
nervous system, 103–104, 103*f*
neurogenic shock, 300, 303, 308

newborn
aftercare of, 376
caring for, 374, 375*f*
premature, 378
resuscitating, 376–377
Next Generation 9-1-1 (NG9-1-1) systems, 5
NHTSA. *See* National Highway Traffic Safety Administration
NIMS. *See* National Incident Management System
nitroglycerin, 215, 218, 218*f*, 219
NOI. *See* nature of illness
nonrebreathing mask, 143, 143*f*
nose, assessment of, 193
nosebleeds, 314, 316, 316*f*
numbers, 443, 443*t*
nutrition, 21–22
diet and hydration, 21–22, 21*f*

O

obstetric (OB) delivery kit, 372, 374*f*
occlusive dressing, 317, 317*f*, 361, 362*f*
older adults, 106
heat and cold injuries, 284
suicide in, 269
on-scene peer support, 24
one-person walking assist, 47, 48*f*
one-rescuer adult CPR, 158–159, 160*f*
one-rescuer and two-rescuer child CPR, 163–164, 164*f*
one-rescuer infant CPR, 162–163, 162–163*f*
open abdominal wounds, 318, 319*f*
bites, 320
extremity wounds, 318, 319*f*
genital wounds, 318
gunshot wounds, 318, 320, 320*f*
open airway, maintaining, 358
open-ended questions, 86
open fracture, 336, 336*f*
open injury of head, 354, 354*f*
open wounds, 310–312
opioid overdose, 251, 253
oral airway, 124–125, 124*f*
organophosphates, 249, 434
oropharyngeal airway. *See* oral airway
oropharynx, 117
orthopaedic stretcher, 52
osteoporosis, 347
ovaries, 104
oxycodone (OxyContin), 251
oxygen, 99, 117
oxygen administration, 141–144, 143*f*
hazards of, 144
nonrebreathing mask, 143, 143*f*
safety considerations, 143

P

PACE mnemonic, 25
pack-strap carry, 45, 46*f*
padded board splints, 341
padded wire ladder splints, 341
paging systems, 81
pain
from heart attack, 219*f*
relievers, 251–253, 253*f*
palpation, 198, 199*f*
pancreas, 104
pandemics, 231, 231*t*. *See also* COVID-19
paralysis, 353–355
paramedics, 4
partial-thickness burns (second-degree burns), 320, 321*f*
PAT. *See* pediatric assessment triangle
pathogens, 28–29
patient assessment. *See individual entries for history taking, primary assessment, scene assessment, secondary assessment, and reassessment*
in behavioral emergencies, 260, 260*f*
for environmental emergencies, 280, 280*f*
of injuries to muscles and bones, 332–333, 332*f*
of limb injury, 337
medical and trauma patients, 204
in medical emergencies, 214–215, 215*f*
for poisoning, 242–243, 242*f*
sequence, 178–180
patient dead at the scene, 71, 71*f*
PCI. *See* percutaneous coronary intervention
PCP. *See* phencyclidine
pediatric assessment triangle (PAT), 201, 201*f*
peer support, 273–274
pelvis, 102, 334
assessment, 195
fractures, 345–346, 346–347*f*
penetrating chest wounds, 361–362, 361–362*f*
penis, 104
percutaneous coronary intervention (PCI), 221
peripheral nervous system, 103
personal exposure, 401
personal protective equipment (PPE), 29*f*, 30–31
petroleum-based products, 244
peyote, 253
pharynx, 117
phencyclidine (PCP), 253
phosgene, 432
physical fitness, 20
physical trauma, 261
physician's orders for life-sustaining treatment (POLST), 70
pillow splint, 344, 344*f*, 351
pin-indexing system, 143, 143*f*
pipe bomb, 432, 432*f*
placards, 246
placenta, 370
delivery of, 374–376
plasma, 101, 154, 298
plastic-laminated glass, 405
platelets, 101, 154, 298
plural endings, 442–443
pocket mask, 125
poisoning, 242
absorption poisons, 248
drug poisoning death rates, 243*f*
ingestion poisons, 242
activated charcoal for, 244, 244*f*
signs and symptoms, 243
treatment for, 243–244
inhaled poisons
carbon monoxide, 245
irritants, 245–246, 246*f*
treatment for, 246
injected poisons
insect bites and stings, 246–247, 247*f*
snakebites, 248
nerve agents, 249–250
patient assessment for, 242–243, 242*f*
signs and symptoms of, 243*t*
POLST. *See* physician's orders for life-sustaining treatment
portable radio, 80, 80*f*
portable stretchers, 49
positioning. *See also* recovery position
cardiopulmonary resuscitation
infant for, 158*f*
switching during, 162
and directions, 443, 444*t*
for ingested poisons, 243
treatment for shock, 301–302
post-run activities, 83*t*
posterior, meaning of, 98
posterior tibial pulse, 197, 197*f*
postimpact fires, 404
postrun activities, 83, 391
posttraumatic stress disorder (PTSD), 269–270
potential targets and risks, 431–432, 431*f*
power of attorney, 70
PPE. *See* personal protective equipment
prefixes, 90, 90*t*, 441, 441*t*
pregnancy
airway obstruction in, 138, 138*f*
anatomy of, 371*f*
and childbirth. *See* childbirth
preincident stress education, 24
premature birth, 378
premature newborn, 378
pressure points, 306–307, 307*f*, 308*f*
pressure regulator/flowmeter, 142, 143
prevention
of violence, 268
of frostbite, 284
primary assessment, 184
airway assessment, 186
breathing assessment, 186, 186*f*
circulation assessment, 186–187, 186–187*f*
general impression, forming, 184
level of responsiveness assessment, 185, 185*f*
rapidly assess the ABCs to identify life threats, 185–186
repeating, 203
update responding EMS units, 187
professional attitude and conduct, 12, 12*f*
prolapsed umbilical cord, 380, 380*f*
prompt transport, 9, 137, 225, 228–230
proximal, meaning of, 98
PSAP. *See* public safety answering point
psychiatric illnesses, 261
psychogenic shock, 300
psychotic behavior, 261
PTSD. *See* posttraumatic stress disorder
public safety answering point (PSAP), 4, 390
pulmonary agents, 432
pulmonary edema, 221*f*
pulse, 101, 152, 153*f*, 197, 197*f*, 298–299
pulse oximeter/oximetry, 144–145, 144*f*
puncture, 310–311, 310*f*
pupil size, 200, 200–201*f*
pursed-lip breathing, 223

Q

quality assurance, 14
quality improvement, 14

R

rabies, 320
raccoon eyes, 354, 355*f*
radial artery, 101, 101*f*, 152
radial pulse, 152, 186, 187*f*, 196, 197, 199, 199*f*
radiation, 435
radiation sickness, acute, 435, 436*t*
radio communications
  arrival at scene, 82
  dispatch, 81
  guidelines for, 83*t*
  postrun activities, 83, 83*t*
  response to scene, 81–82, 82*f*
  transfer of patient care to other EMS personnel, 82–83
  update responding EMS units, 82
radio report, initial, 425
radio systems, 80, 80*f*
radiologic agents, 435–436, 436*f*, 436*t*
radius bone, 102, 333–334
rapid transport, 9
reactivity, 200, 200–201*f*
reassessment
  chief complaint, 203
  effectiveness of treatment, 203
  handoff report, 204, 204*f*
  identify and treat changes, 203
  patient, 203
  primary assessment, repeating, 203
  vital signs, 203
recovery position, 40–41, 40*f*
  airway management, 124, 124*f*
  for seizures, 217
red blood cells, 101, 154, 298
redirection, 263
reflective clothing, 32*f*
refusal of care, 70
regurgitation, 165
religious activities, 24
remorse, 262
repeater, 80
reportable events, 73
reporting, emergency, 4–5, 5*f*
rescue breathing, 129
  mouth-to-barrier, 130–132, 131*f*
  mouth-to-mask, 130, 130*f*
  mouth-to-mouth, 131
rescue throw bag, 408
residential carbon monoxide detectors, 245
respiration, 196–197
respiratory arrest, 124–125
  causes of, 129
  signs and symptoms, 125
respiratory burn, 322
respiratory conditions
  epidemics and pandemics, 231, 231*t*
  infectious diseases, 230–231
respiratory distress, 129
respiratory failure, 129
respiratory rate, 196
respiratory system, 99–100, 99–100*f*, 117–118, 118–119*f*
responding to scene, 31–32
  functions of radio communications, 81–82, 82*f*
  workforce safety
    dispatch, 31
    parking vehicle, 32, 32*f*
    response, 32
responsiveness, check for, 120, 120*f*
restatement, 263
resuscitating newborn, 376–377
ribcage, 102, 102*f*, 333–334, 334*f*
ribs
  floating, 102, 334
  fractures, 164, 360
rigid splints, 341, 341*f*
rigid suction tip, 123, 123*f*
rigor mortis, 71, 156
riptide, 409
road rash, 310
roller gauze bandage, 305, 313, 313*f*
routes of administration, medication, 232
rug burn, 310
rule of nines, 321

S

sacral vertebrae, 102*f*
sacrum, 102, 333, 334*f*
saline solution, 316
SAM splints. *See* structured aluminum malleable splints
SAMPLE history, 189–190, 189*t*, 215, 280
sarin (GB), 249, 434
SARS. *See* severe acute respiratory syndrome
scalp wounds, 314, 314*f*
SCBA. *See* self-contained breathing apparatus
scene assessment, 180, 400–401, 401*f*
  additional resources, 183
  animals, 34
  crime or violence, 33
  crowds, 33
  dispatch information, reviewing, 180, 180*f*
  electrical hazards, 33
  environmental conditions, 34
  fire, 33
  hazardous materials, 33
  mechanism of injury or nature of illness, 182, 182*f*
  number of patients, 182–183
  scene safety, ensuring, 181, 181*f*
  sharp objects, 34
  special rescue situations, 34
  standard precautions, 183
  traffic, 32
  unstable objects, 33–34
scene safety, 31, 181, 181*f*
scene size-up, 82, 242, 250
scene/control hazards, stabilize, 401, 401*f*
  bystanders, 402
  downed electrical wires, 402–403
  electric vehicles, 402
  motor vehicle batteries, 402
  personal exposure, 401
  spilled fuel, 402
  stabilization, 401
  traffic hazards, 401–402
  vehicle fires, 404, 404*f*
  vehicle stability, 403–404, 403*f*
school-aged children, 106
scoop stretchers, 52, 52*f*
scope of practice, 68
scrapes, 310
scuba gear, 409
seasonal influenza, 25
secondary assessment, 191
  appearance, 201, 202*t*
  blood pressure. *See* blood pressure
  capillary refill, 197–198, 198*f*
  circulation to skin, 202
  of entire body, 192–196
  focused exam of specific area of body, 196
  level of responsiveness, 201
  pediatric assessment triangle, 201, 201*f*
  pulse, 197, 197*f*
  pupil size and reactivity, 200, 200–201*f*
  respiration, 196–197
  signs and symptoms, 191
  skin condition, 200
  systematically assessing patient, 191
  vital signs assessment, 196
  work of breathing, 202, 202*t*
seizure, 216–218, 355
  factors causing, 217
  treatment for, 217
self-contained breathing apparatus (SCBA), 33, 245, 246*f*
self-inflating bag, 131–132
self-introduction, 84, 84*f*
senile dementia, 272
sense of helplessness, 261–262
sepsis, 300
septic shock, 303, 308
severe acute respiratory syndrome (SARS), 25
severe airway obstruction, 137
sexual assault, 270–271
sharp objects, 34
shock, 296, 378. *See also specific shocks*
  by blood loss, treatment for, 303
  causes of, 299*t*
  children, traumatic shock in, 303–304
  by fluid loss, 300–301, 301*f*
  general treatment for
    airway, breathing, and circulation, maintaining, 301–302
    arrange for transport, 302
    assist with other treatments, 302
    body temperature, maintaining, 302
    cause treatment, 301
    control external hemorrhage, 302
    not allowing patient to eat or drink, 302
    patient positioning, 301
  by internal blood loss, 303
  patient assessment for, 297, 298*f*
  by pipe failure, 299–301
    treatment for, 303
  by pump failure, 299
    treatment for, 302
  signs and symptoms of, 301
short backboard devices, 53–54, 54*f*
shoulder, dislocation of, 343, 343*f*
shoulder blade (scapula), 333
shoulder girdle, 102, 333, 343, 343*f*
SIDS. *See* sudden infant death syndrome
signs, 191, 201
sign language, 86
Simple Triage And Rapid Treatment (START) triage, 415, 426–428, 428*f*
  algorithm, 429*f*

breathing, 427
categories of, 426–427
circulation, 427–428
mental status, 428
to sort patients, 428*f*
steps in, 427
tagging, 426–427, 427*f*
sirens, 390
situational awareness, 180
situational crisis
defined, 261
phases of
anger, 261–262
denial, 261
high-anxiety or emotional shock, 261
remorse or grief, 262
situational stresses, 261
skeletal muscle, 103, 335, 335*f*
skeletal system, 101–103, 102*f*, 333–334, 333–334*f*
skin, 105, 105*f*
color, 187
condition, 200
skull, 101, 333, 353–356
sleep, 22
sling, 343, 343*f*
SLUDGEM mnemonic, 249
smartphones, 81
smooth muscle, 103
snakebites, 248
SOF-T tourniquet, 305*f*
soft splints, 341, 341–342*f*
soft-tissue injuries. *See also* wounds
patient assessment for, 297, 298*f*
standard precautions and, 297
soman (GD), 249, 434
special rescue situations, 34
spilled fuel, 402
spinal motion restriction, 336
spinal injuries
cervical spine, stabilizing, 358
mechanisms of injury, 356–357, 357*f*
motorcycle and sports helmets, 357–360
signs and symptoms of, 357
treatment of, 357
types of, 357*f*
spine, 101–102, 333–334
splinting, 312
additional considerations, 350–351
general principles of, 340
improvised sling
using belt, 343, 343*f*
using magazines, 344
using safety pins, 343, 344*f*
materials used for
rigid splints, 341, 341*f*
soft splints, 341, 341–342*f*
traction splints, 341–342
specific injury sites
ankle and foot injuries, 350
elbow injuries, 344, 344*f*
forearm injuries, 344
hand, wrist, and finger injuries, 344–345, 346*f*
hip injuries, 347, 347*f*
knee injuries, 348, 350, 350*f*
leg injuries, 350
pelvic fractures, 345–346, 346–347*f*
shoulder dislocation, 343, 343*f*
shoulder girdle injuries, 343, 343*f*
thigh injuries, 348, 348*f*, 350*f*
straightening injured leg for, 348*f*
spontaneous abortion, 378
spontaneous nosebleed, 314
sports helmets, 357–360
sprains, 337
spring-loaded center punch, 405, 406, 406*f*
stabilization of scene and hazards, bystanders, 402
stages of labor, 371, 371*f*
stages of life, growth and development, 105–108
vital signs, 106–108, 106*t*, 108*t*
stair chairs, 49, 50*f*
standard of care, 68
standard precautions, 25, 28, 29*f*, 183
and bleeding control, 309, 309–310*f*
and childbirth, 372, 373
and musculoskeletal injuries, 337
and soft-tissue injuries, 297
standing orders, 68
Staphylococcus aureus (staph), 25
START triage. *See* Simple Triage And Rapid Treatment (START) triage
status epilepticus, 227
sterile dressings, 312
sterile gloves, 373
sternum (breastbone), 102, 334
stethoscope, 199, 199*f*
stillborn delivery, 380–381
stoma, 145, 145*f*
strains, 337
straps and strapping techniques, 57–58, 58*f*
stress, 23–24, 24*f*
stretchers
bed to, transferring patient from, 47
portable, 49
wheeled ambulance, 49, 49*f*
portable stretchers, 49
stair chairs, 49, 50*f*
stridor, 129
stroke
Cincinnati Prehospital Stroke Scale, 224, 225*t*
risk factors for, 224
signs and symptoms of, 224
structured aluminum malleable (SAM) splints, 341, 341*f*, 344, 344*f*
submersion, 285–287
substance misuse
alcohol, 250
amphetamines, 251
drugs, 250–254, 251*f*
hallucinogens, 253
inhalants, 253–254
pain relievers, 251–253, 253*f*
toxic injection from drugs, 254
suctioning, 122–123, 124*f*, 374
sudden infant death syndrome (SIDS), 271
sudden unexpected infant death. *See* sudden infant death syndrome
suffixes, 90, 441, 442*t*
suicide, 268–269, 269*t*
sulfur mustard, 434
superficial burns (first-degree burns), 320, 320*f*
superior, meaning of, 98
supplemental oxygen. *See* oxygen
surgical mask, 27, 28*f*, 29
swathe, 343, 343*f*, 348, 350, 351
symptoms, 191
syphilis, 27
systolic pressure, 198, 199

T

tabun (GA), 249, 434
talk group, 80
targets and risks, terrorism, 431–432, 431*f*
TB. *See* tuberculosis
TBI. *See* traumatic brain injury
teamwork, in serious entrapment situations, 407*f*
telemetry, 81
telephone systems, 81
tempered glass, 405, 405*f*
tendons, 102, 103
terrorism, 34, 431
agents and devices, 432
biologic agents, 435
chemical agents, 432–435, 434*t*
explosives and incendiary devices, 432, 432*f*
radiologic agents, 435–436, 436*f*, 436*t*
WMD safety considerations, 432
potential targets and risks, 431–432, 431*f*
response to, 436–437, 437*f*
weapons of mass destruction, 431, 432
testes, 104
thermal burn, 322, 322*f*
thigh injuries, 348, 348*f*, 350*f*
thighbone, 334
thoracic spine, 102, 333, 334*f*
thoracic vertebrae, 102*f*
thready pulse, 197
tibia, 334
tissue decomposition, 71, 156
tobacco, 22
tongue, 117, 120
topographic anatomy, 98, 98*f*
touching, as part of communication, 87
tourniquet application, 305–309, 305*f*, 307–309*f*
toxic injection, 246, 254
toxic substance, 245
trachea, 117
traction splint, 341–342, 348–349
traffic control, adequate, 425
traffic hazards, 32
traffic incident management
advanced warning area, 425
buffer space, 425
protection vehicle, 425
termination area, 425
transition area, 425
work space, 425
training, cardiopulmonary resuscitation, 170
transfer of patient care, 82–83, 391
transport operations
call, preparing for, 390
EMS call, phases of
arrival at scene, 391
dispatch, 390
perform patient assessment and provide emergency care, 391
postrun activities, 391
response to scene, 390

transport operations *(Continued)*
transferring care of patient to higher-level EMS personnel, 391
helicopter operations. *See* helicopter transport
trauma, 182, 204, 261, 347
head, 126
multisystem, 324
and pregnant patients, 381
traumatic amputation, 311, 311*f*
traumatic brain injury (TBI), 355
traumatic shock. *See* shock
triage, 426
triangular bandages, 313, 313*f*
trunked communications system, 80
tuberculosis (TB), 25, 230
turning patient in water, 410
twisting force, 335
two-person chair carry, 44–45, 45*f*
two-person extremity carry, 44, 44*f*
two-person seat carry, 44, 45*f*
two-person walking assist, 47–48, 48*f*
two-rescuer adult CPR, 159–160, 161*f*
two-rescuer infant CPR, 163, 163*f*

U

ulna, 102, 333–334
umbilical cord, 370
prolapsed, 380, 380*f*
unbroken bag of waters, 378, 380
unequal pupils, 200, 201*f*
unstable objects, 33–34
unzippered air splint, 342, 346*f*
upper extremities, 102, 192, 333
upside-down vehicle, 404
urethra, 104
US Centers for Disease Control and Prevention (CDC), 7, 27
US Department of Agriculture (USDA), 21
uterus (womb), 104, 370

V

V agent (VX), 249, 434
V-fib, 166
vacuum splint, 341–342
VAD. *See* ventricular assist device
vagina, 370. *See also* birth canal
vaginal bleeding, 378
vehicles
emergency drag from, 43–44, 44*f*
fires, 404, 404*f*
stability of, 403–404, 403*f*
on wheels, 403, 403*f*
veins, 298
venous bleeding, 304, 304*f*
ventilation/ventilator, 152
ventricles, 100, 152, 153*f*, 298, 298*f*
ventricular assist device (VAD), 233
ventricular fibrillation, 6, 152, 166
verbal communication, 84
guidelines for effective, 84–86, 84*f*, 87*f*
patients with special needs, 86
developmental disability, 89
disruptive behavior, 89–90
geriatric patients, 88
hard of hearing or deaf patients, 86–87
non–English-speaking patients, 88
pediatric patients, 88–89, 89*f*
visually impaired patients, 87–88
vertebrae, 101, 102*f*, 333
vest-type device, 54*f*
Vicodin. *See* hydrocodone
violence against EMRs, 268
violent patient management, 266, 266*f*
visual survey, 424, 424*f*
vital signs, 106–108, 106*t*, 108*t*
reassessment, 203
secondary assessment, 196
values based on age, 200*t*
voice systems
radio systems, 80, 80*f*
telephone systems, 81
voluntary/skeletal muscles, 335, 335*f*
VX. *See* V agent

W

warm zone, 422
water rescue, 34, 408–409, 409*f*
diving emergencies, 409–411
go, 409
initial treatment of person in water, 409, 410–411*f*
reach, 408, 409*f*
row, 408
throw, 408, 409*f*
weapon of mass destruction (WMD), 431, 432
wellness. *See* workforce safety and wellness
wheeled ambulance stretchers, 49, 49*f*
white blood cells, 101, 154, 298
windchill factor, 282, 283*f*
windows, access through, 405–406, 405–406*f*
WMD. *See* weapon of mass destruction
womb. *See* uterus
wooden cribbing, 403
word roots, 90, 441, 441*t*
work of breathing, 202, 202*t*
assessment, 194
workforce safety and wellness
crew resource management, 25
general wellness principles, 20
emergency medical care, emotional aspects of, 22–24, 22*f*
nutrition, 21–22
physical fitness, 20
sleep, 22
infectious diseases. *See* infectious diseases
responding to scene, 31–32, 32*f*
scene assessment. *See* scene assessment
stress. *See* stress
wounds
abrasions, 310, 310*f*
avulsions and amputations, 311–312, 311–312*f*
bandaging, 313–314, 313*f*
closed wounds, 310
dressing, 312–313, 312*f*
laceration, 311, 311*f*
open abdominal wounds, 318, 319*f*
bites, 320
extremity wounds, 318, 319*f*
genital wounds, 318
gunshot wounds, 319, 320, 320*f*
open wounds, 310
principles of treatment, 312, 312*f*
puncture, 310–311, 310*f*
specific wound treatment
chest and back wounds, 317, 317*f*
closed abdominal wounds, 317–318
eye injuries, 316, 316*f*
face and scalp wounds, 314, 314*f*
impaled objects, 317, 318*f*
neck wounds, 316–317, 316*f*
nosebleeds, 314, 316, 316*f*
wrist, 333–334
artery, 101, 101*f*, 152
injuries, 344–345, 346*f*

X

XABCs. *See* exsanguinating bleeding, airway, breathing, or circulation
xiphoid process, 102, 334

Z

zippered air splint, 342*f*, 345